COMPREHENSIVE
MEDICAL
ASSISTING
ADMINISTRATIVE
&
CLINICAL
PROCEDURES

COMPREHENSIVE MEDICAL ASSISTING

ADMINISTRATIVE

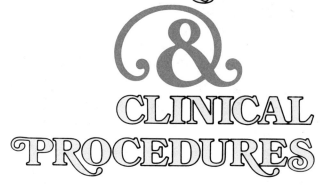

& CLINICAL PROCEDURES

MARY ANN FREW, M.S., R.N., CMA-C

Director, Medical Assistant Program
Gannon University
Erie, Pennsylvania

DAVID R. FREW, M.A., D.B.A.

Professor of Organizational Behavior
Director, M.B.A. Program
Gannon University
Erie, Pennsylvania

 F. A. DAVIS COMPANY • Philadelphia

Library of Congress Cataloging in Publication Data

Frew, Mary Ann.
    Comprehensive medical assisting.

    Includes bibliographies and index.
        1.   Medical assistants.   I.   Frew, David.   II.   Title.
[DNLM: 1.   Allied health personnel.   2.   Physicians'
assistants.   W 21.5 F892c]
R728.8F74   610.69′53   81-9820
ISBN 0-8036-3858-2   AACR2

FOREWORD

In 1969 the first set of "Essentials for an Accredited Educational Program for the Medical Assistant" was adopted by the Council on Medical Education of the American Medical Association. These "Essentials" established minimum educational standards for medical assistant training. They were also an attempt to define career-entry medical assisting through the identification of courses and learning experiences critical to safe job performance in the physician's office.

In 1975 and 1979 studies were done by the American Association of Medical Assistants to determine the competencies of medical assistants. These studies have provided the basis for the current definition of the role of the medical assistant and for the structuring of medical assisting education on competency-based format. These studies have also set the tone and guided the content of this textbook.

I believe that with the publishing of this textbook, medical assisting is taking another significant step forward in its growth as an allied health profession. The theories and principles that undergird the tasks of the profession are presented at a depth that will foster conceptual understanding and provide a sound foundation for medical assistants to identify and solve problems within the scope of their duties. The learning experiences have been carefully designed to lead to student development and demonstration of the actual skills that they will use on the job as competent practitioners.

This is truly a textbook for the times. It is written at a level appropriate for medical assistant students in any academic setting of higher learning. The content is relevant and pragmatic with regard to today's medical assistant competencies, while, at the same time, providing a comprehensive content basis for changes that will occur in the future. I am proud to have this small part in introducing this fine publication to medical assistant educators and students.

Mary Lee Seibert, Ed.D.
Dean of the College of Allied Health Professions
Temple University
Philadelphia, Pennsylvania

PREFACE

We initiated this project several years ago because we realized the need for a comprehensive text in medical assisting, one which would direct the student toward the achievement of the highest levels of professional skill and would adhere to the accountability of competency-based education techniques. We envision the medical assistant as a highly skilled and multifaceted member of the health care team, whose diversity and flexibility are perhaps the most valuable assets in coping with the complexities of medical office practice. We hope that the students who use this text will share our vision and raise their professional sights. We hope that they will strive to achieve the sense of fulfillment and contribution that medical assisting can provide.

We are certainly not alone in feeling a commitment to provide a competency-based approach to the study of medical assisting. In this regard we wish to make special mention of those individuals whose shared expertise and caring have contributed to the development of this text.

We first gratefully acknowledge to each other our coauthorship as a husband and wife team. After more than two years of collaboration, disagreement, and editing each other's work, we still love and respect each other. We recognize that a project such as this could not have been executed by either of us alone. It is fortunate that we possessed the appropriate combination of skills for such an endeavor, as well as the capacity to work with one another and the understanding and support of our children.

Second, we wish to express our appreciation to the entire administrative staff of Gannon University, not only for providing an environment conducive to the creation of scholarly work, but also for courageous "risk-taking" in allowing a husband and wife team to work within the same institution.

Several individuals gave of their technical expertise and so allowed us to add critical dimensions to the project that were clearly beyond our own capabilities. These include Susan Longo, Assistant Professor of Accounting at Gannon, who developed the chapter on accounting procedures; Margaret Watkins, Medical Technologist, who developed the chapter on medical technology laboratory procedures; and Juanita Wilkerson, Physician's Assistant, who supervised the writing of the chapter on electrocardiography and assisted us in the development of the clinical section. We are also indebted to Laverne Dreizen, who skillfully reviewed the entire manuscript, and to Mary Lee Seibert, who made many helpful suggestions based on her analysis of our work.

The unsung heroes of any writing project are the typists who must labor through mountains of scribbled pages, providing not only typing services, but also deciphering, spelling, and editorial skills, as well as patience and emotional support. We are therefore very grateful to Sandy Leonardi and her assistants, Judy Kissman, Kay Wroebel, and Sally Schmidt. We also extend our appreciation to Betty Topezer, M.D., and Sal Sellaro, D.O., for their gracious cooperation and advice.

Finally, we wish to acknowledge the kindness, creative intelligence, and enthusiasm that Bob Martone, Allied Health Editor; Brad Fisher, Production Editor; and Phyllis Spagnolo, Art Director at the F.A. Davis Company, shared with us from the beginning.

We, in turn, share our vision and accomplishment with all of you.

Mary Ann Frew

David R. Frew

CONTENTS

PART 2   THE CLINICAL MEDICAL ASSISTANT: THEORY AND PRACTICE

THE ADMINISTRATIVE MEDICAL ASSISTANT: THEORY AND PRACTICE

1

HUMAN RESOURCES MANAGEMENT

As a medical assistant, you will soon discover the fact that the physician's office is a complex human interaction system consisting of patients, their families and friends, the office staff, and the physician. As coordinator of much of this activity, you will have to be a skilled and dedicated professional who is devoted to the maximization of human resources. Unit 1 deals with the activities of the medical assistant as counselor, coordinator, and manager.

UNIT OBJECTIVES

Upon completion of this unit you will be prepared to:

1. Describe the role of the medical assistant in promoting positive interactions with patients and staff members.

2. List techniques for determining the concerns of patients and their families.

3. Describe several positive approaches for meeting patients' needs.

4. List the potential roles of the medical assistant as a manager of office personnel.

5. Enumerate the other major health care occupations and their functions.

1

UNDERSTANDING PATIENTS AND THEIR FAMILIES

SPECIFIC OBJECTIVES

Upon completion of this chapter you will be able to:

1. Describe the needs of the patient.

2. Define empathy and patient dynamics.

3. List useful skills toward the development of positive interactions with patients and their families.

4. Respond to simulations which represent the patient's needs.

INTRODUCTION

To patients and their families, you symbolize "the doctor's office" and thus lay the foundation for their reactions to the medical care they receive. Whether they will feel comfortable and confident or misunderstood and unwelcome will depend to a very large measure on you and the image that you project.

The patient brings to the office a unique personality that will in some way be affected by this visit. A special set of concerns along with specific kinds of coping behavior, understanding, and cooperation belong to each patient. It is important, then, to understand what happens when a person becomes a patient and the impact that you have on that process.

In many ways, the medical assistant (MA) who works in the physician's office will create the patient's image of the entire medical operation. Do you remember a time when you went to visit your own physician? How often did you walk into the office, report to the receptionist (perhaps an MA), and then sit down to wait? Perhaps you sat for an hour or more. During the time that you waited, you probably watched and listened as the MA handled other patients, phone calls, delivery services, and problems. It's likely that you, and other patients, judged the entire office, including the physician, by your observations of the MA. You may also have observed that during the examination room visit you had more interaction with the medical assistant than with the physician.

THE MEDICAL ASSISTANT AS AN ATTITUDE TRANSMITTER

From the patients' perspective, you are the expert in charge of things. If you appear to be disorganized, the patients will perceive the whole office to be disorganized. If you are grouchy or rushed, hostile or pushy, this attitude will reflect upon the overall operation.

Thus the first and perhaps most important task of the MA, one which is amplified in every unit to be covered in this book, is to project the proper professional image to clients. The MA needs to be kind, empathetic, gentle, knowledgeable, thorough, concerned, and interested in each individual patient. Whether the patient has to make a telephone call, get a glass of water for a child, or put money in an overdue parking meter, the MA needs to be tuned into the problem and willing to offer assistance. It is assumed that you chose this profession because you enjoy working with and helping people. Patients are people who need your help.

PATIENT DYNAMICS

If you were employed as a ticket-taker at a concert, you would have to deal with some pretty unpleasant folks. But if healthy people who are able to have a great time can sometimes be difficult to cope with, consider how much more of a potential there is for problems of interaction in a medical office. Research has shown quite clearly that when people are sick, their capacity to be friendly falls quite rapidly. In addition, patients are likely to be disturbed about their condition and worried about the financial burden of being ill and losing time from work. These are not the best circumstances for establishing a successful relationship.

Even when the visit is for the purpose of a "checkup," the patient will probably have some anxiety about the outcome. The way a patient copes with the visit, the examination, and the illness itself, and the way the medical office personnel cope with the patient, will establish what is called patient dynamics.

Two potential situations can evolve. Either the attitude of the patient is absorbed and magnified by the MA, or the attitude of the MA is absorbed and magnified by the patient. Whichever event takes place there will be a significant repercussion. Between patient and office staff a relationship will evolve that influences even the ability of the physician to diagnose the patient accurately. If the patient is upset when he enters the office, and becomes more so as the interaction in the office unfolds, the vital signs may be affected and his cooperation and willingness to confide in the physician may be hampered. There are several important guidelines to follow in an effort to influence positive patient dynamics:

1. Consider the patient and his needs to be of prime importance.
2. Listen carefully to what the patient has to say.
3. Help patients to ask their questions in a clear and understandable way.
4. Make every effort to minister to the needs of patients.
5. Answer all questions honestly and thoroughly.
6. Make an effort to understand the concerns of the patient.

Skill Development in Patient Dynamics

To be an effective human relations agent, you yourself must be well-adjusted. You may need to examine your own personality and explore positive ways to cope with anger, frustration, and other feelings you are sure to encounter. If you are meeting your own needs successfully and if you feel good about yourself, then you can concentrate on the patient's needs.

To understand the patient and his family you must learn to listen carefully to what is said. You may have to help the patient ask questions or express himself more clearly. Often patients become confused by the vocabulary, the equipment, the entire newness of the experience. They may also have concerns that they will have difficulty in verbalizing.

1. Listen to what is being said and then if appropriate rephrase the statement or question to check for accuracy. (*Example*: Patient: "I'm a little late in coming for a checkup. I should have come months ago." MA: "You think you should have had the checkup earlier?")

2. Listen for feelings about what is being said. In the above example the patient may be expressing concern about the outcome of the examination and may want to discuss this with the physician.

3. While listening, look for signs that indicate how the statement is being reflected in the patient. In the example above, the patient may have a wrinkled brow and look worried and tense, or he may be smiling and simply making conversation. Your own reaction will be influenced by the interpretation you make of the patient's behavior.

To express to patients that you understand their needs, you must minister to them. The development of empathy—putting yourself in the patient's place—facilitates this process. What does the patient need? We have already established that each patient has different needs, but there are also some needs that patients have in common. The need for security, warmth, and well-being is universal. To meet the different needs of each patient, however, empathy is important. Equally important is anticipation of needs. If a patient has just been told that he has cancer, the use of empathy helps us to understand the patient's feelings. You would be upset, obviously. You might cry or become noncommunicative. You might need to call home or be helped out of the room to the doctor's private office. As the medical assistant, you can anticipate and develop a plan for meeting the patient's needs, based on the situation being presented and the patient's age, occupation, and condition.

GUIDELINES FOR EFFECTIVE PATIENT APPROACHES

The following strategies will help you to develop a productive approach to the patient:

1. Assume that the patient will be cooperative. When you sound confident, you appear competent. The patient feels comfortable and secure. (*Example*: "Mr. Jones, please step on the scale. The doctor requires all patients to be weighed at each visit." You have expressed several things to the patient: (a) he does not have a choice; (b) this is routine—there is no cause for alarm; and (c) you expect that he will be cooperative.)

2. Praise correct patient behavior when appropriate. Positive feedback helps the patient to develop a sense of well-being. She is liked; she is worthwhile. (*Example*: "Mrs. Kenyon, you really did a great job keeping that dressing clean." You have expressed (a) that you think she is intelligent and worthwhile; (b) that you have motivated her to continue this behavior; and (c) that you have shown approval.)

3. Give opportunity for negative expression. The patient will make judgments that may be threatening to you. You may feel defensive. Nevertheless, affording the patient the opportunity for negative expression without retaliation helps the patient to feel that you understand and accept him. (*Example*: Patient: "These appointment times are never convenient." MA: "Perhaps we can do better with the next appointment." [Instead of, "Well, you made the appointment, you should have said something then."] With a positive response you have expressed (a) your acceptance of the patient's annoyance; (b) your desire to resolve the difficulty; and (c) that you will not attack or punish the patient for his feelings.)

4. A sense of belonging is important to the patient and will be of assistance in developing a positive relationship. This can be accomplished by (a) giving immediate attention to the patient when he arrives by acknowledging his presence; (b) using the patient's name when talking to him; (c) informing the patient of delays; and (d) explaining procedures. (*Example*: "Good morning, Mrs. Rose. It's good to see you. Your appointment will be delayed about 15 minutes. Please have a seat and I will call you when the doctor is ready." You have (a) expressed a warm welcome; (b) given correct information and helped to prevent the patient's anxiety from developing; and (c) indicated what the patient can expect. Thus anxiety is alleviated and positive dynamics are established.)

Communications between the patient and the medical assistant can be most effective when the medical assistant understands how to integrate the behaviors discussed in the foregoing section. Since the ultimate goals are to develop a professional attitude and positive interaction skills in communications with the patient and his family, it is clear that every encounter should be goal-oriented.

There are objectives or goals to be accomplished in all communications initiated by the medical assistant—that is, in all message-sending. When messages are received by the medical assistant—that is, whenever another individual is initiating the communication—the MA should focus not only on what the patient is saying, but also on what the patient is feeling.

SUMMARY

The person entering the physician's office becomes a patient. As a patient he enters a new and foreign environment. He is now dependent on others, concerned for his welfare, shouldering perhaps special problems related to his well-being.

The medical assistant plays a major role in controlling the office atmosphere. The MA's own personality must be conducive to working with people and the demands of the profession. The medical assistant must acquire an awareness and understanding of the needs of patients and their families and must work toward developing those skills that best produce a positive relationship.

APPLICATION EXERCISES

Role-Playing

The class will divide into work groups of three. Within each group students will assume the role of the medical assistant, the patient, and the observer. (Your teacher will assign the roles.) Try to formulate the best possible response. The observer will lead the group in discussing the response. Keep in mind the principles set forth in the chapter.

1. The MA is to prepare a 7-year-old for examination and comes into the waiting room to announce that it is his turn. (*Remember*: Assume the patient will be cooperative.)

2. While preparing for examination, the patient states that the gown is "absolutely ridiculous." (*Remember*: Give opportunity for negative expression without retaliation.)

3. The patient has completed the visit and stops at the front desk where the MA is sitting. (*Remember*: Establish a friendly atmosphere.)

4. The patient is being accompanied to the examining room by the MA and states, "I'm almost certain it couldn't be cancer." (*Remember*: Listen and look for feelings.)

5. The MA has been instructed to obtain a urine specimen from the patient. (*Remember*: Assume the patient will do as you wish and explain the procedure and the need for the specimen.)

6. The patient enters the waiting room and is seated. (*Remember*: Give immediate attention to the entering patient.)

7. The patient is sitting in the examining room, awaiting the physician. The MA enters and notes that the patient is crying. (*Remember*: The patient's needs are your prime concern.)

8. The MA is weighing a patient who has been placed on a diet and notes that there has been weight loss. (*Remember*: Praise correct behavior.) With the aid of your teacher, make up additional situations to role-play.

Problem-Solving

Before responding to the problems given, try to think about the objectives that you want to accomplish in your response.

> *Example*: The patient comes to the desk and begins criticizing the physician.
> *Objective*: Refer the patient to the physician and try to prevent a disturbance at the front desk.

> *Example*: The patient is about to have x-rays and states that she doesn't like x-rays.
> *Objective*: Reassure the patient. Accept her feelings.

1. Patient: "I don't want Dr. Jones to examine me—I want Dr. Smith." (The two are partners and she is scheduled for Dr. Jones.)
2. Patient: "I can't understand how you would enjoy working in a doctor's office."
3. Patient's relative: "My nephew has been in the examining room for one hour. What could be wrong?"
4. Patient: "I am concerned about paying for all this."
5. Patient: "That woman waiting to see the doctor is quite ill."

COMPLETING THE LEARNING LOOP

You should now have a realization of your role in helping to create the medical office climate. The MA with human relations skills will be of primary importance to the medical delivery system, and will help the patient to feel more at ease, to understand what is happening in terms of the diagnosis and treatment, and to recover more rapidly.

The medical office climate is also influenced by the work relationships of its staff. The following chapter will focus on an introduction to the potential members of the office health team and will serve to further clarify the roles and responsibilities of a medical assistant.

BIBLIOGRAPHY

Benson, H.: *The Relaxation Response*. Avon Books, New York, 1975.
Dixon, S. L.: *Working with People in Crisis*. C. V. Mosby, St. Louis, 1979.
Dyer, W. M.: *Your Erroneous Zones*. Avon Books, New York, 1976.
Rogers, C., and Stevens, B.: *Person to Person*. Pocket Books, New York, 1974.
Selye, H.: *Stress without Distress*. Signet Books, New York, 1974.
Shostrom, E. L.: *Man the Manipulator*. Bantam Books, New York, 1968.
Thompson, D. W.: *Managing People: Influencing Behavior*. C. V. Mosby, St. Louis, 1978.

2

THE PROFESSIONAL STAFF

SPECIFIC OBJECTIVES

Upon completion of this chapter you will be able to:

1. Recognize and describe the functions of the most common members of the health care team.

2. Recognize and describe the most common physician specialties.

3. List the basic role functions of health team members.

4. Describe and utilize the elements of positive interaction.

INTRODUCTION

One of the most difficult problems for any new medical assistant is to begin to develop an understanding of the many different but highly specialized members of the health care team. Like many other careers, health care is quite dynamic. What this means to you is that the number and complexity of different jobs within the field are growing very rapidly.

The typical physician of past decades operated from a modest office, which may in fact have been attached to his home. He probably had a nurse or a medical secretary as his only assistant. Today's physicians may be attached to a large, diversified unit and have several health care professionals or paraprofessionals to assist them.

The MA must be familiar with each of the functions within the office in order to understand how the staff members interact in the delivery of health care services. In addition, the MA may find the opportunity to deal with persons outside of the office who provide ancillary services, such as x-ray technicians and physical therapists. Therefore the MA's understanding of health care roles must extend well beyond the typical office operation.

THE PHYSICIAN

The physician is a doctor of medicine and occupies the highest position in the health team's organizational chart. The term "doctor," however, while often connected to physicians, has a much broader connotation. A doctorate is an advanced degree which may be awarded to a wide variety of individuals. Lawyers are given a J.D., which stands for Doctor of Jurisprudence. Psychologists as well as many college professors earn a Ph.D., or Doctor of Philosophy degree. In addition there are osteopathic doctors, chiropractic doctors, doctors of veterinary medicine, and doctors of dental surgery, among many others. Thus doctoral degrees signify the greatest expertise achieved in a given area. A physician, therefore, is a particular type of doctor—one who practices medicine.

There are two widely recognized approaches to training physicians in the United States: the allopathic and the osteopathic. Allopathic medical schools, which award the medical doctorate (M.D.), are currently in the majority, so that most MAs will find themselves working for an M.D. However, the osteopathic schools are increasing quite rapidly, and consequently many MAs will go to work for a doctor of osteopathy (D.O.). Generally speaking, D.O.s and M.D.s maintain separate offices, clinics, and hospitals. Therefore, it would be unusual for an MA to work with osteopaths and medical doctors at the same time.

In either case the training of a physician is both lengthy and sophisticated. Following four years of college, the aspiring physician must complete medical school (three to four years), an internship, and if he or she is to specialize, a residency (two to three additional years). It is then imperative that the physician obtain a license to practice in a particular state, and become licensed to dispense narcotics and other medications. If physicians achieve board certification, they are then able to practice as medical specialists. Board certification is sponsored by a specialty organization. Specific preparation and successful completion of the examination are required for recognition of the physician as a specialist.

Specialized Types of Physicians

Many physicians choose to take advanced training so that they can become "specialists." A specialist is a doctor who confines his practice of medicine to a particular body system or type of problem. Medical assistants need to be aware of the most common specializations for at least two reasons. First, they may be working for a specialist. Second, they may find themselves dealing with patients who are being referred to specialists by their own physicians.

The list below includes the more common specialties practiced by medical and osteopathic physicians:

Allergy and Immunology
Cardiology
Dermatology
Family Medicine
Internal Medicine
Neurology
Obstetrics and Gynecology
Oncology
Ophthalmology
Orthopedics
Otorhinolaryngology
Pediatrics
Pulmonary Disease
Reconstructive and Plastic Surgery
Urology

NURSES

A second major category which you will encounter in the delivery of health care is the nursing profession. At one time nursing was a relatively simple and undifferentiated field, but the past decade has witnessed significant changes in nursing education and practice. The basic types of nursing personnel are described below.

1. *Practical Nurses*: Individuals who have attended a limited training course, usually one year in length, to learn basic nursing procedures. With additional training, the licensed practical nurse (L.P.N.) may administer medication.

2. *Diploma School Nurses*: Persons who have completed a two- to three-year program of "live-in" training in association with a hospital. A diploma is awarded upon graduation. Diploma schools are decreasing in number because of the growing trend in nursing education favoring four-year college programs for professional nurses and two-year college programs for nurse-technicians.

3. *Associate Degree Nurses*: Persons who complete a two-year college program for nurse-technicians, leading to an Associate in Science (A.S.) degree.

4. *Baccalaureate Nurses*: Individuals who complete a four-year college program leading to a Bachelor of Science (B.S.) degree in nursing.

5. *Nurse Practitioners*: Licensed nurses who receive additional background in a specific health area, usually requiring a year of academic study and training.

6. *Postgraduate Nurses*: Baccalaureate nurses who earn master's and doctoral degrees in nursing education or in clinical specialties.

Nurses are required to pass state registry examinations in order to obtain licensure as a practical (L.P.N.) or registered (R.N.) nurse.

OTHER HEALTH CARE PROFESSIONALS

As an MA you will soon become aware of a virtual explosion in types of allied health care professionals. New occupational titles are evolving every year, and all of this specialization requires you to stay in touch with the newest technological developments in the field.

You will probably not work in an office which includes all these professionals on its staff. But even if you don't work with them directly, you will still need to have an understanding of their functions, since your office will be interfacing with almost all of these allied health specialties at one time or another.

The list below, although incomplete, includes the allied health personnel most likely to be encountered by an MA.

1. *ECG Technologist*: A person who is trained to operate an electrocardiograph machine.

2. *Medical Records Technician*: A person who has specialized training in organizing and maintaining medical records.

3. *Medical Secretary*: A secretary with specialized training in medical office procedures of an administrative nature.

4. *Medical Technologist*: A person who performs routine and specialized tests in the clinical laboratory.

5. *Mental Health Counselor*: A person who is trained in counseling those who are experiencing emotional or psychological problems.

6. *Nuclear Medicine Technologist*: A person who is trained to assist the physician in the operation of equipment employing radioactive nuclides in diagnosis and treatment.

7. *Surgical Technician*: A person who assists the doctor and nurses in the operating room.

8. *Physical Therapist*: A person who specializes in using exercise therapy to assist patients in the recovery process.

9. *Physician's Assistant*: A person with specialized training who assists the physician and carries out supervised diagnostic procedures such as the physical examination.

10. *Radiologic Technologist*: A person who operates x-ray and associated equipment and produces radiographs.

11. *Respiratory Therapist*: A person who assists in the therapy of persons with serious respiratory problems.

Table 2-1 provides further information about the training processes for the major allied health care occupations.

You will note that the term "technician" refers to an individual who has obtained basic skills and knowledge in a particular area and has limited responsibilities. The term "technologist," on the other hand, refers to an individual who has mastered the skill and knowledge required to function with full responsibility in a particular area.

After just a few short months of studying and learning administrative or clinical techniques, you will probably begin to identify very strongly with the concept of being a profes-

TABLE 2-1.   Common Allied Health Care Occupations and the Training Required

Title	Entrance Prerequisites	General Program Length	Credentials*
ECG technologist	High school	6 months	ABRET or ECG certificate
Medical record technician	High school	2 years	ART (Associate degree)
Medical record technologist	High school	4 years college	ART (Bachelor's degree)
Medical secretary	High school	2 years	Associate degree
Certified laboratory assistant	High school	1 year (hospital affiliation)	Certificate
Medical laboratory technician	High school	2 years (hospital affiliation)	M.L.T. (Associate degree)
Medical technologist	3 years college	+ 1 year (hospital affiliation)	M.T. (Bachelor's degree)
Mental health counselor	High school	4 years college	Bachelor's degree
Nuclear medicine technologist	Med. tech., radiologic tech. or R.N. + 3 years college	+ 1 year (average hospital affiliation)	N.M.T. (Bachelor's degree)
Surgical technician	Mixed	1 year	C.S.T. (certificate)
Physician's assistant	College requirements vary	2-4 years college	P.A. (Associate or Bachelor's degree)
Physical therapist	College requirements vary	4 years college + 2 years post.	L.P.T. (May also be Bachelor's degree until 1985)
Radiologic technician or technologist	High school	2-4 years college	R.T. (Associate or Bachelor's degree)
Respiratory therapist	High school	2 years (hospital affiliation)	R.R.T.

* In addition to certificate or degree status, further state and national registry or certification is usually required in most of the allied health professions.

sional. Thus you will soon expect other people to understand and respect your own areas of expertise.

Each person who works in the health care system feels exactly as you do. Whether physicians, nurses, or laboratory technicians, health care personnel feel that they have a specific function to perform and that their function is an important one.

One of the basic problems in our understanding of the health team and the various roles each member takes involves the rapid growth and the "newness" of many of these occupations. Perhaps most difficulty lies in understanding how these roles differ from one another and how they interact.

Because of the dynamic nature of health care, individual offices have often evolved their own unique interaction systems based upon the physician's preferences and the personalities of the individual staff members.

Obviously the medical assistants seeking employment will discern their role with the physicians involved and ask questions about how the office responsibilities are divided. A clear idea of your role expectations will be necessary if you are to become a valuable asset to the office practice.

If a particular office includes only you and the doctor, your duties will almost certainly be more varied than they would be if there were also a nurse, a physician's assistant (PA), and a medical secretary. It is not uncommon to medical office practice to find an MA, a PA, a nurse, and a medical secretary in one office. However, the staff will most often count on the medical assistant in both the administrative and clinical areas of office practice. Medical assistants are perhaps the only health care professionals who are specifically trained to assist the physician in the procedures peculiar to the office setting.

Once employed, you will find that you are the hub of many activities in the office. Almost all of the staff members will interact with you on a continuing basis. Some of your responsibilities may overlap. Thus it is enormously important that you understand and respect the positions of these individuals, as well as your own, and that you strive to maintain harmonious relationships. An office staff whose members know, respect, and like each other will function smoothly and efficiently, but an office which is experiencing problems between staff members will benefit neither the physician nor the patient. Coursework in psychology may be useful to assist you in dealing with others and understanding yourself.

Because differences in the understanding of role responsibilities are perhaps the single most common cause of staff tension, an attempt has been made to define and clarify the various allied health professions. Other problems that may also develop often originate in personality differences. Skill development in the area of coping with others is a life-time process. Coping behavior basics, however, are introduced here.

GUIDELINES TO THE DEVELOPMENT OF POSITIVE INTERACTION

Positive interaction is the goal in all interpersonnal relationships. It assumes that the outcome of interaction will be beneficial or constructive, rather than negative or destructive.

1. Understand your own role expectations—those perceived by yourself and those perceived by others.

2. Confront tense situations between staff members by:

   a. Analyzing and identifying any of your own behavior which may be contributing to the tension.

   b. Confronting the difficulty with the assumption that it is resolvable.

   c. Discussing the difficulty in a professional manner with the individuals involved in the interaction.

   d. Discussing the behavior rather than the personality. (*Example*: Being late in coming back from lunch break poses certain questions: Was the lateness avoidable? Was the lateness selfish? The latter question is subjective and inappropriate.)

   e. Involving the physician only in those matters in which he would play a major role in resolution, and only as a last resort.

APPLICATION EXERCISES

Discussion

The class will be divided into three- or four-person discussion groups. Each group will discuss the three issues which follow:

1. Reference is made in this chapter to two approaches in physician education. Explain the difference between them.

2. Included in this chapter is a list of common specialties for physicians. Briefly describe each of these specialties as well as some of the common diseases with which the specialty is concerned. You may consult a medical dictionary.

3. Discuss what your reaction would be to each of the situations given below, as well as the goal and possible consequences of your response. Try to apply the guidelines for developing positive interaction in each case.

   a. An individual in the office appears to be acting in such a way as to shed some doubt on your competence.

   b. The doctor raises his voice and blames you for an error for which you are not responsible.

   c. The doctor raises his voice and blames you for an error for which you are responsible.

   d. A fellow staff member is listening to the doctor's private telephone conversation.

   e. A staff member tells you how to perform a procedure. The instructions differ from what you have been taught.

Self-Awareness

The following exercises will help you to analyze basic personality traits as well as your frustration and anger patterns and coping mechanisms. These are vehicles for self-awareness and will be useful in clarifying some areas of potential interpersonal difficulty. The exercises are designed as a private activity.

Rate yourself on each of the questions below. One is the highest rating and five is the lowest. Respond honestly to each item. Your instructor will help you to analyze your results.

	High				Low
1. I make friends easily.	1	2	3	4	5
2. I look forward to the future.	1	2	3	4	5
3. I am outgoing in crowds.	1	2	3	4	5
4. I experience boredom often.	1	2	3	4	5
5. I most usually like myself.	1	2	3	4	5
6. I dwell on concerns.	1	2	3	4	5
7. I am usually happy.	1	2	3	4	5
8. I can relate well to authority figures.	1	2	3	4	5
9. I often feel that I may explode.	1	2	3	4	5
10. I feel confident in most situations.	1	2	3	4	5
11. I am very tolerant of differences in others.	1	2	3	4	5
12. I feel there are a number of things about me I'd like to change.	1	2	3	4	5
13. I like meeting other people.	1	2	3	4	5
14. I feel that things are going well for me.	1	2	3	4	5
15. I am certain of my career choice.	1	2	3	4	5

The following self-analysis exercises are designed to help you understand anger and frustration: (a) respond honestly; (b) think about the response yourself and draw some conclusion; (c) discuss with others (friends, family counselors) if desired. Your instructor will help you to analyze your results.

1. How often do you feel frustrated?
2. Can you think of at least three occasions when you were frustrated?
3. Are there any common factors that caused your frustration? Events or people?
4. What was your response in these instances?
5. Were there any common factors in your response? Were all instances handled in similar fashion?
6. How could your frustration have been prevented?

7. How often do you feel angry?
8. What are some things you find really provoking?
9. Remember a time when you were extremely angry. What were the circumstances?
10. How did you respond?
11. Could your anger have been prevented?
12. How would you have liked to respond?
13. How would you rate your temper? Very quick? Slow?
14. What are the prime thoughts of your anger?
15. What factors, if any, would you change in your coping behavior?
16. Decide how you will proceed. Test out your own behaviors. Evaluate.

COMPLETING THE LEARNING LOOP

You should now have acquired an understanding of the basic components of the health care team. If there are any questions, the class discussion and suggested readings given below may be of some assistance. Medical assistants *must* understand the various functions within their scope if they are to effectively coordinate or supervise office personnel. Equipped with this understanding, the theory and practice of coordinating and supervising techniques can be presented.

BIBLIOGRAPHY

Allied Medical Education Directory, 1979. American Medical Association, Chicago, 1979.
Cotton, H., and Martin, N.: *Managing the Doctor's Office.* Medical Economics Company, Oradell, N.J., 1975.
Schwarzrock, S.P., and Ward, D.F.: *Effective Medical Assisting.* ed. 2. Wm. C. Brown, Dubuque, Iowa, 1976.
Winning Ways with Patients. American Medical Association, Chicago, 1966.

CHAPTER 3

COORDINATING AND SUPERVISING OFFICE PERSONNEL

SPECIFIC OBJECTIVES

Upon completion of this chapter you will be able to:

1. Explain the difference between traditional and contemporary styles of management.

2. Describe the management model most useful in the health environment.

3. Differentiate the manager-coordinator and manager-supervisor roles that the medical assistant may assume.

4. List and describe the skills necessary in coordinating and supervising office personnel.

INTRODUCTION

As a medical assistant, you may find yourself involved in a large office or clinical setting. Beyond the awareness of understanding the functions of your coworkers there is a good chance that you may find yourself in the position of supervising or coordinating these functions. We will focus on accomplishing two goals:

1. To help you to understand how to coordinate the specific duties of the office staff.
2. To build a foundation of supervisory skills related to the health setting.

Naturally the subjects here will be most applicable to the medical assistant who works in a reasonably large office or a clinic. But all MAs, even if they choose to begin their careers in a small office, should be prepared to function in a coordinating or supervisory capacity. The ideas that will be discussed fit into the general framework of management, but they may differ substantially from preconceived ideas of what management is all about.

THE TRADITIONAL MANAGEMENT MODEL

Many of us have come to think of managing as a supervisory function which is something like being a drill sergeant or a football coach. We may have a simplified view of being a boss which suggests that someone has given us complete authority over a particular operation and its employees, and that we make and enforce all decisions. The administrative aspects of being the person in charge within this kind of system include the making of *all* the decisions. Supervision consists of a series of techniques for explaining what we want to our subordinates, and watching to be sure that our wishes are carried out.

There are two explanations for this view of management. First, we have all participated in or least observed this kind of system. You may have experienced it as a student or as a part-time employee. Second, and perhaps more important, is the fact that an authoritarian management system such as this can be quite comforting for participants as well as supervisors. Workers are told what to do and how to do it, and supervisors receive a kind of respect as well as obedience.

Another interesting aspect of authoritarian management systems is their traditional effectiveness. The "listen and do what I tell you" approach to managing evolved over a number of years in response to the Industrial Revolution, and it served us well. For years it was the undisputed "best" approach to being a supervisor—and it worked. In fact it worked so well that teachers, football coaches, and parents borrowed ideas from this traditional style of management. By now many of us have seen this authoritarian approach used so often and by so many that we may be ready to adopt it ourselves. Nevertheless there are alternatives.

A MANAGEMENT MODEL FOR THE HEALTH CARE ENVIRONMENT

As persons who were working in the health care field began reporting their supervisory experiences to the researchers and theorists of management, it became quite obvious that the older methods were not working quite as well as they had in the factory. Hospital administrators, for example, found that it was nearly impossible to decide what a physician or a nurse should do, much less to tell them how to do it. It appeared that the management of the health care professional presented a whole new set of problems.

There are several aspects of health care management or supervision which differ from the old ideas of industrial management. Most obvious is the fact that as a health care manager you will be dispensing a service to people rather than producing a product. Moreover, you will be providing a service which is of prime importance—good health. And while not every decision made in the physician's office will be of "life or death" importance, even treating a sore throat—at least to the person with a sore throat—is of tremendous significance. As consumers we have learned to accept crooked lines on writing paper, fenders that rust on new cars, and an assortment of other factory management problems, but poor quality health care is unacceptable to everyone because of the dire consequences.

The second special aspect of health care management concerns the problem of managing professionals. In the traditional factory system you "worked your way up" and learned the entire operation. By the time you began to manage or supervise, you probably knew more than your subordinates about their jobs. But in the health care environment you will find yourself dealing with professions which may be a great mystery to you. You may find yourself managing x-ray technicians, but you may not have knowledge of how their job really should be done.

Situational approaches to management dictate that the approach be tailored to the particular job. When a job is simple, clearly outlined, and predictable, the old factory management or authoritarian approach is useful. But when the work is complicated, ever-changing, and unpredictable, a more democratic approach is required. Table 3-1 contains a survey of the precepts of situational management.

THE MANAGER-COORDINATOR

In the typical principles of management textbook, managing is described as the process of planning, organizing, and directing the activities of a group. And in the past when a great many people went to work in factories, they could be sure that it would be years before they would be called upon to perform the various functions of a manager. But as a medical assistant you will probably be expected to become a manager-coordinator (in the modern sense) almost immediately.

You may be called upon to manage and coordinate staff members and their activities

TABLE 3-1.   Situational Management

Type of Task Performance	Examples	Best Management Approach
Very simple and repetitive	Assembly line, punch press	Very autocratic
Moderately simple and repetitive	Assembly work, maintenance	Moderately autocratic
Average	Complex assembly, office work	Mixed
Moderate degree of complexity and unpredictability	Delivery of medical care, supervisory work	Democratic
High degree of complexity and unpredictability	Research, marketing, and advertising	Very democratic

as well as patient flow. It should be clear, however, that the authoritarian style of managing has no place in a sophisticated health care environment.

You may find yourself functioning as a scheduler, a coordinator, or an organizer—one who must create order and logic by cooperation rather than by decree. In the past the manager took the position of "owner," even if he was simply a hired employee. He tended to make decisions based on the classic "if this were my company" idea. Thus your first expectation of the physician who "owns" the office might be that he or she will be the traditional manager, making all decisions and supervising the staff. But this will usually be a false presumption. The physician is the owner of the office and is ultimately responsible for decision-making, but the primary interest of the typical physician is practicing medicine. It is presumed that a staff member will handle most of the day-to-day managing so that the physician can concentrate on delivering quality medical care.

Perhaps the main source of confusion for new medical assistants is that they may be asked to manage the owner or physician: to schedule appointments; to keep track of projects, commitments, and deadlines; and to coordinate the physician's activities. It should be obvious to you that you will not be able to manage a physician, nurse, or physician's assistant in the same way that a factory foreman supervises a machine operator.

Planning and Organizing

The bulk of your managerial responsibilities as an MA revolve about the everyday problems of coordinating the roles of other office staff members. You will not be in "charge" of them in the traditional sense. In fact, some if not all of these professionals may be staff members, such as physicians, who are, "professionally speaking," more than your equal. You may find, as in the case of physicians, that you cannot accurately predict when they will be coming to the office, or how long it will take them to perform various office procedures. Thus your job will primarily consist of planning the day's work, organizing it into logical modules, then maintaining a communications flow with the professional staff and the patients.

In the following chapters we will discuss each facet of the medical office tasks in great detail. Here the problem of staff interaction and the MA's role as an integrator are our prime concerns.

As an integrator and coordinator, you must realize that you are responsible for creating and maintaining a logical flow of activities within the office, without having the ultimate authority (in a traditional sense) over the people whose tasks you are coordinating. In classic management terms, you will have responsibility without authority. If you don't learn to accept and deal with this situation you will soon become frustrated and begin taking out your anxieties on patients and staff members. This will compound an already difficult problem.

A very typical problem occurs in patient scheduling. As a medical assistant you may be in charge of setting up the physician's office hours and accepting appointments. You will probably be given some working guidelines by the physician, who may tell you that he is going to stop at the hospital to make his "rounds" first thing in the morning and then begin appointments at 9:30 a.m. You will perhaps respond to this by having the first office patient come in to see the doctor at 9:30. What happens, however, when one of the hospital patients has a complication which holds the physician at the hospital until 10:30, and your first patient is a businessman who has been waiting patiently since 9:30, and then informs you that he has another appointment at 10:30? Another typical situation may exist in staff inter-action. The doctor asks you to get Miss Jones and have her come to the examination room immediately, and you will have to use all of your human relations skills to do that without ir-ritating her as she is extremely busy.

Typical office situations require you to be a democratic coordinator. You must be pos-itive, supportive, creative, and sensitive to the needs of others. Throughout your coordinat-ing efforts it is imperative that you understand and respect the various functions of the staff members. This requires constant effort. Daily conversation with every member of the staff will keep you in touch with their work schedules and with problems that they may be en-countering.

How you handle these kinds of situations is critical to your success as a medical assis-tant because, unlike a factory assembly line where the worker may not experience such problems, in the physician's office these types of difficulties are expected and accepted. Since you can't design the problems out of the system, attacking each of the problems that arise with creative judgment and with a democratic managerial style is essential.

Skill Development Guidelines for the Democratic Manager-Coordinator

1. Organize and plan your work:
   a. List tasks to be performed.
   b. Assign priorities to the tasks.
   c. Understand how tasks are to be divided, who is responsible for their performance, and how they will be coordinated.
   d. Know the time schedule in which the tasks are to be performed.

2. Demonstrate thoughtfulness and consideration for your colleagues:
   a. Become sensitive to their needs and concerns.
   b. Demonstrate a willingness to help others to complete their tasks if able.

3. Handle errors made by yourself or others in a constructive manner:
   a. Accept errors by colleagues by joining with them in the resolution, without fostering blame or guilt.
   b. Accept errors made by yourself by placing them in realistic perspective, acknowledg-ing your error, and accepting the responsibility.

4. Demonstrate flexibility regarding your plans:
   a. Be open to the suggestions of the staff.
   b. Anticipate changes and have alternative approaches ready.

5. Be clear in explaining important objectives and time tables to others:
   a. Demonstrate an understanding of the importance of the tasks and time tables of others.
   b. Explain, when necessary, the objectives and time tables related to your task so that others will understand their importance.

6. Become a willing communicator:
   a. Be aware of the needs and concerns of others.

    b. Respond to questions and comments.

    c. Be available or open for communication.

7. Develop and maintain a positive work climate:
   a. Identify your own sources of frustration and cope with situations as they arise and with directness.
   b. Accept the frustration of others and attempt positive solutions.
   c. Accept that each work day provides new challenges and new sources of frustration and that calmness is an ever-present goal.
   d. Encourage the input of others.

8. Develop and maintain an effective communications system in the office:
   a. Speak clearly and precisely.
   b. Listen attentively to what is being said.
   c. Check for accurate interpretation, if necessary, by repeating what is said.
   d. Demonstrate and mobilize an appreciation for your fellow-workers' cooperation.

THE MANAGER-SUPERVISOR

In addition to being the office coordinator, it is conceivable that you may supervise one or more members of the office staff. The likelihood of this added responsibility will probably depend upon the size of the operation, the length of your experience, the relationship that you develop with the doctor, and, of course, your own skills. Thus the role of manager-supervisor is not a position you would assume immediately upon employment. It requires advanced skills, experience, and knowledge.

It is difficult to predict who you will be supervising. It may be a temporary employee such as a student on an externship or a Kelly girl. It may also be a regular staff member such as a secretary or receptionist. But if and when you do become a supervisor, you will need to follow some basic management prescriptions.

There are several possible approaches to being a manager, but these are often organized within the framework shown in Table 3-2. The set of management styles shown in the table ranges from autocratic (1) and moderately autocratic (2) to democratic (5). The "old-fashioned factory manager" is representative of an autocratic leadership style. The moderately democratic and democratic styles are shown to be approaches which are quite distinct from the autocratic standard, and are more appropriate in a health care environment.

Modern Management Theory

Situational management theory would suggest that the effectiveness of a particular management approach is linked to at least two different factors: (1) the task to be performed, and (2) the staff and their personalities.

If you were doing an uncomplicated and predictable job, such as running a machine shop or assembly line in a factory, the autocratic or moderately autocratic style of management would probably be best. You could carefully analyze the work, which you know will be repeated thousands of times, design the best approach, and teach it to the staff. However, running a medical office is a different kind of responsibility. Often the medical office provides

TABLE 3-2. Basic Supervisory Approaches

Style	Description
1 Autocratic	Supervisor decides exactly what will be done, then dictates how to do it
2 Moderately autocratic	Supervisor makes slightly flexible decisions, then discusses them with staff
3 Mixed	Supervisor makes a tentative decision, consults with the staff, then comes to a final decision
4 Moderately democratic	Supervisor presents the problem and assists the staff in coming to a decision
5 Democratic	Supervisor allows the staff to define both problems and solutions, and serves as a coordinator and facilitator

unpredictable tasks and emergencies that require full cooperation and democratic supervision.

As a medical assistant you will be dealing with a relatively high level of complexity; thus your approach to persons whom you supervise should be an open-ended one, presuming, of course, that you can live and work with such flexibility.

Complicating the task of supervising is the fact that those being supervised are of differing types. Some individuals do very well in a flexible environment where supervisors provide guidelines rather than directives and advice rather than orders. They seem to be able to define problems and develop excellent solutions with little or no difficulty. Others, however, seem to be overwhelmed in this kind of environment. They seem to wander aimlessly about, without being able to decide how to proceed. Organizational psychologists describe this personality dimension as embodying "followership needs." It seems that some workers are most comfortable with a high degree of direction, while others perform best with less direction and more autonomy. Given the relatively complex nature of the physician's office, it would seem logical to hope for staff members who can comfortably cope with moderately democratic leadership patterns.

Skill Development Guidelines for the Democratic Manager-Supervisor

1. Organize and plan the work day:
   a. Solicit input from others.
   b. Ascertain agreement concerning what is to be accomplished, by whom, and when.
   c. Accurately inform everyone concerning common objectives and goals.

2. Provide opportunity for input by staff members on important decisions:
   a. Hold regular staff meetings.
   b. Encourage openness and a willingness to listen.

    c. Encourage and praise independent thinking.

    d. Be willing to modify approaches and procedures where possible.

3. Demonstrate concern for staff members:
   a. Become sensitive to their needs and concerns.
   b. Be supportive when a mistake is made, rather than critical and degrading.
   c. Provide positive feedback when appropriate.
   d. Become aware of changes in office climate and attempt to anticipate and resolve these situations when necessary.

4. Maintain effective communications:
   a. Give clear directions.
   b. Provide opportunity for teamwork.
   c. Listen to what is being said and felt by others.
   d. Demonstrate flexibility in decision-making.

5. Individualize management style when needed:
   a. Attempt to learn which approaches are best with each staff member.
   b. Ask questions of staff members and participate in evaluation of your own leadership style.

SUMMARY

As a medical assistant, most of the managerial work for which you are responsible will come under the broad heading of planning and organizing. To be an *effective planner/organizer*, the key is to understand the objectives and approaches that will be used by the members of the staff. This process demands constant attention on your part in terms of asking questions and helping to determine objectives. You must approach each staff member in a positive and constructive manner and on a routine basis.

    Ask the staff for their input and advice in helping to define the objectives, the problems, and the solutions. When a particular individual appears unable to cope with this approach, adjustments are necessary in the sense of becoming more directive and therefore more capable of individualizing your leadership style.

APPLICATION EXERCISES

Since your primary experience to date in observing supervisory styles has been as a student, begin the following exercise by recalling some of your "best" and some of your "worst" teachers in elementary and secondary school. Make an attempt to relate their teaching styles to their effectiveness as teachers. Management theory would suggest that the choice of the "best" teacher depends upon several factors, including the subject being taught, individual teaching styles, and the student group.

Class Discussion Exercise

1. Break the class into several groups of five or six students.

2. Each student should describe a few cases of good learning and a few cases of bad learning styles and analyze the reasons for supporting those choices.

3. The group should attempt to describe these cases in terms of management vocabulary and the principles set forth in this chapter (*Example*: simple, straightforward classes such as algebra, as opposed to complex classes such as philosophy; autocratic versus democratic teaching methods.) Compare task complexity with teaching method.

4. Through group discussion make an attempt to reach a consensus regarding those subjects which are better presented in a democratic style or an autocratic style. Have your group spokesman share group findings with the class.

5. With this understanding of the differences of management style, apply the concepts presented to the medical office situation.

Coordinating Exercise

1. (a) Determine if "appointment scheduling" is a simple or complex task. Your teacher will explain some of the basic components of scheduling. (b) Determine the appropriate management style.

2. Miss Jones, the clinical medical assistant, is scheduled to perform a blood pressure check on Mr. Adams. The doctor will see Mr. Adams following the procedure. Inform Miss Jones and proceed with the coordination of these activities. Discuss how it would be handled. Role-play your approach to Miss Jones.

Supervising Exercise

1. Imagine that you are holding a meeting with staff members. The topic is the doctor's schedule. He continually runs late, and personnel must remain at the office after closing hours. Role-play the supervisor's leadership of the group. Role-play and discuss how the meeting would proceed.

2. Miss Jones has made a serious error. Role-play the supervisor's approach.

COMPLETING THE LEARNING LOOP

You have just completed a very brief overview of management, one which was tailored to the kind of problems you will encounter in a physician's office. You will probably still have some important questions about your role as a manager. We will be dealing with some of these in the chapters on scheduling and communications. Becoming an effective manager is a long and tedious process which requires years of experience—the prime requirement is interest and willingness to learn.

Subsequent chapters will describe in detail the tasks pertaining to medical office practice. Of prime importance to organizing and planning is the procedure manual, which will be discussed in the following unit.

Keep in mind that the ultimate goal is to provide the best possible total care to the patient. A well-managed office will facilitate that objective.

BIBLIOGRAPHY

Dyer, W. D.: *Team Building*. Addison-Wesley, Reading, Mass., 1977.
Frew, D. R.: *The Management of Stress*. Nelson-Hall, Chicago, 1976.
Gellerman, S. W.: *The Management of Human Relations*. Holt, Rinehart & Winston, New York, 1966.
George, C. S.: *The History of Management Thought*. Prentice-Hall, Englewood Cliffs, N.J., 1972.
Haimann, T., and Hilgert, R.: *Supervision: Concepts and Practices*. South-Western, Cincinnati, 1977.
Nadler, D. A., et al.: *Managing Organizational Behavior*. Little, Brown, Boston, 1979.

CHAPTER 4

SELF-MANAGEMENT

SPECIFIC OBJECTIVES

Upon completion of this chapter you will be able to:

1. Describe the unique characteristics of the medical office environment.

2. Describe the rationale for making a written list of all unanticipated tasks.

3. Describe how time and tasks may be effectively managed.

4. Apply organized tools of self-management to present life situations.

INTRODUCTION

As a medical assistant you will discover that the environment in a medical office is unique. There are certain characteristics of this environment which differ from most other work environments. The pace, the nature of the work, and the people all provide the type of environment which is mentally, physically, and emotionally taxing, as well as challenging and rewarding.

To operate successfully in this situation, self-management skills are required. An understanding of the needs and expectations peculiar to the medical office environment is necessary before these skills can be applied. In earlier chapters the needs and characteristics of the patient and the staff were identified; in this chapter needed characteristics of a medical assistant and methods of managing these are introduced. The work environment demands that medical assistants act creatively and autonomously, while at the same time refraining from making decisions or performing procedures beyond their own professional scope.

Another perplexing demand inherent in the medical environment is the lack of predictability and order. Unlike a factory where workers perform a particular job, uninterrupted until completed, the medical office is characterized by emergencies and a series of sidetracks and interruptions.

These expectations for the MA contribute to a potentially frustrating work environment. A high degree of confusion can result, and important tasks can be forgotten or neglected. Therefore, self-management skills are essential in coping successfully with the demands of the medical office.

THE MEDICAL ASSISTANT IS AN ASSISTANT

Perhaps the most useful first step in dealing with the frustration inherent in a medical office environment is to approach the work with a specific philosophy. You must remember that you are an assistant. Your essential role is that of a facilitator, acting to make things easier for the physician.

There will be many times when you will become irritated and frustrated because you set goals for yourself or begin projects only to find that you are unable to accomplish them as expected. This frustration and anxiety can provoke irritability, which in turn reduces the likelihood of being able to carry out your major role expectation in the office—assisting.

The highest priority for the medical assistant is to assist the physician in meeting the goals he determines. This sometimes necessitates reordering your personal priorities and substituting the physician's goals for your own. This is the challenge and skill of assisting—retaining composure and flexibility when personal goals are blocked or delayed.

The physician is already subjected to a staggering amount of stress. The MA who has acquired this awareness will cooperate with and support the physician in achieving reasonable goals, even when occasionally her own are subordinated. Continually questioning assignments and expressing concerns related to the physician's approach are usually unproductive exercises. Again, good judgment is the chief criterion for action. Internalization of the philosophy that the primary function of medical assistants is to assist—to act as physician-facilitators—will enable MAs to perform both effectively and comfortably.

THE TASK OF DAILY ORGANIZATION

The manner and philosophy by which you personally approach medical assisting are extremely important. Beyond these, however, there are other techniques that can be helpful in simplifying an otherwise complicated work environment.

Don't Trust Your Memory

The most serious errors made by medical assistants and others who work in dynamic environments are usually errors of omission rather than of execution. For example, the physician may suggest in passing that you "order some plastic gloves, we're almost out." You are busy filing and you think, "I'll do it right after lunch." But then Mrs. Jones has a ruptured appendix in the office, and by the time things calm down it's break time. As the day's responsibilities continue to unfold, the request is forgotten. Then two or three days later the physician comes storming out of the examination room because there are no gloves and he can't proceed.

This vignette illustrates the typical error made and the consequences that can ensue when an attempt is made to rely on memory for retention of information. Thus the first and most critical technique for the assistant is to *write down* all messages or self-reminders. Although a seemingly simplistic exercise, errors of omission are avoided when items to be acted on are written.

Create a Job-List System

Developing a system for recording tasks to be achieved and checking them off as they are accomplished can serve as an important organizational tool. A cork board may be used and notes attached, or a blackboard or notebook may suffice. Perhaps the best approach is to utilize a plain form (Fig. 4-1), or a form designed to meet the particular need categories of the office (Fig. 4-2).

The job-list serves as a planning guide and reminder for those tasks that are unanticipated in the daily routine. Such a form may be attached to a clipboard or placed on the desk, and whenever an assignment is given which cannot be carried out immediately, it can be recorded. Include on the list any pertinent information that you will need, such as telephone numbers and due dates.

Usually this recording system is an ongoing process. One day's list may be planned the day before just prior to leaving the office or early in the morning when arriving.

Acquiring a habit of recording assignments and proper use of the job-list are the major objectives; the design of the form and the location are secondary.

How to Use the Job-List

Effective use of the job-list requires that principles of time management be applied, for another major source of errors stems from spending time on the wrong assignments. The objective here is to continually be working on the item assessed to be most critical.

It is assumed that most of the workday will be spent reacting to emergencies or immediate concerns. The phone rings, the doctor calls for your assistance, a patient asks a question. Such occurrences demand immediate response and full attention.

It is the remainder of the workday which needs to be managed logically. During periods when direct assisting duties are not being performed, consult the job-list. Determine which of the listed items is most important, then act on the decision. The determination is not made on how easily or quickly the job can be completed, because this logic leads to

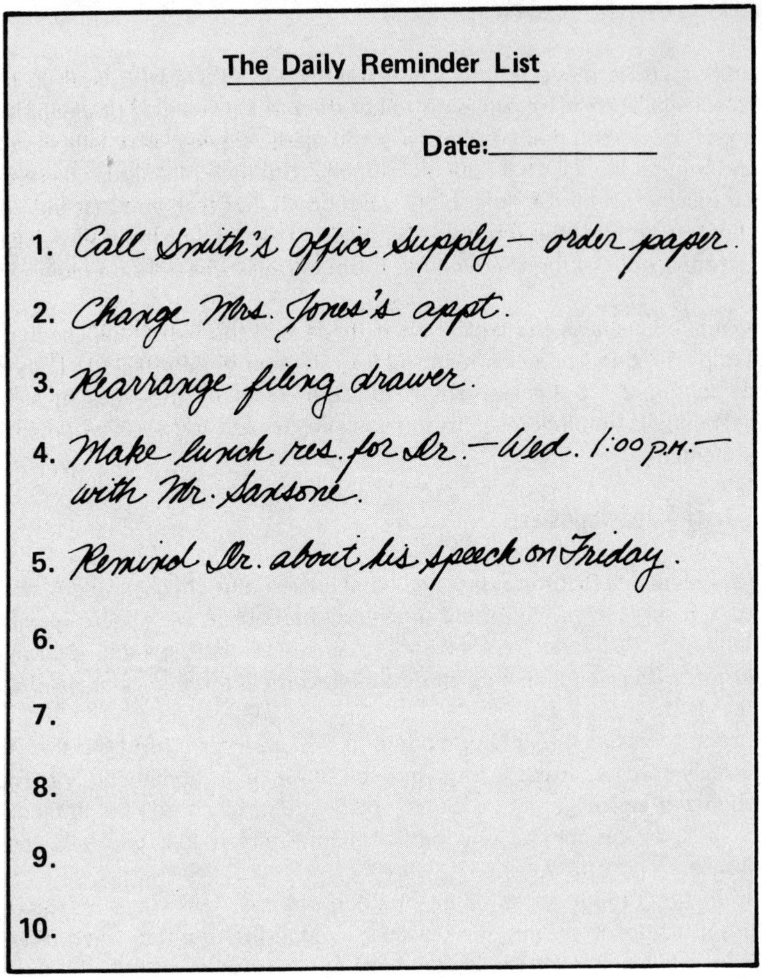

The Daily Reminder List

Date:_____

1. *Call Smith's Office Supply — order paper.*

2. *Change Mrs. Jones's appt.*

3. *Rearrange filing drawer.*

4. *Make lunch res. for Dr. — Wed. 1:00 p.m. — with Mr. Sansone.*

5. *Remind Dr. about his speech on Friday.*

6.

7.

8.

9.

10.

FIGURE 4-1.   A simple reminder form.

delaying critical projects. It is usually more productive to initiate an important project than to complete one of lesser importance.

　　　If it becomes apparent that a task may not be completed on time, let the doctor know in advance. This courtesy prevents the possibility of an uncomfortable situation for both the medical assistant and the physician.

Avoid Double Work

Many times the temptation to procrastinate is so great that persons end up hurriedly performing twice the amount of work which should be necessary. You may open the mail and find a letter that requires a response. After reading the letter and thinking what the reply should be, you then put the letter in a drawer and write a note on your job-list. A day later,

Things to Do

Office Projects:

1. *Rearrange drug cabinet and label shelves.*
2. *Magazine subscription check.*
3. *Check laundry supplies.*
4.
5.
6.
7.
8.
9.
10.

Calls to Make:

1. *Smith's Office Supply — order paper — 891·7740*
2. *Lunch res. for Dr. — Wed. 12 noon at University Club — 896·5431*
3.
4.
5.
6.
7.
8.
9.
10.

Physician Reminders:

1. *Luncheon today — should leave by 11:30 AM*
2. *Respond to Dr. Walter's call from yesterday.*
3.
4.
5.

FIGURE 4-2. A categorized reminder form.

when you have a few moments, you refer to the job-list. You have carried this letter-writing task over to a second day. Now you must find the original letter and again think through what you are to do before proceeding. Double-processing should be avoided when a task can be done without risking completion of another important project.

An excellent guideline in this regard is: *Always follow through with what you have in your hand if at all possible.* Putting the job-list to this use — as a guide for establishing time and task priorities — results in more productive use of the time available in the workday.

SUMMARY

From the physician's perspective, the true value of medical assistants is clearly related to their capacity to anticipate needs and facilitate the physician's goals harmoniously. These expectations require the self-management techniques and role philosophies outlined in this chapter.

Medical assistants must be cheerful, warm, cooperative, and friendly, creatively pursuing ways to be of service to the physician as well as the patient. In addition, if MAs strive to be well-organized, self-motivated, and efficient, they will prove to be a most valuable asset in the operation of the physician's practice.

GUIDELINES FOR EFFECTIVE SELF-MANAGEMENT

1. Accept the changeable and unpredictable nature of the medical office.

2. Continually reflect on the philosophy of assisting: your role is to facilitate goal fulfillment as defined by the physician.

3. Record all important tasks on a job-list.

4. Refer to your job-list often, use it to organize and establish priorities for tasks in the daily work schedule.

5. Avoid procrastination—complete the task in hand whenever possible.

6. Determine the importance of a project and proceed with tasks evaluated to be high on the list of priorities.

APPLICATION EXERCISE

To participate in the class exercise, you need a blank piece of paper and a pencil or pen. This assignment requires that you develop an individualized job-list arranged according to priority. Since you are a student, the application of the principles contained here can be applied to your present situation. Choose a school day.

1. List the tasks which you must complete between now and the end of the day (prepare for exams, write papers, etc.). Include personal life tasks in the list, such as cleaning your apartment or getting your car fixed.

2. After you have developed this list, take a moment to mark the items which are of greatest importance (+), least importance (−), and medium importance (0).

3. Form groups of three or four persons and share your lists with each other. Discuss the lists you have each written. Evaluate the following:
   Are expectations realistic?
   Is time well managed?

Are efficiency and organization apparent?

Have difficult projects been put off in favor of easier or more appealing tasks?

4. Modify your own list according to recommendations.

5. Select a representative group to report to the class on any common denominators, patterns, or general impressions.

COMPLETING THE LEARNING LOOP

As a student you are constantly faced with some of the same types of self-management decisions confronting the medical assistant, including a large number of seemingly unrelated projects, such as papers and tests whose due date is known in advance, as well as many other unanticipated assignments that are given daily. If you begin to use some of the organizational skills which are useful to the medical assistant, two important benefits will emerge: (1) you will be a better organized student, and (2) you will gain organizational experience needed for your later professional work.

For anticipated and routine functions, a necessary organizational tool for the medical assistant is the procedure manual to be discussed in the next chapter.

BIBLIOGRAPHY

Close, C. C.: *Work Improvement.* John Wiley & Sons, New York, 1960.
Dayton, E. R.: *Time Saving Tools.* Zondervan, Grand Rapids, Mich., 1974.
McCay, J. T.: *The Management of Time.* Prentice-Hall, Englewood Cliffs, N.J., 1959.
Zinck, W.: *Dynamic Work Simplification.* Reinhold, New York, 1962.

UNIT 2

OFFICE PROCEDURES MANAGEMENT

The medical assistant will serve as the business manager for the medical office, thus allowing the physician to concentrate on day-to-day clinical responsibilities. As office managers, MAs will not be called upon to make major policy decisions; rather their responsibility will be the administration of normal business procedures. They will be asked to oversee the general office management, to schedule appointments, to maintain the accounting systems, and to process insurance claims.

UNIT OBJECTIVES

Upon completion of this unit you will be prepared to:

1. List and describe the procedures required for administering a medical office.

2. Design and maintain an appointment book.

3. Make proper entries in an appointment book.

4. List and describe the components of an accounting system.

5. Recognize and complete all of the major types of insurance forms.

CHAPTER 5

BASIC OFFICE MANAGEMENT PROCEDURES

SPECIFIC OBJECTIVES

Upon completion of this chapter you will be able to:

1. Describe the components of basic office management procedure.
2. Understand the nature of personnel policies and procedures.
3. Maintain and control office records.
4. Perform filing operations appropriate to the medical office.
5. Design effective office layouts, including equipment and supply requirements.
6. Prescribe office maintenance procedures.

INTRODUCTION

As a medical assistant, your job description extends to various administrative functions. The ability to create a well-planned and well-organized office structure will create an atmosphere in which both the physician and the MA can maximize time spent on their primary function—patient health care. Planning and designing an efficient work station and records management system and assigning priorities to office procedures provide the tools by which the medical assistant translates the goals and objectives of quality health care into effective management practices and specific administrative task responsibilities.

THE PROCEDURES MANUAL

A major mainstay of efficient office management is the office policies and procedures manual. The manual has four primary functions: (1) it serves as a chronicle of the tasks to be performed; (2) it is a training device to be referred to by all members of the office unit, as an aid to the standardizing of procedures; (3) it is utilized as a reference source for the description of job titles and responsibilities for members of the office staff; and (4) it serves as a "how to" document when personnel are introduced into the office unit on a temporary basis.

    A loose-leaf notebook format is preferable for the manual, since it allows for additions and deletions of material with a minimum amount of effort. This design encourages frequent updating and revision. The manual should be divided according to appropriate administrative and clinical subjects, and indexed by major headings and subheadings. Cross-referencing within the body of the manual will enable the reader to easily cover all relevant material concerning a particular subject.

    The first major division within the manual should consist of a checklist of tasks to be performed and their respective due dates. This can best be organized on a daily, weekly, and monthly basis. Below are some suggestions as to the contents of such a checklist: *

Daily	Weekly	Monthly
1. Mail routine	1. Payroll duties	1. Payroll register
2. Review appointment book	2. Physician's practice correspondence	2. Payroll deposit
3. Check medical supplies	3. Inventory medical and administrative supplies	3. Summarize daily receipts and disbursements
4. Complete previous day's patient records	4. Review technical journals for professional developments	4. Patient billing
5. Complete insurance forms		5. Collection letters
6. Complete filing		6. Accounts receivable and accounts payable summaries
7. Correspondence		7. Bank reconciliation
8. Record patient receipts		8. Financial statements
9. Summarize daily earnings record		
10. Prepare bank deposits		
11. Prepare disbursements		
12. Reconcile petty cash		
13. Complete office maintenance procedures		

* Details as to the proper procedures to be followed under each topic are outlined in various sections of this chapter and Chapter 7.

Personnel Policies

With respect to the training function, the contents of the procedures manual should outline specific personnel policies enforced in the office practice. If the ground rules are detailed, questions as to authority and responsibility, as well as accrued benefits, are not left to chance, nor do inconsistent applications occur. The following is a checklist for such a personnel policies subdivision:

Administrative: Job definitions and descriptions
Hours of work
Lunch and break periods
Pay periods
Job evaluation policy
Discipline
      probation period
      disciplinary actions
      grievance procedures
      termination procedures

Compensation: Basic pay scale and pay increments
Overtime pay
Holidays
Vacations
Leaves of absence
Sick pay
Fringe benefits
      medical insurance
      workers' compensation
      social security
      unemployment
      retirement
      profit-sharing
Professional development and training

Personnel file: Outline of contents
Equal employment opportunity and affirmative action policies
Accessibility to the files

As a source for the description of job titles and role responsibilities for the individual members of the staff, the procedures manual serves as a valuable reference for the physician and the medical assistant. With respect to the administrative functions of the MA, the following should serve as a basic checklist for inclusion in the manual:

Office Equipment and Supplies: Inventory of medical maintenance and office equipment and supplies; details as to manufacture, frequency and quantity of ordering, last price paid, and evaluation of the quality of the product and servicing.

Office Procedures: Description of the physical layout of the office; the records control and management system; office maintenance and equipment review procedures.

Outside Services: Referral services for patients; professional services utilized by the physician, such as attorneys, accountants, and insurance agents; equipment deadlines and repair services; medical supply houses, drug and pharmaceutical concerns.

Patient Policies: Billing procedures for each physician; patient ledger cards and medical histories, progress reports, laboratory reports, and correspondence.

Personnel Policies: As outlined above.

Physicians: Resumes and professional vitae on each doctor; policies as to office hours and hospital hours; personal data such as addresses and call services; hospital and medical society affiliations; outside services and medical consultants utilized on a referral basis.

Record-keeping: Basic forms needed, such as those related to medical insurance, medicare payroll, licensing, patient care, and financial records; procedures to fill out the documents and to perform the record-keeping.

The keys to the success of the procedures manual are (1) that details should be specific and inclusive; (2) that extensive cross-referencing is done; and (3) that the information contained therein is up-to-date and complete. In other words, within each division and subdivision, each subtopic would be covered in sufficient detail to train office personnel and to serve as a future reference source. For example, the "Basic Forms" section under the heading of "Record-keeping" would contain a list of all forms utilized by the office together with a sample of each. Procedures for completion of forms would be outlined; names and addresses for filing instructions would be included, as would an audit trail to the final location of each copy completed. Finally, a checklist of due dates would be compiled and placed at the beginning of the subsection. Then the entire subsection would be referenced to (1) the daily routine outline; (2) the office procedures section; (3) specific subsections within "Record-keeping" where each form is utilized; and (4) the topic subsection which refers to the usage of each form of medical insurance for insurance forms.

Another example might involve "Patient Procedures," subheading "Billing." A detailed schedule of each physician's fees for service would be provided and summarized in the individual patient records. The subheading would be cross-referenced to outside services where referral fees would be discussed. The subheading would also be referenced to "Record-keeping," where the subheading "Basic Forms" would illustrate the proper billing format and procedures, and to financial record-keeping procedures where the "one-write" billing, receipt, and accounts receivable process would be illustrated.

The loose-leaf procedures manual format is designed to allow for ease of modification. The MA must be sure to (1) spend time each month reviewing the manual; (2) revise or remove outdated material; (3) make additions of current concern and interest to members of the office staff; (4) check that details are up-to-date and accurate; (5) delete material which is unnecessary; and (6) translate sections of the manual to "tickler" (reminder) files or rotary wheel devices to provide for easier and more frequent assessibility to all members of the professional staff.

Organizing and Composing the Procedures Manual

Initiating the use of a procedures manual may be the responsibility of the medical assistant. Therefore the actual organization and writing of the manual may require the utilization of the medical assistant's skills in these areas. The following stepwise approach to the writing of a procedure sheet will be helpful to the assistant in the completion of this task.

WRITING MANUAL STATEMENTS

Procedure	*Principle*
1. Adopt a heading to be used for all procedure sheets which: a. identifies the topic; b. determines who is responsible.	1. A standardized approach facilitates ease in reading and announces the beginning of the task directions.
2. Before beginning the rough draft, jot down, in outline form, the major points to be included.	2. This steps helps to organize the topic and subtopics into a logical sequence.
3. Begin the rough draft from the outline. Isolate the first step and clearly express it in writing as though giving specific directions. Specific direction: Always answer the telephone politely: "Good morning—Dr. Jones' office, Cindy speaking."	3. Specific direction as opposed to general information is essential to clarify steps to be taken in performing a given task if the approach is to standardize. General information will produce a variety of responses since interpretations can be individualized.
4. Proceed with each step, rereading the statement for clarity and precision.	4. If each step is precisely and clearly described with as few words as possible, the main idea will be more easily understood and remembered.
5. When all statements are written, reread for errors and cohesiveness. Then begin final typed copy upon physician's approval.	5. A procedure sheet should not contain grammatical errors. A consistent pattern of writing will promote comprehension and retention of the material presented.

Examples of Office Procedure Formats

On the following pages the student will find examples of the five basic parts of a comprehensive office procedures system: a job description which would be included in the personnel policies section, a bank reconciliation, a patient file procedure instruction, a supply inventory card, and a records retention procedure sheet.

PERSONNEL POLICIES

Job Description: Office Manager

Reports to: Physician

Supervises: Assigned staff

Basic Function:

Under the direction of the physician, performs related clerical and administrative duties and relieves assigned staff of office detail when practical.

Major Duties:

1. Prepares correspondence related to the physician's practice.
2. Schedules physician's patient appointments.
3. Maintains inventory records related to medical and administrative supplies.
4. Completes patient record files.
5. Prepares patient billing forms.
6. Records daily earnings summaries.
7. Handles bank responsibilities related to deposits, check disbursements, payroll depositories, and bank reconciliations.
8. Controls petty cash disbursements and reimbursements.
9. Supervises office maintenance procedures.
10. Reviews office procedures manual to update and upgrade.

BANK RECONCILIATION*

Format: Bank Reconciliation   Date _____

Balance per bank statement and date above $ _____a

Add: Deposits in transit   _____
     Service charge not on books   _____
     N.S.F. (not sufficient funds) check   _____
     Note/payment paid by bank not recorded   _____
     Bank error   _____
                                   Total   _____b

Subtract: Outstanding checks   _____
        Note payment collected by bank not recorded   _____
        Bank error   _____
                                   Total   _____c

Balance per physician's records and date above.   _____a + b − c

Completed by   _____

Reviewed by   _____

Date   _____

---

*The procedure must be completed on a monthly basis to be reviewed by the office manager and/or accounting service. Any discrepancies should be promptly reported to the physician.

Procedure:

Preparing a bank reconciliation means determining those items which make up differences between the amount shown on the current month's bank statement and the balance in the cash account in the physician's accounting records. The specific steps to prepare such a reconciliation are as follows:

1. Compare the deposits on the bank statement with deposits shown in the physician's records. Place check-marks in the physician's cash records and on the bank statement beside the items which agree. Any unchecked item in the physician's records of deposits will be deposits not yet recorded by the bank (see "Deposits in transit") and should be added to the balance reported by the bank on the bank statement. Be sure to determine that any deposits in transit listed on last month's bank reconciliation are included in the current month's bank statement.

2. Arrange the checks returned with the bank statement in numerical order and compare each with the corresponding entry in the physician's disbursements records, placing a check-mark beside a returned item. The unchecked entries should be listed in the bank reconciliation as outstanding checks to be deducted from the amount indicated on the bank statement. Determine whether the checks listed as outstanding on last month's bank statement have been returned and add those which have not to the list on current reconciliation.

3. Adjust the physician's records for bank debit or credit memoranda which have not been recorded on the physician's accounting records.

4. Prepare a bank reconciliation similar to the format illustrated above.

5. Make journal entries in the general journal for items on the bank statement which have not yet been recorded in the physician's accounting records.

PATIENT FILES

Policy: Filing procedures must conform to the system utilized, either alphabetic or numeric.

Procedure:

1. Prepare file folders for all patients for whom a medical history is kept.

2. File folders should contain copies of medical history, progress reports, laboratory reports, insurance records, billing records, medicare records, and correspondence with the patient's hospital or other physicians.

3. File all the material pertaining to each patient in his own individual file. Arrange the documents within the folder in chronological order.

4. Prepare a miscellaneous file for records of patients whose treatment is not extensive enough to warrant an individual file folder.

5. Prepare a file folder label utilizing the tools outlined in the "files management" section of this manual.

6. Place folders numerically or alphabetically in a separate file cabinet.
7. Patient files must be updated on a daily basis.
8. Prepare any cross-referencing indexes where necessary.
9. Review patient's files to see that the documents within them are current and that the file folder itself is properly classified as active, permanent, or inactive.

SUPPLIES INVENTORY

Procedure:

A separate inventory card should be maintained for each item or group of similar items utilized by the physician's office with respect to clinical, clerical, and administrative supplies. The standardized card (Fig. 5-1) should be completed in detail, reviewed, and updated on a daily or weekly basis as a matter of office routine.

RECORDS RETENTION

Policy: Records retention refers to determinations as to what, where, and for how long documents will be stored, and when and how outdated documents will be destroyed.

Procedure:

1. Documents are to be classified as active, permanent, or inactive.
2. Active files referring to records of patients currently under a physician's care and to financial records concerning the physician's practice should be filed and stored, utilizing the procedures outlined in the "files management" section of the manual.

	Description	Purchases			Vendor	Date of Invoice	Inventory			Total Inventory	Condition
Item		Qty	Cost	Invoice Amount			Qty / Date	Cost	Amount		
Vendor A: ______ ______											
Vendor B: ______ ______											
Completed by____ Date____ Checked____											

FIGURE 5-1. A supply inventory card.

3. Permanent files refer to patient or administrative records of ongoing importance and may be stored with current records or filed in separate storage facilities.

4. Inactive files concern discharged patient records or financial records older than one year. These documents should be removed from the current files, microfilmed, and stored separately.

5. Files are to be reviewed on a quarterly basis in order to update the above classifications.

6. Legal requirements of local, state, and federal agencies should be posted in the manual and referred to when reviewing financial records.

7. Case histories constituting research documentation should be removed from the files and stored separately.

8. Inactive files older than seven years may be removed from storage and destroyed by shredding.

RECORDS MANAGEMENT

The orderly and efficient maintenance of a physician's office unit depends on obtaining information quickly and easily. The information required for records must be controlled and stored in such a manner as to protect their integrity and yet provide accessibility when needed. To achieve that end there are four main areas of concern within records management:

1. *Files management:* the design of effective filing systems with respect to methods and equipment to be used.

2. *Information retrieval:* the development of effective and rapid recall and replacement methods.

3. *Records protection:* the classification of documents by importance and the designation of storage methods for each classification.

4. *Records retention and storage:* the determination of what, where, and for how long documents will be stored, as well as when and how outdated documents will be destroyed.

This section will provide details and methodologies with respect to each of the four areas of records management.

Files Management

Filing may be defined as a system of classifying, arranging, and storing documents in an orderly and efficient manner. Files must be systematized and kept up to date. A deviation from the prescribed procedures results in lost documents, wasted time due to inefficient retrieval methods, outdated documents used as reference materials, and the inability of all office personnel to utilize the records management system.

EQUIPMENT AND SUPPLIES

The first step in designing a well-planned and well-organized records management system is to determine the most efficient records control equipment and the supplies necessary for the physician's office. Efficiency should be measured by (1) the size of the materials to be filed; (2) the number of items to be filed; (3) the physical limitations of the office and clinical practice work areas; and (4) the physical demands to be placed on the medical assistant. Again, systemization and standardization are key elements.

Standard file cabinets are available for storing documents of the two most common sizes: letter size ($8^{1/2}$ × 11 inches) and legal size ($8^{1/2}$ × 14 inches). Other cabinets are available to house card files, visible records, punched cards, and computer printouts.

The typical "pull-out drawer" file cabinet (vertical file) is manufactured with multiple drawer units. False economy should be avoided and the best heavy-duty equipment purchased because it provides maximum protection for patient records and financial documents. Physical efficiency for the medical assistant who must operate the equipment is achieved as well. The physical layout of the physician's office will determine the number and arrangement of the file cabinets. Often consultants are employed to design the office layout as well as the records management system. If possible, questions with respect to designing or revising an efficient system should be directed to the manufacturers of the equipment or supplies, since they have experience in dealing with physicians' practice problems on a broad scale.

Because of the increasing numbers of patient-related and financial documents that must be kept by the physician, many practice units are now utilizing lateral and shelf files. Lateral cabinets look like a chest of drawers and are often used for documents which must be retrieved quickly and frequently in the medical assistant's work unit. In shelf filing, records are held in file folders in an upright position and stacked seven or eight units high for maximum space efficiency. However, retrieval efficiency tends to be reduced with shelf files unless the files are well indexed.

In addition to the standard filing equipment cited above, special equipment is available for card files in various sizes, for visible files where a portion of the patient record becomes a key point of the indexing system, for rotary files, for microfilm and microfiche, and for electronic data processing records.

FILING AIDS

The efficiency of the filing system is enhanced by the use of specific filing aids, such as guides, folders, and labels. Guides subdivide the drawer of the file cabinet for ease of referencing; file folders further subdivide the drawer as well as physically protecting the documents within the drawer; and labels identify the records within the drawer, guide units, or folders.

GUIDES

Guides are heavy cardboard sheets which are the size of the file folders. A caption indicating the alphabetic range of materials filed behind the guide is printed on the top, or tab, of the guide. Primary guides indicate major divisions—alphabetic, numeric, subject, or geographic. Secondary or special guides are subdivisions of primary guides and highlight special sections of subjects within the filing system. For an efficient system, frequent use of guides is recommended.

FOLDERS

File folders are made of heavy manila paper and measure slightly larger than the letter-size or legal-size documents they will contain. The back cut of the folder contains tabs for captions or reference indexes and may number two, three, or five cuts or sections per folder width. Folders should never be overcrowded but should be subdivided when the bottom scores or creases are filled. The subdivision of file folders should be as follows: "miscellaneous" for less than six documents; individual captions for more than six items per reference index; and "special" for patients or organizations with a large quantity of frequently used material. If an individual file folder contains more than 1 inch of material, it should be subdivided by date or subject and indexed as part 1, part 2, and so on.

LABELS

Labels identify the contents of the file cabinet and the individual folders. Captions should be consistent in terms of indexing order, capitalization, and punctuation. Color-keying often makes referencing and retrieval much easier. The best way to maximize efficient retrieval is to make sure that labels are current, accurate, and in good condition, and that they specifically identify contents with respect to index discription, date (current or inactive), and the particular filing system in use (Fig. 5-2).

Having designed the physical layout of the filing system, the next step is the identification of the documents to be handled by the system. Records pertaining to the physician's practice will include medical correspondence of various types: letters from patients and other physicians and from organizations such as hospitals, medical societies, and insurance companies. Records pertaining to business will include formal correspondence; purchase requisitions, orders, and invoices; patient bills and receipts for payment; records of income and expenses; financial statements; tax records; payroll records; bank deposits, checks, and statements; and insurance records. Specific medical and technical materials also will be accumulated. All of these documents should be classified on a scale from active to permanent to inactive, and the specific filing system chosen should enhance efficient retrieval of the required materials.

FILING PROCEDURES

The filing process should stress the regular, orderly, and reliable collection of all retainable documents, whether generated in-house or deriving from external sources. The process

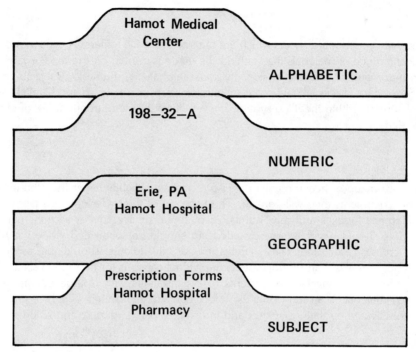

FIGURE 5-2.   Examples of commonly used forms of labeling.

should affix responsibility for the flow and deposition of all materials, usually by means of a time stamp and routing index. Finally, the filing process should provide for document release (usually indicated by initials), which designates that the transaction has received the required processing and that the document may be filed.

A five-step filing process is recommended for efficient and orderly document flow, consisting of inspecting, indexing and cross-referencing, coding, sorting, and storing. The steps are outlined and compared in Table 5-1.

The first step in the filing process is to inspect the document for the necessary release marks which indicate that the document is cleared for filing. Documents without the necessary clearance should be rerouted to the last indicated work unit on the routing index.

The second step is indexing and cross-referencing, which is the process of choosing the file folder caption under which the document will be filed. The most frequent recall pattern is determined by reference to the name on the letterhead, the name of the person to whom the letter is addressed, the signature on the letter, the subject of the contents, and the name of the location. Cross-referencing by means of photocopies or a cross-reference sheet indicating the location of the original document is done when frequent recall for the document may occur under more than one index caption.

The third step is coding, which is achieved by marking the index caption on the document to be filed. A color-key system is employed either by underlining or by indicating the caption in the upper right hand corner of the record and by placing an X with an underlined or written index for cross-referencing to emphasize the indexing which has been completed in step 2. This will ensure accuracy in both the original filing process and during filing.

TABLE 5-1. The Five-Step Filing Procedure

Step	Alphabetic System	Subject System	Geographic System	Numeric System
Inspecting	File release by initials	Same	Same	Same
Indexing	Individual folder caption	Alphabetic or numeric	First by location, then by name or subject	Alpha index and code followed by cross-reference code (or) alphabetic sort
Coding	File caption underscored; cross-reference underscored and placed at end	Subject classification or numeric index in upper right hand corner; various cross-reference captions indicated	Name underscored, location circled, cross-reference indicated with separate note for permanent cross-reference	Numeric code as indicated by relative index file
Sorting	Alphabetic by underscored caption	First by main headings (either alpha or numeric), then by divisions of main headings, finally by subdivisions	First by main geographic divisions, then by geographic subdivisons	Numeric by hundreds, tens, then units; miscellaneous file has alpha sort
Storing	Proper file cabinet placement	Alpha or numeric file cabinets; relative index cited for captions and cross-references	First by city, then state, then name; cabinets have alpha section and miscellaneous folders within subdivisions; relative index done alphabetically by name	Numeric files for numeric document code; separate alpha file for miscellaneous records; relative index done alphabetically by name and subject

The fourth step, sorting, is merely the alphabetizing of documents to be filed. The key to efficiency here is to arrange the documents in small alphabetic divisions such as A-C, D-G, H-L, M-R, and S-Z; to resort each division (A, B, C); and finally to alphabetize the sections within each division.

The final step, storing, is the placement of the documents in file folders for vertical filing. Care in this terminal step is imperative. A final document check should be made for agreement of the filing index, the file folder caption, and the index on the first document already contained in the folder. Documents should be filed neatly, with the heading to the left as you face the file, and without overcrowding the folder. Documents should be inserted while the folder is raised and resting on the side of the file cabinet drawer to ensure correct folder selection and proper document preservation.

Standards for Filing Systems

Developing an orderly, efficient filing system requires that standardized rules and procedures be followed. The following basic rules are of use when closing the index captions:

1. Individual names are indexed by surname, then given name, then middle name or initial.

2. Each unit letter is alphabetized by letter, starting with the order indicated above.

3. A surname, when used alone, precedes the same surname with a first name or initial. A surname with a first initial only precedes the same surname with a complete first name beginning with the same letter as the initial.

4. A surname prefix is not a separate indexing unit.

5. Firm and institutional names are indexed in the order written when they do not contain the complete name of an individual.

6. When the firm or institution name includes the complete name of an individual, indexing order follows rule 1 above.

7. "The" is always disregarded in indexing.

8. Hyphenated words in a firm name are indexed as separate units. Hyphenated surnames of individuals are considered as *one* indexing unit even when part of a firm name.

9. Abbreviations are indexed as though the words were written in full.

10. Conjunctions and prepositions (such as and, for, in, of) are disregarded in indexing.

11. Names that may be written as either one or two words are indexed as one unit.

12. Parts of compound geographic names are indexed separately except when the first part of the name is not an English word.

13. Titles and degrees are disregarded except when it indicates seniority or when the title is the initial word of the name.

14. "Apostrophe s" causes the "s" to be disregarded; "s apostrophe" is indexed including the "s."

15. U.S. government and foreign government names are indexed and subdivided by department, bureau, division, commission, and board.

16. Political divisions are indexed by classification, state, county, and city, and then subdivided as in rule 15.

17. A number in a name is considered as though written in words and is indexed as *one* unit.

18. Addresses are indexed by name, city (state, if a duplication), street, and lowest to highest street number.

19. Banks are indexed by city, bank name, and state.

20. Married women are indexed as in rule 1, with husbands' given and middle names parenthetically noted.

21. Cross-referencing or indexing is done if more than the first word in the name can identify the organization; if the surname is not easily identified; if abbreviations can be readily identified; and if subject identification is possible.

THE BASIC FILING RULES ILLUSTRATED

Rule	Concerning	Name	Index Order of Units		
			Unit 1	Unit 2	Unit 3
1	Individual names	Larry M. Stewart	Stewart	Larry	M
		Mary Ann Pasquale	Pasquale	Mary	Ann
		J. V. Dickey	Dickey	J	V
2	Alphabetic order	Donald C. Lundgren	Lundgren	Donald	C
		Robert Lundgren	Lundgren	Robert	
		Robert A. Lundgren	Lundgren	Robert	A
3	Surnames	Schneider	Schneider		
		A. Schneider	Schneider	A	
		A. Mary Schneider	Schneider	A	Mary
4	Surnames with prefixes	James V. MacDonald	MacDonald	James	V
		Richard E. McClain	McClain	Richard	E
		Gordon M. VanAse	VanAse	Gordon	M
5	Firm names	Dispatch Printing Co.	Dispatch	Printing	Company
		Marquette Savings Assn.	Marquette	Savings	Association
		Tanner Office Supply Co.	Tanner	Office	Supply
6	Firm names containing individuals' names	Bracken Funeral Home	Bracken	Funeral	Home
		Chet Taft, Realtor	Taft	Chet	Realtor
		R. Collins, Signs	Collins	R	Signs
7	"The"	The Greenery	Greenery	(The)	
		The Ace Drawing School	Ace	Drawing	School
		Check the Plumber	Check	(the) Plumber	
8a	Hyphenated names	Mulligan-McCloskey Heating	Mulligan	McCloskey	Heating
8b	Hyphenated names	Joyce-Jean Ceramics	Joyce	Jean	Ceramics
		Link-Belt Power Tools	Link	Belt	Power
9	Abbreviations	AAA Rental Service	A	A	A
		St. Peter's Cathedral	Saint	Peters	Cathedral
		Chas. Moore Printing	Moore	Charles	Printing
10	Conjunctions, prepositions and firm endings	Moped Sales & Service	Moped	Sales	Service
		Sterrett & Co., Inc.	Sterrett	Company	Inc.
		A. Susol & Sons	Susol	A (&)	Sons
		Lutheran Church in America	Lutheran	Church	America

			Index Order of Units		
Rule	Concerning	Name	Unit 1	Unit 2	Unit 3
11	One or two words	North East Coop. Assn.	North East	Cooperative	Association
		Northeast High School	Northeast	High	School
		Down Town Garage	Downtown	Garage	
12	Compound geographic names	New Mexico Publishing Co.	New	Mexico	Publishing
		San Francisco Publishing Co.	San	Francisco	Publishing
		East Rutherford Mills	East	Rutherford	Mills
13	Titles or Degrees	Dr. Salvatore Longo	Longo	Salvatore	(Dr)
		John Price, Jr.	Price	John	(Jr)
		Prince Edward Island	Prince	Edward	Island
14	Possessives	Frank's Cleaners	Franks	Cleaners	
		Mitchells' Grocery Store	Mitchells	Grocery	Store
15	U.S. and foreign government names	U.S. Dept. of the Air Force	United	States	Govt. (1)
		Internal Revenue Service	United	States	Govt. (2)

			Unit 4	Unit 5	Unit 6
		(1)	Air	Force	Dept.
		(2)	Internal	Revenue	Service

			Unit 1	Unit 2	Unit 3
		Canadian Trade Office	Canadian	Trade	Office
16	Other political subdivisions	Erie County Courthouse	Erie	County	Courthouse
		Mayor's Office, City of Erie	Erie	(Pa)	Mayor
		Environmental Resources Dept., Commonwealth of Pennsylvania	Pa	Common-wealth	Environ-mental
17	Numbers	The 9th St. Plaza	Ninth	Street	Plaza (The)
		5th Ave. Hotel	Fifth	Avenue	Hotel
		Restaurant at 66 Park Plaza	Restaurant	Sixty-Six	Park
18	Addresses	Stride-Rite Bootery	Stride	Rite	Bootery
		Millcreek Mall, Erie, Pa.			
		2174 W. 8th, Erie, Pa.			

			Unit 4	Unit 5	Unit 6
			Erie	Pa	Millcreek Mall
			Erie	Pa	West 8th (2174)

Rule	Concerning	Name	Index Order of Units		
			Unit 1	Unit 2	Unit 3
19	Banks, churches, organizations	First National Bank of Erie, Pa.	Erie (Pa)	First National	Bank
		Trinity Lutheran Church	Lutheran	Church	Trinity
		Fraternal Order of Eagles	Eagles	Fraternal	Order (of)
		Iron Workers' Union	Iron	Workers	Union
20	Married women	Mrs. Greg Horgan (Mary Ann)	Horgan (Greg)	Mary	Ann (Mrs)
		Mrs. Jennifer L. Smith (Mrs. Theodore)	Smith (Theodore)	Jennifer	L (Mrs)
		Mrs. Carol Rogers Miller (Mrs. James C.)	Miller (James C)	Carol	Rogers (Mrs)

Information Retrieval

Filing system designs which apply to the standard rules may be classified into four main combinations: alphabetic, subject, geographic, and numeric. Each of these systems will be outlined below, and several diagrams have been provided for a comparison of the different approaches.

ALPHABETIC FILING

Alphabetic filing follows indexing rules with respect to names of business firms, persons, or organizations. Folder captions are restricted to only one correspondent or subject, and documents within the folders are arranged chronologically with the most recent in front. File guides are prepared using alphabetic captions with a single letter reference to indicate documents beginning behind that caption, or double-letter references which indicate the beginning and the end of the document range. Most alphabetic systems utilize primary captions, special captions, individual captions, and miscellaneous captions. For ease of retrieval color-keys may be used for the guide tabs and the folders filed behind these guides. Commercial filing systems use colors related to vowels in the position of the filing unit and a separate color for index units whose second letter is not a vowel. Miscellaneous files are attached to the color corresponding to the guide with individual folders for the appropriate sections (Fig. 5-3).

SUBJECT FILING

Subject filing systems designate document retention and retrieval by topic rather than by alphabetic or numeric reference. These systems may be employed (1) if the document does

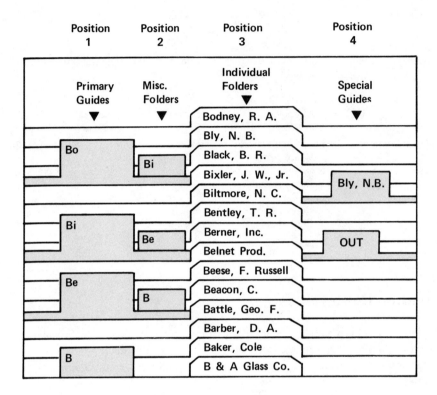

Variadex System by Remington Rand

If 2nd letter of first unit of name is	Section Guide tab color is	Example
a, b, c, d	orange	Baker
e, f, g, h	yellow	Bellow
i, j, k, l, m, n	green	Bixler
o, p, q	blue	Bodney
r, s, t, u, v, w, x, y, z	violet	Brayton

FIGURE 5-3. Alphabetic filing with a color-key scheme.

not refer to the name of a person or organization, (2) if retrieval is more likely to be by subject than by name, (3) if rational grouping of documents may be achieved by activities or products, or (4) if too many small subdivisions would occur if records were not grouped by subject.

There are two main types of subject systems (Fig. 5-4). A combination alpha-subject system is used when the main body of the files has a nominal alphabetic reference and a small number of files are indexed by subject. Alpha-subject systems utilize subject headings for main file divisions and alphabetic divisions within the subject headings. This system requires a cardex or similar index to identify all heading divisions and subdivisions as well as strong referencing to maximize retrieval efficiency. By way of reference, such systems often look like dictionary or encyclopedia catalogs. The second system is a numeric-subject com-

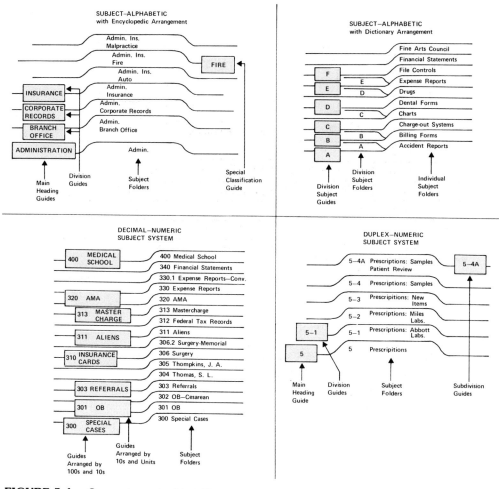

FIGURE 5-4.   Comparison of subject filing systems.

bination whereby number captions are assigned to each subject heading with a relative index as the key to entry into the filing system.

GEOGRAPHIC FILING

Geographic filing systems employ an alphabetic arrangement of the document location index. Primary guides indicate large geographic divisions, and special guides are used for subdivisions of the main geographic units. Individual folders list city and state references and are indexed in accordance with the standardized rules. A cardex is used to identify each document's geographic location and is referenced on an alphabetic basis. Cross-referencing is necessary if the index reference has more than one geographic location or when the recall reference may be made either by name, subject, or location (Fig. 5-5).

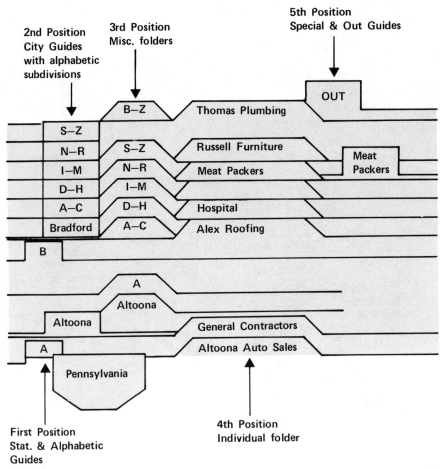

FIGURE 5-5. Geographic filing system.

NUMERIC FILING

Numeric filing systems utilize numbers as index captions on guides and folders. This is an indirect retrieval system since the user must refer to an alphabetized code to find the number assigned to the document name or subject. Numeric systems are maintained when record retention is by case history, contract, or project for an indefinite time period. While the system requires extensive cross-referencing to be effective, it does preserve the anonymity of the documents should that be a major goal of the files management system.

In a numeric system the individual folders bear consecutively assigned numeric captions, and the folders are filed in numeric sequence. Documents which have not accumulated sufficient quantity to warrant a numeric index are filed in miscellaneous alphabetic folders which are stored separately. A cardex which is filed on an alphabetic basis identifies the assigned numeric indexes by name and subject and accounts for all unassigned numbers.

There are several file drawer arrangements for numeric filing systems, including consecutive number, terminal-digit, and alpha-numeric. In consecutive number filing, documents are assigned a numeric index which is cross-referenced in the cardex for subsequent document additions, and records are filed by their numeric sequence. Consecutive number filing is appropriate when the individual patient folders are large enough to warrant subdivision by subject. For example:

607 John W. Roger	607-1 case history	607-2 surgery
	607-3 health insurance	607-4 referral services

Terminal digit filing is based on numeric digits read from right to left. Files are assigned consecutive numeric indexes, but the file guides are prepared by groupings beginning with the terminal group. The digit read is by pairs—the primary reference equally 01-99, the secondary reference equally 100 to 9900, the tertiary reference equally 10000 to 90000, and so on. Terminal digit file storage keys right to left and codes the primary pair as the file cabinet drawer number, the secondary pair as the special guide number or individual folder number, and the third pair as the sequence within the file folder or the patient case identification number. A master file with alphabetic name indexing must be maintained in order to create rapid and efficient entry into the filing system.

Alpha-numeric filing systems assign numeric sequencing to the records and alphabetic codes to the documents by name or subject. This method allows for maximum expansion of the filing system and is utilized when document files number in the millions. Commercial systems of this type require extensive training, and their applicability to the medical field is directed more to hospitals than to individual private practices.

CHARACTERISTICS OF VARIOUS FILING SYSTEMS

Methods	Advantages	Disadvantages
Alphabetic	1. Direct filing and reference 2. No index required	1. Misfiling of common names 2. Related records scattered throughout the files

3. Record groupings by name

3. Cross-referencing may be either too simple or too extensive

4. Record management by guides, folder colors
5. Miscellaneous files easily identified

Subject

1. Records grouping which establishes statistical or technical relationships
2. Unlimited expansion

1. Difficulty in classifying records for filing

2. Extensive-cross-referencing necessary
3. Miscellaneous records difficult to classify
4. Frequent reference to index to determine subject heading or subdivision

Geographic

1. Direct filing and reference by location—indirect by individual
2. Records grouped by location

3. Provision for miscellaneous records

1. Location as well as name required for document retrieval
2. Triple sort—state, city, alphabet—increases error rate and raises labor costs
3. Reference to card index necessary to find document
4. Fold labels required and extensive information and maintenance

Numeric

1. Accuracy
2. Unlimited expansion
3. Cross-referencing permanent and extensive
4. Index is complete list of documents by name and subject
5. Document retrieval by specific numeric identification with reference to name or subject (Same numeric ID can provide uniform system for all department and company files)

1. Indirect filing and reference
2. Cumbersome index
3. Miscellaneous documents requiring separate files
4. High labor cost with specialized training required

SPECIAL FILING SYSTEMS

Special filing systems are available for specific document material problems within the physician's practice. These systems utilize one filing design or a combination of the basic designs enumerated above and arrange the physical storage and document flow procedures to maximize efficient accessibility. The specific files of concern to the medical assistant are card files, vertical files, visible files, microfilm and microfiche files, and electronic data processing (EDP) files.

Card files are utilized for material which is frequently referenced, as an index for the main filing system and as a guide to the cross-referencing system. A well-organized card file system is a miniaturization of the full-blown system and as such can be used to revise, rearrange, or redesign the main body of files on a trial basis before the original documents become physically involved. In addition, the same process may be employed to reclassify documents from active to permanent to inactive or to purge the files of outdated materials.

Vertical files are used extensively for posted card records of patients and financial matters. Records such as patient ledger cards can be indexed on a separate card containing the name, address, subject, case history, billing, and payments. These cards can then be organized in drawers or open file cabinets with file guides for every 25 to 50 cards.

Visible files have the advantage that separate file guides become unnecessary since part of the card is visible and therefore provides its own guide. The indexed card records are stored in an overlapping vertical drawer or in rotary racks, tubs, wheels, or loose-leaf visible books.

Microfilm and microfiche files are utilized to reduce (1) file space requirements, (2) the number of files needed, and (3) the labor required for file retrieval. Additionally, protection and storage efficiency for individual documents are enhanced since the accuracy, condition, and sequencing of the records are preserved indefinitely and unalterably. To maintain these file systems, standard filing procedures are designed for use with one of the four main classifications (alphabetic, numeric, subject, or geographic).

Records Protection

Effective and efficient retrieval methods create conditions conducive to control over document flow, assuring that all records are accounted for and easily accessible and that a standard routing schedule for document movements has been designated and is maintained. A charge system is the methodology by which (1) requests for filed materials are initiated through a requisition slip; (2) document materials are charged to the individual collecting the records; and (3) followup procedures are instituted until such time as the documents have been returned to the files.

Charge-out systems (a transfer process) utilize either out-guide or out-folder records to indicate who removed the individual file folder and when it was removed. Substitution cards may be inserted to indicate individual documents which have been removed. Either form of charge-out record should specify the nominal index of the borrowed record, the subject of the record, the name of the borrower, the signature of the borrower, the date of the record, the date borrowed, the date when the materials are to be returned, and the borrower's department or work unit. The charge-out records are removed when materials are returned or when a notation is made showing that the documents have been reclassified and filed as permanent or inactive records (Fig. 5-6).

A cardex system should be utilized as a reminder file so that followup procedures are instituted when the borrowed records have been kept beyond the time stated on the charge-out record. A systematic followup procedure reduces the possibility of document loss, as do definite loan periods of short duration.

Records Retention and Storage

No matter how small the physician's office operation, the same essential standardized file maintenance procedures are necessary to maximize efficiency and minimize the chance of error or document loss. The essential ingredients of an effective information system are fourfold: document flow, document accountability, frequent initial and replacement filing, and efficient storage.

Documents under discussion in this chapter can be classified as incoming, outgoing, or office-generated. The medical assistant should see to it that documents keep moving

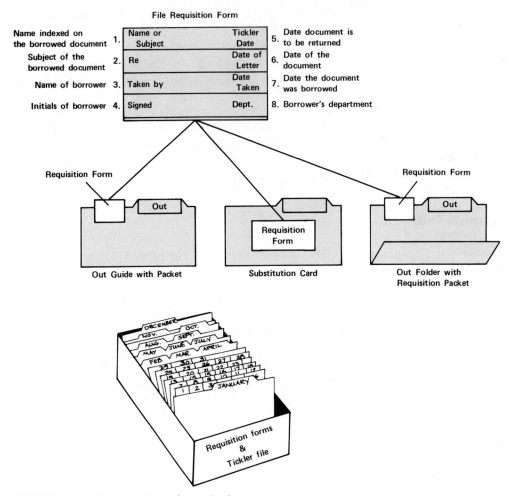

FIGURE 5-6.   Charge and transfer methods.

through the use of time stamps and routing indexes. In addition a transfer process should be instituted to reclassify documents for active, permanent, or inactive storage. Periodic review of the files will reduce file space needs and will confine the contents of active files to current recallable materials.

Only records of patients currently under the physician's care should be maintained in the active files. The records of discharged patients are generally transferred to inactive files. If a patient dies, moves, or terminates health care, the individual folder should be micro-filmed and placed in storage for retrieval when research practice review or family history referencing is required.

Document accountability is achieved through the charge-out system outlined above. The value of such a method will become all too apparent should the medical assistant have to institute document search procedures for lost, misfiled, or unfiled records. Additionally, a well-designed, standardized system will provide for easy identification of a document's terminal location for either the initial filing process or replacement filing.

Frequent initial and replacement filing preserves the integrity of the documents themselves, protects the records from misplacement or loss, and provides for accurate and up-to-date information systems. Information accessibility is imperative for all members of the physician's office, but the materials contained in the records management system must be current and accurate.

Efficient storage minimizes physical strain and maximizes information retrieval methods. Equipment and supplies design and layout should follow the procedures outlined throughout this chapter. Standardization and systemization are the key elements of effective records management.

RECORDS RETENTION POLICIES

Records retention policies determine what, where, and for how long documents will be stored as well as when and how outdated documents will be destroyed. The physician's information requirements dictate the classification of files as to active, permanent, or inactive status. Requirements imposed by federal, state, and local agencies will identify specific documents which must be retained as well as the required retention period. Historical documents concerning the physician's practice provide valuable documentation for scientific and medical research as well as for legal purposes. Finally, vital patient records need to be preserved and stored for case history referrals at subsequent dates and for their research potential.

OFFICE SUPPLIES AND EQUIPMENT

Planning and organizing the physical aspects of the physician's office are important responsibilities of the medical assistant. The administrative functions required include (1) the efficient structuring of the work unit; (2) the acquisition of basic equipment and responsibility for its smooth operation; (3) the keeping of a basic inventory of office and maintenance supplies and determination of reordering needs; (4) the determination of maintenance schedules for both administrative and health care facilities; and (5) the provision or supervision of office cleaning needs.

The office procedures manual should provide the medical assistant with a basic equipment list for the work unit. The actual physical layout may be at the discretion of the MA or may be dictated either by patient traffic flows or office architectural considerations. Office policy will determine the nature and extent of decorating possibilities both in the work unit and more generally in the office. The medical assistant should consult with professionals whenever possible to see that the efficiency of the administrative and health care functions of the office is enhanced by the spatial arrangements without neglecting the value of an aesthetic atmosphere. Certain guidelines can be recommended. Remember that you and your colleagues must work in the office environment and that patients who make frequent visits need to find the atmosphere inviting, cheerful, tasteful, and well-kept. Colors can be used to create desired moods. Music can be employed when appropriate, and the transition spaces of the office can be accented with well-tended plants. While standardization is required in office procedures, your creativity can be utilized to its fullest in the planning and design of the physical requirements of the facility.

A checklist approach similar to that introduced earlier provides for maximum efficiency in designing the medical assistant's work unit. Equipment and supplies inventory records should include detailed descriptions of each item, the supplier's name and address, the quantity purchased and price paid, routine and special maintenance procedures, maintenance contracts and the names and addresses of service personnel, evaluations of the quality of the products purchased, and an evaluation of the current condition of equipment and supplies in inventory. Separate inventory cards should be maintained for each item or group of items so that the daily or weekly review process can be indicated on the records and the inventory updated as a matter of routine. The following is a suggested list of basic office supplies and equipment:

Office Equipment:

Desks
File cabinets
Telephone system
Lighting system
Desk trays for incoming and outgoing recordkeeping
Transcribing machine
Tape recorder
Copier equipment

Office Supplies:

Filing folders, guides, labels, charge and transfer records
Rotary files
Card files
Vertical files
Visible files
Microfiche files
Appointment book
Calendar
Stapler
Pencil sharpener
Message pads
Telephone directories
Reminder pads
Paper (letterheads, blank stationery, envelopes, announcement cards, business
    cards, appointment cards, carbon paper)
Basic steno tools (staples, paper clips, pens, pencils, tape, stamps, ruler, correction
    fluid)
Forms for recordkeeping
        bills and invoices

payroll records
bank deposit tickets and checks
insurance forms
petty cash reimbursement forms
pegboard "one-write" systems
collection aids
charge and third-party billing forms
"truth-in-lending" forms
prescription forms and drug envelopes
medical questionnaires
patient history forms, lab record forms, consent forms, hospital care record
   forms, ledger cards

Maintenance Supplies:

Laundry items (uniforms, gowns, sheets, towels, pillows—either of disposable or non-
   disposable types)
Cleaning items (cleansers, detergent, soaps, paper towels, toilet tissue, drain cleaner,
   deodorizer, floor wax, rags, window and mirror cleaner, metal and furniture polish,
   mops, scrub brushes, sponges, light bulbs, stain remover)

OFFICE MAINTENANCE

Part of the administrative task assigned to the medical assistant is the supervision of
maintenance for the office and waiting room areas and for the health care facility. Utilizing
the checklist approach and the equipment and supplies inventory discussed earlier, the MA
should include in the office procedures manual daily, weekly, and monthly maintenance
procedures specific to each area of the office unit and the clinical practice. The procedures
would, of course, be modified if the physician used an outside professional cleaning service.

	Work Unit	*Office and Waiting Room*	*Clinical Area*
Daily:	1. Organize desk top 2. Organize desk drawers 3. Inventory supplies 4. Dispatch rubbish 5. Dust and polish 6. Instruct professional cleaning service	1. Dust and polish 2. Clean bathroom frequently 3. Straighten and/or replace reading materials 4. Replenish supplies 5. Empty ash trays 6. Provide childrens' toys and books 7. Tend plants 8. Mop spills and provide special flooring for inclement weather	1. Dust and polish frequently 2. Remove soiled linen 3. Replace used instruments 4. Straighten and restock medical supplies 5. Review supplies in physician's bag

Weekly: 1. Dust bookshelves and files
              2. Vacuum furniture and rugs
              3. Clean lighting systems
              4. Clean mirrors and pictures
              5. Scrub and wax floors

Monthly: 1. Clean windows, blinds, and curtains
              2. Clean upholstered furniture
              3. Polish metal fixtures
              4. Clean and check office equipment

In addition to the maintenance of the physical layout of the physician's office, the medical assistant will undoubtedly be in charge of the library of scientific, medical, and technical materials which the doctor and the office personnel use as reference documents. A cardex system is the most efficient means of indicating the books, journals (including those kept in the waiting room), technical monographs, pamphlets, and other materials which are housed in the library. The cardex should include the following information: author, title, subject, publisher, year of publication, and number of pages, as well as editor, volume, and issue number for journals. For ease of access the cardex should be indexed and cross-referenced by author, title, and subject in a manner similar to a Library of Congress listing or the Dewey decimal system utilized by many medical societies. The MA should review both the cardex and the library materials to see that they are current and in good condition. Subscriptions subject to renewal should be compiled and located in a "tickler" file in the front of the cardex. Professional development materials should be added to the library, and facilities should be provided for a charge-out system so that they may be utilized frequently. As the library increases in sophistication it may be necessary to obtain special equipment such as tape recorders, microfiche readers, and document reducers so that audio-visual materials which become part of the library holdings may be used with ease.

GUIDELINES FOR EFFICIENT RECORDS MANAGEMENT

1. Keep the system simple—the emphasis is on speed, accuracy and reliability.

2. Use standardized procedures and use them without variation—the emphasis is on organization, efficiency, and consistency.

3. Train others in your system—be sure everyone with access to the files maintains them with the same care and concern as you do.

4. When in doubt, cross-reference—be sure the document trail is obvious from alphabetic to numeric to subject files and within each area.

5. Set aside a definite time in the daily office routine for filing duties. A disciplined approach will guarantee that the files are current and that you are not overwhelmed with the paper flow.

6. Use proper filing tools and supplies—the physical document flow through the office and the physical energy you expend related to it can be minimized with preplanning and efficient work-unit organization.

7. Use the right supplies for the right records and *don't* economize. Design your system and carefully purchase quality supplies and you will minimize file maintenance activities. (Documents of substandard size should be attached to standard-size paper and then filed.)

8. Examine all folder contents each time the file is retrieved and before it is returned to the file. Being totally familiar with the normal document contents reduces file search time and the chances of misfiling.

9. Maintain all facets of your system. Keep tabs and guides neat and current. Mend torn documents before refiling.

10. Organize your system for easy accessibility. Active files should be front and center within a file cabinet and the cabinets in the most active section of the work area.

11. File cabinets are for document files—don't use them for storage of other office items.

12. Physical safety should be emphasized. Open one drawer at a time and reclose immediately after use.

13. Don't cram—subdivide and cross-reference bulging files. Don't fill the drawer to capacity or the neatness, order, and ease of accessibility of your system will be diminished.

14. Classify documents and regularly review them. Separate permanent files from active and inactive files. Regularly purge the current files of inactive records.

15. Use a well-designed color-key system. Retrieving speed and accuracy can be enhanced by file folders, guides, and labels that aid in establishing a document flow trail.

SUMMARY

As a medical assistant you will be expected to relieve the physician of the day-to-day mechanical responsibilities of operating the office. To effectively carry out this task, MAs must perceive their role to be more comprehensive than that of a secretary. They must act more in the capacity of a manager and systems designer.

While approaching this challenge, medical assistants must try to remind themselves from time to time that office procedures interact in many instances with the delivery of good medical care. MAs must constantly strive to develop office practices which facilitate the provision of quality medical care. They must also learn how to relieve physicians of the needless burdens of the office without removing them from active participation in important policy decisions.

As a new MA you will have to prove yourself to the physician before he or she will be willing to relinquish the role of manager to you. Thus new MAs will have to learn the virtue of patience while convincing the physician of their competence.

APPLICATION EXERCISES

The first step in preparing for the classroom application exercise work will be to complete an assignment at home. The student should obtain a generous supply of standard index cards and carry out the following procedures:

1. The names and addresses given below are to be properly and consistently indexed and filed—first alphabetically, then geographically.

2. Using the indexed entries, design a numeric filing system.

3. Using the indexed entries, design a subject filing system, where possible.

1. Jayman Printing Service, 7804 N. Michigan Ave., Chicago, Ill. 60626
2. "Kitchens by Mead," 2401 Klein Bldg., Erie, Pa 16505
3. Mlle. Jeanette Marie Curie, Rue de la Pais 5, Paris, France
4. E-Sac Builders, 3201 Amherst Rd., Akron, Ohio 4434?
5. Edward Klean Trucks and Heavy Equipment, 4919 Wm. Flynn Hwy., Allison Park, Pa. 15352
6. Barchony and Federcwicz, Attorneys at Law, G Daniel Baldwin Bldg., Cleveland, Ohio 44141
7. Robert P. Vander Meen, 221 Waterleet St., Detroit, Michigan 48217
8. Jerome Labelson, Apt. 3B, 60 Fulton Place South, New York, N.Y. 10022
9. Morgan E. Jacox and Co., Tax Consultants, Suite 12, Hotel Baltimore, Baltimore, Md. 21202
10. Karoll Tieberkrob, Chalfonte Hall, Campus Station, Durham, N.C. 27707.
11. Scriptomatic Addressing Systems, 801 East Ave., Omaha, Nebr. 68108
12. Melfax-Dayton, 210 N. Park Row, Albany, N.Y. 12210
13. Paragen Packaging Products, 625 Buckhill Rd., N.W. Atlanta, Georgia 30308
14. Raymond L. Eckerson and Associates Advertising, 3511 Post Ave., Los Angeles, CA 90035
15. Flying Tigers Airfreight, 117 McLaughlen Rd., Lufken, TX 75901
16. Product Demand Tele-Productions, Junction State Routes 7&9, Osburn, Id. 83849
17. Youman & Barties Mfg. Company, Inc., 1848 Greentree Road, Columbus, Ohio 43201
18. The World-Telegram News, Dallas, Texas 78421
19. Aer Lingus-Irish Airlines, 2000 Market, Philadelphia, Pa. 18781
20. Bronson's Air Conditioning Service, 1119 West 26th St., St. Joseph, Mo. 64504
21. North American Amusement Corp., 1010 Pacific Boulevard, Portland, Ore. 97220
22. Perry Plaza Bowling Center, 2230 Broad, Erie, Pa., 16515
23. John C. Veenschoten Gallery, 5020 N. Ridge E., Ashtabula, Ohio 45750
24. Craft-N-Flower Ltd., Monroeville Mall, Oak Park, Ill. 60403

25. Dalton-Dalton-Newport, A-5 Commerce Bldg., Sarasota, Fla. 33580
26. Buzz n' B's Aquarium and Pet Shop, Reading and Vine Sts., Camden, Ohio 45311
27. Northview Heights Apartments, 2324c 43rd, Wilmington, Del. 19810
28. Maybro Asphalt Company, Inc., 654 W. French, Louisville, Ky. 40218
29. American Heart Assn. Northwestern Pa. Chapter, 806 Masonic Temple Building, Erie, Pa. 16501
30. Physician's Planning Service Corp., 69-75 Ompi Plaza, Miami, Fla. 33839
31. GECAC, First St. at B & O R.R., Camden, N.J. 08105
32. House of Cars Body Shop, 1667 Edgewood Dr., Richmond, Va. 23223
33. McQuillen Oldsmobile-Pontiac Inc., 2606 Zuck Rd., Yuma, Arizona 72901
34. Northeast Ohio Bank & Trust Co., Forty-seven N. Center, Marietta, Ohio 45750
35. Sal's Barber & Beauty Salons, 225 E. Main, Titusville, Fla. 32742
36. Hi Skippen' Marina Inc., Ft. of Cranberry, New Orleans, La. 70130
37. Allegheny Reproductive Health Center, 5530 Forbes Ave., Pittsburgh, Pa. 15221
38. Cook's Industrial Crating, Danow Rd., Bethel, CT 06253
39. The Duchesse Shoppe, 2214 Powell Ave., Girard, Pa. 16417
40. Eastland Bowl Inc., 3109 Collins Ave. Houston, Tex. 77007
41. Erie Hard Facing Industries Inc., 5601 Great Detroit, Me. 48217
42. J & E Welding Service, 6610 East Lake Rd., St. Louis, Mo. 63155
43. Christian & Missionary Alliance (Church), 1016 State, Denver 80214
44. Plastic Coating & Molding Inc., Rt. 505, Sante Fe, N.M. 87501
45. Twaney's Cleaners & Decorators, 412 Jodie Lane, Seattle, Wash. 98112
46. Lawrence Park Athletic Club, 4130 Old French Rd., Syracuse, N.Y. 13271
47. The Disabled American Veterans Club, 1404 K. ST. N.W., Washington, D.C. 20005
48. Rite Light Family Optical, Plaza 9, Memphis, Tenn. 38122
49. R.A. Greig Equipment Co., 3202 Sterratania Rd., Cincinnati, Ohio 45201
50. Hemtens & Trappers Supply, 1406 W. 26th St., Cicero, IL 60650
51. Offerle The Florist, 3034 Elmwood Ave., Colorado Springs, CO 80904
52. Villa Medical Supply, 22 Medical Arts Bldg., Seattle, WA 98121
53. Modern Machinery Sales Co., 11758 Valley Rd., Cleveland, OH 44141
54. The Art School, 941 West 36th St., Albany, N.Y. 12210
55. Pennsylvania Artificial Limb & Brace Co., Inc., 5530 Peach, Erie, Pa.
56. Kuhn's Picture & Gift Shop, 154 West Twentieth St., Portland Oregon 97220
57. Service Master by Hewitt, 435 Guand, Alexandria, Va. 22313
58. LW Preece Inc., 9181 Foothill Rd., Springfield, Ill. 62701
59. Elk Valley Golf & Recreation Inc., 8965 Tippecanoe Rd., Indianapolis, Ind. 42625
60. The Housing Authority of the City of Baltimore, City Hall, Baltimore, MD 21202
61. Federal Public Defender, 129 Federal Building, Saint Louis, Mo. 63166
62. NOAA National Weather Service, O'Hare Int'l. Airport, Chicago, Ill. 60611

63. Wate Rajhma, Room 2100, United Nations Secretariat, New York, N.Y.
64. Carlson's Industrial Grinding, 6340 Firman Rd., Minneapolis, Minn. 55413
65. MA Bornand Co. Inc., 1418 Buffalo Rd., Buffalo, N.Y.
66. Fuhrman-Brown Precision Tool & Mfg. Corp., 5630 Perry Highway, Dallas, Texas 75221
67. Norton Grinding Wheels, 4650 W. Ridge Road, Little Rock, Ark. 72214
68. Special Delivery, 2717 Greencrest Dr., Charleston, W. Va. 25303
69. Abercrombie's General Store, East Center, Mill Village, Pa. 16427
70. Depcraft Manufacturing Co., 722 Nevada, Reno, Nevada 89504
71. General Medical Home Healthcare Center, 11885 Main East, Phoenix, AZ 85041
72. Great Lakes Behavioral Research, 9015 Station Rd., Nashville, Tenn. 37202
73. Li'l Shopper Store No. 411, 5414 Cherry, Lexington, Ky. 40507
74. Olympiad Gymnastic Academy, 2215 West 12th, Chase Hotel, St. Louis, Mo. 63166
75. Kraus Department Store, 7700 South Wells St., Roune, Wisc. 53401
76. Terra Natural Foods, 5229 Crest Drive, Baton Rouge, La. 70821
77. Medical Oxygen Dio Raimy Corp., 21-01 19th St., Long Island, N.Y. 11105
78. Coordinated Health Accident Life Pension Benefits Inc., Prudential Center, Boston 01432
79. LoCastro-Giacomelli-Domino Inc., 3819 Meadow Dr., Los Angeles, Calif. 90053
80. Drug Counseling Center, 4210 Burton Ave., Tallahassee, Fl. 32302
81. Bloxdorf's Presque Isle Pharmacy, 1600 Peninsula Dr., Fairview, Pa. 16415
82. Medicine Shoppe, 1039 Newton Ave., Columbus, Ohio 43201
83. Ken Lockbaum Physical Therapy Clinic, 5125 Exeter Ave., Springfield, Ill. 62701
84. Consultants in Cardiology Inc. 10765 W. Main Rd., Fargo, N.D. 58102
85. Iroquois Medical Center, 4313 Conrad Rd., Sante Fe, N.M. 87501
86. Dept. of Urology—Erie Clinic, SS. Peter & Paul Memorial Hospital, Erie, Pa. 16512
87. Fairview Medical Associates Inc., 2704 Washington Ave., Milwaukee, WI. 52140
88. Dr. Gary Pasqualicchio, Professional Bldg., 1615 W. 26th, San Diego, Ca. 90291
89. Northwest Cardiovascular Surgery Inc., 104 E. 2nd St., Cincinnati
90. L.M. Verdecchio, M.D., Inc., 3317 Liberty, Providence, R.I. 02909
91. MEDICOR Associates, Inc., 3815 Field Ave., Boston Mass. 01432
92. Larson Laboratories, Inc., Highpoint Tower Suite 25, N.Y.C., N.Y.
93. McGee Women's Hospital, Pittsburgh, Pa. 15221
94. St. Vincent Drug & Poison Information Center, St. Vincent Hospital, 232 West 25th St. Atlanta, Ga. 30308
95. Community Blood Bank, IBM Building, 1654 W. 18th St., Omaha, Ne. 68108
96. Family Crises Intervention Inc., Medical Center Bldg., Dallas, Tx 78421

97. Hermitage House, 3822 Wayne, Richmond, Va. 23223
98. Hispanic-American Health Counseling Services, 4348 La Cienaga Blvd., Los Angeles, Calif. 90035
99. Minority Health-Education Delivery System, 1104 Marshall Dr., Lufken, Tx. 75901
100. TEL—MED, 2005 Southern Dr., Miami, Fla. 33839

After your instructor has had an opportunity to check over the filing systems which the students have designed, she will organize the class into groups to discuss the issues listed below.

Discussion Issues

1. Describe and illustrate each of the four main areas of records control and management.

2. Describe the cross-referencing process and apply it to each of the four main filing systems.

3. Why is indexing so important?

4. How are documents arranged in individuals folders? In miscellaneous folders? In special folders?

5. What is the purpose of the charge-out process?

6. Describe a "tickler" file and its uses.

7. What factors affect the retention policy of a business firm?

8. Describe the five-step filing process and compare and contrast its application in alphabetical, numeric, subject, and geographic filing systems.

9. Why is standardization necessary in filing?

10. Describe the document search procedure.

11. Describe a possible physical arrangement of a work unit to maximize filing efficiency.

12. What basic questions must be asked when planning a filing system?

13. Discuss the similarities and differences of required filing systems in a small office and those a large business organization.

14. Design an efficient filing system utilizing commercial color-key schemes in each of the four principal filing procedures.

15. Take the system you designed in answering questions 11 and 14 and discuss how you would train someone totally unfamiliar with filing procedures. Describe the strengths and weaknesses which you discovered about your system and how you would revise and improve the design.

COMPLETING THE LEARNING LOOP

As a result of study and discussion of the material contained in this chapter, you should have developed competencies in the following areas:

1. Preparation and use of an office procedures manual
2. Physical design of a medical assistant's work unit
3. Planning and design of an efficient central records system
4. Specific files management procedures
5. Basic functions of specific types of office equipment and supplies
6. Basic office maintenance procedures

Another office management responsibility of the medical assistant is the scheduling of appointments, which is discussed in the following chapter.

BIBLIOGRAPHY

Bredow, M.: *Medical Office Procedures.* McGraw-Hill, 1973.

Dennis, R. L., and Doyle, J. M.: *Complete Handbook for Medical Secretaries and Assistants*, ed. 2. Little, Brown, Boston, 1978.

Foster, M.: *Medical Office Practice.* Bobbs-Merrill, Indianapolis, 1975.

McCormick, J., and Grayburn, D. W.: *The Management of Medical Practice.* Ballinger, Cambridge, Mass., 1978.

McFadden, M. S.: *Medical Office Management Handbook.* Career Publishing, Orange, Cal., 1977.

Steward, J. R., et al.: *Progressive Filing*, ed. 9. McGraw-Hill, New York, 1980.

6

ORGANIZING AND COORDINATING APPOINTMENTS

SPECIFIC OBJECTIVES

Upon completion of this chapter you will be able to:

1. Organize and administrate a complete office appointment system.

2. Schedule appointments and enter these in the appointment book.

3. Assist in the organization of office activities which are related to the day's appointments.

INTRODUCTION

Not long ago the physician's organization of appointments consisted of displaying a sign which read: "Office Hours M-F, 12 to 4 P.M." Patients soon learned to appear during the times indicated. They were usually treated on a "first come, first served" basis.

Over the past several years, however, the increasing complexity of medical practice, coupled with the great demand for the services of physicians, has created the need for a more orderly and efficient system. The emphasis in appointment scheduling is on optimal utilization of office resources and on the efficient management of the physician's and patient's time. The basic problem in scheduling revolves around the conflict of interest between these objectives.

The "blocking" of time for the scheduling of individual appointments has become the most widely accepted practice. This method facilitates the attainment of the major objectives of scheduling and is shaped by the physician's scheduling preferences, the type of specialty, the facilities, the size and type of staff, and the needs of the typical patient.

THE APPOINTMENT BOOK

The most logical first step in the design of an efficient appointment system is to find or create an appropriate appointment book. While there are many alternatives available, the medical assistant must attempt to determine the approach which is best suited for her or his particular office. There are a large number of different appointment books available from stationery supply houses. If the decision has been made to purchase one of these standard books, several factors should be considered.

An example of a standard appointment book sheet is shown in Figure 6-1. If special needs are present, such as scheduling appointments for a large number of physicians or unique information requirements, the MA might consider designing a book which reflects these individualized needs (Fig. 6-2).

Before moving ahead with the finalized design of a specialized appointment book, MAs should put together a rough draft format, then talk over their ideas with the physician. Once the final design has been developed, a master can be reproduced to provide pages for the appointment book. These may, in turn, be bound in a loose-leaf notebook. If several physicians are involved in a practice, appointment books can be color-coded for ease in identification.

Whether the MA utilizes a standardized appointment book or a special design, several basic requirements must be met.

The Matrix System

A matrix system provides for the inclusion of basic or "core" information:

1. *Who*—the person making the appointment.

2. *Why*—the purpose of the appointment.

3. *When*—the time designated for the office visit.

4. *How much*—the length of time needed for the visit.

5. *Additional information*—the patient's telephone number is needed when the patient is visiting the office for the first time (if a cancellation were necessary, no reference could otherwise be made).

Size and Placement

Appointment books should open flat for ease in recording and ready access. Desk size is an important consideration, as is proximity to the telephone. The interval spaces allotted on the appointment sheet should be of ample width to record the necessary information.

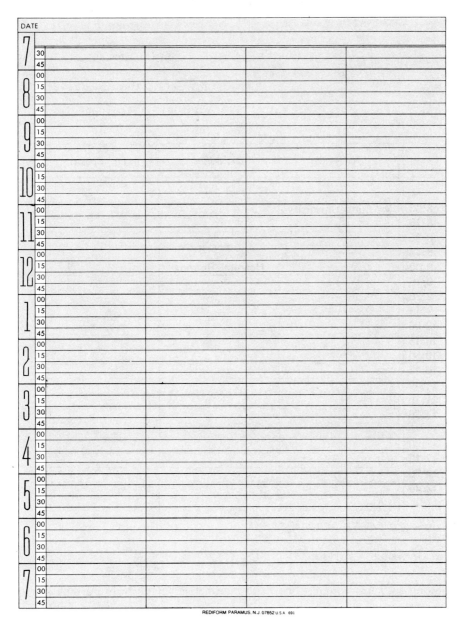

FIGURE 6-1. A standard appointment sheet.

Recording

If appointments are scheduled in pencil, erasures can be made neatly and changes easily accomplished. However, many physicians prefer that pen be used and erasures avoided as protection against potential legal problems. Accountability for all time intervals during the day is provided on the appointment sheets.

Month _____

Date _____

Day _____

	Dr. Smith	Dr. Jones	Dr. Brown
8:00	At State University		
8:15	— — —		
8:30	— — —		
8:45	— — —		
9:00	— — —	Hospital Rounds	
9:15	— — —	— — —	
9:30	— — —	— — —	
9:45	— — —	— — —	
10:00			
10:15			
10:30			
10:45			
11:00			
11:15			
11:30			
11:45			
12:00			
12:15			
12:30			
12:45			
1:00			

FIGURE 6-2.   A specialized appointment sheet.

Making Proper Entries

The following six items comprise the basic information units which are required for any scheduling system:

1. *Space for Entries.* The appointment book must contain the space required to make all of the entries necessary for each appointment.

2. *Patient's Name.* Full names should be entered clearly, the last name first. There may be several patients with the same surname, particularly in family medical practices:

> 9:30—Evans, Ralph (Sr.)
> 9:45—Evans, Raymond
> 10:00—Evans, Ralph (Jr.)

3. *Time of Appointment.* The patient's name should be entered next to the appropriate time in the book.

4. *Length of Appointment.* Knowledge of office procedures is required to estimate the time needed for a particular appointment. A schedule guide for procedures, observations, and the approximate time required should be inserted in the inside cover of the appointment book for convenient access. (It may be helpful to refer to the Guide to Estimated Times for Common Medical Office Procedures, found in the Appendix.)

> *Example:* P&P (pelvic examination and pap smear—15 minutes)
> Drsg. chg. (dressing change—30 minutes)
> 9:15—Jones, Mary—P&P
> 9:45—Roberts, Bob—Drsg. chg.

5. *Reason for Visit.* The purpose of the visit should be noted in the book, using standard abbreviations only.

6. *Telephone Number.* For the new patient, both home and work numbers should be listed in case of the need to adjust the appointment. In offices where cancellations by the physician are frequent or appointment waiting lists occur, phone numbers for all patients are advised.

Figure 6-3 provides an illustration of the "blocking" of appointment entries on a specially designed sheet. Mrs. Jones is going to need 30 minutes for her annual physical examination, and Mr. Brown is coming in for a post-surgical checkup. Mr. Brown's visit will take only 15 minutes.

PLANNING THE DAY'S APPOINTMENTS

It is important to gather and evaluate some basic information prior to organizing the day's appointments:

1. The different types of appointments made in the office must be assessed (physical exams, treatments, tests). The medical practice will dictate the variety of appointment types.

2. An estimate of the time required for each of the common types of appointments is pertinent to effective planning (complete examination: 30 min.; treatment: 15 min.; etc.). The physician will estimate time allotments for procedures.

3. The physician's preferences must also be taken into consideration. (For example, some doctors like to perform complete physicals in the morning and see new patients later in the afternoon.)

4. The handling of emergencies also requires planning. (It is quite common for patients to call with problems requiring immediate attention. Most physicians have some open appointment times for these individuals.)

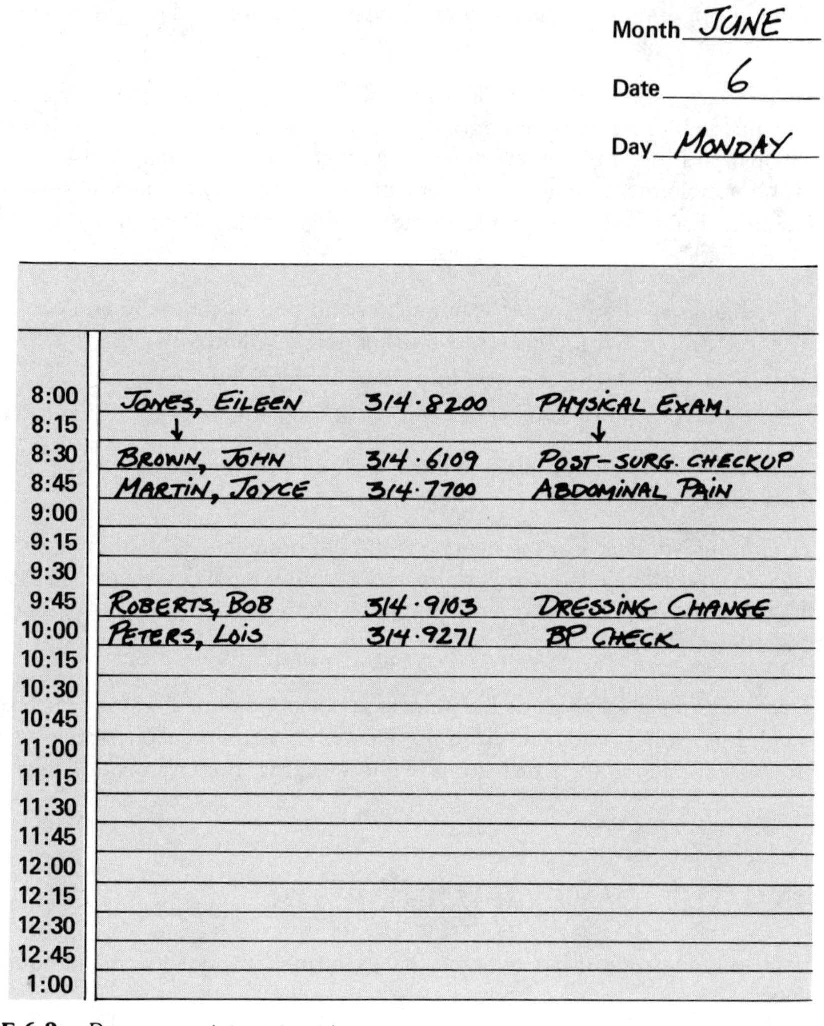

Month _JUNE_

Date ___6___

Day _MONDAY_

8:00	Jones, Eileen	314·8200	Physical Exam.
8:15	↓		↓
8:30	Brown, John	314·6109	Post-Surg. Checkup
8:45	Martin, Joyce	314·7700	Abdominal Pain
9:00			
9:15			
9:30			
9:45	Roberts, Bob	314·9103	Dressing Change
10:00	Peters, Lois	314·9271	BP Check
10:15			
10:30			
10:45			
11:00			
11:15			
11:30			
11:45			
12:00			
12:15			
12:30			
12:45			
1:00			

FIGURE 6-3. Proper appointment entries.

These considerations should be discussed with the physician prior to the adoption of a scheduling plan. Specifics will then be entered in the procedures manual.

In addition to beginning the appointment system with a basic knowledge of these factors, the medical assistant assumes the responsibility for monitoring the system. Continuous daily monitoring of the established appointment scheduling plan is necessary since adjustments may be required. Determinations of the length of time each appointment is taking and of whether the time allotted for emergency cases is adequate or excessive are examples of monitoring. This procedure is particularly important if there are apparent problems related to the office appointment system. Patients may be routinely waiting longer than is reasonable for their appointments. There may be frequent time lags in the doctor's day when no appointments are scheduled. Actual time required for various kinds of appointments may differ from predicted time. The physician will depend on feedback from the medical assistant concerning these conditions. Collaboration of the office staff with the physician is essential to resolving these scheduling difficulties.

The harmonious interaction of the physician's preferences, the available staff and facilities, and the patient's needs is achieved through the adoption and continuous monitoring of the appointment plan.

PATIENT SCREENING

While organization is essential to appointment scheduling, patient screening skills ultimately determine the successful implementation of the plan.

Patient screening is fundamental to all medical office functions. Every aspect of office practice demands competent patient screening. The medical assistant responsible for administrating the office is usually the first person to communicate with the individual patient. Patient screening is most often exercised when the patient telephones for an appointment, at which time the medical assistant assesses the need and urgency of the visit.

Perhaps the greatest challenge in patient screening is the skill of information processing. Most often when the patient phones to schedule an appointment for a routine physical examination or predetermined treatment, screening techniques are not applied. The information to be processed by the medical assistant is straightforward. Almost all calls for appointments, however, require techniques that attempt to facilitate the sorting and processing of information and decision-making.

Sorting Information

The information communicated by the patient to the medical assistant must be carefully scrutinized. Most frequently, one of the following messages is involved:

1. The patient wants to speak to the physician.
2. The patient wants to make an appointment.
3. The patient requests information without asking for an appointment or a return call from the physician.

One problem in sorting information is that the patient's verbal expression does not always reflect his real intent. A patient asking to speak to the physician may actually want to make an appointment for an office visit. There are many possible variations of the disparity between the verbalized message and the actual need or desire.

Expressing Empathy

The real purpose of the patient's telephone call must be established in a manner which expresses concern for the needs and feelings of the caller.

Often patients call the physician's office and expect to be seen immediately. The great demands placed on the physician's time necessitate some questioning of the urgency of the visit.

Listening skills and interviewing techniques uncover the needs and symptoms of each patient and provide the data needed to make an accurate determination of when the patient should be seen.

HANDLING SPECIAL APPOINTMENTS

There are certain categories of appointments which require special handling. Appointments for new patients, unscheduled or acute illness, and nonroutine treatments require discretion and special management. The procedure manual should provide guidance for proper action in these situations.

The Physical Examination Appointment

A great many appointments will be requested for routine physical examinations. While this type of appointment will not take precedence over those required for an emergency or acute condition, the patient should not be made to wait for an unreasonable length of time. Understanding the motive for the physical examination request is important to the assignment of an appointment time. The request for a physical examination appointment may represent the patient's interest in obtaining regular checkups or a concern related to a particular problem the patient feels must be diagnosed, or perhaps a return visit suggested by the physician.

If the patient is not experiencing any specific problem and has not been asked by the doctor to return during a certain time period, the scheduling of an appointment within a 6- to 12-week period is an accepted practice.

Revisits and Treatments

Occasionally, as a result of a diagnosis revealed during an emergency visit or a physical examination, a patient is put on a schedule of return office visits by the physician. One or more followup visits with a complex instruction such as "see us every two weeks for the next few months" may be advised. The patient will need assistance in making these appointments. Appointments of this nature are usually made for the same weekday and the same time during the day to promote the patient's retention of the appointment times. Failing to schedule the followup appointments as directed by the physician results in a tendency to reduce the quality of the medical treatments, either because the doctor will have to spend time becoming familiar with the case, or because systematic treatment procedures are interrupted.

Unscheduled Visits

Most offices reserve several blocks of 15-minute intervals for dealing with acute illness or emergencies. The medical assistant should consult the physician to determine how many appointment openings to schedule and when during the day such openings should be scheduled. Emergency cases may, of course, preempt existing appointments.

Once you have determined how much time is to be blocked and when to schedule the blocks, the process of patient screening for need and urgency is begun. Several objectives must still be accomplished. You must help patients to describe the problem fully, assure them that you are concerned for their welfare, and still guide as many patients as possible toward their future scheduled appointments.

To a large extent the approach taken should be dictated by the type of practice involved and by the guidelines obtained from the physician. The patient and his description of symptoms will often make for an easy decision. In situations which are questionable, and when the day's appointments are already fully scheduled, the physician must be consulted.

PROCEDURES FOR UNSCHEDULED APPOINTMENTS

In the event of questions concerning a particular patient's need for an appointment on the same day requested, a number of solutions are available:

1. A brief note including the patient's name and symptoms will bring the problem to the attention of the doctor. The patient can then be called and informed of the physician's decision. The appointment can be scheduled accordingly.

2. A relatively detailed guide of common acute problems and symptomatology might serve as a reference. This guide could be placed in the procedures manual described in the previous chapter.

3. Assuming that the physician has entrusted full responsibility for decisions regarding appointment scheduling to the medical assistant, her experience will serve as the basis for discretionary judgment.

A Four-Step Approach to Appointment Handling

Procedure	Principle
1. Ask patient when he is not available for appointments.	1. Demonstrate willingness to accommodate the patient's needs. The patient can more clearly and easily relate time restrictions.
2. Offer at least two choices if available, stating the day, date, and time.	2. This enables the patient to realistically choose from alternatives and demonstrates to the patient the importance of his own input.
3. Repeat the time desired to the patient.	3. This provides confirmation and avoids confusion.
4. Close with an expression of anticipation of the next visit.	4. Closure expresses appreciation for advanced scheduling and provides further verification of the date.

AN EXAMPLE OF THE FOUR-STEP APPROACH

Medical Assistant: Mr. Jones, when would you *not* be available for an appointment?
Mr. Jones:　　　Well, I work from 7:00 to 3:30 every day.
Medical Assistant: Mr. Jones, the earliest appointment I have then would be 4:00 on Mon-

day, December 9th. There is also an opening on Thursday, December
12th at 4:15 pm.

Mr. Jones: I'll take the December 12th appointment.

Medical Assistant: Okay, Mr. Jones, that's December 12th at 4:15. Thank you for calling and
we'll see you on the 12th. Goodbye.

The efficiency of the four-step approach in terms of time saving and its effectiveness in expressing concern for patient needs are perhaps best reflected in an example of the *wrong*
approach.

Medical Assistant: Mr. Jones, when would you like to come in?

Mr. Jones: Well, as soon as possible. How about next Monday in the afternoon?

Medical Assistant: No, I'm sorry, Mr. Jones, we don't have an opening then. How about
Tuesday at 2:30?

Mr. Jones: I work till 3:30.

Medical Assistant: Oh, I see. Well that presents a problem. Hmm . . . how about on Thursday
at 4:15?

Mr. Jones: That would probably be okay.

Medical Assistant: Okay. Come in on Thursday, December 12th then.

Mr. Jones: Okay. Was that 4:15?

Medical Assistant: Yes.

Mr. Jones: Thank you. Goodbye.

Medical Assistant: Goodbye.

ACCOMMODATING PATIENT NEEDS

Although a logical system of appointments may be established, flexibility and an understanding of the needs of individual patients should govern its application. There will be instances
when patients cannot be scheduled within the structured appointment times. The physician
will need to make a decision as to his own willingness to accommodate the patient's schedule.
The physician should provide guidelines that are applicable in such situations, and these
should be contained in the procedures manual.

Patients should be directed in their choice of an appointment time through careful
management by the medical assistant. When visits are arranged by appointment only, it is appropriate, whenever possible, to follow certain steps which ensure the efficient and effective
handling of appointment scheduling.

MAINTAINING AN APPOINTMENT FLOW

Maintaining an even flow of appointments is a challenging responsibility. Patients may not appear on time. Emergencies or acute disease may warrant some juggling of appointments.
Cancellations by the physician or patient represent unplanned disruptions in the desired appointment flow. It is the reaction to these interruptions in flow that will either sustain the
perception of controlled management or inject chaos.

A new patient, for instance, should be encouraged to come approximately 15 minutes early to complete the preliminary paperwork and receive an orientation to the office. If appointment delays are a pattern, "time-constrained" patients should be encouraged to phone the office approximately one hour before the scheduled appointment time to determine whether office visits are running late. Initiating this service presumes that the medical assistant will be willing to provide accurate information to the inquiring patients. A patient who, through no error on his part, sits in the waiting room for an extra hour or two will be rightfully irritated.

Patients should be encouraged to notify the office as soon as possible when cancellations are necessary. The physician may prefer that patients be reminded by phone in advance of their appointment, especially those patients who seem to have a history of forgetting or being late.

It is helpful to keep a list of those patients with scheduled appointments who had preferred an earlier time. Reference to this list will provide willing patients with appointments on brief notice as can happen when cancellations occur. Often, however, a cancellation is welcomed as an opportunity for physicians who are running late to catch up or pause in their labors.

RESOURCE LIMITATIONS

The office may possess a particular resource (such as a special examination room or a therapeutic device) which, because of constant use, is the cause of problematic disruptions in the flow of appointments. This is particularly relevant when the medical assistant manages the scheduling of appointments for several physicians who share both office facilities and equipment.

If the sharing of facilities becomes a recurring problem, anticipation and prevention of the difficulty can best be achieved by designing a separate scheduling category into the appointment book. Figure 6-4 provides an illustration depicting a satisfactory scheduling arrangement involving limited facilities.

In addition to clearly designating an appointment time for equipment use, a review of the doctor's orders after each patient's visit will enable the medical assistant to plan the appointment well in advance. The MA can apply this approach to any scheduling problem, including special treatments or diagnostic tests. In a one-physician office where there may be several patients at different stages of the office process at any given time, special appointment categories can be constructed to maintain accurate control over the patient flow.

THE PHYSICIAN'S PROFESSIONAL COMMITMENTS

The physician's involvement in professional societies and community organizations places demands on appointment time management. The physician may leave the office regularly to attend meetings, conferences, and other professional functions. These commitments must be noted in the appointment book to avoid scheduling patients during this time and to serve as a reminder for the physician concerning obligations.

The physician may prefer to use a personal appointment book in addition to the office book. In the personal appointment book, hours throughout the evening are scheduled. In

Month _____

Date _____

Day _____

	Dr. Smith	Dr. Jones	Ultrasound Machine
8:00			
8:15		GREEN, LOIS 412-6190	
8:30		(BACK PAIN)	DR. JONES: MRS. GREEN
8:45			
9:00			
9:15			
9:30			
9:45			
10:00			
10:15			
10:30	BROWN, JIM 417-2014		
10:45	(TENNIS ELBOW)		DR. SMITH: MR. BROWN
11:00			
11:15			
11:30			
11:45			
12:00			
12:15			
12:30			
12:45			
1:00			

FIGURE 6-4.   A limited facilities appointment sheet.

some instances the medical assistant may also be responsible for the management of the physician's time after office hours.

It is a good practice to review the appointment book with the physician at least once each week in order to advise him in advance of upcoming commitments and to allow for adjustments and facilitate better organization. When the physician is aware of his own personal commitments and those of the medical practice a week in advance, shared objectives can be identified and mutual cooperation established.

THE NEXT APPOINTMENT

At the conclusion of the office visit and prior to the patient's departure, the medical assistant should schedule the next appointment if one is necessary. When the next appointment is not contemplated for more than six months, most physicians prefer patients to phone for an appointment at a later time as the office schedule may not be planned beyond several weeks in advance. Many physicians have adopted the use of a small card, such as the one shown in Figure 6-5, for the purpose of reminding patients of their next appointment.

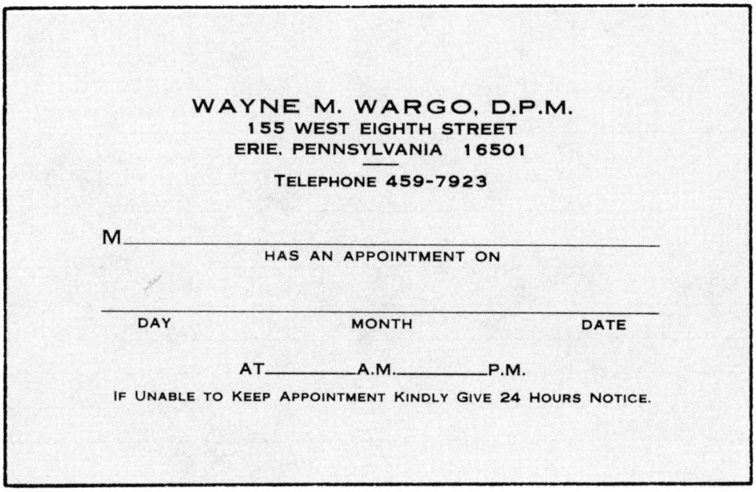
WAYNE M. WARGO, D.P.M.
155 WEST EIGHTH STREET
ERIE, PENNSYLVANIA 16501

TELEPHONE 459-7923

M____________________
HAS AN APPOINTMENT ON

DAY MONTH DATE

AT________A.M.________P.M.

IF UNABLE TO KEEP APPOINTMENT KINDLY GIVE 24 HOURS NOTICE.

FIGURE 6-5. A typical appointment card.

SUMMARY

The task of managing the physician's office appointment schedule is clearly one of the most important jobs of the medical assistant. To properly carry out the full range of responsibilities which are associated with appointment scheduling, MAs must view this assignment in a broad manner. They must see themselves not simply as people who answer the phone and fill in the book. Instead, they should regard themselves as managers of a system, a support-system for the physician. Medical assistants must identify with the entire process of appointment scheduling, including the design of the physical system, patient screening, and information updating. And most important, MAs must see themselves as the guardians of this system.

APPLICATION EXERCISES

Use the list on page 89 to complete the practice appointment sheet. Consider the patient's preferences for appointment time and the physician's scheduled hours. Select patients for appointment times on the basis of urgency. Assume the calls are received in the order given in advance of the dates specified (March 8 to 17). Note that calls will also be received on the dates scheduled. This simulation offers six appointment day alternatives. The physician anticipates a fair number of patients with acute illnesses and affords half an hour of unscheduled time in the afternoon. Specific time designation is left to the medical assistant's discretion.

Note that the physican usually has hours on Thursdays and Fridays but will be attending

Month_____

Date_____

Day_____

8:00	
8:15	
8:30	
8:45	
9:00	
9:15	
9:30	
9:45	
10:00	
10:15	
10:30	
10:45	
11:00	
11:15	
11:30	
11:45	
12:00	
12:15	
12:30	
12:45	
1:00	

a convention of the American Medical Association on Thursday and Friday of the first week and will be delivering a paper on Thursday and Friday of the next week. Therefore the appointments listed must be scheduled during the hours indicated:

Monday: 9 a.m. to 12 noon and 2 p.m. to 4 p.m.
Tuesday: 2 p.m. to 6 p.m.
Wednesday: 9 a.m. to 12 noon

Use this work and allotted time guide to complete the exercise:

Patient's Name	Purpose of Visit	Requested Time
1. Amos, James R.	Checkup	Early morning
2. Colby, Mrs. Virginia	Injection and consultation	Morning
3. Zenith, William	Removal of warts, right hand	Monday, late afternoon
4. Benz, Mrs. Amelia	Exam and consultation regarding gastric surgery	Wednesday, 4 p.m. or later
5. Morris, Karen	Exam, complaint—pain in both legs	Late Wednesday
6. Free, Kathy	Sore throat	Received complaint March 8, 11:00 a.m.
7. Jacobs, Stanley	Check leg cast	Afternoons
8. Deslatte, Paula	Possible vaginal infection	Afternoons after 4 p.m.
9. Taraski, Sandra	Menstrual problems	Morning
10. Leonardi, Thomas	Hemorrhoids	Tuesday morning
11. Wallace, Tasha	Teacher examination	Mondays after 3 p.m.
12. Wunsch, Walter	Stomach pain	Wednesday, anytime
13. Hetterman, Patrick	Stepped on nail	Emergency phone in on Tuesday at 2:30 p.m., March 9
14. Balczon, Lee	Pap smear check	Tuesdays
15. Hopkins, Robert	Chest cold	Mornings
16. Andera, John	Premarital exam and blood test	Late afternoon
17. Herbstritt, Richard	Headaches and sinus trouble	Anytime
18. Borg, Mary	Desires weight reduction	Mondays
19. Volpe, Ronald	Vaccination—travel abroad	Tuesday after 3:30
20. Coffey, Emilia	BP check	Early afternoons
21. Hanson, Rose	Small growth on toe	After 4 p.m. any day
22. Brown, George	Sores in mouth	Morning
23. Hopkins, Richard	Swelling, left groin	Anytime
24. Askims, Margaret	Annual physical exam and pap test	Morning
25. Felder, Sally	Shortness of breath, dizziness	Early afternoons
26. Reynolds, Mary	Suture removal	Monday, Tuesday, or Friday
27. Parks, Albert	Fell down steps—dazed	Call received Monday, March 15 at 10:00 a.m.
28. Denver, Joseph	Consultation regarding radiation therapy	Near noon any day
29. Hampton, Mrs. Amy	Dressing and check—facial surgery	Anytime
30. Leonard, Craig	College exam, urinalysis	After 2:30 p.m., Tuesday and Thursday

31.	Geisler, Chris	New patient appointment	Morning
32.	Palmisano, John	Pain in left ear	Morning
33.	Allfield, Mrs. Kay	Bleeding, urinary tract	Emergency call received Tuesday, March 9, 3:30 p.m.
34.	Shields, Chris	New patient examination	Anytime
35.	Adolph, Mrs. Ruth	Influenza vaccination	Anytime
36.	Swanson, Sally	Lump in breast	Early afternoon
37.	Abraham, Mrs. Betty	Cough for 2 weeks	Early afternoon, prefer Tuesday
38.	Johnson, Cathy	Loss of weight, fatigue	Anytime but ASAP
39.	Jackman, Ann	Vomiting, fever 102°	Call received Wednesday, March 19, at 9:30 a.m.
40.	Kelvington, Paul	Exam for driver's license	Anytime

Complete the blank appointment cards for the following patients:

1. The doctor indicates that Mrs. Jones should return for recheck in two weeks. The patient is given two alternatives: Monday, March 26 at 2:00 p.m., and Thursday, March 28 at 4:00 p.m. She chooses the March 28 appointment.

2. The doctor indicates that Mr. Leonardi should return for a recheck in 10 days (April 4). You have checked the appointment book and no appointment times are available in 10 days. However, there are two appointment time possibilities: Thursday, March 31 at 10:00 a.m., and Monday, April 11 at 2:00 p.m. You schedule Mr. Leonardi on March 31.

3. The doctor indicates that Mrs. Taraski should return in three months for repeat blood work and examination. The date selected is Wednesday, May 17 at 3:30 p.m.

Patient Screening Role-Playing Exercise

Two student roles are required: one student assumes the patient role; the other student takes the role of the medical assistant. To determine the urgency of the visit, apply patient screening techniques to the following situation:

A call is received and the individual wants to speak to the doctor. The caller has not identified himself.

Problem-Solving Exercise

The roles of patient and medical assistant can be simulated prior to classroom discussion and a critique of the problem-solving methods applied.

1. Mrs. Sims has called to cancel her appointment for the third consecutive time.

WAYNE M. WARGO, D.P.M.
155 WEST EIGHTH STREET
ERIE, PENNSYLVANIA 16501
TELEPHONE 459-7923

M_____

HAS AN APPOINTMENT ON

_____ _____
DAY   MONTH   DATE

AT _____ A.M. _____ P.M.

IF UNABLE TO KEEP APPOINTMENT KINDLY GIVE 24 HOURS NOTICE.

WAYNE M. WARGO, D.P.M.
155 WEST EIGHTH STREET
ERIE, PENNSYLVANIA 16501
TELEPHONE 459-7923

M_____

HAS AN APPOINTMENT ON

_____ _____
DAY   MONTH   DATE

AT _____ A.M. _____ P.M.

IF UNABLE TO KEEP APPOINTMENT KINDLY GIVE 24 HOURS NOTICE.

WAYNE M. WARGO, D.P.M.
155 WEST EIGHTH STREET
ERIE, PENNSYLVANIA 16501
TELEPHONE 459-7923

M_____

HAS AN APPOINTMENT ON

_____ _____
DAY   MONTH   DATE

AT _____ A.M. _____ P.M.

IF UNABLE TO KEEP APPOINTMENT KINDLY GIVE 24 HOURS NOTICE.

WAYNE M. WARGO, D.P.M.
155 WEST EIGHTH STREET
ERIE, PENNSYLVANIA 16501
TELEPHONE 459-7923

M_____

HAS AN APPOINTMENT ON

_____ _____
DAY   MONTH   DATE

AT _____ A.M. _____ P.M.

IF UNABLE TO KEEP APPOINTMENT KINDLY GIVE 24 HOURS NOTICE.

2. The doctor is running an hour behind schedule. It is now 2:00 p.m., and the doctor is scheduled to attend a very important hospital staff meeting at 4:30 p.m.

3. A patient calls requesting an appointment as soon as possible. You determine that this is desirable but are booked for the next three days. The patient has a lump on her breast and is quite concerned.

4. A patient calls for an appointment and is unable to come to the office during regular hours.

5. The doctor has been allotting an hour a day for calls received as unscheduled appointments from patients with emergency or acute illness needs. However, there is frequently a 15-minute period of unscheduled time and the physician finds this undesirable.

COMPLETING THE LEARNING LOOP

As a student you can begin to apply the principles of scheduling to your own activities. Purchase a date book at your college store and begin to keep a record for yourself. If you do this you will not only improve your own efficiency as a student, but you will gain important experience for later use in the physician's office.

BIBLIOGRAPHY

Baker, K. A.: *Introduction to Sequencing and Scheduling.* John Wiley & Sons, New York, 1974.
Ewing, D. W.: *The Human Side of Planning.* Macmillan, New York, 1969.
Le Breton, P. P., and Henning, D. A.: *Planning Theory.* Prentice-Hall, Englewood Cliffs, N.J., 1961.

CHAPTER 7

MAINTAINING THE ACCOUNTING RECORDS

SPECIFIC OBJECTIVES

Upon completion of this chapter you will be able to describe:

1. The procedures of flowcharting and be able to construct a basic flowchart for any required office procedure.

2. The three main forms of medical practice organization.

3. The billing cycle, cash receipts/daily earnings summaries, and accounts-receivable control procedures.

4. The medical disbursements cycle and cash payments procedures.

5. Petty cash procedures.

6. Banking procedures including check preparation, deposits, and a bank reconciliation.

7. The required payroll records, payroll calculations, and related federal, state, and local tax laws.

8. The advantages of a pegboard "one-write" system and the procedures for its use.

9. The basic accounting equation and its relationship to the financial accounting/recordkeeping function.

10. The types of data processing equipment available and their effect on the accounting procedures in the medical practice unit.

INTRODUCTION

The physician is concerned with the completeness and accuracy of the medical treatment afforded to patients. He or she must also be concerned with the completeness and accuracy of the financial records which summarize the medical practice. Just as the medical assistant was required to master a vocabulary and standardized methodology when instituting and utilizing an office files management system, so in this chapter the medical assistant will be introduced to accounting terminology and standardized accounting/recordkeeping as the means by which the physician's financial transactions are summarized.

The accounting process presented here is the means by which business information is analyzed, recorded, classified, summarized, and reported. By this process business events, called transactions, are expressed in monetary terms, grouped into related categories, and summarized into financial reports which indicate the physician's financial position at a particular time or the operating results of the practice during a specific period which created the aforementioned financial position. The accounting process becomes the means by which the physician measures the profitability and solvency of the practice, weighs alternative courses of action, discovers significant trends in practice treatment, and estimates which events may have significance for the practice in the future.

While the medical assistant will be familiar with and responsible for the basic source document preparation and summarization, it will be assumed that the physician relies upon an external accounting service to review that initial accounting process and to prepare the final financial reports and tax summaries. As the legal and financial requirements placed upon physicians have increased, they have turned more frequently and more extensively to business management and consulting services which are available from a certified public accountant, a medical management consultant, a tax advisor, or a data processing service center. Any or all of these professionals may be called upon to familiarize the medical assistant with extensive areas of the accounting cycle or to provide the actual training necessary for the preparation of the documents within that accounting cycle. The MA should be sure that such instructions and training are clear and concise and that the professionals are available to evaluate performance, answer questions, or make procedural changes which will update and upgrade the physician's financial records.

Before the discussion of the accounting process is presented, an explanation of flowcharting may prove useful. The specific method by which the physician's financial transactions will be recorded may be defined as the accounting cycle. Within the cycle are systems of accounting procedures, each requiring documents, preparation, calculation, summary reports, and filing procedures. In order to make clearer the steps within the procedures, symbolic representations of each step will be presented. A written explanation and a numerical example will accompany the flowchart or symbolic representation.

The symbols used on the flowcharts in this chapter are outlined in Figure 7-1. To read a flowchart, start at the top and follow the directions, normally top to bottom and left to right. The flowchart will graphically break down each step of the accounting procedure and detail the required operations. The flowchart will indicate the data and documents necessary. It will also show the direction in which both flow. If the flowchart has been prepared, corrected, and followed by the medical assistant, the physician may be assured of complete and accurate financial records.

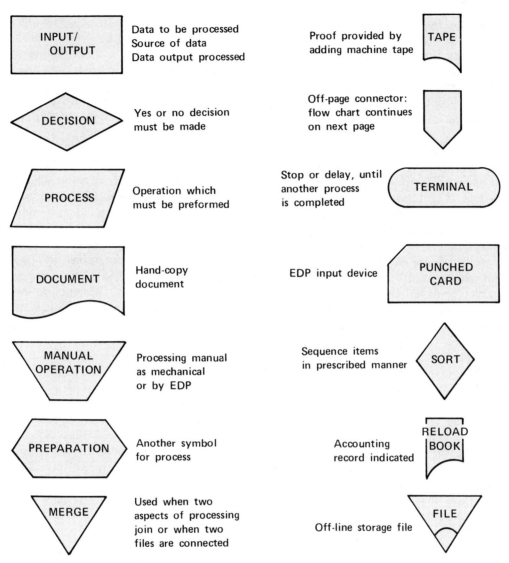

FIGURE 7-1. A symbolic flowchart key.

PRACTICE ORGANIZATION

There are three main forms of business organization from which a physician may choose: a single proprietorship or single practice owned by one physician, a partnership, or a professional corporation which involves two or more practicing physicians. The form of organization determines how the profits are distributed, who makes management and financial decisions, and who assumes the legal responsibilities and liabilities.

The simplest form of medical practice to organize and operate is the single proprietorship or single-physician practice. The physician is in full control and makes all decisions—financial, administrative, and medical. If the practice is successful, he reaps all the benefits. If the practice fails, the physician suffers the total loss. When operating a single-proprietor practice, the physician is exposed to unlimited liability; that is, the physician is personally liable for all debts incurred by the practice unit. If the practice cannot pay the debts, the personal assets of the physician may have to be liquidated to do so. The life and vitality of the practice unit is therefore limited to the life, financial resources, and talents of that single physician.

In a partnership, the ownership of the medical practice is divided between two or more physicians who agree to share their financial resources and talents. A partnership agreement will provide the legal framework by which decisions as to financial contributions, distributions, and practice management structure are made. By pooling resources in a group practice the physicians are able to extend their medical skills and financial resources beyond what each could do individually. However, this form of business organization has one distinct disadvantage. Each member of the partnership has unlimited liability for the debts of the group practice and thus may have that member's personal resources marshalled to pay partnership debts. Additionally, since one partner speaks for all in a legal sense, the partnership may be required to assume liability for an individual partner's debts. Coupled with the fact that the partnership arrangement terminates each time a member physician enters or leaves the group, the changing circumstances of the practice can lead to management disagreements.

The third form of medical practice organization is the professional association or corporation. A corporation is formed under state law and has a legal identity distinct from the physicians involved in the medical practice. It has the right to buy and sell property, make contracts, borrow money, and go to court, all in its own name. A corporation has liability only for the debts it incurs itself, not for the debts of its managers or its owners. Physicians are turning to this form of practice organization as a way of limiting personal liability and as a means by which they may benefit from a more advantageous tax structure. Under a corporate arrangement certain pension, profit-sharing, life insurance, and health insurance benefits are more extensive for both the physician and the practice unit employees. As a result the use of the designation "P.C." (Professional Corporation) or "P.A." (Professional Associate) after a physician's name has become an increasingly common practice.

BILLING PROCEDURES

While questions concerning medical treatment are part of the physician-patient relationship, the matter of fees for such medical treatment may be extended to involve the medical assistant. Fees for service are set for each procedure by the physician. The fees may be fixed per office visit or for specific procedures, or they may extend for definite periods of time or be subject to modification to accommodate the financial circumstances of the patient.

The details of the physician's fee schedule (Fig. 7-2) must be thoroughly known by the medical assistant since she provides the communication link between the physician and patient and may be called upon to explain the charges to inquiring patients. Explanations should include exactly what treatment is covered by the fee in question.

The medical assistant will also be responsible for communicating the methods of pay-

```
90005 — Brief Office Visit — $ 15.00                    94010 — Spirometry — $ 50.00
90020 — Inter-Office Visit — $ 18.00                    95000 — Allergy Testing — $ 99.00
90030 — Extended Office Visit — $ 50.00
90400 — Nursing Home Visit — $ 25.00                    Reapplying Cast — $ 25.00
90110 — Home Visit, brief (limited) exam, evaluation and/or   Subclavian Catheter — $ 75.00
         treatment — $ 25.00
                                                        IUD — $ 30.00
11420 — Excision and Cautery — $ 75.00                  IUD and PAP — $ 45.00
11482 — Excision of Lipoma — $ 75.00                    Diaphragm — $ 25.00
                                                        Diaphragm and PAP — $ 30.00
20551 — Lumbosacral — NOT COVERED                       PAP — $ 23.00
20605 — Arthrocentesis, Inter-Joint — $ 30.00           Polypectomy — $ 150.00
20610 — Arthrocentesis, Major Joint — $ 40.00           MMR — $ 18.00
21800 — Fractured Rib — $ 75.00                         Pneumovac Injection — $ 18.00 (good 3–5 yrs.)
25505 — Fractured Radius — $ 125.00                     Flu Vac with Office Visit — $ 5.00
26400 — Repair Tendon, hand or fingers, single, primary — $ 175.00   Flu Vac walk-in — $ 8.00
26605 — Fractured Metacarpal, fixation/casted — $ 75.00
26750 — Fractured Phalanges, no reduction — $ 50.00
27532 — Fractured Tibia — $ 150.00
27780 — Fractured Fibula — $125.00
28475 — Fractured Metatarsal — $ 75.00
29405 — Ankle Strain and Ligamentous Tear,              PHYSICALS — Charges must be put through for all
         casting of lower extremity — $ 35.00                       physicals on day of visit.

30904 — Epistoxis (Nasal Hemorrhage), Cautery and Packing — $ 75.00   ATTORNEY AND COURT FEES
31525 — Laryngoscope (biopsy), indirect — $ 25.00       Depositions — Min. Fee
                                                           Mail or Telephone — $ 150.00
42860 — Infected Tonsil Tag, surgical excision of tag,     In-person — $ 250.00
         treatment and biopsy — $ 75.00                    To Court — $ 350.00
                                                           Letters to Attorneys — $ 50.00 per letter
53660 — Urethral Dilatation (2nd time) — $ 35.00
53661 — Urethral Dilatation (1st time) — $ 50.00        AUTO ACCIDENTS
57500 — Excision Neoplasm, Cervical Area — $ 75.00
                                                        First Visit — $ 35.00
64420 — Intercostal Nerve Block — $ 40.00               Remaining Visits — $ 15.00 to $ 20.00 per visit
64420 — Spinal Tap — $ 50.00
                                                        Price changes/dates
                                                        Arthrocentesis, Inter and Major — 4/10/79, 6/13/80
```

FIGURE 7-2. A typical physician's fee schedule.

ment which are available. Patient charges should normally be paid in cash at the time the procedure is performed, but for major services or treatments which extend over a considerable period of time, the total fees may be so great that partial payment arrangements will have to be made. Weekly payment schedules can be suggested as well as payment assistance through financial institutions.

Payment arrangements can also be scheduled so that fees are billed at the end of the month following treatment or as soon as the patient has been discharged from care. These two methods for handling patient accounts require a knowledge of the credit rating of the patient and his willingness to pay the medical expenses. Problems related to credit and collection of patient accounts will be discussed in a later section of this chapter.

The basis for recording patient charges for medical treatment is the patient charge slip (Fig. 7-3), which is an itemized summary of the medical services provided to the patient. This source document is the method by which physicians' earnings, patient billing, and patient medical histories are recorded in the permanent records of the practice unit. It is vitally important, therefore, that the medical assistant prepare these patient charge slips accurately and that they be reviewed and approved by the attending physician. Although the method for completing such slips may vary among practice units, the normal procedure is to attach the charge slip to the medical history to be completed by the physician while attending the patient. The physician then requests that the patient discuss the financial arrangements with the medical assistant. If cash payment is made at this time, it is noted on the charge slip. If other arrangements are made for payment, these are also noted.

For those patients whose charges have not been remitted in cash, a monthly state-

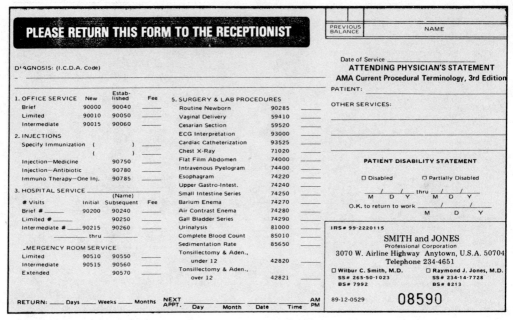

FIGURE 7-3. A patient charge slip. (Courtesy of Control-o-fax)

ment must be sent. This statement (Fig. 7-4) summarizes the medical treatment provided and should be as detailed as possible to avoid misunderstanding. The charge slip will provide the data necessary to list all services rendered: physician's visits, office visits, injections, examinations, laboratory tests, x-rays, physical therapy, or other special procedures.

Patient bills are normally sent out on the first day of the month following treatment. Occasionally the patient requests to pay upon discharge or at a specific point in the succeeding month. If possible, this request should be honored. Additionally, medical offices with large patient billings may utilize cycle billing. Under this system patient accounts are billed in staggered sequence throughout the month, based upon an alphabetic division. For example, patients with names beginning A through D would be billed on the first of the month, letters E through J on the tenth, and so forth.

As noted above, the patient charge slip is the source document for both the physician's earnings record and the patient's medical history. Charge slips accumulated during the day should be posted daily to both of these financial records. The patient's ledger card (Fig. 7-5) records all charges, payments, and balances due the practice unit. All details from the charge slip should be entered completely so that both the medical treatment and the financial consequences are noted. The patient ledger card should indicate all data received during the registration process on the first visit: name, address, telephone number, social security number, business address and telephone, party responsible for the account, special billing instructions, and third-party reimbursement procedures. When the patient receives services, those charges are transferred to the ledger card, and when the patient pays for such services, these remittances are entered on the ledger card. Charges and payments should be posted on a current basis so that the physician may refer to the ledger and be assured that the account reflects a current status.

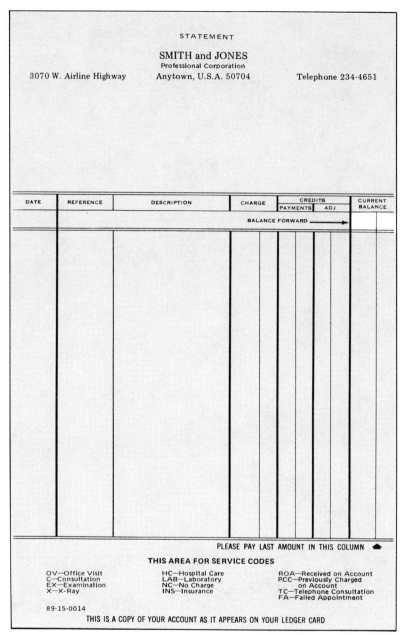

FIGURE 7-4. A patient billing statement. (Courtesy of Control-o-fax)

The physician's earnings will be recorded on a daily basis. This summary should detail the names of patients, the services rendered, and the fees charged as they have been entered on the charge slips. At the close of the day the medical assistant should total all recorded amounts.

STATEMENT

LEONARD S. TAYLOR, M.D.
2100 WEST PARK AVENUE
CHAMPAIGN, ILLINOIS 61820

TELEPHONE 367-6671

RECEIPT NUMBER	DATE	PROFESSIONAL SERVICE	CHARGE	PAID	NEW BALANCE

1631   PAY LAST AMOUNT IN THIS COLUMN △

OC - OFFICE CALL	INS - INSURANCE	PE - PHYSICAL EXAMINATION
HC - HOUSE CALL	OB - OBSTETRICAL CARE	EKG - ELECTROCARDIOGRAM
HOSP - HOSPITAL CARE	PAP - PAPANICOLAOU TEST	XR - X RAY
L - LABORATORY	OS - OFFICE SURGERY	M - MEDICATION
I - INJECTION	HS - HOSPITAL SURGERY	NC - NO CHARGE

FIGURE 7-5.   A patient ledger card.

When patients pay for medical services, a written acknowledgment must be given. A receipt (Fig. 7-6) should be completed with a carbon copy, indicating the amount of cash received, the date, by whom the cash was received, from whom, and for what services. Because this document becomes a source of data for recording in the patient accounts and the daily log, completeness and accuracy are imperative.

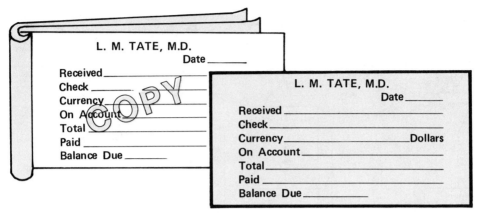

FIGURE 7-6. A physician's receipt book.

Mail payments must also be opened, totaled, and entered in the daily log. It is not usually necessary to make out a receipt form for mail payments since the paid check will serve as a receipt when it is returned to the patient in his bank statement.

At the close of the day all receipt forms should be totaled together with the adding machine tape of the mail payments received. This figure must equal the total monies actually received during the day, and represents the funds to be deposited in the physician's bank account that evening.

The payments recorded in the daily summary log need to be transferred to the patient ledger card. Utilizing the receipt form as a source document, the monies paid should be indicated on the account card. A current balance is then computed such that the previous balance plus current charges minus payments constitutes the account balance for which a statement of account must be mailed during the month's end billing cycle.

The billing cycle must be verified by reference to the patient ledger cards. All ledger cards with current amounts due should be listed by patient name and amount. This constitutes the physician's total accounts receivable. This total must equal the total of the statements or bills to be sent. The total listing of all balances on patient ledger cards and the total amounts on all billing statements must be equal. If there is a discrepancy, the error may be found in mathematics or in posting. The statements should be reviewed and compared to the patient ledger accounts, and patient ledger cards should be retotaled. If mistakes are still not located, the entire recording process must be reviewed from the original source documents, charge slips, and receipt forms. A "one-write" system in which the daily log, patient ledger cards, and bills are prepared simultaneously from a charge/receipt form eliminates the wasted time necessary to find such mechanical errors. It also eliminates the need for a separate receipt.

Flowcharts illustrating the billing procedure and the patient receipts procedure are provided in Figures 7-7 and 7-8. These diagrams should be examined closely as they provide a graphic summary of the operations discussed in this section.

MEDICAL PRACTICE DISBURSEMENTS

As will be noted throughout this chapter, for complete and accurate accounting of the financial aspects of the physician's medical practice, the medical assistant must control all

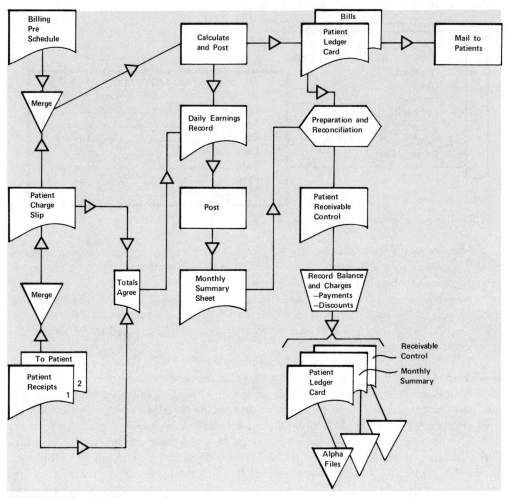

FIGURE 7-7. A billing procedure.

transactions. That control is based upon the single promise that all receipts must be deposited in the bank and all payments will be disbursed by check.

Petty Cash

It is not practical to use checks for unusual or small cash transactions. As a result the physician will want to set up a petty cash fund for such payments. The physician will decide the types of payments to be made from petty cash, such as postage or office supplies, as well as the dollar amount of the purchases and the total amount of the petty cash fund.

A petty cash fund is an imprest account, which means that at any time the total cash or cash value of the fund must remain the same. This provides the necessary control over the cash as well as insuring accountability for the medical assistant when the fund is used for

103

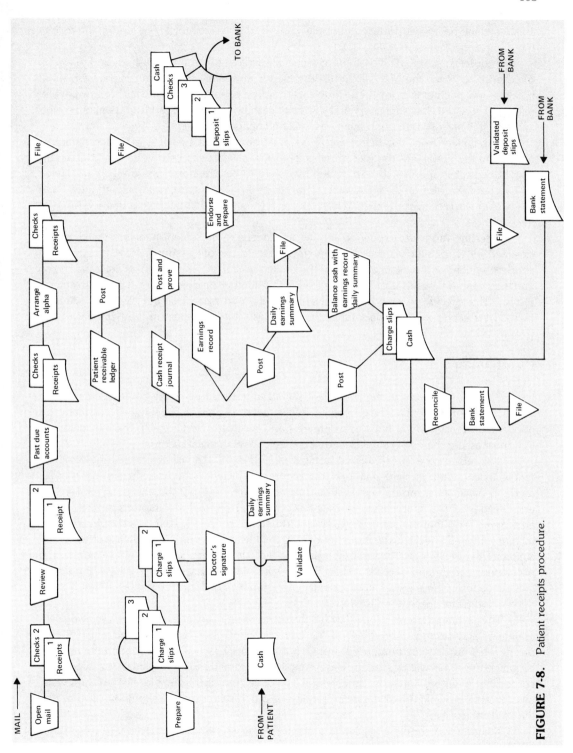

FIGURE 7-8. Patient receipts procedure.

small, routine payments. Refer to the petty cash fund flowchart (Fig. 7-9) during the following discussion.

In order to start a petty cash fund, a check is written to the fund, cashed, and placed in a locked box. Since the MA will be responsible for a separate accounting of the cash fund, receipts and payments from these monies should be separate from those that are patient-related. Therefore, it is suggested that the petty cash box be kept apart from patient receipts and that it is not used for such things as making change for patients.

A payment from the petty cash fund must be covered by some evidence regarding who spent the funds and the reason. Special forms, called petty cash vouchers (Fig. 7-10), should be kept in the locked box. When funds are to be expended, these forms are signed by two persons—the medical assistant, who has authority to approve the expenditure, and the person who receives the cash. The voucher is then placed in the box to provide proof of the expenditure.

After the fund has expended money and needs to be replenished, the vouchers are classified by type, such as delivery expense, postage, or office supplies and expenses. A check is written for the exact amount of the totaled vouchers. The vouchers are canceled so that they cannot be used again and are filed with the other paid vouchers in a disbursements system. The checks are then cashed and the funds used to replace the cash. A systematic method for keeping a running total of the petty cash fund is shown in the petty cash book (Fig. 7-11).

Purchasing

Part of the management of the physician's financial transactions is the control of cash payments, or disbursements. The physician needs to be assured that payments are made for goods and services which have been ordered and received. Additionally, the medical assistant must assure the completeness and accuracy of the financial records.

The basic procedures outlined in Figures 7-12 and 7-13 will assure that the disbursements (accounting) system will provide accurate, efficient, and speedy payment of all amounts owed. First, no payments should be made without proof that the goods or services have been received, that a bill or invoice has been received, that the amounts on the invoice are correct, and that payment has been authorized. Second, all payments should be made by prenumbered checks with a voucher or stub to indicate the underlying details of the transaction. This voucher will become a source document for recording the transaction in the permanent accounting records. Third, the responsibility for cash transactions should be divided between the medical assistant and other members of the office staff such that no one person completes the entire function.

The actual purchase procedure involves four main functions: ordering, receiving, accounting, and storing. Regardless of the size of the practice, an authorized person must decide what needs to be purchased, from whom the purchase will be made, and the manner by which the order will be placed. Basic supplies for administrative or clinical use will be recorded on inventory cards, as described in a later section of this chapter. When these supplies need to be replenished, a written request or purchase requisition should be filled out by the medical assistant.

Next the MA should complete a purchase order which indicates a detailed description

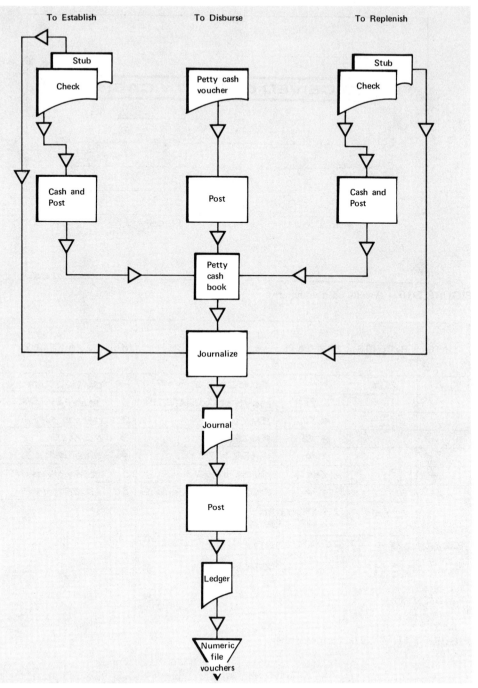

FIGURE 7-9. A petty cash fund.

No._____   Amount $_____

RECEIVED OF PETTY CASH

_____19____

For_____

Charge to_____

_____

_____   _____
        Approved by   Received by

FIGURE 7-10.   A petty cash voucher.

DATE	RECEIPTS	PAYMENTS	EXPLANATION	NO.	ACCOUNT
JUNE 1	25.00		ESTABLISHED FUND	—	CHECK #159
4		6.95	LYONS TRANSPORTATION	1	DELIVERY EXP.
10		4.50	ENVELOPES	2	OFFICE SUPP.
12		3.75	POSTAGE	3	POSTAGE
15		2.00	RAFFLE TICKET	4	MISC. EXP.
18		1.49	PAPER TOWELS	5	CLEANING SUPP.
25		5.00	PROGRAM AD—East High Schl.	6	ADVERTISING
	25.00	23.69 TOTAL			
		1.31 CASH ON HAND			
SUMMARY	25.00	25.00			
JULY 1	23.69		REPL. FUND		

FIGURE 7-11.   A petty cash worksheet.

of the goods or services, the quantity, the stock number if known, the unit price, the terms for paying, the bill, and shipping instructions. An authorized signature should be obtained before the order is placed. When the goods are received, they should be unpacked, counted, and inspected. Each item should be checked against the purchase order to verify agreement as to description, quantity, and condition.

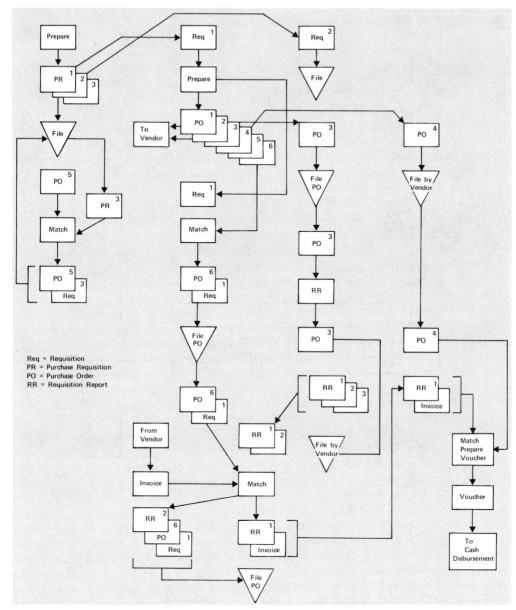

FIGURE 7-12. A purchasing procedure.

An invoice, or bill (Fig. 7-14), will be sent from the supplier requesting payment for the goods or services purchased by the physician. The invoice also includes a computation of the amount owed. When the invoice is received it should be compared with the purchase order and the receiving report and any differences in description, quantity, or price noted. If the invoice is correct it may be processed for payment.

The terms shown on the purchase order and on the invoice indicate when the physi-

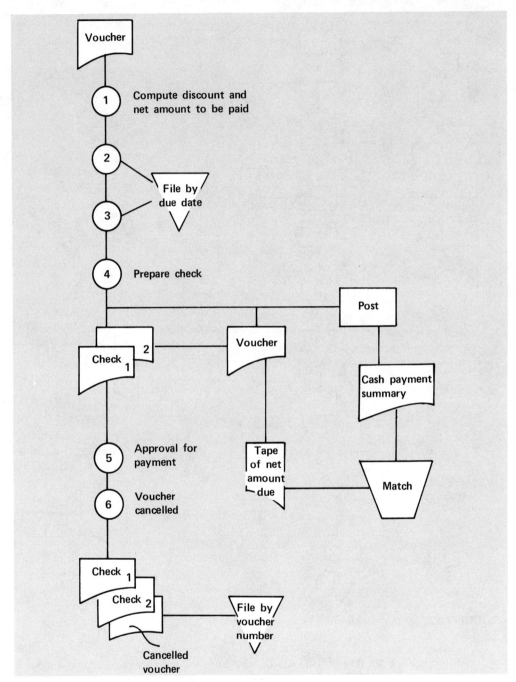

FIGURE 7-13. A payment procedure.

ABC	ABC SUPPLIES COMPANY 106 Main Street Anytown, Illinois 60521	INVOICE ORIGINAL
SOLD TO	SHIP TO	

CUST. NO.	CUSTOMER ORDER NO. AND DATE	INVOICE NO.	ABC ORDER DATE	MKT.	SLSM.

TERMS:	SHIPPED FROM	CTNS.	WEIGHT	INVOICE DATE

SHIP VIA

THIS ORDER IS SUBJECT TO CONDITIONS PRINTED ON THE ACCEPTANCE COPY OF THE ORDER FORM

QUANTITY BACK ORDER	QUANTITY SHIPPED	PART NUMBER AND DESCRIPTION	PRICE	AMOUNT

"X" INDICATES COMPLETE SHIPMENT

E=EACH
M=THOUSAND

AMOUNT SUBJECT TO DISCOUNT	FREIGHT ALLOWANCE	SHIPPING CHARGES	TAXES			TOTAL

FIGURE 7-14. A typical invoice form.

cian must make payment. If the invoice calls for payment in cash when the goods are delivered, the terms on the invoice will be "cash" or "net cash." If the physician has been extended credit, the amount, terms, and exact period of time will be noted on the invoice.

When an invoice is to be paid, a check is made out for the exact amount of the invoice. Should a discount be offered and payment made within the discount period, that amount is subtracted from the gross invoice amount and a check is written for the net amount. Invoices which have been paid should be marked accordingly so that they cannot be paid a second time. The paid invoice together with the requisition, purchase order, and receiving report should be filed in a paid invoice file.

All cash payments are recorded in a cash payments journal. Multicolumn cash payments journals are frequently used to make the recording process more accurate and efficient. Cash payment should be listed in detail, noting the date, the check number, the payee (supplier's name), and an explanation of the source and reason for payment. The amount of the payment is recorded twice: once in the column headed "cash" and once in the column whose heading most nearly corresponds to the explanation of the reason for payment. At the end of the month all the columns in the journal are totaled. To verify that the recording has been done correctly, the sum of all the specially headed columns must equal the total in the cash column. If agreement is not found, the transactions during the month must be rechecked to see that each one has been listed, or posted, correctly.

At any one time the physician may be able to calculate his expenses by a review of the cash payments journal. The information contained in it will indicate not only the total payments up to that point in the year, but also the total of various categories of expenses, such as medical or office supplies, by reference to the totals for the specially headed columns. The physician should be able to keep a record of practice income by subtracting patient receipts in the receipts journal from patient-related expenses in the cash payments journal.

Additionally, however, the medical assistant or office manager may be requested to prove the physician's calculations with the total of the outstanding bills or invoices owed. Coupled with the accounts receivable control explained previously, this information will provide the physician with the means by which he or she can plan, or manage, the cash flow.

The simplest method for a cash payment control system is an "accordian" file organizer. These files are alphabetically separated units in a self-contained folder.

BANKING PROCEDURES

In order to ensure that the physician's financial records provide a complete and accurate summary of all monies received and spent, all of the transactions must flow through normal banking activities. All cash or checks received by the physician must be deposited promptly in the bank, and all payments, for whatever purpose, should be made by check.

In order to open a checking account, each person who is authorized to sign checks on that account must fill out a signature card (Fig. 7-15). The signature on the card must be exactly as it will appear on the checks. The bank keeps the signature card on file for purposes of comparison when a check is presented for payment.

A check is a written order from the physician, telling the bank to deduct a specific sum of money from the depositor's checking account and to pay that amount to the patient, company, or organization named on the check. The advantages of check payment are that it provides (1) a record of cash paid out, (2) proof that money has been paid to the person legally entitled to it, and (3) a safer delivery system as checks are less subject to theft or loss than cash.

(1)_____   (2)_____
    Social Security Number   Social Security Number

(3)_____   (4)_____
    Social Security Number   Social Security Number

EMPLOYER IDENTIFICATION NUMBER _____

BUSINESS OR OCCUPATION _____

BUSINESS ADD. _____

RESIDENCE _____

REMARKS _____

DATE OPENED   INITIAL DEPOSIT   INTRODUCED BY   OPENED BY

_____ $_____   _____   _____

Regular Checking--INDIVIDUAL--PARTNERSHIP--FIRM

Acct.
Title _____   Attach Account No.

                                               Label Here

The depositor fully understands these regulations and agrees
to them, and so designates his acceptance thereof by his
signature on this card.   Form 5013

Authorized Signature (1) _____

Authorized Signature (2) _____

Authorized Signature (3) _____

Authorized Signature (4) _____

THE FIRST NATIONAL BANK OF PENNSYLVANIA _____, PA. Sigs.
                                                          Req. ____

In receiving items for deposit or collection, this bank acts only as depositor's collecting agent and assumes no responsibility beyond the exercise of due care. All items are credited subject to final payment in cash or solvent credits. This bank will not be liable for default or negligence of its duly selected correspondents nor for losses in transit, and each correspondent so selected shall not be liable except for its own negligence. This Bank or its correspondents may send items, directly or indirectly, to any bank including the payor, and accept its draft or credit as conditional payment in lieu of cash; it may charge back any item at any time before final payment, whether returned or not, also any item drawn on this bank not good at close of business on day deposited. The bank also may charge to the account service and other charges, whether it is active or dormant (an account shall be considered dormant when no deposit shall have been made or check drawn for a period of one year) with or without notification to the depositor of such action, and it shall not be liable in any way for any consequences that may arise therefrom.

FIGURE 7-15. A bank signature card.

Check Preparation

Before writing a check, bring the checkbook up to date to make sure there is enough money on deposit in the bank to cover the check. Add each deposit to the balance previously shown in the checkbook and subtract each check as it is written, then carry that total to the next stub in the checkbook. This running total represents the amount remaining in the bank account against which checks may be written.

First fill out the check stub, indicating the check number, the date, the person to whom the payment is being made, and the reason for which payment is being made. The stub should also contain the information, deposits, and check amounts necessary to calculate the running total in the checkbook. All information on the stub must be complete and accurate since it becomes the source document for recording and transaction in the physician's accounting records.

To prepare the check itself, first write the check number if the check has not been prenumbered, being sure to account for all check numbers in sequential order. If any errors are made in preparing a check, write VOID in large letters across the face of the check *and* the stub as well and staple the check into the checkbook. At all times it is necessary to maintain the sequential order of the checks and to account for all consecutively numbered checks so that the canceled checks are properly returned from the bank.

Next indicate the date on which the check is being issued and the payee or person to whose order the check is to be paid. Be sure to fill all space provided, either with the payee's name or with a line, so that it is not possible for any alteration to be made.

In the space beside the payee's name write the amount of the check in the numerical format of dollars followed by cents as a fraction of 100. Again, be sure to completely fill the space provided so that no alterations can be made to the check. This same amount is entered in words on the face of the check, immediately under the payee's name. Start at the extreme left in order to utilize all space provided and separate the dollar amount from the fractional cents amount by the word "and." If any space remains, draw a line to the end of the space as was done above with the payee's name. Be sure that the amount beside the payee's name and the amount written under the payee's name are exactly the same. If the two sums are different, the bank will either pay the amount in words or choose not to process the check at all.

Finally, while the check may be prepared by anyone in the office, only a person authorized to do so may sign the check. The signature used must be exactly that of the signature on the signature card on file with the bank. After the check has been signed, it may be processed through a check-writing machine which punches five holes in the check as it prints the amount of the check. This makes it impossible for anyone to alter the name of the payee or the amount of the check.

In addition to the standard check described above, the physician may use voucher checks or certified checks. A voucher check consists of two parts. The first part is the standard check and the other part, the voucher, describes the purpose for which the check has been written. The voucher portion of the check is kept by the payee. A record of payment received and a carbon copy of the voucher replaces the check stub to prove that payment has been made by the physician. A certified check carries the bank's guarantee that the depositor has enough funds on hand in the checking account to pay the check when it is presented. To have a check certified, the depositor prepares the check in the normal manner and presents it to the bank where it is stamped "Certified" across the face. Immediately, the amount of the check is deducted from the depositor's bank account.

Occasionally, a check may be lost or stolen after it has been issued. When this occurs, the bank should be notified immediately and a "stop payment" order, authorizing the bank not to make payment if the check is presented, should be executed. The notice should be attached to the checkbook stubs and the amount of the check added to the current checkbook balance. A new check can then be issued to replace the former.

Deposits

The physician should deposit all cash received (whether in coins, currency, checks, or money orders) promptly at the close of each business day. Currency and coins are sorted by denominations and wrapped in bands provided by the bank. A check or money order must be endorsed before it can be deposited. To endorse a check or money order, write or stamp the physician's name across the left end of the reverse side. The endorsement creates a legal responsibility on the bank's part to deposit the face amount in the physician's account and to collect payment from the drawer.

When the deposit ticket (Fig. 7-16) and cash items are presented for deposit, the bank teller gives the depositor a receipt indicating the date of the deposit and the total amount. These two pieces of information must correspond exactly with what appears on the deposit ticket. The bank receipt should be attached to the duplicate deposit ticket as further proof of the transaction for the physician's accounting records. Duplicate deposit tickets should be accounted for in numerical sequence in the same manner as are the physician's checks.

Bank Reconciliation

Once a month the bank sends the physician a bank statement indicating the balance at the beginning of that monthly period, deposits made during the month, checks and other charges subtracted during the month, and the balance in the checking account at the end of the month. As soon as the bank statement is received it should be checked to verify that the balance shown by the bank agrees with the amount indicated in the physician's checkbook. Bank statements do not ordinarily agree exactly with the checkbook due to delays either by the physician or by the bank in recording deposits, checks, or other bank charges.

In order to account for the differences between the amount indicated as the cash balance on the bank statement and the amount indicated as the cash balance in the checkbook, calculations must be made of all items for which there has been a delay in the recording process. Outstanding checks will cause the bank statement to have a higher balance than the checkbook because the amount of these checks has been subtracted from the physician's checkbook balance but has not been subtracted from the physician's bank account, since the checks have not been presented by the payee for payment. Deposits in transit occur when the physician mails deposits to the bank and adds those amounts to the checkbook balance but the bank does not receive them in time to add them to the monthly bank statement. In this case the physician's checkbook will indicate a higher balance than will the monthly bank statement. Bank fees or service charges for handling the physician's checking account will be computed by the bank and deducted directly from the physician's bank balance. Evidence of such charges will be provided in the monthly bank statement and will reduce the balance indicated on that statement. However, because the physician will not have been notified of such charges prior to the end of the month, they will not be deducted from the checkbook balance. Such charges cause the bank statement amount to be lower than the physician's checkbook balance.

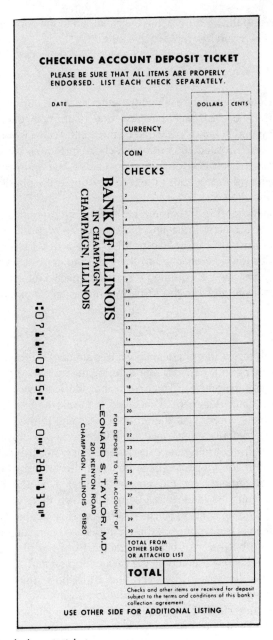

FIGURE 7-16. A bank deposit ticket.

A dishonored check is one that is not paid when properly presented to the bank. This may occur when the drawer does not have sufficient funds (NSF) to cover the check, when the signature on the check does not match the signature card, when a "stop payment" order has been executed, when an endorsement is missing or improper, or when it appears that the check has been altered, predated or postdated. When the deposited check is dishonored, the bank subtracts that amount from the physician's bank balance, in effect reducing the amount of total deposits made into the account during the month. However, the physician's checkbook deposit totals have not been reduced by these amounts unless prior notice has been received. Therefore, the checkbook balance will be higher than the bank statement balance.

Finally, mathematical errors on the part of the bank or in the physician's records may create differences. The check face and the check stub may not be in agreement. Checks may not have been entered on the stub or in the disbursements ledger. Deposit amount may have been omitted from either the checkbook or the receipts ledger. The bank may accept a check with the physician's signature forged, or may charge the physician's account with another depositor's transactions. In any of these events notice must be given immediately to those persons responsible for complete and accurate record-keeping at the bank or at the physician's office.

A formal procedure for determining the causes of the differences in the checkbook balance and the bank statement balance is known as reconciling the bank statement. Bank reconciliations may be completed by utilizing the format on the back of the bank statement or by preparing a separate statement. For purposes of completeness and accuracy, and to verify that all transactions have been properly recorded, the individual who prepares either the deposit tickets or the checks should not be the same person who prepares the bank reconciliation.

The steps for completing a bank reconciliation are as follows:

1. Enter the heading, physician's name, title of the format, and date of the reconciliation.

2. Record the bank statement balance at the end of the period.

3. Compare the amounts of the deposits listed on the bank statement with those listed in the checkbook and indicate with check marks those that agree. Any deposit listed in the checkbook which is not found on the bank statement is a deposit in transit and is added to the bank balance amounts. A review of last month's bank reconciliation should verify that deposits in transit at that time have been received by the bank and recorded on this month's bank statement. If any discrepancies exist, notify the bank immediately.

4. Review all canceled checks and debit memoranda enclosed with the bank statement. Any discrepancies in amount between the documents and the listings on the bank statement should be reported to the bank.

5. Arrange the canceled checks in numerical order and account for the sequence, being sure to include voided checks and "stop order" payments in the process.

6. Compare each check (canceled or voided) with the checkbook agreement as to payee and amount. Those check stubs without a check mark represent outstanding checks.

7. Prepare a list of all check numbers and amounts of the outstanding checks. Review

last month's bank reconciliation in order to include on the list previous outstanding
checks which still have not been returned.

8. The adjusted bank balance amount is the calculation performed by adding deposits
   in transit and subtracting outstanding checks from the end of the month bank statement balance.

9. Calculate an adjusted checkbook balance which agrees with the adjusted bank statement balance. List any mathematical or computational errors and any bank charges
   which have been recorded on the bank statement but which have not as yet been
   recorded in the physician's checkbook. Subtract the total of these deductions from
   the checkbook balance to compute the adjusted checkbook balance. The bank
   reconciliation is complete and the underlying financial records are accurate if the adjusted bank statement balance and the adjusted checkbook balance are identical. If
   they do not agree, all the details must be rechecked until the error is located and the
   balances reconciled. Common errors which will create an imbalance in the reconciliation process include omissions of deposits or checks in the checkbook, duplicate
   recordings of deposits, omissions of service charges or fees, disagreement in amount
   between the paid check and the checkbook stub, omissions of the previous month's
   outstanding checks, or errors in addition or subtraction.

After the bank reconciliation has been completed, the physician's records must be updated to reflect the differences between the bank statement amount and the checkbook
amount. The deductions listed in step 9 above must be recorded in the checkbook and any
adjusting journal entry prepared and posted to the cash account in the physician's general
ledger. When the entry is posted, the cash account in the ledger and the adjusted checkbook
balances will be in agreement, and the amount indicated will reflect the actual amount
available in the checking account against which checks may be drawn in the future. The
reconciled checkbook balance should be so noted for reference as a beginning balance in the
succeeding bank reconciliation process.

PAYROLL PROCEDURES

Federal, state, and local laws require that the physician keep records of all salaries and wages
paid to employees. The payroll records must provide data on (1) the amount of wages or
salaries paid; (2) amounts deducted from the employee's earnings; (3) expenses involved with
the payroll; and (4) the payroll taxes owed by the physician and the employees to the
government.

Employee earnings may take the form either of salaries or wages. Salaries are fixed
amounts paid to employees on a regular basis, whereas wages are amounts paid to employees
at a certain rate per hour, day, or week. The total earnings of all employees for a pay period
(weekly, biweekly, semi-monthly, or monthly) is called the payroll.

The Fair Labor Standards Act regulates the number of hours employees may work and
the rate of pay. Employers who are covered by the Act must pay a minimum hourly wage
($3.35 as of January 1, 1981). In addition, the Act requires employers to pay overtime at a

minimum rate of $1\frac{1}{2}$ times the regular rate for hours in excess of 40 hours worked in any week.

The Fair Labor Standards Act also requires that a complete record be kept of the hours worked by each employee. This record can be in the form of a time book or a time card. Gross earnings for the employee are computed by totaling the weekly hours worked and multiplying that total by the employee's wage or salary rate.

The employee's gross pay, as computed above, differs from the actual amount paid to the employee. These differences, or deductions, include those required by law, such as income tax and social security (FICA), or those of a voluntary nature, such as group life insurance and hospitalization insurance premiums.

Any physician is required to withhold (deduct) federal, state, and city income taxes and the employee's share of social security taxes from an employee's gross earnings. The amount of federal income tax withheld depends upon the employee's gross earnings, marital status, and number of exemptions. The tax is determined by using wage-bracket tables provided by the Internal Revenue Service.

The second required federal deduction is FICA, or social security. The FICA tax is paid by both the physician and the employee. The tax is based on annual gross earnings up to a certain maximum amount paid between January 1 and December 31. The Internal Revenue Service provides a social security tax table which computes the amount of social security tax to be withheld from an employee's gross wages.

City and state income tax withholdings are determined in a manner similar to federal income tax. The tax amount is usually a certain percentage applied to the employee's gross wage earnings.

An employee's net or take-home pay is calculated by subtracting all taxes withheld as well as all voluntary deductions, such as medical insurance or life insurance premiums, from gross wage earnings. In other words, gross pay is what is earned by the employee and net pay is the amount actually given to the employee.

A flowchart of the payroll procedure as well as illustrative payroll calculations have been provided in Figures 7-17 and 7-18. Refer to these and review the foregoing discussion before proceeding to the next section.

By law the physician is required to keep payroll data for at least four years, and must provide each employee with an employee pay statement for each pay period. This statement is frequently the stub of the employee's payroll check. In effect the check provides the employee with monetary reimbursement for services rendered, and the stub provides the employee with information as to how that reimbursement was calculated. The data contained on the stub will be exactly what has been recorded in the payroll register and in the employee's earnings record. The income taxes and FICA taxes withheld from the employee's earnings and the employee's FICA tax contribution must be remitted to the Internal Revenue Service and the state or local taxing authorities.

Once a year the physician is required to give each employee a wage and tax statement (Form W-2). Form W-2, which must be prepared and distributed to the employee no later than January 31 of each year, contains summary earnings data for the preceding calendar year. The employee's gross wages, the amount of federal income tax withheld, the FICA tax withheld, the total amount of earnings subject to FICA taxes, the state and local income taxes withheld, and all voluntary deductions will be indicated. The information for Form W-2 is ob-

REGULAR HOURS   × RATE =
          40   × $3.75 = $150.00

OVERTIME HOURS   × RATE =
          8   × $5.625 = $45.00
_____

TOTAL GROSS $195.00

DEDUCTIONS
     FEDERAL INC. (TABLE)   17.40
     FICA   ON $100.00 = 6.13
             ON $95.00 = 5.82   11.95
     STATE TAX   2% GROSS   3.90
     CITY TAX   1% GROSS   1.95
     LIFE INS.   3.00
     GROUP HEALTH   3.50
     UNIFORMS   5.00
_____

GROSS ($195.00) − DEDUCTIONS $46.70

              = NET WAGE $148.30

FIGURE 7-17. Payroll calculation.

tained from the employee's earnings records. Multiple copies of the form are prepared: one to be sent to each taxing authority, one for the employee's permanent records, and one for the physician's records. Additionally, the physician sends copies of the W-2 forms for all employees to the Internal Revenue Service. As a final note, the physician must calculate and remit federal and state unemployment compensation taxes. These are taxes which only the employer must pay and which do not affect the employee's earnings.

PEGBOARD/"ONE-WRITE" SYSTEMS

The pegboard or "one-write" system (Fig. 7-19) is a mechanical accounting technique which makes it possible to complete more than one step at a time in the process of recording the

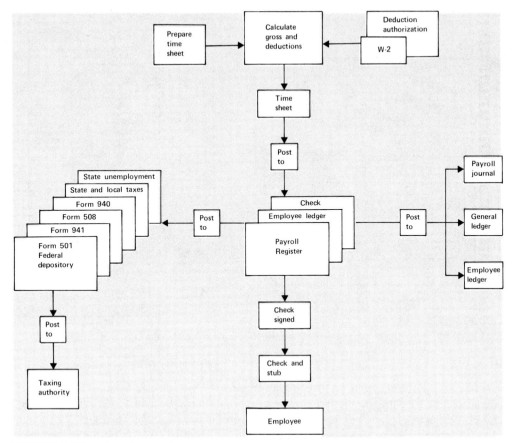

FIGURE 7-18. Payroll procedure.

physician's financial data. Because more than one operation is completed concurrently, speed and accuracy are improved. Additionally, because specialized forms are utilized, each requiring detailed completion, the underlying or source documents for the physician's record-keeping are standardized.

The pegboard system consists of a flat writing surface and a series of evenly spaced metal pegs along the edge of the board. Specially provided forms with punched holes fit over the pegs in such a manner as to line up all writing surfaces concurrently. When the form on top is completed, the information is transferred simultaneously to those forms lying underneath it.

Basic pegboard systems are available for receipts, payments, and purchases. Each is outlined below, complete with a description of the specific permanent records which will be generated concerning the physician's practice unit.

The use of the pegboard system for patient accounts involves the simultaneous generation of a patient account or ledger card, a daily earnings summary, and a patient billing card. Thus, in one process, the recording will be completed for patient records, daily earnings and

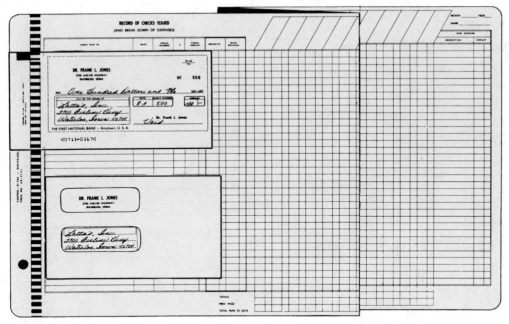

FIGURE 7-19.   A "one-write" bill-paying record. (Courtesy of Control-o-fax)

receipts, and patient accounts control. To assemble the form for use, mount the daily summary sheet first, next line up the billing charge/receipt slip on the side peg in such a manner that only one entry is made per line, and finally insert the patient ledger card such that an entry on the charge/receipt slip will simultaneously enter a correct amount on the ledger card. As a result, an entry will be made recording the proper data on all three source documents.

For use as a payments system, the "one-write" or pegboard device allows the physician to record a cash payment journal, a voucher, and a check simultaneously. The same method is used as was noted for patient charge/receipts. In this case the cash payments summary sheet is attached to the side page first, followed by the voucher and then the check. The medical assistant draws the check, and the proper entries are made simultaneously on the voucher and in the payments journal. In this manner it is possible to provide complete and accurate accounting for all of the physician's expenditures and in one process to write checks and to provide voucher-file proof of the expenditures for the supplier and a disbursements record to categorize cash expenditures for use in the formal accounting process which is described in the next section.

As was noted earlier, conventional payroll procedures require the use of time sheets, a payroll journal, an employee earnings record, an employee earnings statement, and a payroll check with voucher stub. Each time one of these forms is completed and the information transferred to the next document, speed and accuracy may be lost. In a pegboard system the payroll register is mounted first, followed by the employee earnings record, and finally the payroll check. As the payroll and its accompanying voucher stub are completed, that information is simultaneously entered on the employee's earnings record and the payroll register. The information is now complete and accurate, and may be transferred to the formal accounting records through the process outlined in the following section.

It should be noted that pegboard systems vary according to the needs of the physician's practice unit and the type of device employed. The basic format and method for use will be the same, but training may be necessary in the various aspects of the system finally chosen.

FINANCIAL RECORDS AND THE ACCOUNTING CYCLE

The formal accounting process is a method by which the financial data collected by the physician's practice unit are systematically summarized into standardized reports. The standardized reports are called financial statements, and the summarization is achieved through the use of books of account. The entire system is based upon the fact that all transactions which occur in conjunction with the physician's practice may be classified as assets, liabilities, or equity. In this case, assets are anything of monetary value which is owned by the physician; liabilities are debts owed by the practice unit; and equity is the residual claim which the owner has against whatever assets remain after the debts have been liquidated. The relationship between assets, liabilities, and equity is expressed by the standard accounting equation:

$$\text{Assets} = \text{Liabilities} + \text{Owner's Equity}$$

If one moves the elements around, one can see that what is owned (assets) must equal the claims against it, either by creditors or by the owner. Alternatively, the assets minus the claims by creditors equal the claims of the owner; or assets minus the claims of the owner equals the claims of creditors. The two sides of the accounting equation always remain equal since any transaction will be summarized in such a manner as to maintain its equality.

All transactions can be related to one or more of the elements of the accounting equation and its effect on that equation measured. To do so, one must fit the elements of the financial event into categories of assets, liabilities, or equity. Assets, defined as resources owned, would include items such as cash, furniture, supplies, buildings, and patient accounts receivable. Liabilities, or debts, would include credit purchases, loans, and mortgages. Equity is the physician's investment in the practice and his residual share of assets at any point in time. Figure 7-20 illustrates several financial transactions and their effect on the accounting equation.

As the basic equation has been presented thus far, the physician can summarize his financial position (assets and liabilities) in a standardized report called a balance sheet. This report is merely the translation of the accounting equation, in its exact order, into a format acceptable to those who have a financial interest in the physician's practice: accountants, lawyers, bankers, and the Internal Revenue Service. The balance sheet indicates the status of the physician's practice at a particular time, an artificial means to stop the clock long enough to see where one has been.

The balance sheet, however, does not indicate how the sum total of the elements of the accounting equation was determined. What is necessary is a report which summarizes the operations of the practice, the revenue earned, and the expenses incurred. This report, called an income statement, summarizes those financial transactions involving revenues or expenses for a specific period of time, for example, a year or a month. The income statement is also based upon the standard accounting equation. As was noted above, equity is

ASSETS =	LIABILITIES	+ EQUITY		
		Investment	+ Revenue	− Expense
DR. SMITH INVESTS CASH IN MEDICAL PRACTICE (50,000-)		CAPITAL (50,000)		
BORROW FROM FIRST NATIONAL BANK (200,000)	NOTE PAYABLE (200,000)			
BUY EQUIPMENT ON CREDIT (10,000)	ACCOUNTS PAYABLE (10,000)			
PATIENT TREATMENT PAID IN FULL (1,000)			(1,000)	
PAY CASH FOR OFFICE SUPPLIES SUPPLIES (+5,000) CASH (−5,000)				
PAY M.A. CASH (−100)				SALARY (100)
PATIENT BILLINGS MAILED RECEIVABLE (7,000)			(7,000)	
PAID UTILITY BILL CASH (−90)				UTILITY (90)
PAID ON EQUIPMENT CASH (−5,000)	ACCOUNTS PAYABLE (5,000)			
COLLECTED BILLINGS CASH (+5,000) PATIENT RECEIVABLE (−5,000)				

FIGURE 7-20. A physician's transaction record.

defined as the physician's investment plus his share of the increase in value of the assets of the practice. Therefore it is possible to expand the basic equation (Assets = Liabilities + Equity) to read:

$$\text{Assets} = \text{Liabilities} + [\text{Equity Investment} + (\text{Revenue} - \text{Expenses})]$$

From this expansion it should be noted that the income statement (Revenue − Expenses) is interrelated for a part of the balance sheet (Assets = Liabilities + Equity) and that the increase in value of the physician's equity in the practice comes in part from the income or profit which that practice generates.

While the medical assistant may not be required to perform all the steps within the accounting cycle in order to prepare formal financial statements, he or she will be expected to summarize the financial transactions upon which these statements are based. Therefore, it is important that the process be explained thoroughly by those individuals responsible for preparing the statements, whether by a bookkeeper or an external accountant. Any questions as to why certain procedures must be followed or what to do with specific data should be asked and answered fully.

By way of summary, the complete accounting cycle is outlined below and in Figure 7-21. It is not expected that the MA will be able to perform all the steps without training, but the following discussion should present an introductory overview.

The *first step* in the accounting cycle is to record the details about each transaction in a standard form or journal. Each transaction must be supported by a source document which serves as a reference when completing the accounting cycle, or when reconstructing the event at a later date.

The *second step* involves the source documents in journal or register form that provide the basis for each transaction to be classified according to its effect on the accounting transaction. Within the practice unit, the medical assistant will be responsible for a receipts journal, a cash payments journal, and a payroll journal. If the reader refers back to the appropriate sections of this chapter, it will be noted that emphasis was placed upon the proof, or balancing, of each journal to see that each transaction had been summarized accurately and completely. This is necessary so that the equality of the accounting equation is maintained. Should an inequality exist, the remainder of the accounting cycle cannot be completed and the financial statements prepared until the error is found.

The *third step* in the accounting cycle involves transferring the data contained in the journal into the formal books of account, called a general ledger. This ledger is a summary of the same transactions contained in the journal rearranged and reclassified into an order which facilitates the preparation of the financial statements. The summary sheet records the increases and decreases in assets, liabilities, or equity which have occurred during the period. The balance, or the increases minus the decreases, will be the amount indicated in the financial reports. For example, the opening cash amount plus the cash increases recorded in the cash receipts journal minus the cash decreases from the cash payments journal will equal the financial statement, or balance sheet, amount listed for the assets in cash.

It should be noted that if we have completed the cycle properly there should be some external evidence or source document to verify that fact. Using cash as an example, it was noted earlier that the cash balance in the checkbook, which is equal to the cash balance in the general ledger, can be compared to the cash balance in the bank as evidenced by the monthly bank statement. If the two cash balances are in agreement, further proof exists that the equality of the accounting equation has been maintained while the individual financial transactions of the practice unit were being summarized.

The use of a general ledger and specialized ledgers for patient receivables and for practice purchases and payables will be determined by the size and sophistication of the accounting system for the practice unit. Training is required in the use of these formal books of account, and they must be coordinated with the required record-keeping of the external accountant and the Internal Revenue Service.

The *fourth step* in the accounting cycle is to summarize the general ledger. A listing is made of each individual asset, liability, equity, revenue, and expense. This listing, or trial balance, is then proved to ascertain that the equality of the accounting equation has been maintained.

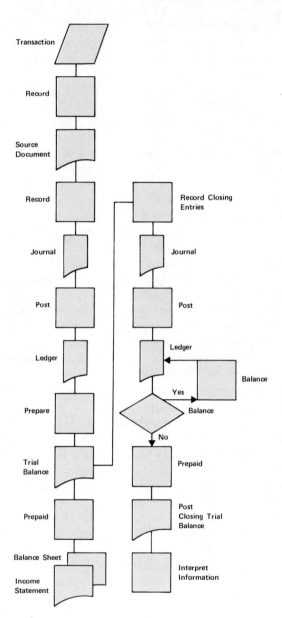

FIGURE 7-21. The accounting cycle.

The *final step* is to rearrange the elements of the trial balance into formal financial statements: transferring the assets, liabilities, and equity accounts to the balance sheet and those of the revenue and expense accounts to the income statement.

The foregoing steps suggest that the medical assistant is the primary link in the accounting cycle. If the source documents utilized or the transaction summaries prepared are incomplete or inaccurate, the rest of the process cannot be completed. Thus it is vital that care, efficiency, and concern be exercised when financial data are being prepared and recorded. Regardless of the accounting system being used, and regardless of the number of outside professionals either completing the process or reviewing what has already been completed, the medical assistant will be expected to be knowledgeable about what was done, how it was done, and why it was done. Therefore, the MA should keep notes, utilize the procedures manual extensively, and ask questions about anything which is not understood or which deviates from what was done previously. The medical assistant will not be expected to handle the entire accounting cycle herself, but she will be expected to know those sections she does handle and to prepare them completely and accurately.

CREDIT AND COLLECTION

The primary concern for the physician is quality medical treatment for his patients. The physician provides a service for those individuals who need to rely upon his training and expertise. Such services should be provided at a rate which will allow the physician to maintain and upgrade the quality of health care which he delivers to the patients.

Concurrently, the patient who requested medical treatment and received it when in need must recognize his financial responsibility to remunerate the physician for his services. To do so the patient must be fully informed as to the services that have been performed, the cost of these services, and the alternative payment methods available to him.

Credit and collection policies, or the formal definition of the fees and payment schedules that are available to patients are the prerogative of the physician. Once the fee schedule has been set and the forms of cash, deferred payment, or third-party reimbursement have been outlined, it is the medical assistant's responsibility to communicate this information to the patient, to prepare the necessary source documents, and to record the events in the summary accounting records.

Credit procedures within the physician's practice unit require complete and accurate information regarding services received by individual patients (charges), payments made by those patients (receipts), and a definite contractual arrangement for future payment of any outstanding charges on the patient's account. Generally speaking, it is good credit policy to have fees and payment policies clearly posted in the office so that all patients may be informed or reminded of their responsibilities regarding the medical treatment they have requested.

The first step in the management of credit procedures is complete and accurate information about each patient, which should be obtained during the first office visit. Obtain details regarding full name, current resident address, and telephone number so that positive identification may be made and the patient can be differentiated from other patients being served by the practice unit. Obtain a business address and telephone number for use if the patient cannot be reached at home, or if the patient moves without notifying the physician, or for emergency notification or assistance in the collection process should that become necessary. Obtain facts concerning the patient's personal history which will assist both in medical treatment and in the credit process. Date of birth, occupation, and the names of former physicians and of those currently providing care are useful diagnostic aids as well as data necessary to establish current and previous credit ratings. References from relatives, friends, and acquaintances provide an additional verification of the patient's credit rating and are a source of information should the physician need to reach the patient in an emergency or should collection problems occur. Finally, obtain information regarding who is responsible for payment of treatment services. The responsible individual should be billed for the patient charges, whether the patient himself, a husband or wife, a parent, or some other legally responsible guardian. Additionally, if the patient qualifies for third-party reimbursement for medical treatment, the proper forms must be completed detailing the insurance carrier, policy number, and type of coverage.

If the first two steps in credit management have been accomplished, education of the patient as to charges and payment options for treatment and the complete and accurate detailing of patient's biographical data on the formal accounting records, then the third step of credit control is much easier. Credit control provides for a prompt followup when collection problems become evident. Ability to pay for the medical treatment has been established through the registration information obtained on the first visit, and the patient has been informed of the fees and payment schedule. The accounting process outlined earlier in this chapter should provide the patient with a prompt and accurate record of outstanding charges which he must remit to the practice unit. Evidence that either the communication process or the accounting process has broken down occurs when patient receipts for specific treatment are not forthcoming. A view of the source documents will establish the veracity of the charges/receipts and the patient ledger balance. A courteous, interested followup will establish satisfaction with the medical treatment, or perhaps dissatisfaction, in which case the physician should be informed of the problem in terms of the financial as well as the medical aspects of the case.

A routine policy of collection followup should be established by the medical assistant as part of the normal patient billing process. The first monthly statement, outlining treatment received and charges for which payments are due, is mailed to patients at the end of the month following treatment. It can be expected that most patients will remit all or a major portion of these charges during the succeeding month. Those patients who do not pay within a 30-day period should be subject to regular collection followup procedures. Beginning with the second or third billing cycle reminder notices should be attached to the patient statements, indicating that the amounts are past due. These reminder notices are usually staggered, starting with a very polite request and progressing, if necessary, to a final notice which indicates that appropriate legal action will be taken if prompt payment is not arranged.

The followup policy must be clearly outlined and strictly applied to all patient accounts so that the medical assistant knows when to start, which reminder notices to use, the order in which they are to be used, the time span over which they are to be used, and what to do when the followup procedure has yielded no payment.

The basis for determining which patient accounts are subject to followup collection procedures and at what stages the notices should follow is an "aging" schedule. To "age" a patient account, reference must be made to the patient ledger card. A simple calculation may be made on the card, indicating which charges for medical treatment have been outstanding for 30 days, which for 60 days, which for 90 days, and which are in excess of 90 days. It is good credit practice to make a summary schedule analyzing the "age" of all outstanding patient accounts at the beginning of each month. To do so, list on a seven-column journal sheet each patient account by name for which there is an outstanding balance. In the first column indicate the total balance due the practice unit. (The total of this column represents both the total billings to be mailed out during this billing cycle and the total accounts receivable owed to the practice unit.) In the second column indicate the portion of the total balance due which has been outstanding for 30 days or less; in the third column, the charges outstanding for 31 to 60 days; in the fourth column, charges outstanding 61 to 90 days; and in the fifth column, charges outstanding more than 90 days. The remaining columns provide space to note the collection procedures being employed (reminder notices, telephone calls, collection agencies, etc.) and the response from patients, including any disputes of the charges. To prove the schedule the footing or total of the first column must equal the sum of the footings of the columns to its right.

An analysis of this aging schedule (Fig. 7-22) should provide the physician with valuable information regarding his patient load. Trends will be evident as to whether payment cycles are increasing or decreasing in terms of total dollars and collection periods as well as the time required for total payment. In addition, trends will be observed for individual patient accounts and promptness of payment. Categories of patient types (income groups, age groups, treatment groups) or a three-part reimbursement format may also reveal particular payment trends.

An analysis of the accounts receivable can also be obtained by determining a collection percentage. The total accounts receivable owed to the practice unit (the first column in the aging schedule) divided by the total amount collected on those accounts during that same monthly billing cycle is the collection percentage. Trends should be noted as to increases or decreases in the collection percentage, and explanations for those trends will be found in the details provided by the aging schedule. Diplomatic, thorough, and accurate followup procedures will maintain this collection percentage at an appropriate level and will assure the soundness of the underlying accounts receivable.

Should an aging analysis and the concurrent routine followup procedures still not yield prompt payment by the patient, alternative collection methods need to be instituted. Because impersonal sticker or stamp reminders are often not successful, a more personal

PATIENT	BALANCE	CURRENT BILLING CYCLE	1–30 DAYS PAST DUE	31–60 DAYS PAST DUE	61–90 DAYS PAST DUE	OVER 90 DAYS PAST DUE	EXPLANATION
ALEXANDER, A.B.	500.00	250.00	250.00				REMINDER NOTICE SENT
BRAGGINS, C.L.	350.00	350.00					
FINNEY, J.P.	675.00	75.00	300.00	300.00			2ND NOTICE
McMULLIN, G.R.	1780.00				1780.00		COLLECTION AGENCY
RANDOLPH, T.E.	925.00	125.00	200.00	300.00	300.00		UNEMPLOYED
TUNNEY, A.S.	1240.00			240.00	1000.00		PROMISE TO MAKE PAYMENT
TOTAL	5740.00	800.00	750.00	840.00	1300.00	1780.00	

FIGURE 7-22. An "aging" schedule.

type of credit collection is necessary. A telephone contact, a formal letter, or a personal interview is the next step in this process.

The telephone is an efficient and speedy method of communicating with patients about treatment charges for which they are responsible. The patient should be reminded that the fee schedule, medical treatments, and payment schedules were outlined on his first visit and that he agreed to them during the registration process. Listen attentively to any explanations as to why the payment is in arrears, when payment might be expected, and if any dissatisfaction exists with either the treatment or the charges. Make detailed notes during the conversation and include them on the aging schedule. Be sure to close the conversation with some form of promise to pay on the patient's part and note this in a tickler file so that the patient is again subject to followup procedures.

An alternative to the telephone is a personal letter outlining the medical treatment fees and payment policies. A polite request for payment together with one or two payment options should be included. The letter should be firm and should not present an ultimatum, but rather the alternative of improved physician-patient relations.

The third approach is a personal interview arranged in private and at the convenience of the patient. Fees and payment options should again be outlined, and the patient should be afforded the opportunity to explain his current financial situation and his reason for delinquency. Alternative arrangements for payment can be made as a result of this interview. Complete notes should be taken, added to the aging schedule, and details verified where possible and noted on the patient ledger card as further references for establishing the patient's credit rating.

When neither the impersonal reminder process nor the personal contact approach has led to the payment of patient accounts, the use of a collection agency is required. Several collection agencies with national ratings are in operation, all with specific expertise in the medical field. The physician will make the final decision as to which agency to use and which patient accounts to turn over to the agency for collections.

Once an account has been turned over to a collection agency, the medical assistant is no longer responsible for monitoring its payment progress. The MA should provide the agency with all appropriate data from the registration form and any additional data that becomes pertinent. Should the patient contact the practice unit, he need only be informed that the collection agency is handling his account and he must deal with them. If the patient remits payments to the practice unit, report them promptly to the collection agency.

The collection system outlined above should provide for an open, honest, responsible relationship between the physician and the patient. The physician takes the responsibility for providing quality medical treatment for which published fees for service must be remitted. The patient accepts such treatment with the promise to remunerate the physician for services rendered. The process should be accurate, prompt, and businesslike. In this manner the patient and physician can benefit from an association marked by mutual appreciation and courtesy.

DATA PROCESSING PROCEDURES

Whatever the business transaction, the physician must process data to provide information about his operation. The series of steps taken to provide basic business information is called the data processing cycle and includes the organization of source documents, the arrangement of that data on an input device or medium for processing, the manipulation or processing of the data, and the production of output, or new information. Four methods may be used in any combination to generate data processing materials: manual, mechanical, punched-card, or electronic.

Manual data processing involves the handwritten journals and ledgers described earlier. Mechanical data processing utilizes adding machines, cash registers, and accounting (posting) machines. Punched-card operations are commonly referred to as automatic data processing to differentiate them from electronic data processing which utilizes the computer.

Whatever processing method is chosen, source documents must be recorded in some permanent, standardized financial description, complete with reference guides (audit trails) which provide a means to reconstruct the transaction at a later date. Secondly, the data must be classified into groups of similar transactions in order to save time in processing and to summarize like kinds of business events. Frequently this classification process requires indexing or coding methods similar to those discussed in connection with the files management system. The classified data are sorted by common characteristics, again utilizing files management techniques, and the computation procedures, or processing, may then be performed. The final step, or summary, results in a printed report that has organized and condensed the data in order to emphasize any decisions which must be made. A schedule of "aged" accounts receivable, for example, will indicate to the physician those patients whose payments are far enough behind to warrant collection proceedings. A payroll register will indicate year-to-date earnings for each employee, as well as providing a basis for recording salary expense and withholding tax amounts which must be posted in the accounting records.

Punched-card or unit record operations are the first step in both automatic and electronic data processing. A standard 80-column card records the source document information in appropriate sections. As the cards are prepared, holes or codes are punched which translate the data into a machine-readable format. The main advantage to this punched-card method of summarizing data is that once the information has been recorded it may be processed over and over again to produce many different types of financial reports which depend on common data. For example, the patient charge card can be utilized to generate a bill, a daily earnings summary, a listing of the types of services performed, a list of clinical supplies utilized, or a listing of accounts receivable.

Punched cards are produced on machines which provide data processing manipulations such as recording, sorting, computing, storing and summarizing. If the physician's practice is sufficiently large, a machine may be set up in the office. If the physician utilizes an external accounting service center, their operations will undoubtedly include a battery of such machines.

Punched-card machines include alphabetical and numerical keyboards not unlike a combination typewriter/adding machine. After the cards drop from a feeding station, the code (or holes) punched as the operator translates the source document information to the card is checked for accuracy, and the cards are then stacked. Certain of these machines may also have the capability to merge, match, sort, or sequence the stack of punched cards.

The punched card is the basis of the processing step or data manipulation which will be done either automatically by an accounting machine, or electronically, by a computer.

Both of these machines are capable of printing a summary report of distribution to the physician for his review.

The most sophisticated forms of data processing are performed by computers which consist of a series of interconnected machines: an input device, a central processor, and an output device. The main advantages to this type of data processing are speed, accuracy, storage or memory, and decision-making. Speed alone would justify a computer's existence when large groups of similar but complex calculations are considered, but the ability to store and reconstruct previous transactions, to retrieve and play back either original or summarized data, and to choose among alternative decisions based upon programmed instructions makes it a valuable tool for analyzing a myriad of financial events.

The computer utilizes source documents and converts them to coded punch cards, tapes, discs, or on-line display units. From there the data are sent to the central processor which translates the information into a machine-readable form and where it is either stored or processed, depending upon the instructions contained in the processor program. Once the central processor has performed the necessary manipulations, the data are summarized and printed on an output device either in a hard copy (paper) format or a display format. The final report becomes the basis for business decisions.

Depending upon the size of the physician's practice, a computer may be located within the office unit, or source documents may be sent to a service center for data processing. In either of these circumstances, extensive, specialized training is required of the physician's staff to learn the operation of the equipment involved or to learn the proper preparation of source documents for processing.

SUMMARY

The accounting system is perhaps the single most abused aspect of the typical physician's office practice. Most doctors are inexperienced and essentially uninterested in designing or maintaining good accounting procedures. Here, then, is another area in which the medical assistant may become an invaluable asset to the medical office. As a knowledgeable resource person, the medical assistant can remove the mechanical burdens of record-keeping and accounting from the day-to-day responsibilities of the physician, and can maintain the quality and efficiency of those functions.

APPLICATION EXERCISES

Problems

This section contains ten exercises involving accounting problems. Your instructor will assign several of these to be completed before the class meets.

EXERCISE 1

On June 30, the cash account shows a balance of $4337. The bank statement received on July 2 indicates a balance in the checking account of $5015. The following information resulted from the bank reconciliation routine:

1. The bank charged a collection fee of $7 for collecting a $1000 patient note and $12 interest. Collection of the note has been recorded in the physician's accounting records.

2. A deposit of $483 made on June 30 did not appear on the bank statement.

3. The following checks are still outstanding:
   No. 473 for $74
   No. 532 for $123
   No. 593 for $73

4. Check no. 321 for $225 for office supplies was recorded as $252.

5. George Mead's check for $39 was returned for insufficient funds.

6. Check no. 370 for office equipment costing $881 was recorded as $818.

7. The monthly service charge amounted to $3.

Prepare a bank reconciliation for June 30 and indicate which items need to be recorded in the physician's accounting records.

EXERCISE 2

Prepare a bank reconciliation for Dr. L. A. Pietro as of September 30, using the following information:

1. As of September 30, cash per the accounting records was $32,199; per the bank statement, $38,729.

2. Cash receipts of $5691 on September 30 were not received by the bank until October 1.

3. Checks outstanding per the accounting records totaled $12,684.

4. A miscellaneous expense check was recorded as $89; the check cleared the bank as $98.

5. A debit memo with a check attached for $596 was returned for insufficient funds.

6. Included in the bank statement was a deposit by Leah Pietro, M.D. for $2561 and a paid check for $1520.

7. Paid checks returned with the statement included an item for $4817, which was

correctly written and entered in the accounting records. The bank charges the Lee Jeans account $4187.

8. A debit memo for September service charges of $29.

9. A debit memo for safety deposit rental of $50.

10. A credit memo for a note receivable collection of $3689 (including $39 interest).

11. A debit memo for mortgage payments of $5139, including $639 interest charges.

EXERCISE 3

Prepare a bank reconciliation for January 31, using the following information:

1. The debit balance of the cash ledger, as of July 1, was $4876.80.

2. The cash receipts journal shows total receipts of $13,115.63 for the month of July.

3. The cash payments journal shows total disbursements of $15,278.43 for the month of July.

4. The bank statement shows a balance of $3,208.51 as of July 31.

5. The following checks are outstanding:
   No. 663 for $64.51
   No. 694 for $210.00
   No. 705 for $345.00
   No. 708 for $445.00

6. The bank returned a check drawn by A. B. Kelly in the amount of $85, stamped "ATF."

7. A night deposit of $485 was made at the close of business on July 31.

EXERCISE 4

Set up a petty cash book to record the following transactions. Rule and balance the petty cash account at month's end and determine the amount of cash necessary to replenish the fund.

1. Establish a $100 petty cash fund.

2. Payments supported by petty cash vouchers:
   A. Office supplies $35.00
   B. Express charges $12.00
   C. Repairs to typewriter $10.00
   D. Postage $15.00
   E. Cleaning supplies $22.50

EXERCISE 5

Establish a petty cash fund of $250 and then indicate how the petty cash book would look at month's end after the following petty cash vouchers were paid and the fund was increased to $300:

> May 1 Purchased 100 fifteen-cent stamps
> 3 Paid UPS $27.50 for delivery charges
> 5 Paid Dugan Office Supply $18.50 for paper supplies
> 12 Purchased a coffee maker and supplies for the office, $42
> 17 Paid the service man $29.98 to repair the plumbing
> 21 Paid Erie Arts Council for advertising
> 25 Paid newsboy $9 for weekly paper delivery

EXERCISE 6

Set up a petty cash book to record the following transactions. Total rule and balance the petty cash account at month's end and determine the amount of cash necessary to replenish the fund.

1. Establish a $200 petty cash fund.

2. Payments supported by petty cash vouchers:

> Nov. 1 Purchased 100 fifteen-cent stamps
> 3 Paid freight on medical supplies, $27.50
> 5 Paid Egan Stationery for typewriter ribbons, $16.75
> 9 Paid Art Craft for gift for physician's wife, $22.50
> 14 Paid printer for physician's personalized bills, $55.00
> 22 Paid $17.80 for window cleaning service
> 28 Reimbursed physician for business lunch, $18.25
> 30 Paid $32.50 for repairs to x-ray machine

EXERCISE 7

From the following information prepare a schedule "aging" accounts receivable. Determine the dollar estimate of bad debts as of April 30:

Patient Name	Amount Due	Invoice Date
R. L. Adams	$ 250	January 1
J. T. Collins	85	February 28
B. K. Edwards	1275	November 30
F. T. Kelly	790	April 30
L. E. McMullen	480	March 31
D. R. Puscano	135	April 30

Experience indicates that rates of uncollectability range as follows:

current = 1%
30 days = 3%
60 days = 5%
90 days = 12%
over 3 months = 20%

EXERCISE 8

From the following information prepare a schedule "aging" accounts receivable. Determine the dollar estimate of bad debts as of January 1:

Patient Name	Total Amount Due	Invoice Billing Date				
		Jan. 1	Dec. 1	Nov. 1	Oct. 1	Aug. 1
B. C. Ackerman	$1375	375	1000			
J. T. Thomas	1500		1000	500		
R. T. Wagner	895	95	400	400		
T. M. Wagner	425	25			400	
P. T. Zimmerman	148	148				
E. F. Zukor	565	35	35	400		95
Rate of Uncollectability		2%	3%	7%	12%	15%

EXERCISE 9

From the following information prepare a schedule "aging" accounts receivable. Determine the dollar estimate of bad debts as of October 31. Review collectors in November and determine the collection percentage.

Patient Name	Amount Due	Billing Date	Subsequent November Payments
C. R. Kelly	$ 675	Sept. 30	$ 375
F. T. Miller	1025	Oct. 31	1025
A. S. Nelson	382	Aug. 31	0
O. M. Primmel	775	Sept. 30	75
T. T. Riker	1365	Aug. 31	365
E. E. Samson	2100	Sept. 30	1000
D. R. Thomas	3625	Feb. 28	0
B. L. Thompson	418	Oct. 31	418
G. M. Venopol	295	June 30	95
H. H. Wicker	80	Oct. 31	0

Experience indicates that the rates of uncollectability range as follows:

current = 1%
30 days = 3%
60 days = 7%
90 days = 15%
120 days = 20%
180 days = 50%
over 180 days = 75%

EXERCISE 10

From the information provided below calculate the gross wages and net pay due each employee. (Be sure to use the appropriate state and local tax rates.)

Employee	Hours Worked	Pay Rate	Exemptions	Deductions
L. K. Adams	40 (M-F) 3 (S)	$3.75 reg. $1^{1}/_{2}$ ×	1	$ 3.50 uniforms 7.50 health insurance 2.50 life insurance
B. J. Collins	40 (M-F)	$3.10 reg.	2	5.00 uniforms
R. J. Kelly	40 (M-F) 8 (S)	$3.50 reg. $1^{1}/_{2}$ ×	3	5.00 uniforms 10.00 health insurance 7.00 United Way
T. K. Mann	12 each day 60 (M-F) 5 (S)	$4.75 reg. $1^{1}/_{2}$ ×	4	7.50 uniforms 12.00 health insurance 10.00 life insurance
E. F. Riley	40 (M-F) 10 (S)	$3.25 reg. $1^{1}/_{2}$ ×	6	5.00 uniforms
S. T. Vaughn	10 each day 50 (M-F) 10 (S)	$4.50 reg. $1^{1}/_{2}$ ×	5	7.50 uniforms 15.00 health insurance 12.00 life insurance 7.50 United Way

Classroom Suggestions

1. The instructor may wish to have the students write their homework assignments on the board for purposes of comparison and discussion.

2. Working in groups of four or five, the class should role-play a personnel interview for a new medical assistant. Complete the personnel file procedure.

3. It would be useful to ask an experienced accountant to speak to the class and answer questions regarding accounting systems.

COMPLETING THE LEARNING LOOP

This chapter should serve as a practical introduction to office business procedures for the prospective medical assistant. If nothing else it should highlight the need for accounting expertise as a part of the MA's skills. Naturally, a brief overview of this kind cannot transform the student medical assistant into a skilled accountant or even a fully qualified resource person. Much more effort will be required.

Most medical assisting programs suggest that the student take one or more courses in accounting. These could be among your most important classes. Attack them with vigor and take every available opportunity to ask questions which will be relevant to medical office practice.

BIBLIOGRAPHY

Anthony, R.N.: *Essentials of Accounting,* ed. 2. Addison-Wesley, Reading, Mass., 1977.
Bauer, R.D., and Darby, P. H.: *Elementary Accounting,* ed. 4. Harper & Row, New York, 1973.
Brock, H. R., et al.: *College Accounting for Secretaries.* McGraw-Hill, New York, 1971.
Chilton, C. S.: *Successful Small Client Accounting Practice.* Prentice-Hall, Englewood Cliffs, N.J., 1976.
Doyle, D. M.: *Efficient Accounting and Record Keeping.* John Wiley & Sons, New York, 1977.
Moore, C. L., and Jaedicke, R. K.: *Managerial Accounting.* South-Western, Cincinnati, 1977.
Myer, J. N.: *Accounting for Non-Accountants,* ed. 2. E. P. Dutton, New York, 1980.
Rossell, J. H., and Frasure, W. W.: *Financial Accounting Concepts,* ed. 2. Charles E. Merrill, Columbus, 1974.

CHAPTER **8**

INSURANCE FORMS AND PROBLEMS

SPECIFIC OBJECTIVES

Upon completion of this chapter you will be able to:

1. List and describe the major types of insurance encountered in the doctor's office.

2. Recognize the forms which are associated with these types.

3. Employ the correct methods of processing insurance claims.

4. Describe the current trends of insurance management in the medical office.

5. Utilize the "super bill" for claim processing.

INTRODUCTION

From the patient's perspective as well as the physician's, insurance adds an immense degree of complexity to the problem of health care delivery. When badly managed, insurance paperwork can become an overwhelming collection of duplicate and triplicate forms, but proper handling of this seemingly complex responsibility can be successfully achieved.

A major source of insurance problems stems from the fact that the patient may not have sufficient experience in the processing of insurance forms to complete them properly. Thus needless delay and aggravation in an already cumbersome system may result. Directions on insurance forms are often difficult to follow. Confusion also occurs in the interpretation of imprecise statements.

The knowledgeable and skillful medical assistant can intervene, impose simplicity, and apply logic to the patient's dilemma. For the MA to become part of the solution, a comprehensive understanding of medical insurance systems must be developed. In addition, medical assistants must be able to effectively communicate their understanding of those systems to patients and provide the necessary assistance.

There are two generic approaches to managing an office insurance system: (1) the MA takes full responsibility for processing insurance forms for the patient, or (2) the patient takes responsibility for dealing with his own insurance processing and the MA simply provides the required medical bills (or receipts) and serves as an information resource person.

In the past the first approach was typical, but the current trend has been toward billing systems which make the patient responsible for his own processing. This places the medical assistant in the unique position of educator. Rather than functioning as a skilled insurance clerk, medical assistants may find themselves in the role of patient teacher. In this capacity, MAs must help patients to understand their responsibility for filling out their own insurance forms with the help of the billing information provided.

THE "SUPER BILL"

The key to the patient-involvement approach is a multi-part "super-bill" system, which is illustrated in Figure 8-1. Before the patient leaves the office the physician fills out the three-part form. Two parts are then given to the patient so that he can process his own insurance forms. The "superbill" forms have been designed to facilitate the needs of all of the major insurance programs. Thus the completed "super bill" provides all of the information which the physician previously included on several separate forms. When patients send the "super-bill" form to their insurance company, they relieve the physician of the responsibility of filling out individual forms. This "super-bill" system is essentially the same as that previously introduced in the discussion of accounting and billing procedures.

Each physician must ultimately decide how to approach the insurance system. Whatever the doctor decides, the function of the medical assistant will be one of providing support in implementing the plan. The remainder of this chapter is devoted to an explanation of the most common types of insurance. Whether the MA will function as an insurance clerk or as an information resource, a basic knowledge of insurance will be required.

INSURANCE TERMINOLOGY

Listed opposite are definitions of the insurance terms most likely to be encountered by medical assistants in the course of their daily office activities. Additional vocabulary can be found in the Appendix to this book.

PLEASE RETURN THIS FORM TO THE RECEPTIONIST

PREVIOUS BALANCE | NAME

Date of Service ______

1 d Revision ADA Dental Procedures and Nomenclature
Tooth No. Refers To Veterans Nomenclature

ATTENDING DENTIST'S STATEMENT

DIAGNOSTIC
☐0110 Initial ☐0120 Periodic
☐0130 Emergency examination $____
0210 Intraoral X-Ray complete ____
0220 Intraoral X-Ray single film ____
0230 Intraoral—add. film #____ ____
0270 Bitewing X-Ray single film ____
0280 Bitewing—add. film #____ ____
0460 Pulp vitality tests ____
0470 Diagnostic casts ____

PREVENTIVE
☐1110 Adult ☐1120 Child prophy ____
12____ Fluoride Treatment ____
1³³0 Oral hygiene instruction ____
1‥____ Maintainer-tooth #____ ____

ORAL SURGERY
07110 Single extraction #____ ____
07120 Ea. add. tooth @ $____ ____
Tooth #'s ____

AMALGAM RESTORATIONS
Code Tooth#'s Ea. Total Code Tooth#'s Ea. Total
21__/____@____=____ 21__/____@____=____
21__/____@____=____ 21__/____@____=____
21__/____@____=____ 21__/____@____=____

ACRYLIC OR PLASTIC RESTORATIONS
23__/____@____=____ 23__/____@____=____
23__/____@____=____ 23__/____@____=____

GOLD INLAY RESTORATIONS
2510 /____@____=____ 2530 /____@____=____
2520 /____@____=____ 2540 /____@____=____

CROWN RESTORATIONS
27__/____@____=____ 27__/____@____=____
28__/____@____=____ 28__/____@____=____

FIXED BRIDGE
62__/____@____=____ 62__/____@____=____
65__/____@____=____ 65__/____@____=____
67__/____@____=____ 67__/____@____=____

PATIENT ______
5100 Complete Dentures—
☐5110 Complete upper ☐5130 Immediate upper $____
☐5120 Complete lower ☐5140 Immediate lower $____
5200 Partial Dentures $____
☐52__ ☐5240 ☐5260
☐5230 ☐5250 ☐5280
OTHER SERVICES: ______

09999 Special Report ______

☐THIS IS A PRE-TREATMENT ESTIMATE
Circled fees are for services performed
Today's Charges $____ Treatment Estimate $____

IRS# 972245
SMITH and JONES
PROFESSIONAL CORPORATION
3070 W. Airline Hwy. Anytown, USA 50704
Telephone 234-4651
☐William T. Smith, D.D.S. SS# 265-50-1023 DP# 33472
☐Raymond D. Jones, D.D.S. SS# 337-10-5678 DP# 33473

RETURN: ____ Days ____ Weeks ____ Months NEXT APPT. ____ Day ____ Month ____ Date ____ Time AM PM

89-12-1509 07329

FIGURE 8-1. A "super bill." (Courtesy of Control-o-fax)

Beneficiary The person who is to receive a sum of money or other benefit in the event of the policyholder's death.

Claim A demand for payment of benefits.

Deductible The amount which a person must pay before the policy will cover the remaining costs.

Dependent A person, usually a child or spouse, who is covered by the policyholder's insurance.

Disability A condition which renders a person unable to carry out his usual duties.

Indigent A person without the means to meet medical expenses.

Lapse Termination of an insurance policy because of failure to make agreed payments.

Liability An outstanding debt.

Premium Payment, often in installments, required to maintain insurance coverage.

Recurrent illness A sickness or injury related to one which was previously reported.

Waiting period The time period during which benefits are not yet extended to a new policyholder.

WHAT IS INSURANCE?

Basically, acquiring insurance is a strategy which minimizes the risk of a large-scale financial disaster. The insurance system is predicated upon the willingness of a very large number of people to pay a certain sum of money on a regular basis for protection against unforeseen calamities. If a disaster occurs, the insurance company will pay most of the sudden and major costs. The system can only operate successfully if, over a projected period of considerable length, most people are paying more in premiums than they are taking in claims. This is sometimes called the "pooled-risk" concept. Millions of people, for example, pay regular automobile insurance premiums but have never had an accident. These persons, in effect, are supplying the monies required to operate the insurance companies as well as facilitating the payment of large settlements when a minority of insured persons do have serious accidents.

Since the costs of all insurance, including health insurance, are rising quite rapidly, and the employees of many large organizations are either partially or fully supplied with health care coverage as a fringe benefit, a definite insurance psychology has developed. The medical assistant's understanding of this psychology should facilitate an ability to assist patients with their insurance questions. The individual patient who has for years paid into a policy with no claims may be thinking that the physician is collaborating with the insurance agencies on pricing and other decisions. The patient must be educated to understand that it is his responsibility to expedite paperwork and process all necessary forms so that the physician will be paid. The medical assistant should take responsibility for communicating to the patient what needs to be done and when, and should stress that it is the patient who must initiate the paperwork and not the company or institution by which he is employed. Many patients assume that since their insurance is a job benefit, the personnel department will be taking care of everything automatically. Clarification of responsibilities is essential to the successful processing of insurance.

KINDS OF HEALTH INSURANCE

As a medical assistant you will probably be encountering several different kinds of insurance problems. Each of these requires specialized approaches, separate forms, and above all, a comprehensive understanding of the coverage. The most common insurance types are as follows:

1. Group health
2. Major medical
3. Blue Cross/Blue Shield
4. Medicare
5. Medicaid
6. CHAMPUS
7. Individual policies
8. Workers' compensation
9. Automobile insurance
10. Capitation programs

Each of these insurance types will be described and the basic methods of completion identified for the purpose of preparing MAs for their role as insurance expeditors.

Group Health Insurance

Most individuals who are members of the work force have, as a fringe benefit, some kind of group health policy. The company may pay all or some of the costs of this insurance coverage. Whether the physician demands payment at the time of the office visit or is willing to wait for a check from the insurance company, it is the person making the claim who must complete and process the necessary forms. There are dozens of major insurance companies. Each of these may require its own slightly different form or completion procedure.

When the MA becomes oriented in a particular office, she will probably find that a relatively small number of insurance agencies account for the largest proportion of the paperwork. These agencies usually have local representatives who will be of assistance in answering questions. With less common policies each case may be a new learning experience, and much care will be needed in following unfamiliar directions.

A typical set of insurance forms for a group policy is illustrated in Figures 8-2 and 8-3. The form shown in Figure 8-2 is to be completed by the employee and sent to the insurance agent. The general purpose of this form is to allow the employee to notify the insurance agent that a claim should be processed and that a certain doctor is the attending physician. The form shown in Figure 8-3 should be initialed and signed by the patient and then completed by the physician, unless he uses a "super-bill" system.

Perhaps the most efficient method of processing these forms is to have the patient bring them along to the office. If the patient has not brought his insurance form with him, he is given a regular insurance receipt for his visit and then instructed to mail the receipt with his insurance form as soon as possible. The completed forms will then be mailed either to the insurance company or the patient, depending upon the particular insurance agent's requirements.

CERTIFICATION OF ELIGIBILITY

When working with the individual patient on the problems of group health insurance forms, it is important to inform him of his own responsibility for expediting the paperwork. Generally, this means that the patient must be certain that his employee claim form is sent to the insurance company.

In the case of some insurance policies, however, the insurance agent makes an agreement which covers a large group of employees. Since the company needs to ascertain that it is not insuring a person who is not currently eligible, an additional form is necessary (Fig. 8-4). The patient should be instructed to complete this form himself and then give it to the insurance clerk at work.

PROCESSING OF GROUP FORMS

As a first step, the medical assistant will need to discuss insurance processing, regardless of type, with the physician, to determine how this facet of medical office practice can be effec-

LIBERTY MUTUAL
LIBERTY MUTUAL INSURANCE COMPANY
LIBERTY LIFE ASSURANCE COMPANY OF BOSTON
HOME OFFICE: BOSTON

GANNON COLLEGE

Mail To
Liberty Mutual
900 State Street
Suite 211 – P. O. Box 2067
Erie, Pennsylvania 16512

FOR LIBERTY MUTUAL USE						
DIAGNOSIS:						
PLANT NO.	M	F	MAT	DISABILITY DATE or D.I.	AGE	REPORT NO.
	1	2	3			
EFF. DATE OF INS.						
EMPLOYEE				DEPENDENT		

TO BE COMPLETED BY EMPLOYEE

EMPLOYEE'S NAME | ☐ Male ☐ Female | Date of Birth
Complete Home Address | Telephone No.
Employed by GANNON COLLEGE | Employee Social Security #
Claim Is Made For ☐ Self ☐ Spouse ☐ Child | Name of Disabled Person | ☐ Male ☐ Female | Date of Birth
Was Disability Caused by Work? ☐ Yes ☐ No | Is or will there be a claim filed with the workers' compensation carrier for this disability? ☐ Yes ☐ No | First Date Unable to Work: Date, Hour ☐ A.M. ☐ P.M. | Date of Return to Work

COMPLETE FOR *ALL* CLAIMS

Date of Accident | Time ☐ A.M. ☐ P.M. | Was claimant at work when accident happened? ☐ Yes ☐ No | For Whom
Place and Details of Accident
Nature of Illness or Injury | Date First Treated for this Illness or Injury?
Treating Physician's Name and Address

ANSWER IN ALL HOSPITAL CASES: Hospital Name and Address | Admission ☐ Entered ☐ Will Enter | Date | Time ☐ A.M. ☐ P.M. | Discharge | Date | Time ☐ A.M. ☐ P.M.

ALL FAMILY MEMBERS EMPLOYED	Name	Relationship	Name and Address of Employer

IS CLAIMANT ENTITLED TO ADDITIONAL BENEFITS UNDER

A. Group Insurance, or any other arrangement of coverage for individuals in a group ☐ Yes ☐ No | C. Any coverage for students? ☐ Yes ☐ No
B. Blue Cross, Blue Shield or any other prepayment arrangement ☐ Yes ☐ No | D. Any Federal, State or other government program? ☐ Yes ☐ No

IF ANSWER TO ANY OF THE ABOVE IS "YES" COMPLETE THE FOLLOWING

Person Insured	Name and Address of Insurance Company or Organization providing benefits or services	Policy No. or I.D. No.

I/We jointly certify that the above information is true and correct. I/We hereby authorize all doctors, pharmacists, hospitals, or other institutions rendering care and treatment to furnish Liberty Mutual Insurance Company/Liberty Life Assurance Company of Boston with full information regarding treatment rendered (including copies of their records.) I/We also authorize any Union, Trust Fund, Employer or Insurance Carrier to furnish Liberty Mutual Insurance Company/Liberty Life Assurance Company of Boston, with any information that it may possess respecting benefits to which I may be entitled, benefits paid to or claimed by me in the past, my own medical history, and the medical history of any dependent whose injury or illness is the basis of an existing claim on my part. (If claim for spouse, spouse also must sign.) A photostatic copy of this authorization shall be considered as effective and valid as the original.

DATE | SPOUSE'S SIGNATURE (If Claim for Spouse) | EMPLOYEE'S SIGNATURE

ASC-2323 R4

FIGURE 8-2. An employee health insurance claim form. (Courtesy of Liberty Mutual Insurance Company)

tively systemized. Some physicians prefer that the insurance paperwork be processed daily; others prefer that it be completed weekly. Obviously, the doctor's preferences are a prime consideration in developing working habits related to insurance handling.

GANNON COLLEGE

LIBERTY MUTUAL
LIBERTY MUTUAL INSURANCE COMPANY
LIBERTY LIFE ASSURANCE COMPANY OF BOSTON
HOME OFFICE: BOSTON

Mail To
Liberty Mutual Insurance Company
900 State Street
Suite 211 — P.O. Box 2067
Erie, Pennsylvania 16512
Phone: 814 — 454-8111

HEALTH INSURANCE CLAIM — GROUP OR INDIVIDUAL

PART A   TO BE COMPLETED BY PATIENT (INSURED)
Spaced for Typewriter — Marks for Tabulator Appear on this Line

EMPLOYER (NAME OF COMPANY)
GANNON COLLEGE

EMPLOYEE (INSURED PERSON) AND ADDRESS

PATIENT'S NAME   DATE OF BIRTH

AUTHORIZATION TO PAY BENEFITS TO PHYSICIANS: I hereby authorize payment directly to the physicians for their services for treatment of the injury or sickness described herein, of the Health Insurance Benefits, if any, otherwise payable to me.

Signed (Insured Person)

Date

AUTHORIZATION TO RELEASE INFORMATION: I hereby authorize the undersigned Physician to release any information acquired in the course of my examination or treatment.

Signed (Patient, or parent if minor)

Date

PART B   ATTENDING PHYSICIAN'S STATEMENT

1. DIAGNOSIS AND CONCURRENT CONDITIONS
   (If diagnosis code other than ICDA* used, give name):

2. IS CONDITION DUE TO INJURY OR SICKNESS ARISING   PREGNANCY?   If yes, approximate date pregnancy commenced.
   OUT OF PATIENT'S EMPLOYMENT?   Yes ☐ No ☐   Yes ☐ No ☐   Date

3. REPORT OF SERVICES (Or attach itemized bill)   (If previous form submitted to this carrier, you need show only dates and services since last report.)

DATE OF SERVICES	PLACE OF SERVICES	DESCRIPTION OF SURGICAL OR MEDICAL SERVICES RENDERED	PROCEDURE CODE IF USED (IF CODE OTHER THAN CPT** USED, GIVE NAME)	CHARGES

tO—Doctor's Office   I H—Inpatient Hospital   NH—Nursing Home
H—Patient's Home   OH—Outpatient Hospital   OL—Other Locations
*ICDA—International Classification of Diseases
**CPT—Current Procedural Terminology (current edition)

TOTAL CHARGES ▶ $_____
AMOUNT PAID ▶ $_____
BALANCE DUE ▶ $_____

4. DATE SYMPTOMS FIRST APPEARED OR ACCIDENT HAPPENED.   5. DATE PATIENT FIRST CONSULTED YOU FOR THIS CONDITION.

6. PATIENT EVER HAD SAME OR SIMILAR CONDITION?   7. PATIENT STILL UNDER YOUR CARE FOR THIS CONDITION?
   Yes ☐ No ☐   If "yes" when and describe.   Yes ☐ No ☐

8. PATIENT WAS CONTINUOUSLY TOTALLY DISABLED   9. PATIENT WAS PARTIALLY DISABLED.
   (Unable to work)
   From   Thru   From   Thru

10. IF STILL DISABLED, DATE PATIENT SHOULD BE ABLE TO   11. PATIENT WAS HOUSE CONFINED.
    RETURN TO WORK.
                                                          From   Thru

12. DOES PATIENT HAVE OTHER HEALTH COVERAGE?
    Yes ☐ No ☐   If "yes" please identify

Date	Physician's Name (Print)	Signature	Degree	Telephone
Street Address	City or Town		State or Province	Zip Code

ASC 2324 R2   EQUAL OPPORTUNITY EMPLOYERS

FIGURE 8-3. A health insurance claim form completed by the physician. (Courtesy of Liberty Mutual Insurance Company)

The primary role of the medical assistant is to facilitate payment to the physician without needless delay. It is expected that the MA can and will attach the insurance form to the patient's file and complete as much of the form as is feasible. At very least, the

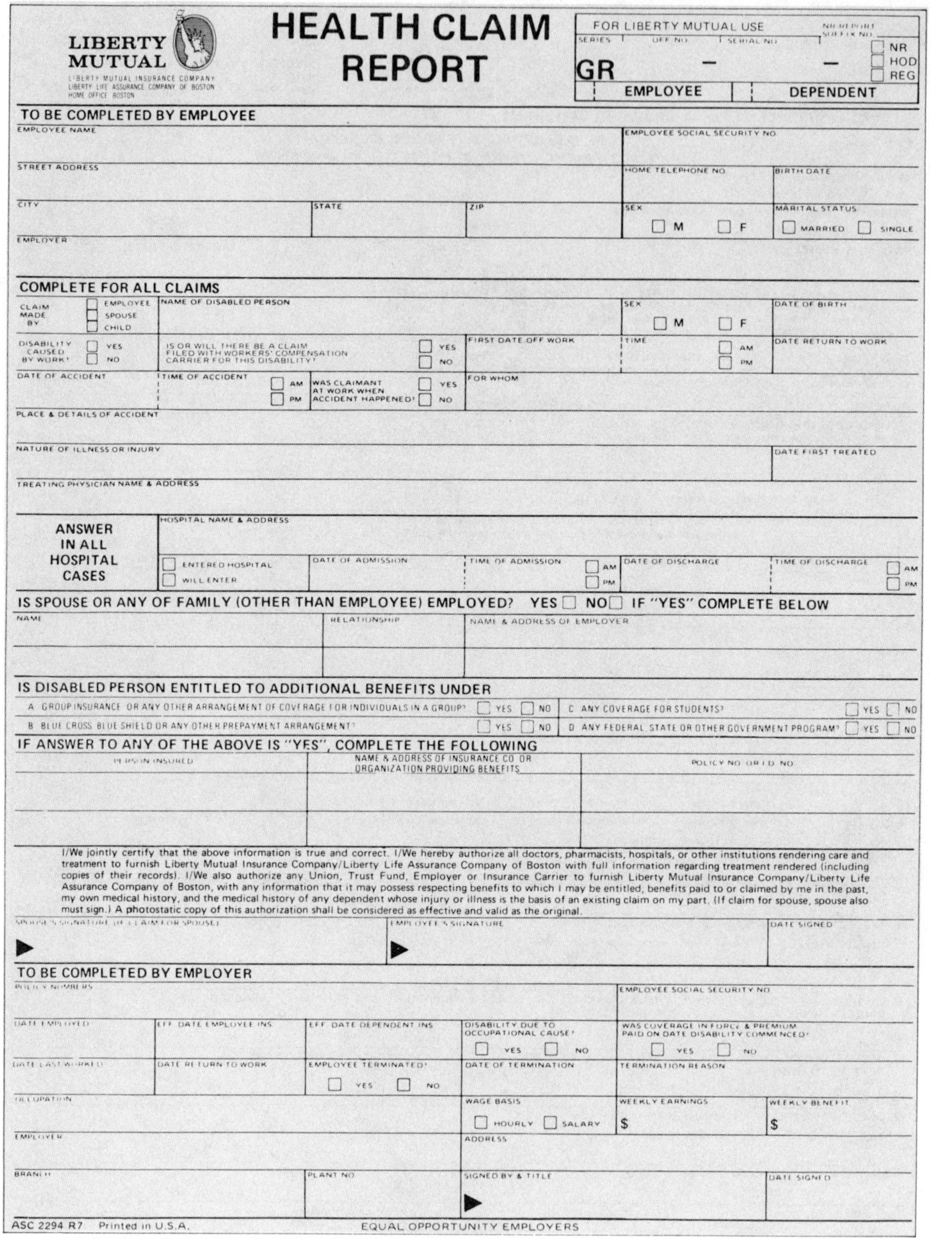

LIBERTY MUTUAL
LIBERTY MUTUAL INSURANCE COMPANY
LIBERTY LIFE ASSURANCE COMPANY OF BOSTON
HOME OFFICE BOSTON

HEALTH CLAIM REPORT

FOR LIBERTY MUTUAL USE
SERIES | OFF NO | SERIAL NO | NR REPORT SUFFIX NO
GR — —
NR
HOD
REG
EMPLOYEE | DEPENDENT

TO BE COMPLETED BY EMPLOYEE

EMPLOYEE NAME | EMPLOYEE SOCIAL SECURITY NO
STREET ADDRESS | HOME TELEPHONE NO | BIRTH DATE
CITY | STATE | ZIP | SEX ☐ M ☐ F | MARITAL STATUS ☐ MARRIED ☐ SINGLE
EMPLOYER

COMPLETE FOR ALL CLAIMS

CLAIM MADE BY ☐ EMPLOYEE ☐ SPOUSE ☐ CHILD | NAME OF DISABLED PERSON | SEX ☐ M ☐ F | DATE OF BIRTH
DISABILITY CAUSED BY WORK? ☐ YES ☐ NO | IS OR WILL THERE BE A CLAIM FILED WITH WORKERS' COMPENSATION CARRIER FOR THIS DISABILITY? ☐ YES ☐ NO | FIRST DATE OFF WORK | TIME ☐ AM ☐ PM | DATE RETURN TO WORK
DATE OF ACCIDENT | TIME OF ACCIDENT ☐ AM ☐ PM | WAS CLAIMANT AT WORK WHEN ACCIDENT HAPPENED? ☐ YES ☐ NO | FOR WHOM
PLACE & DETAILS OF ACCIDENT
NATURE OF ILLNESS OR INJURY | DATE FIRST TREATED
TREATING PHYSICIAN NAME & ADDRESS

ANSWER IN ALL HOSPITAL CASES | HOSPITAL NAME & ADDRESS
☐ ENTERED HOSPITAL ☐ WILL ENTER | DATE OF ADMISSION | TIME OF ADMISSION ☐ AM ☐ PM | DATE OF DISCHARGE | TIME OF DISCHARGE ☐ AM ☐ PM

IS SPOUSE OR ANY OF FAMILY (OTHER THAN EMPLOYEE) EMPLOYED? YES ☐ NO ☐ IF "YES" COMPLETE BELOW

NAME | RELATIONSHIP | NAME & ADDRESS OF EMPLOYER

IS DISABLED PERSON ENTITLED TO ADDITIONAL BENEFITS UNDER

A. GROUP INSURANCE OR ANY OTHER ARRANGEMENT OF COVERAGE FOR INDIVIDUALS IN A GROUP? ☐ YES ☐ NO | C. ANY COVERAGE FOR STUDENTS? ☐ YES ☐ NO
B. BLUE CROSS, BLUE SHIELD OR ANY OTHER PREPAYMENT ARRANGEMENT? ☐ YES ☐ NO | D. ANY FEDERAL, STATE OR OTHER GOVERNMENT PROGRAM? ☐ YES ☐ NO

IF ANSWER TO ANY OF THE ABOVE IS "YES", COMPLETE THE FOLLOWING

PERSON INSURED | NAME & ADDRESS OF INSURANCE CO. OR ORGANIZATION PROVIDING BENEFITS | POLICY NO. OR I.D. NO.

I/We jointly certify that the above information is true and correct. I/We hereby authorize all doctors, pharmacists, hospitals, or other institutions rendering care and treatment to furnish Liberty Mutual Insurance Company/Liberty Life Assurance Company of Boston with full information regarding treatment rendered (including copies of their records). I/We also authorize any Union, Trust Fund, Employer or Insurance Carrier to furnish Liberty Mutual Insurance Company/Liberty Life Assurance Company of Boston, with any information that it may possess respecting benefits to which I may be entitled, benefits paid to or claimed by me in the past, my own medical history, and the medical history of any dependent whose injury or illness is the basis of an existing claim on my part. (If claim for spouse, spouse also must sign.) A photostatic copy of this authorization shall be considered as effective and valid as the original.

SPOUSE'S SIGNATURE (IF CLAIM FOR SPOUSE) ▶ | EMPLOYEE'S SIGNATURE ▶ | DATE SIGNED

TO BE COMPLETED BY EMPLOYER

POLICY NUMBERS | EMPLOYEE SOCIAL SECURITY NO
DATE EMPLOYED | EFF. DATE EMPLOYEE INS | EFF. DATE DEPENDENT INS | DISABILITY DUE TO OCCUPATIONAL CAUSE? ☐ YES ☐ NO | WAS COVERAGE IN FORCE & PREMIUM PAID ON DATE DISABILITY COMMENCED? ☐ YES ☐ NO
DATE LAST WORKED | DATE RETURN TO WORK | EMPLOYEE TERMINATED? ☐ YES ☐ NO | DATE OF TERMINATION | TERMINATION REASON
OCCUPATION | WAGE BASIS ☐ HOURLY ☐ SALARY | WEEKLY EARNINGS $ | WEEKLY BENEFIT $
EMPLOYER | ADDRESS
BRANCH | PLANT NO | SIGNED BY & TITLE ▶ | DATE SIGNED

ASC 2294 R7 Printed in U.S.A. EQUAL OPPORTUNITY EMPLOYERS

FIGURE 8-4. A health claim report form. (Courtesy of Liberty Mutual Insurance Company)

physician's name, address, and telephone number should be completed by the assistant. In addition, dates of visits, diagnosis, and fees may be required and completed for the physician.

Major Medical Coverage

The relatively high cost of insurance policies has popularized a unique type of coverage called major medical. Many group or individual policies are accompanied either by a separate major medical policy or a major medical clause.

There are two common applications for major medical coverage: (1) large or catastrophic medical bills which extend beyond the limits of normal coverage, and (2) the possibility of a long sequence of small but uncovered procedures, such as repeated office visits, which can add up to a large overall bill. For example, presuming that the regular policy does not cover a visit to the physician's office, and that a family finds it necessary to take a child to the office twice a week for a year, the 104 visits at ten dollars per visit would add up to $1040. This may be an oppressive expense for many families.

Major medical policies usually stipulate that "uncovered" medical expenses beyond a certain limit (the limits vary with different policies) will pay a given percentage of the costs. A typical policy might require that the patient pay the first $200 per year. After that the policy might cover 80 percent of the costs up to $3000, and 100 percent of the costs beyond $3000.

If the patient does have major medical coverage, detailed itemized receipts for each visit must be provided. The patient should be advised to retain these for later reference when applying for new coverage. If the patient has a major medical policy along with his group insurance, he must be encouraged to process all the physician's charges on the appropriate insurance forms. In this way the insurance agent will automatically record the major medical expenses.

The "super-bill" system will assist the patient in maintaining records for his major medical coverage and for later purposes. He should simply send all "insurance claim" copies to the insurance company, together with copies of the insurance company's individual forms. If these procedures are not immediately covered under the basic policy, they will be recorded under major medical. This process will further relieve the physician of the problem of providing receipts to patients at year's end for major medical or income tax purposes.

Blue Cross/Blue Shield

The Blue Cross/Blue Shield insurance plan is sponsored by the Blue Cross/Blue Shield organization, a giant nonprofit agency which operates in the United States and Canada. As a nonprofit agency its primary responsibility is to provide insurance services rather than to return profits to investors. Most doctor's offices will serve a large number of patients who are covered by one or both of these plans.

Because Blue Cross is a hospitalization plan, patients will involve the physician in Blue Cross processing on a secondary basis, as when a patient making arrangements to go into the hospital needs answers to certain insurance questions. Blue Shield coverage, however, is exclusively concerned with doctor's office visits and thus will require the medical assistant's full attention.

The primary difference between Blue Shield and a typical group policy is that Blue Shield coverage depends upon the patient's income. Beyond a certain income level (which changes periodically) Blue Shield coverage is exactly the same as that of any group policy.

The physician charges his normal fees for services, the insurance company then pays the amount which it has determined for that particular service, and the patient is liable for the difference. If the patient's income is below that particular level, then the physician must charge only what Blue Shield will pay. Blue Shield refers to these as "service benefits."

There are several practical implications for the medical assistant. When insurance coverage is first discussed with the patient, a determination must be made as to the category in which the patient is to be placed. Once the MA has determined that a patient falls within the "low-income" category, for example, a list of Blue Shield coverage fees will act as a guide in billing the patient for services. The MA enters the patient's insurance policy number and includes a notation relating to his income status on the medical record.

There are several additional considerations in implementing a Blue Shield program. Obviously, each individual physician must make a decision about participating in the program. If the doctor has agreed to participate, he or she will periodically receive an updated schedule of fee allowances. The medical assistant will need to have access to this information for billing purposes. If the doctor does not participate, new patients will need to be advised. Blue Shield also makes available a guide which can be used to interpret the kind of insurance coverage which a patient has by reading his identification card.

As a unique service for persons 65 years of age or older, Blue Shield provides a program of coverage for fees which are not paid by Medicare. Since this is a relatively obscure policy, the medical assistant should discuss this possibility with patients of this age.

PREPARING THE BLUE SHIELD FORM

The newly revised Blue Shield claim form is illustrated in Figure 8-5. Since such forms will eventually find their way to a large regional office rather than a local sales agent, there is a much larger potential for form rejection and needless duplication of effort if errors have been missed. The medical assistant should make every effort to be sure that each form is filled out in a complete and accurate manner. Since forms are to be filed within 30 days of the service which has been provided, the doctor must review and sign them promptly.

Medicare

Medicare is a program of health insurance sponsored by the federal government. Persons who are 65 years of age or older, disabled or insured under the social security retirement system, or in need of kidney dialysis or replacement, are eligible. Under the Medicare system, the patient pays a nominal monthly fee, and the program provides both hospital and medical coverage. To be eligible for Medicare coverage the patient must register with the Social Security agency in his area. Patients who are approaching 65 should be encouraged to take advantage of this coverage and make application in advance of their birthday.

Because of interest in containing the basic costs of this program, there have been frequent changes in both the payment procedures and in the nature and extent of coverage. It is to be expected that Medicare will not cover all of the fees which the physician normally charges.

A fiscal agent is appointed by the government to administrate a geographic area.

HEALTH INSURANCE CLAIM FORM

☐ MEDICARE ☐ CHAMPUS ☐ BLUE SHIELD ☐ OTHER
(CHECK ONLY ONE)

READ INSTRUCTIONS BEFORE COMPLETING OR
SIGNING THIS FORM

PATIENT & INSURED (SUBSCRIBER) INFORMATION — Form Approved OMB No. 09-38008

1. PATIENT'S NAME *(First name, middle initial, last name)*
2. PATIENT'S DATE OF BIRTH
3. INSURED'S NAME *(First name, middle initial, last name)*

4. PATIENT'S ADDRESS *(Street, city, state, ZIP code)*
5. PATIENT'S SEX — MALE / FEMALE
6. INSURED'S I.D. or MEDICARE NO. *(include any letters)*

7. PATIENT'S RELATIONSHIP TO INSURED — SELF SPOUSE CHILD OTHER
8. INSURED'S GROUP NO. *(Or Group Name)*

TELEPHONE NUMBER

9. OTHER HEALTH INSURANCE COVERAGE - Enter Name of Policyholder and Plan Name and Address and Policy or Medical Assistance Number

10. WAS CONDITION RELATED TO
   A. PATIENT'S EMPLOYMENT — YES / NO
   B. AN ACCIDENT — AUTO / OTHER

11. INSURED'S ADDRESS *(Street, city, state, ZIP code)*

12. PATIENT'S OR AUTHORIZED PERSON'S SIGNATURE *(Read back before signing)* I Authorize the Release of any Medical Information Necessary to Process the Claim and Request Payment of MEDICARE CHAMPUS Benefits Either to Myself or to the Party Who Accepts Assignment Below

SIGNED ___ DATE ___

13. I AUTHORIZE PAYMENT OF MEDICAL BENEFITS TO UNDERSIGNED PHYSICIAN OR SUPPLIER FOR SERVICE DESCRIBED BELOW NOT APPLICABLE TO BLUE SHIELD

SIGNED *(Insured or Authorized Person)*

PHYSICIAN OR SUPPLIER INFORMATION

14. DATE OF — ILLNESS (FIRST SYMPTOM) OR INJURY (ACCIDENT) OR PREGNANCY (LMP)
15. DATE FIRST CONSULTED YOU FOR THIS CONDITION
16. HAS PATIENT EVER HAD SAME OR SIMILAR SYMPTOMS? YES / NO
16A. IF AN EMERGENCY CHECK HERE ☐

17. DATE PATIENT ABLE TO RETURN TO WORK
18. DATES OF TOTAL DISABILITY — FROM / THROUGH
DATES OF PARTIAL DISABILITY — FROM / THROUGH

19. NAME OF REFERRING PHYSICIAN OR OTHER SOURCE *(e.g., public health agency)*
20. FOR SERVICES RELATED TO HOSPITALIZATION GIVE HOSPITALIZATION DATES — ADMITTED / DISCHARGED

21. NAME & ADDRESS OF FACILITY WHERE SERVICES RENDERED *(If other than home or office)*
22. WAS LABORATORY WORK PERFORMED OUTSIDE YOUR OFFICE? YES / NO — CHARGES

23A. DIAGNOSIS OR NATURE OF ILLNESS OR INJURY RELATE DIAGNOSIS TO PROCEDURE IN COLUMN E BY REFERENCE NUMBER 1, 2, 3, ETC. OR DX CODE
1
2
3
4

23B.
EPSDT — YES / NO
FAMILY PLANNING — YES / NO
PRIOR AUTHORIZATION NO. ___

24. A DATE OF SERVICE FROM TO	B* PLACE OF SERVICE	C T O S	D FULLY DESCRIBE PROCEDURES, MEDICAL SERVICES OR SUPPLIES FURNISHED FOR EACH DATE GIVEN PROCEDURE CODE (IDENTIFY) *(EXPLAIN UNUSUAL SERVICES OR CIRCUMSTANCES)*	E DIAGNOSIS CODE	F CHARGES	G DAYS OR UNITS	H. LEAVE BLANK

25. SIGNATURE OF PHYSICIAN OR SUPPLIER *(I certify that the statements on the reverse apply to this bill and are made a part hereof.)*
SIGNED ___ DATE ___

26. ACCEPT ASSIGNMENT (FOR GOVERNMENT CLAIMS ONLY SEE BACK) YES / NO
30. YOUR SOCIAL SECURITY NO.

27. TOTAL CHARGE
28. AMOUNT PAID
29. BALANCE DUE

31. PHYSICIAN'S OR SUPPLIER'S NAME, ADDRESS, ZIP CODE & TELEPHONE NO. & I.D. NO.

32. YOUR PATIENT'S ACCOUNT NO.
33. YOUR EMPLOYER I.D. NO.

*PLACE OF SERVICE CODES ON THE BACK
REMARKS

APPROVED BY AMA COUNCIL ON MEDICAL SERVICE
APPROVED BY THE HEALTH CARE FINANCING ADMINISTRATION & CHAMPUS

Form HCFA - 1500 A
Form CHAMPUS - 501   6/81

FIGURE 8-5. A multi-use health insurance claim form.

Generally this will be the Blue Cross/Blue Shield office for that area. The medical assistant should record the agent's name and refer to the agent any questions which she is unable to answer in the processing of Medicare patients.

It is important to remember that it is possible to subscribe only to Medicare "A" coverage (hospitalization), which does not cover the physician and his office expenses. Only persons who *purchase* Medicare "B" will be covered for medical expenses incurred in the doctor's office.

COMPLETING MEDICARE FORMS

When a particular patient has been identified as a Medicare client, this information must be entered on the medical record. The identification card number must also be included. This consists of the social security number and a suffix letter, as for example 172-32-9542A. A supply of Medicare payment request forms (Fig. 8-6) should be on hand. Complete instructions for the patient are included on the reverse side of this form (Fig. 8-7).

SECURING MEDICARE PAYMENT

Under 1980 Medicare regulations there are several alternatives available for payment. If the amounts which are being charged by the physician are reasonably small, it would be sensible, at least from the physician's perspective, to ask for payment at the time of treatment. The completed Medicare form can be given to the patient with the doctor's signature. The patient can then hold his various bills until he has accumulated more than the required $50 deductible amount. At this time the patient can send all of the signed forms in one group to the Medicare agent for reimbursement.

If the fees are quite extensive, or if the patient seems unable or unwilling to begin processing the forms, it is then more effective to have the patient sign them and the medical assistant assume the responsibility for mailing them to the local agent. If the physician has accepted a patient on the basis of "assigned care," the Medicare regulations require that he accept the standard charges which are determined by the Medicare agent. In all cases the Medicare patient will be responsible for paying the difference (generally 20 percent) between the fixed-fee-payment schedule and the Medicare coverage.

Medicaid

Title 19 of the Medicare Act of 1965 provides for the medical care of persons who live below the poverty level. While it is often assumed that such indigent persons are a small minority, the fact is that most physicians will receive a significant number of requests for their services from persons who are covered by Medicaid. Sometimes a family tragedy such as the death of the sole "bread-winner" will cause the surviving relative to become a Medicaid client.

Dealing with a Medicaid recipient calls for the utmost in diplomacy and tact on the part of the medical assistant. This is especially true in the case of a person who will be using Medicaid coverage for only a short time. The patient should be reassured that he is going to receive quality care and that he will be treated as well as the "paying" patient.

The mechanics of Medicaid are directed by each state rather than the federal govern-

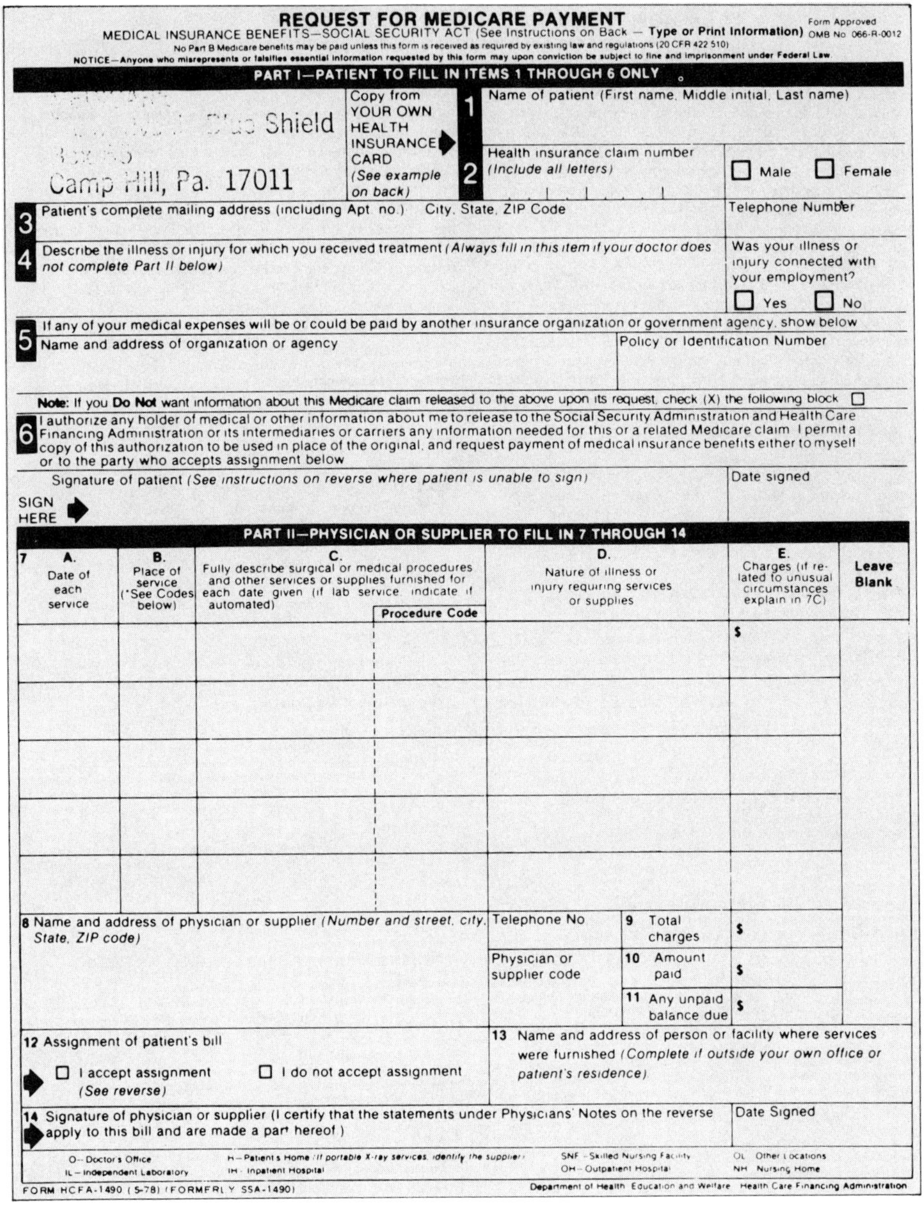

FIGURE 8-6.   A request for Medicare payment form.

ment. The regional director of the plan, usually the state Department of Welfare, will be helpful in clarifying the state's particular regulations.

Although procedures vary from state to state, the patient usually must go to the local welfare office and apply for Medicaid benefits. Once accepted for the plan, the patient

HOW TO FILL OUT YOUR MEDICARE FORM
There are two ways that Medicare can help pay your doctor bills

One way is for Medicare to pay your doctor.—If you and your doctor agree, Medicare will pay the doctor directly. This is the assignment method. You do not submit any claim; the doctor does. All you do is fill out Part I of this form and leave it with your doctor. Under this method the doctor agrees to accept the charge determination of the Medicare carrier as the full charge for covered services; you are responsible for the deductible, coinsurance, and non-covered services. Please read Your Medicare Handbook to help you understand about the deductible and coinsurance.

The other way is for Medicare to pay you.—Medicare can also pay you directly—before or after you have paid your doctor. If you submit the claim yourself, fill out Part I and ask your doctor to fill out Part II. If you have an itemized bill from the doctor, you may submit it rather than have the doctor complete Part II. (This form, with Part I completed

by you, may be used to send in several itemized bills from different doctors and suppliers.) Bills should show who furnished the services, **the patient's name and number,** dates of services, where the services were furnished, a description of the services, and charges for each separate service. It is helpful if the diagnosis is also shown. Then mail itemized bills and this form to the address shown in the upper left-hand corner. If no address is shown there, use the address listed in Your Medicare Handbook—or get advice from any social security office.

Notice: It is important to keep a record of your claim in case you ever want to inquire about it. Before you send it in, write down the date you mailed it, the services you received, the date and charge for each, and the name of the doctor or supplier who performed the services. Have this information available when you inquire about a claim.

SOME THINGS TO NOTE IN FILLING OUT PART I
(Your doctor will fill out Part II.)

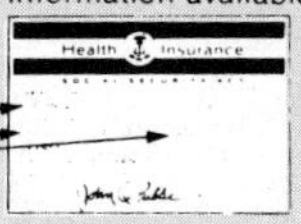

1 & 2 Copy the name and number and indicate your sex exactly as shown on your health insurance card. Include the letters at the end of the number.

3 Enter your mailing address and telephone number, if any.

4 Describe your illness or injury. Be sure to check one of the two boxes.

5 If you have other health insurance or expect a welfare agency to pay part of the expenses, complete item 5.

6 Be sure to sign your name. If you cannot write your name, sign by mark (X), and have the signature witnessed. The witness's signature and address must also be shown in item 6.
If you are filing the claim for a Medicare beneficiary, in item 6 enter the patient's name and write "By," sign your name and enter your address in this space, show your relationship to the patient, and explain why the patient cannot sign. (If the patient has died, the survivor should contact any social security office for information on what to do.)

COLLECTION AND USE OF MEDICARE INFORMATION

We are authorized by the Health Care Financing Administration to ask you for information needed in the administration of the Medicare program. Authority to collect information is in section 205(a), 1872 and 1875 of the Social Security Act, as amended.

The information we obtain to complete your Medicare claim is used to identify you and to determine your eligibility. It is also used to decide if the services and supplies you received are covered by Medicare and to insure that proper payment is made.

The information may also be given to other providers of services, carriers, intermediaries, medical review boards, and other organizations as necessary to administer the Medicare program. For example, it may be necessary to disclose information about the Medicare benefits you have used to a hospital or doctor.

With one exception, which is discussed below, there are no penalties under social security law for refusing to supply information. However, failure to furnish information regarding the medical services rendered or the amount charged would prevent payment of the claim. Failure to furnish any other information, such as name or claim number, would delay payment of the claim.

It is mandatory that you tell us if you are being treated for a work related injury so we can determine whether workmen's compensation will pay for the treatment. Section 1877(a)(3) of the Social Security Act provides criminal penalties for withholding this information.

IMPORTANT NOTES FOR PHYSICIANS AND SUPPLIERS

Item 12: In assigned cases, the physician agrees to accept the charge determination of the Medicare carrier as the full charge, and the patient is responsible only for the deductible, coinsurance, and noncovered services. Coinsurance and the deductible are based upon the charge determination of the carrier, if this is less than the charge submitted. If the physician or supplier does not want Part II information released to the organization named in item 5, the physician or supplier should write "No further release" in item 7C following the description of services.

SIGNATURE OF PHYSICIAN (OR SUPPLIER): I certify that the services shown on this form were medically indicated and necessary for the health of the patient and were personally rendered by me or were rendered incident to my professional

service by my employee under immediate personal supervision, except as otherwise expressly permitted by Medicare regulations.

For services to be considered as 'incident to' a physician's professional service, 1) they must be rendered under the physician's immediate personal supervision by his employee, 2) there was a covered physician's service rendered of which the other services are an integral, although incidental part, 3) they must be of kinds commonly furnished in physicians' offices, and 4) the services of nonphysicians must be included on the physicians' bills.

Notice: Anyone who misrepresents or falsifies essential information to receive payment from federal funds requested by this form may upon conviction be subject to fine and imprisonment under applicable federal laws.

FIGURE 8-7. Directions for filling out a Medicare payment form.

generally brings an official authorization form to the physician's office. Each state's plan dictates the fees which are to be covered.

Each participating physician will probably be asked to certify his willingness to comply with the Medicaid regulations (Fig. 8-8). In addition the medical assistant will need to complete a form for each client, such as the one illustrated in Figure 8-9.

I AGREE TO COMPLY WITH THE MEDICAL ASSISTANCE LAW AND REGULATIONS AND TO KEEP SUCH RECORDS AS NECESSARY TO FULLY DISCLOSE THE EXTENT OF SERVICES AND MAKE AVAILABLE TO DPW, OR ITS AGENTS, RECORDS PERTAINING TO PAYMENTS FOR SERVICES TO MA PATIENTS. I UNDERSTAND THAT PAYMENT BY DPW REPRESENTS PAYMENT IN FULL AND ADDITIONAL CHARGES MAY NOT BE IMPOSED ON THE PATIENT AND/OR OTHERS ON HIS/HER BEHALF FOR COVERED SERVICES.

I CERTIFY THAT SERVICES HAVE BEEN PROVIDED WITHOUT DISCRIMINATION AS TO RACE, CREED, OR NATIONAL ORIGIN (TITLE VI OF THE CIVIL RIGHTS ACT OF 1964).

I UNDERSTAND THAT PAYMENT AND SATISFACTION OF THESE CLAIMS WILL BE FROM FEDERAL AND STATE FUNDS AND THAT I MAY BE PROSECUTED FOR FALSE CLAIMS, STATEMENTS, OR DOCUMENTS, OR CONCEALMENT OF MATERIAL FACTS.

I CERTIFY THAT THE INFORMATION SHOWN ON THE ATTACHED INVOICE(S) IS TRUE, ACCURATE AND COMPLETE.

SIGNATURE OF PROVIDER (STAMP NOT ACCEPTABLE) — DATE

SOCIAL SECURITY OR EMPLOYER ID NO.

YOUR NAME, ADDRESS AND ZIP CODE (Type or Print)

THIS FORM IS USED TO MAIL PAYMENT CHECK

Commonwealth of Pennsylvania — Department of Public Welfare

FOR DPW USE ONLY

VOUCHER TRANSMITTAL NO.	SUFFIX NO.

PROVIDER—ANY REFERENCE TO PAYMENT MUST INCLUDE THE NUMBERS SHOWN ABOVE

PROVIDERS SECTION	
D.P.W. I.D. NUMBER	
COUNTY	
NO. OF INVOICES	

DEPT. OF PUBLIC WELFARE USE	
NO. OF INVOICES PAID	
NO. OF INVOICES RETURNED	
NO. OF INVOICES HELD	

PA 259S 6-75

INVOICE TRANSMITTAL

FIGURE 8-8. An invoice transmittal.

STANDARD MEDICAL INVOICE

CASE NUMBER	COUNTY CODE

PATIENT'S NAME	AGE	SEX	TECHNICAL DIAGNOSIS
1.			
2.			
3.			

NAME AND ADDRESS OF PERSON RECEIVING ASSISTANCE CHECK

EXPLANATION

PROVIDER'S RECORDS AND CERTIFICATION

I HEREBY CERTIFY THAT SERVICES WERE PROVIDED AS SHOWN AND UNDER CONDITIONS 1 THROUGH 5 AS SHOWN ON THE REVERSE OF THIS FORM

Certification No.

Social Security or Employers I D Number

Signature of Provider or Clinic Officer

Name and Address of Provider or Clinic

RECIPIENTS OR AGENT'S SIGNATURE (DO NOT SIGN UNTIL MEDICATION AND/OR SERVICES LISTED ARE RECEIVED)

Practitioner's Report

PAT. NO.	DATE	TYPE VISIT		AMOUNT INC. MILEAGE
		OFFICE	HOME	
Totals				

DISTANCE BORO LIMITS TO PATIENT'S HOME — MILES

Commonwealth of Pennsylvania — Department of Public Welfare — PA 259 - 10-77

FIGURE 8-9. A standard medical invoice.

CHAMPUS Coverage

Most members of the armed services and their dependents, including some additional government employees, receive insurance coverage under CHAMPUS, the Civilian Health and Medical Program of the Uniformed Services Act of 1956. As in the case of Medicare, CHAMPUS plans are administrated by a local or regional agent, usually Blue Cross/Blue

Shield. Under CHAMPUS coverage all medical expenses must be preauthorized, except for emergency treatment. Thus when a CHAMPUS patient comes to the office he or she should have a completed authorization form.

The local agent will establish a schedule of fees. The physician may charge only the fee which is authorized, otherwise the payment will not be made. A CHAMPUS form is

CHAMPUS/CHAMPVA CLAIM FORM

For services or supplies provided by civilian sources except Institutions

Read cover instructions and the back of this form before completing and signing!

Form Approved OMB No. 022-RO[illegible]

Patient/Sponsor Information (Items 1 through 18 to be completed by the beneficiary patient or sponsor)

1. PATIENT'S NAME (Last name, First name, Middle initial)
2. PATIENT'S DATE OF BIRTH MONTH DAY YEAR
7. SPONSOR'S NAME (Last name, First name, Middle initial)
3. PATIENT'S ADDRESS (Street, city, state, ZIP code)
4. PATIENT'S SEX ☐ MALE ☐ FEMALE
8. SPONSOR'S SOCIAL SECURITY NO. OR VA FILE NO.
9. VA STATION NO.
6. PATIENT'S RELATIONSHIP TO SPONSOR ☐ SELF ☐ SPOUSE ☐ NATURAL or ADOPTED CHILD ☐ STEPCHILD OTHER (Specify)
10. SPONSOR'S DUTY STATION OR ADDRESS FOR RETIREES

PHONE NO. (Include area code)
5. MILITARY VA IDENTIFICATION CARD

CARD NO.

ISSUE DATE MONTH DAY YEAR | EFFECTIVE DATE MONTH DAY YEAR | EXPIRATION DATE MONTH DAY YEAR

15. IS CONDITION WORK RELATED? ☐ YES ☐ NO MILITARY SERVICE RELATED? ☐ YES ☐ NO AUTOMOBILE ACCIDENT RELATED? ☐ YES ☐ NO

PHONE NO. (Include area code)
11. SPONSOR'S BRANCH OF SERVICE ☐ USA ☐ USAF ☐ USMC ☐ USN ☐ USCG ☐ USPHS ☐ NOAA ☐ VA
12. SPONSOR'S GRADE RANK
13. SPONSOR'S STATUS ☐ ACTIVE DUTY ☐ RETIRED ☐ DECEASED

14. DO YOU HAVE OTHER HEALTH INSURANCE? ☐ YES ☐ NO
IF YES, ENTER NAME OF OTHER PLAN OR PROGRAM

ADDRESS

CITY STATE ZIP

14a. TYPE OF COVERAGE ☐ EMPLOYMENT (GROUP) ☐ MEDICAID ☐ STUDENT PLAN ☐ PRIVATE (NON-GROUP) ☐ MEDICARE ☐ OTHER

14b. OTHER IDENTIFICATION NUMBER
14c. EFFECTIVE DATE MONTH DAY YEAR
14d. OTHER PROGRAM THROUGH EMPLOYMENT? EMPLOYER NAME

16. INPATIENT OUTPATIENT CARE ☐ OUTPATIENT ☐ INPATIENT-EMERGENCY ☐ INPATIENT HOSPITAL OUTSIDE 40 MILE RADIUS ☐ INPATIENT-SKILLED NURSING FACILITY ☐ INPATIENT-OTHER ☐ INPATIENT HOSPITAL-WITHIN 40 MILE RADIUS (ATTACH DD FORM 1251)

17. DESCRIBE CONDITION FOR WHICH YOU RECEIVED TREATMENT. IF AN INJURY, NOTE HOW IT HAPPENED

18. SIGNATURE OF PATIENT OR AUTHORIZED PERSON CERTIFIES CLAIM INFORMATION AND AUTHORIZES RELEASE OF MEDICAL OR OTHER INSURANCE INFORMATION. READ INSTRUCTIONS AND BACK OF THIS FORM BEFORE SIGNING

SIGNED DATE RELATIONSHIP TO PATIENT

Physician / Other Provider (Items 19 through 33 are to be completed by the physician or other provider.)

19. NAME, ADDRESS & PHONE NO. OF REFERRING PHYSICIAN
20. NAME & ADDRESS OF FACILITY WHERE SERVICES RENDERED (other than home or office)

☐ PRIVATE PRACTICE or ☐ UNIFORMED SERVICES

21. PROVIDER OF SERVICES ☐ ATTENDING PHYSICIAN ☐ OTHER
22. HOSPITALIZATION INFORMATION MO DAY YEAR ADMITTED MO DAY YEAR DISCHARGED
23. LAB WORK OUTSIDE YOUR OFFICE? ☐ YES ☐ NO CHARGES

24. DIAGNOSIS, SYMPTOM OR NATURE OF ILLNESS OR INJURY. RELATE DIAGNOSIS TO PROCEDURE IN COLUMN D BY REFERENCE TO NUMBERS 1, 2, 3, or DX CODE

1.
2.
3.

25 A DATES OF SERVICE MO/DAY/YEAR	B PLACE OF SERVICE	C PROCEDURE CODE IDENTIFY	D DESCRIBE PROCEDURES SUPPLIES FOR EACH DATE. SUBMIT REPORT EXPLAINING UNUSUAL SERVICES OR CIRCUMSTANCES	E DIAGNOSIS CODE	F CHARGES	LEAVE BLANK

26. PATIENT'S ACCOUNT NO.
29. PHYSICIAN'S OR OTHER PROVIDER'S NAME, ADDRESS, ZIP CODE & PHONE NO. (INCLUDING AREA CODE)
G. TOTAL CHARGES $
30. AMOUNT PAID BY BENEFICIARY $
31. AMOUNT PAID BY OTHER INSURANCE $
27. PROVIDER'S SOCIAL SECURITY NO.
32. AGREEMENT TO PARTICIPATE (READ BACK OF THIS FORM) ☐ YES ☐ NO
28. PROVIDER'S EMPLOYER I.D. NO.
33. SIGNATURE OF PHYSICIAN OR OTHER PROVIDER (READ BACK OF THIS FORM BEFORE SIGNING)

PROVIDER NO. SIGNED DATE

FIGURE 8-10. CHAMPUS claim form.

illustrated in Figure 8-10. This form must be signed by the patient and then submitted by the physician to the Blue Cross/Blue Shield agent who represents the local or regional CHAMPUS program.

Individual Policies

A large number of individuals do not work in an organization which provides group insurance coverage. Many of these persons choose to purchase health coverage for themselves from private insurance agents. There are so many different companies and policies available that it would be impossible to include a "typical" form in this discussion.

As a medical assistant, you will generally find that with private policy customers the claim is paid to the patient and then the patient pays the physician. It is usually a good practice to ask patients to pay their bills before the doctor completes the forms. This motivates the patient to expedite the insurance payment.

If a patient has a private policy, discuss his insurance with him so that you will both understand how to process the paperwork properly.

Workers' Compensation

Workers' compensation insurance laws are in effect in every state. While the states may vary in some of the details of the plan's execution, workers' compensation is generally implemented as follows. Workers who are injured during the time that they are working, or who become ill as a result of the work that they have done or are doing, are covered by the workers' compensation laws. Individual employers insure themselves with various agents, who, in turn, pay the physicians for treatment rendered.

The individual physicians enrolled in the various state workers' compensation plans are usually required to register with the state Workers' Compensation Board on an annual basis. A code number will be assigned which will limit the physician's certification, in workers' compensation cases, to his particular medical specialty. The state board will then supply the physician with a schedule of fees which may be charged for various services.

Workers' compensation cases are initiated in most states by the employer who completes a multi-part form. Copies of this form will be sent to the state (usually the state Department of Labor and Industry), the employee, and the physician. The physician's copy serves as authorization to provide medical care under the Workmen's Compensation Act and as a format upon which the physician can submit his bill to the insurance carrier. An example of an employer-physician report form is shown in Figure 8-11.

In the event that a medical problem prevents a person from continuing employment, workers' compensation coverage will provide wage benefits. The physician will be asked to certify the employee's inability to continue working, using the form shown in Figures 8-12 and 8-13. If the disability persists, he may also be required to complete a supplementary form such as the one shown in Figure 8-14.

For both permanently and temporarily disabled patients, the proper processing of forms is essential to the issuing of benefit payments. The forms must be carefully completed and the requested information precisely recorded. Since the various states may operate

COMMONWEALTH OF PENNSYLVANIA
DEPARTMENT OF LABOR AND INDUSTRY
BUREAU OF OCCUPATIONAL INJURY
AND DISEASE COMPENSATION
HARRISBURG, PA. 17120
TELEPHONE 787-3715
LONG DISTANCE (TOLL FREE) 800-932-0580

EMPLOYER'S REPORT OF OCCUPATIONAL INJURY OR DISEASE

INJURED'S SOCIAL SECURITY NUMBER

EMPLOYER'S IRS REPORTING NUMBER

INSURANCE POLICY NUMBER

DATES

1. Date of Report
2. Date of injury and Time AM PM
3. Normal Starting Time AM PM
4. If Employe Back to Work Give Date:
5. At Same Wage? Yes ☐ No ☐
6. If Fatal Injury, Give Date of Death:
7. Date Employer Knew of Injury
8. Date Disability Began
9. Last Full Day Paid - Date

EMPLOYER

10. Employer | Location #
11. Person Making Out This Report
12. Address - Include County and Zip Code
13. Employer Telephone Number (Include Area Code)
14. Mailing Address - If Different Than Above
15. Nature of Business - Type of Mfg., Trade, Construction, Service, etc.

EMPLOYE

16. Employe: First Middle Last
17. Male ☐ Female ☐
18. Employe Telephone Number (Include Area Code)
19. Address - Include County and Zip Code
20. Married Yes ☐ No ☐
21. Number of Children Under 18
22. Date of Birth
23. Age
24. If Under 18, Certificate Number
25. Occupation for Which Issued
26. Occupation
27. Department or Division Regularly Employed
28. How Long Employed

OCCURRENCE

29. Place of Injury: Employer's Premises Yes ☐ No ☐
30. If No - Exact Location - Street, City, County, and State
31. What Was Employe Doing When Injured? (Be Specific. If Using Tools or Equipment or Handling Material - Name Them and Tell What He Was Doing with Them.)
32. How Did Injury Occur? (Describe Fully the Events Which Resulted in Injury or Disease. Tell What Happened and How It Happened. Name Any Objects or Substances Involved and Tell How They Were Involved. Give Full Details on All Factors Which Led or Contributed to Injury or Disease.)

Did Injury or Disease Occur Because of: →
33. Mechanical Defect ☐ No ☐ Yes (Describe Above)
34. Unsafe Act ☐ No ☐ Yes (Describe Above)
35. CHECK IF AMPUTATION ☐

INJURY OR DISEASE

36. Nature and Location of Injury or Disease (Describe Fully, Including Parts of Body Affected.)
37. Attending Physician and Address (If Hospital Involved - Indicate)

DO NOT WRITE IN THIS COLUMN

DATE
HOURS WORKED
REPORT LAG
DISABILITY
INDUSTRY
SEX
AGE
OCCUPATION
COUNTY
ACCIDENT TYPE
OCCUPATIONAL DISEASE
UNSAFE ACT
MECHANICAL DEFECT
NATURE
LOCATION
INSURANCE
PAYMENT LAG
COMPENSATION RATE

DISTRIBUTION OF THIS REPORT:

1. ORIGINAL MUST BE SENT IMMEDIATELY TO WORKMEN'S COMPENSATION INSURANCE CARRIER
2. COPY TO BUREAU - SEE INSTRUCTIONS
3. EMPLOYER'S COPY - RETAIN AS RECORD
4. MEDICAL COPY MUST BE SENT IMMEDIATELY TO TREATING PHYSICIAN OR DELIVERED BY INJURED EMPLOYE
5. CHANGE OF STATUS REPORT - SEE INSTRUCTIONS
6. INJURED EMPLOYE'S COPY

WORKMEN'S COMPENSATION INSURANCE COMPANY AND ADDRESS
(Preprint or Stamp - Include Bureau Code)

Liberty Mutual Insurance Company
First Federal Savings Building
1202 State Street
Box 2067
Erie, Pa. 16512

BUREAU CODE #025

SIGNATURE OF PERSON IN 11 ABOVE

OFFICIAL POSITION

OIDC-344 (8 72) 839C-1 R9

FIGURE 8-11. A workers' compensation report form.

SURGEON'S REPORT   C

PLEASE COMPLETE AND RETURN TO

LIBERTY MUTUAL INSURANCE CO.   EMPLOYEE

                                                          EMPLOYER

The Patient	1. Name of patient if other than above .... Age: .... Sex: ....
The Accident	2. Date of accident: .... Hour .... M. Date disability began .... 3. State in patient's own words where and how accident occurred: ....
The Injury	4. Give accurate description of nature and extent of injury and state your objective findings: .... 5. Is accident above referred to the only cause of patient's condition? If not, state contributing causes: .... 6. Will the injury result in (a) Permanent defect? If so, what? .... (b) Disfigurement? .... (Permanent disability such as loss of whole or parts of fingers, disfigurement, etc., must be accurately marked on chart on reverse side of this report.) 7. Is patient suffering from any disease of the heart, lungs, brain, kidneys, blood, vascular system or any other disabling condition not due to this accident .... Give particulars: .... 8. Has patient any physical impairment due to previous accident or disease? .... Give particulars: .... 9. Has normal recovery been delayed for any reason? .... Give particulars: ....

Treatment	10. Date of your first treatment: .... Who engaged your services? ....
	 11. Describe treatment given by you: ....
	
	 12. Were X-Rays taken? .... By whom? .... When? ....
	     Number of views ( ) (Name and Address)
	 13. X-Ray diagnosis: ....
	 14. Was patient treated by anyone else? .... By whom? .... When? ....
	                                    (Name and Address)
	 15. Was patient hospitalized? .... Name and address of hospital: ....
	 16. Date of admission to hospital: .... Date of discharge: ....
	 17. Is further treatment needed? .... For how long? ....

Disability	18. Patient was/will be able to resume regular work on: .... 19. Patient was/will be able to resume light work on: .... 20. If death ensued give date: ....
	REMARKS: (Give any information of value not included above) .... I am a duly licensed physician in the State of .... I was graduated from .... Medical School in .... Year .... Date of this report: .... (Signed) .... This report must be signed personally by physician Address .... Telephone .... (Include Zip Code Number)

ASC-1482 R7   Printed in U.S.A.

FIGURE 8-12.   A surgeon's report form. (Courtesy of Liberty Mutual Insurance Company)

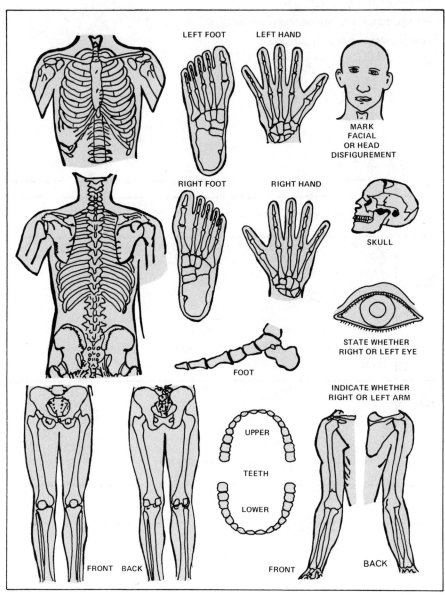

FIGURE 8-13. Reverse of surgeon's report detailing site of injury. (Courtesy of Liberty Mutual Insurance Company)

LIBERTY MUTUAL

LIBERTY MUTUAL INSURANCE COMPANY
LIBERTY LIFE ASSURANCE COMPANY OF BOSTON
HOME OFFICE: BOSTON

PHYSICIAN'S SUPPLEMENTARY STATEMENT

Claim Number...

Policyholder ....

Dear

The following supplementary medical report must be completed and returned to us in order that any further Benefits due may be paid promptly. It is important that if disability or treatment continues, the best estimate possible of that further disability and/or treatment should be made by the physician.

Very truly yours,

....

....

....

(1) Patient's name ....Age...............

Patient's Address ....

(2) Nature of sickness or injury (Describe complications, if any)...

....

....

(3) (a) Are you now treating patient?...

(b) Frequency of treatments...

(c) Date of most recent treatment...................................19........

(4) The patient has been continuously disabled (unable to work) from.............19........ through.............19........

If still disabled, when should patient be able to return to work?...19........

(5) Remarks: ....

....

....

....

Date...................19........   Signed ....M.D.
                                          (Attending Physician)

Address ....

....

Phone ....

A.S.C. 1794 R12

FIGURE 8-14. A physician's supplementary medical report form. (Courtesy of Liberty Mutual Insurance Company)

their programs somewhat differently, a regional representative of the state Department of Labor should be contacted to clarify particular procedures.

Automobile Insurance

Patients who require medical attention as a result of an automobile accident will have to enlist their physician's assistance in submitting a claim form such as the one shown in Figure 8-15. In states with "no-fault" insurance coverage, the costs will be paid by the patient's insurance agent. In states without a "no-fault" law, these costs may be covered by the carrier of the person judged at fault.

It is common practice for the insurance agent to withhold payment until treatment is completed. If a patient is involved in long and expensive treatment, the method of payment should be discussed with the physician and the patient.

Capitation Programs

Some physicians have organized themselves into groups of varying degrees of complexity. Many of these groups include the most common specialties along with x-ray and laboratory services. Patients or their employers pay a monthly fee to the "group" in return for which the physicians provide all of the person's medical care requirements. Usually, some practical limitations are associated with these services. There may be a maximum allowable number of office calls or a list of disorders which are not covered.

If the physician is a member of the capitation group, a knowledge of the paperwork procedures and the regulations of this group will be required. It should be understood that for some patients a capitation system is an alternative to group insurance.

SUMMARY

Since there are many different kinds of insurance policies, and variations of each basic type, there is a high potential for confusion and error in insurance processing. The medical assistant can greatly reduce these problems by becoming familiar with current medical insurance practices. Continuous awareness of the latest developments in insurance is essential. Some insurance organizations have educational representatives whose function is to keep insurance processors in the medical office informed of changes through seminar presentations and office visits. Questions concerning insurance practices can be directed to these individuals.

When the medical assistant is well-informed and confident, discussion of insurance coverage and procedures with patients becomes an easier and more efficiently completed task. It is also important to advise all patients to inform the office of any changes in their coverage.

Insurance processing can seem at first to be an overwhelming project. Application of knowledge and patience in following specified procedures will result in yet another useful accomplishment for the medical assistant.

ATTENDING PHYSICIAN'S STATEMENT

LIBERTY MUTUAL

CLAIM NUMBER

| SERIES/OFFICE NO. | SERIAL NO. | SUFFIX | C.D. |

☐ HOLD ☐ REG.

| DATE | PATIENT'S NAME | ACCIDENT DATE |

THIS PHYSICIAN'S STATEMENT MUST BE COMPLETED BY THE ATTENDING PHYSICIAN BEFORE BENEFITS THAT MAY BE DUE THE PATIENT CAN BE DETERMINED. PLEASE RETURN THE COMPLETED FORM TO:

CLAIMS DEPT.

FOLD HERE

1. PATIENT'S NAME AND ADDRESS

2. AGE 3. SEX 4. OCCUPATION (IF KNOWN)

5. HISTORY OF OCCURRENCE AS DESCRIBED BY PATIENT

6. DIAGNOSIS AND CONCURRENT OR CONTRIBUTING CONDITIONS*

7. WHEN DID SYMPTOMS FIRST APPEAR?
DATE:

8. WHEN DID PATIENT FIRST CONSULT YOU FOR THIS CONDITION?
DATE:

9. HAS PATIENT EVER HAD SAME OR SIMILAR CONDITION?
YES ☐   ☐ NO   If "YES" state when and describe *

10. IS CONDITION SOLELY A RESULT OF THIS ACCIDENT?
YES ☐   ☐ NO   If "NO", EXPLAIN °

11. IS CONDITION DUE TO INJURY OR SICKNESS ARISING OUT OF PATIENT'S EMPLOYMENT?
YES ☐   ☐ NO

12. WILL INJURY RESULT IN PERMANENT DISFIGUREMENT OR DISABILITY?
YES ☐   ☐ NO   If "YES", describe

13. PATIENT WAS DISABLED (Unable to work)
FROM: THROUGH:

14. IF STILL DISABLED, DATE PATIENT SHOULD BE ABLE TO RETURN TO WORK:

15. REPORT OF SERVICES

DATE OF SERVICE	PLACE OF SERVICE	DESCRIPTION OF SURGICAL OR MEDICAL SERVICE RENDERED	CHARGES
			$
			$
			$
		TOTAL CHARGE TO DATE	$

16. IS PATIENT STILL UNDER YOUR CARE FOR THIS CONDITION?
YES ☐   NO ☐

ESTIMATED FUTURE CHARGES $

| DATE | PHYSICIAN'S NAME (PRINT) | PHYSICIAN'S SIGNATURE | IRS/TIN IDENTIFICATION NO. |

| NO | STREET | CITY OR TOWN | STATE | ZIP CODE |

* Use reverse side if additional space is needed.
ASC 2286 R3 Printed in U.S.A.

EQUAL OPPORTUNITY EMPLOYERS

FIGURE 8-15. An attending physician's statement form. (Courtesy of Liberty Mutual Insurance Company)

APPLICATION EXERCISES

The medical assistant must be very familiar with the use and processing of insurance forms. Perhaps the best approach to developing this skill is to practice completing actual insurance forms. The following exercises are designed to provide experience with several different representative forms.

Using the information provided, complete both the insurance company and Medicare report forms which follow. (Omit procedure codes where they are requested.)

Mr. Jones, a college professor who is single and has no friends, has broken all of the fingers on both hands in a work-related accident. As he leaves Dr. Brown's office, he gives you his insurance form and asks you to fill it out for him. Use the following information:

1. On January 12, Mr. Jones slammed a drawer on both hands.

2. The next day, Dr. Brown, who met Mr. Jones in the emergency room on the 12th, had him stop at the office.

3. Dr. Brown's fees are as follows:

Met patient in emergency room	$50.00	1/12
Examined and set broken fingers	30.00	1/12
Followup office visit	20.00	1/13

4. Mr. Jones, who was born on March 27, 1944, lives at 25 State Street, and even though he is in some pain, he says that he will be able to return to work.

5. Mr. Jones has not yet paid any of his charges.

Mrs. Banini was born in Italy and cannot read or write English. Her husband, who is eligible for Medicare, has had a heart attack and is recuperating at home. Mrs. Banini has just come to the office to ask you to help her with the Medicare form.

1. The Banini's live at 2400 Orchid Drive, Cleveland, Ohio 44240.

2. The patient's name is Alfredo P. Banini. His telephone number is (216) 414-8240.

3. Their claim number is 413 AA6123.

4. The Banini's have no other insurance.

5. Use today's date.

6. Mr. Banini is retired.

7. Dr. Brown's office is at 200 East Euclid Avenue, Cleveland, Ohio 44245, and his supplier code is BR 158600. His office telephone number is (216) 413-8105.

8. Dr. Brown's policy is to accept Medicare assignments.

HEALTH INSURANCE CLAIM – GROUP OR INDIVIDUAL

PART A — **TO BE COMPLETED BY PATIENT (INSURED)**
Spaced for Typewriter – Marks for Tabulator Appear on this Line

EMPLOYER (NAME OF COMPANY)
GANNON COLLEGE

EMPLOYEE (INSURED PERSON) AND ADDRESS

PATIENT'S NAME	DATE OF BIRTH

AUTHORIZATION TO PAY BENEFITS TO PHYSICIANS: I hereby authorize payment directly to the physicians for their services for treatment of the injury or sickness described herein, of the Health Insurance Benefits, if any, otherwise payable to me.

Signed (Insured Person)

Date

AUTHORIZATION TO RELEASE INFORMATION: I hereby authorize the undersigned Physician to release any information acquired in the course of my examination or treatment.

Signed (Patient, or parent if minor)

Date

PART B — **ATTENDING PHYSICIAN'S STATEMENT**

1. DIAGNOSIS AND CONCURRENT CONDITIONS
   (If diagnosis code other than ICDA* used, give name):

2. IS CONDITION DUE TO INJURY OR SICKNESS ARISING OUT OF PATIENT'S EMPLOYMENT? Yes ☐ No ☐
   PREGNANCY? Yes ☐ No ☐
   If yes, approximate date pregnancy commenced. Date

3. REPORT OF SERVICES (Or attach itemized bill) (If previous form submitted to this carrier, you need show only dates and services since last report.)

DATE OF SERVICES	PLACE OF SERVICES†	DESCRIPTION OF SURGICAL OR MEDICAL SERVICES RENDERED	PROCEDURE CODE—IF USED (IF CODE OTHER THAN CPT** USED, GIVE NAME)	CHARGES

TOTAL CHARGES ▶ $_____

AMOUNT PAID ▶ $_____

BALANCE DUE ▶ $_____

†O—Doctor's Office   IH—Inpatient Hospital   NH—Nursing Home
H—Patient's Home   OH—Outpatient Hospital   OL—Other Locations
*ICDA—International Classification of Diseases
**CPT—Current Procedural Terminology (current edition)

4. DATE SYMPTOMS FIRST APPEARED OR ACCIDENT HAPPENED.

5. DATE PATIENT FIRST CONSULTED YOU FOR THIS CONDITION.

6. PATIENT EVER HAD SAME OR SIMILAR CONDITION?
   Yes ☐ No ☐   If "yes" when and describe.

7. PATIENT STILL UNDER YOUR CARE FOR THIS CONDITION?
   Yes ☐ No ☐

8. PATIENT WAS CONTINUOUSLY TOTALLY DISABLED (Unable to work)
   From _____ Thru _____

9. PATIENT WAS PARTIALLY DISABLED.
   From _____ Thru _____

10. IF STILL DISABLED, DATE PATIENT SHOULD BE ABLE TO RETURN TO WORK.

11. PATIENT WAS HOUSE CONFINED.
    From _____ Thru _____

12. DOES PATIENT HAVE OTHER HEALTH COVERAGE?
    Yes ☐ No ☐   If "yes" please identify

Date	Physician's Name (Print)	Signature	Degree	Telephone

Street Address	City or Town	State or Province	Zip Code

ASC 2324 R2   EQUAL OPPORTUNITY EMPLOYERS

REQUEST FOR MEDICARE PAYMENT

MEDICAL INSURANCE BENEFITS—SOCIAL SECURITY ACT (See Instructions on Back — Type or Print Information)

Form Approved OMB No 066-R-0012

No Part B Medicare benefits may be paid unless this form is received as required by existing law and regulations (20 CFR 422 510)

NOTICE—Anyone who misrepresents or falsifies essential information requested by this form may upon conviction be subject to fine and imprisonment under Federal Law

PART I—PATIENT TO FILL IN ITEMS 1 THROUGH 6 ONLY

_____ Blue Shield

Camp Hill, Pa. 17011

Copy from YOUR OWN HEALTH INSURANCE CARD (See example on back)

1 Name of patient (First name, Middle initial, Last name)

2 Health insurance claim number (Include all letters)

☐ Male   ☐ Female

3 Patient's complete mailing address (including Apt no.)   City, State, ZIP Code

Telephone Number

4 Describe the illness or injury for which you received treatment (Always fill in this item if your doctor does not complete Part II below)

Was your illness or injury connected with your employment?

☐ Yes   ☐ No

5 If any of your medical expenses will be or could be paid by another insurance organization or government agency, show below

Name and address of organization or agency

Policy or Identification Number

Note: If you **Do Not** want information about this Medicare claim released to the above upon its request, check (X) the following block ☐

6 I authorize any holder of medical or other information about me to release to the Social Security Administration and Health Care Financing Administration or its intermediaries or carriers any information needed for this or a related Medicare claim. I permit a copy of this authorization to be used in place of the original, and request payment of medical insurance benefits either to myself or to the party who accepts assignment below

Signature of patient (See instructions on reverse where patient is unable to sign)

Date signed

SIGN HERE ➧

PART II—PHYSICIAN OR SUPPLIER TO FILL IN 7 THROUGH 14

7 **A.** Date of each service	**B.** Place of service (*See Codes below)	**C.** Fully describe surgical or medical procedures and other services or supplies furnished for each date given (if lab service, indicate if automated) Procedure Code	**D.** Nature of illness or injury requiring services or supplies	**E.** Charges (if related to unusual circumstances explain in 7C)	**Leave Blank**
				$	

8 Name and address of physician or supplier (Number and street, city, State, ZIP code)

Telephone No

Physician or supplier code

9 Total charges	$
10 Amount paid	$
11 Any unpaid balance due	$

12 Assignment of patient's bill

➧ ☐ I accept assignment   ☐ I do not accept assignment
(See reverse)

13 Name and address of person or facility where services were furnished (Complete if outside your own office or patient's residence)

14 Signature of physician or supplier (I certify that the statements under Physicians' Notes on the reverse apply to this bill and are made a part hereof)

Date Signed

O— Doctor's Office	H—Patient's Home (If portable X-ray services, identify the supplier)	SNF - Skilled Nursing Facility	OL - Other Locations
IL—Independent Laboratory	IH— Inpatient Hospital	OH— Outpatient Hospital	NH - Nursing Home

FORM HCFA-1490 (5-78) (FORMERLY SSA-1490)

Department of Health, Education and Welfare Health Care Financing Administration

9. Services to date have included:

A house call to examine the patient	$12.00	11/6
Visiting the patient in the hospital	12.00	11/7
Visiting the patient in the hospital	12.00	11/8
Examining the patient at home	12.00	11/12

Class Exercise

Your teacher will organize the class into groups of five or six students. Once you have been placed in these groups, compare your insurance forms. Do any of you have entries which are different? Which entry is correct? Compare the forms and check for accuracy and thoroughness.

At the end of this exercise, one person from each group should give a short synopsis of what the group learned to the entire class. Your instructor will lead a class discussion dealing with the most common errors or pitfalls in filling out the forms and suggesting solutions to problems encountered in the exercise.

COMPLETING THE LEARNING LOOP

Some of the aspects of managing insurance paperwork must be determined by the doctor's preferences. Thus, no matter who the medical assistant chooses to work for, she or he will need to discuss specific procedures in a thorough and detailed way. Some physicians will prefer that the MA simply makes sure that the insurance forms are in a handy place and that such mechanical items as the patient's name and address are clearly and properly listed. In this case, the physician will usually fill out the descriptions and costs of services which he or she has provided. Other physicians will expect the MA to complete much or all of the treatment information in addition to the basic duties of filling out and checking the patient information.

If this is the case, the MA's practical office training will include an introduction to the physician's fee schedule, specialized insurance fees, Blue Cross/Blue Shield schedules, and the various sources for identifying procedure and diagnosis codes. In all cases, an enthusiastic and energetic approach to insurance processing will provide the basic difference between failure and success.

BIBLIOGRAPHY

Denenberg, H. S.: *The Insurance Trap.* Western Publishing, Racine, Wis., 1972.
Law, S. A.: *Blue Cross: What Went Wrong?* Yale University Press, New Haven, Conn., 1974.
Levy, M. H.: *A Handbook of Personal Insurance Terminology.* Farnsworth, Rockville Centre, N.Y., 1968.
McCay, J. T.: *The Management of Time.* Prentice-Hall, Englewood Cliffs, N.J., 1959.
Pfeffer, I., and Klock, D.: *Perspectives on Insurance.* Prentice-Hall, Englewood Cliffs, N.J., 1974.

UNIT 3

COMMUNICATIONS MANAGEMENT

Medical assistants are expected to serve as office communications managers. In this regard they assist the physician by coordinating, summarizing, and integrating both incoming and outgoing information. In their capacity as message processors, MAs oversee the use of the telephone, assist with the writing of business letters, instruct patients, and help the physician to carry out research functions.

UNIT OBJECTIVES

Upon completion of this unit you will be prepared to:

1. List and describe the major components of a telephone system and the proper ways to utilize them.

2. Compose and prepare the basic types of business letters.

3. Describe the basic parts of a patient information system and the ways in which they should be utilized.

4. List the typical responsibilities of assisting the physician in research activities.

CHAPTER 9

DEVELOPING TELEPHONE SKILLS

SPECIFIC OBJECTIVES

Upon completion of this chapter you will be able to:

1. Describe proper telephone reception.

2. Apply patient screening techniques in appointment scheduling.

3. Effectively utilize telephone hardware and software systems.

4. Describe the different types of telephone systems which are available to the medical office.

5. List the most basic errors committed by telephone receptionists.

INTRODUCTION

Although the tasks of the administrative medical assistant are many and varied, there are certain underlying principles which remain constant. In this unit the principles of effective verbal communication are presented and in this chapter applied to telephone handling procedures.

167

The telephone is a communications tool essential to the operation of the medical office. The importance of the telephone receptionist's role in managing the telephone cannot be overemphasized. It is the telephone voice that creates expectations and images of the office staff and the physician. Since it is the most common link between patient and doctor, the telephone is the focus for the greatest frequency of interaction and therefore has the greatest potential for mismanagement.

To highlight proper use and management of the telephone, this chapter begins with a discussion of frustrations common to all phone users, and then moves from this common ground to positive techniques of effective telephone communication.

The telephone provides the chief initial connection between doctor and patient in the practice of office medicine. Thus it is imperative that medical assistants learn to use it effectively. MAs must sharpen and refine their daily use of the telephone, and avoid common pitfalls.

The origin of many telephone problems consists in the fact that the telephone is an instrument over which very little control can be exercised. Just when you are about to complete a sentence in the letter you are writing, or when you are speaking to a patient, the phone rings. Telephone interruptions are a major source of frustration partly because they cannot be planned or anticipated. The only alternative is use of an answering service. Another source of frustration consists in placing calls. Dialing the phone number often results in receiving a busy signal. The time taken to place the call is lost and the work goal temporarily aborted.

Many of the skills involved in using telephone systems are related to the art of self-control. Frustration is rapidly conveyed from the speaker to the listener, who then reacts negatively to the attitude being projected. Tone of voice, word choice, and telephone manners are extremely important tools in preventing the spread of frustration. The call will be productive only when self-control is maintained.

NONVERBAL COMMUNICATION PROBLEMS

Adding further complexity to telephone management is the most immediate functional problem of physical separation. The person on the other end of the conversation cannot be visualized. Therefore, nonverbal behaviors which would be helpful in understanding the message are denied.

To test this process, close your eyes momentarily while talking with a friend or listening to a classroom lecture. When you reopen your eyes, you will be amazed at the diversity and quantity of information being transmitted. When your eyes are closed, communication awareness is lessened. Facial expression, hand and body movements, and other nonverbal cues all help us to interpret the spoken word. Interpretation of the message received is based not only on what is being *said*, but also on judgments made concerning *feelings* about what is spoken.

Advertisers learned this lesson when they extended their focus from radio to television audiences. It is now rare for an advertising agency to design a commercial which can be used both on radio (without nonverbal cues) and on television (with nonverbal cues).

The medical assistant must learn to function without the aid of nonverbal cues in accurately giving and receiving messages.

Clear speech, a projection of positive attitudes, and awareness of the limitations of the telephone are other variables to be considered in developing an effective telephone technique and a pleasant telephone personality.

TELEPHONE ANSWERING TECHNIQUES

Whenever possible, answering the telephone during the first few rings is desirable. The immediate response to the call should include an appropriate greeting. The major telephone companies, most of whom provide phone etiquette courses for their clients, prescribe the following basic techniques in the order given.

1. Identify time of day and express cordiality. When you pick up the phone, begin by saying "Good morning" or "Good afternoon."

2. Identify the office by name. (*Examples:* "Dr. Smith's office," "Drs. Smith and Jones," or "Orthopedic Associates")

3. Identify the person speaking. (*Example:* "Miss Black speaking")

These three opening statements provide callers with clearly useful information. They know that they have reached the proper office and to whom they are speaking.

OBTAINING THE CORRECT MESSAGE

The next logical step in the process is to ascertain the purpose of the call. Usually, after the initial identification procedure, the caller will state the purpose of the call. The message is clear when the caller states the purpose as appointment scheduling. Very often, however, the message is embedded in verbiage that must be sorted. Screening techniques are necessary to interpret the appropriate message. These will be discussed in detail later in this chapter.

There are certain guidelines of telephone usage which set the conversational tone and are essential to the accuracy of message interpretation.

1. *Establish calmness.* When either responding to or initiating the call, a calm voice will be reassuring to the patient and will prepare you to receive the message accurately.

2. *Project calmness.* The caller may be agitated and in a hurry to tell you something. Gently slow down the conversation. Don't interrupt. The caller will then know that you are not in a hurry, and are intently listening.

3. *Maintain patience.* Callers make errors, contradict themselves, and sometimes become unjustly angry with you. You must be prepared and willing to accept that the caller may be troubled and is not focusing on you personally.

4. *Restate the question.* An attempt to summarize the issue should be made so that it can be clarified in both the mind of the caller and your own. A good approach is to summarize by restating the major points. The patient will correct you if in error.

(*Example:* "Mrs. Jones, I will leave a message for the doctor that you are still having headaches, that you have finished your medication, and that you wanted to ask the doctor if your prescription should be refilled.")

5. *Record the message.* The medical assistant should always have a message pad close to the phone so that the patient's name, phone number, message, and directions to the physician can be recorded without delay. Don't trust your memory—write it down!

6. *Obtain the correct name and number.* If you miss one or two of the critical numbers or letters in a message you may pay dearly in time and energy later. Be certain to repeat these items carefully. When recording names which may be confusing, repeat the letters as you are writing in this manner, "R" as in Robert, "P" as in Paul, etc.

TELEPHONE SCREENING

Acting as the telephone receptionist is a major responsibility for the medical assistant. A qualified telephone receptionist may well be the key member of the office team as she or he is the liaison between the physician and all office contacts. Receptionists are the public relations representatives who create and reflect the mood of the practice. Their attitude toward patients can promote either anticipation or dread of an upcoming visit. Their approach can inspire patient trust or foment patient anger. They can instill confidence or a reluctance to call again. Thus, as receptionist, the MA plays a role that is of vital importance in establishing the attitudinal climate of the office.

To add complexity to this responsibility, the medical assistant must screen all calls to determine how each call should be handled. This task requires a tremendous degree of skill in public relations. The assistant needs to achieve the objective of correct call response and categorization while avoiding patient alienation.

The guidelines for effecive telecommunication presented in this chapter can be applied to patient screening techniques. Consistent applications of the guidelines and techniques will help the MA to accomplish the objectives of telephone interaction successfully.

Screening Calls to the Physician

Perhaps the single most common problem in telephone screening is dealing with the caller who, regardless of purpose, requests to speak to the physician.

The medical assistant's response to the caller must initially convey the message: "The doctor is with a patient, may I help you?" Word choice is extremely crucial. Note the difference between the foregoing response and the statement, "The doctor is busy now." Both responses carry the same meaning. The first, however, allows the individual to gracefully accept the situation, rather than prompting such reactions as, "The doctor is busy doing what? He's too busy for me? Maybe I shouldn't bother him." Responses that are nonthreatening to the patient produce the best results.

Screening can be defined as a procedure whereby the patient is asked questions which will lead to the determination of the individual's *real* need to speak to the physician and whether the need is immediate or can be postponed. Calls that are usually put through immediately include:

1. Calls from other physicians.

2. Calls from family members.

3. Calls that appear to be of an urgent nature.

4. Calls from a pharmacy, other medical centers, or hospital departments.

Calls that can be postponed are relayed to the physician at an opportune time. A message is taken and the return call can be made by the physician or, if he directs, by the medical assistant. Examples include:

1. A change in a condition that is not serious but requires the physician's judgment and response.

2. Requests for medication change or prescription refills.

3. Requests by the patient for laboratory results. Most physicians permit medical assistants to handle phone calls when the results are normal, but reserve the responsibility to inform patients when results are abnormal or questionable, or when a discussion may be required.

4. Calls that are nonmedical in nature but require the physician's response.

Calls that the medical assistant can handle independently usually relate to appointment scheduling. It is in this area of office practice that screening techniques are most often employed. The MA must make a decision as to when the patient needs to be seen. Judgments are made according to the urgency expressed and the availability of open time. Routine physical examination scheduling is not problematic. Acute conditions and appointments requested on the day of the call necessitate screening.

Table 9-1 presents a feasible guide for determination of urgency. The restricted time factors are assumed.

The medical assistant will often be in doubt regarding the urgency of the request. In these situations, the MA's responsibility is to consult the physician.

The Screening Interview

In order to successfully determine the urgency of a visit when a judgment cannot be readily made, obtaining the answers to key questions will facilitate the screening exercise by establishing the severity and duration of the symptoms.

Key Questions	Objectives
1. When did these symptoms begin?	1. Determine the time of onset and duration of the illness. If symptoms have existed unchanged for some time, the urgency of scheduling is usually diminished.

2. Have you been on medication or are you currently taking medication?

2. Determine if medication is being taken or has already been prescribed. The physician may then decide to change medication rather than to schedule the patient for re-examination.

3. How severe are the symptoms?

3. Determine the degree of symptoms. Severity of pain, presence of fever, and persistence of vomiting will suggest the level of urgency.

4. How often have you experienced the symptoms?

4. Determine the sequence and frequency of symptoms. The answer to the question will also be a clue to the persistence of the symptoms and therefore the urgency involved.

You will remember that screening techniques were discussed in the chapter on appointment scheduling. They are reviewed here for further emphasis and clarification.

In addition to the patient screening techniques discussed, there are certain other considerations pertinent to telecommunications that will be helpful to the medical assistant in handling calls independently of the physician whenever possible:

1. The patient may have been recently examined, or may be currently undergoing treatment and expressing a need for reassurance. You may be able to help the pa-

TABLE 9-1. Urgency Scale*

Variables	Most Urgent	Urgent	Margin- ally Urgent	Not Urgent
Acute illness (sudden onset of symptoms; fever, vomiting, etc.)		X		
Bleeding	X			
Chronic condition (change in condition may be suspected)			X	
Patient expresses health concerns (lump discovered, fatigue, etc.)			X	
Requests for routine physical examination				X
Routine checks (medication, blood pressure, etc.)				X
Sudden change in condition	X			
Sudden onset of critical symptoms (difficulty in breathing, severe pain)	X			

*Most urgent: possible emergency visit; doctor should be consulted.
Urgent: visit on same day as call may be necessary.
Marginally urgent: appointment as soon as possible, not necessarily on day of call.
Not urgent: scheduling at convenience.

tient to reassure himself by becoming a sympathetic listener. The patient isn't always seeking answers to questions, but often requires the opportunity to check the validity of his concerns.

2. Perhaps the patient does need a routine answer to a problem which you could solve yourself. "Yes, Mrs. Smith, it is important to take your medication right after each meal as directed. The medication will not irritate your stomach when taken following a meal." Again, the patient is seeking reassurance coupled with accurate information.

3. Sometimes you may refer the question to another member of the office staff. Often questions may be handled by you or another staff member independently of the physician. Be certain that the question is answerable by the staff member before referring the call. Never attempt to guess at the answer.

4. Many times a problem can be written on a memo pad and presented to the physician. Assure the patient that the call *will* be returned and give some reasonable expectation of when.

5. Occasionally, you will perceive the situation to be serious enough to interrupt the doctor. "Mrs. Brown is on the phone. You treated her husband for his heart condition yesterday and he is having severe pains. Would you like to talk to her, or should I have her take him to the hospital?" It is imperative to the patient's well-being that the physician have the opportunity to express his expert judgment in such situations. At times it will appear that you were overly cautious. However, errors attributed to conservative judgment are excusable.

6. The medical assistant may have to help make emergency decisions. "I'm sorry Mrs. Brown, the doctor won't be in until later this afternoon. Perhaps you should take your husband to the emergency room to be checked. I'll tell the doctor what happened." Again, when in doubt concerning the urgency of the visit, refer the patient to the emergency room or another physician on call. Never diagnose or prescribe treatment. Always act well within the boundaries of your professional role.

In reference to patient screening, the task of the medical assistant is to divert as many interruptions and unscheduled tasks as possible from the physician's routine without making decisions which assume responsibility for extending the medical care itself. While the MA's responsibility is to reduce the number of trivial tasks which face the physician, she or he must also engineer all responses so as not to leave patients feeling that they have been ignored or mistreated.

Another broad category in which telephone screening duties are performed relates to non-patient callers. Physicians are constantly burdened with calls from salesman, civic groups seeking contributions, and other sundry persons. Your function as the telephone manager is to set up a gentle barrier between these individuals and the physician.

Once you have established that a particular individual is not a patient, you should directly request information regarding the purpose of the call. A judgment is then necessary as to how the call will be handled. Several options are available. Here are some examples of acceptable responses:

1. "The doctor will review the message and will contact you."

2. "Please send literature for the doctor to review."

3. "I will call you back if the doctor would like an appointment scheduled."

Treat all calls with care. Never speak rudely to a caller, even when you yourself do not approve of the purpose of the call. Record all calls, including the phone number and the caller's purpose or request. Review all non-patient calls with the physician before discarding the messages.

TELEPHONE COURTESY

Good manners are necessary in all service-oriented professions. A medical assistant must possess an awareness of the forms of polite behavior. Courtesy is essential to telephone communications.

Most major telephone companies offer free courses in telephone courtesy to their clients. These courses usually emphasize the simple "do's" and "don't's" of telephone usage, including general answering procedures and specific telephone language found to be effective. It is extremely helpful to utilize the practical experiences of these resource individuals, since their experiences with the use of telephone systems are specialized and extensive.

The guidelines given below appeared in a recent pamphlet issued by General Telephone and Electronics for the use of office personnel.

1. Make the first impression a favorable one by answering at the first ring, if possible, and be ready to talk with the caller.

2. Identify the office and yourself—"Mr. Smith's office, Ms. Brown." This is time-saving and businesslike and gets the confidence of the caller for it indicates that you are a responsible person ready to be of service.

3. The term "office" is preferable to "desk," "line," "wire," or "telephone" as it adds prestige to your boss and the organization. Proper identification prompts callers to identify themselves.

4. Always keep your message forms handy and record the details accurately and completely while they are being given by the caller. Making a mental note often results in the message being incomplete or forgotten.

5. Request, rather than demand, information. Such phrases as "What's your name?" or "Repeat that, I didn't get it" sound abrupt when compared to "May I have your name please?" or "Would you mind repeating that information?"

6. If the name is an unusual one or contains letters which sound alike, verify the spelling through the technique of key-letter spelling. Also be certain to obtain the initials if it is a name like "Smith," "Jones," etc.

7. It is especially important to be accurate if the message requires action on the part of your boss. Repeat the information to assure the caller that you have the correct message.

8. When you leave your desk, advise the person who is to answer for you, where you are going, the telephone number where you can be reached, and when you will return. Give prompt attention to your telephone messages when you return.

9. None of us likes the proverbial "run-around," so transfer calls only when necessary. Begin by telling the caller why and where you are transferring the call. Then transfer the call using the method prescribed for your telephone system.

10. End your call in the same sincere and agreeable way you began it by saying "good-bye" pleasantly. Let your telephone visitor know that you were glad to be of service or sorry you were unable to help. Let the caller hang up first. Hang up gently and make sure the telephone rests securely on its base.

11. You will be best understood if you hold the mouthpiece as close to your lips as possible without touching and speak directly into it in a normal tone of voice. Your voice should always be warm, friendly, and sincere. Only you have complete control over what you say and how you say it. Always remember—what comes out of the telephone depends on what you put into it. Have a voice that always smiles!

12. Whether you are making a telephone call for yourself or your boss, be sure you have the right number before you make the call. Keep a list of frequently called numbers and up-to-date directories.

13. Plan your call before you make it. Knowing beforehand what you are going to discuss will make your call brief but effective. Planning saves time and money.

14. When your boss does not wish to place his/her own calls it is your responsibility, not the attendant's, to place them. You can take the time to announce the call in a more diplomatic fashion than the attendant who is usually too busy to concentrate on the secretarial aspects of a call.

15. If your boss is the type who disappears or makes another call after you have placed one, you will want to give him/her some training. Your boss may not be aware that these habits are discourteous and irritating to the called person and imply that the other person's time is not as valuable as his/hers.

16. Always stay on the line when you place a call. This will prevent irritation to the called person, tying up equipment unnecessarily, additional work for the operator, and a waste of money by lengthening the call. By staying on the line you can take immediate action if the number is busy or does not answer.

17. If you are connected to the called person's secretary advise him/her who is calling, for example: "Ms. Smith of Blank Company is calling Mr. Jones." If you reach the called person, announce your boss, for example: "Ms. Smith of Blank Company is calling you, Mr. Jones."

ORGANIZING TELEPHONE MESSAGES

Among the most commonly used office tools of medical assistants are the telephone log and the message pad.

A telephone log is a comprehensive record of incoming, and usually outgoing, phone calls. The use of a telephone log is often a choice made by the physician. If a record of calls is considered valuable, an ordinary spiral notebook will usually suffice. For each telephone transaction, the MA lists the caller's name, telephone number, and basic message.

Most offices will also benefit from the use of a telephone message form. Several types are available from commercial stationery stores. A standard form is shown in Figure 9-1. In most instances physicians will purchase a general, all-purpose message form; however, since medical assistants are the office management resource persons, their suggestions for improvements to the form may well be sought and implemented.

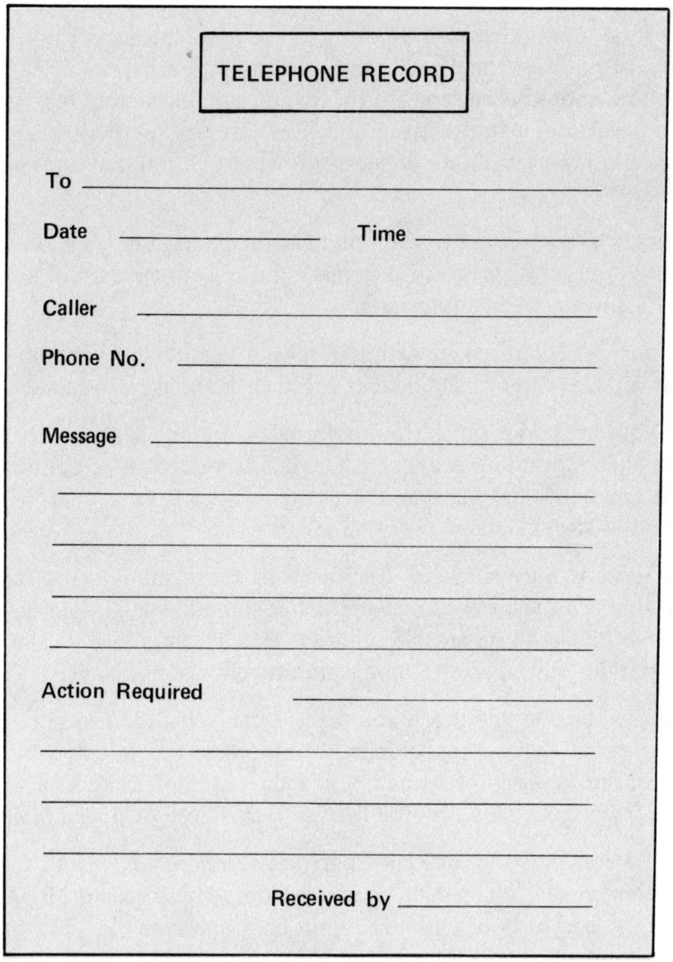

TELEPHONE RECORD

To ______________________________

Date ______________ Time ______________

Caller ______________________________

Phone No. ______________________________

Message ______________________________

____

____

____

____

Action Required ______________

____

____

____

Received by ______________

FIGURE 9-1. A standard message pad.

An effective telephone message form should contain the following items:

1. A heading, so that you will be able to send messages to various persons, including other staff members.

2. Date and time, so that the physician will know precisely when the message was received.

3. A notation of who received the call, so that the physician can obtain further information when desired.

4. Name and telephone number for quick identification.

5. A message space for listing the purpose of the call.

6. The action required, which will guide the physician in his response by indicating whether a call-back is expected or the call will be returned, or other special instructions.

To be effective the message pad system must also have two other attributes:

1. The pad must be close to the telephone at all times so that it can be utilized by the assistant.

2. A systematic procedure must exist for getting the message to the doctor for review.

To help the doctor process these messages, you might divide them into categories:

Emergency messages. These should be delivered immediately. If the doctor is not in the office, an alternative judgment is required.

"A" (most importance). These should be reviewed daily, perhaps in the early afternoon, so that calls can be returned during office hours.

"B" (medium importance). These should usually be given to the doctor at the end of the day or early the next morning.

"C" (least importance). These can be stored in a convenient place and allowed to "stack up" for several days. The doctor can go through them as time permits.

In any case you should discuss your ideas concerning message systems with the physician in an effort to develop an approach which satisfies the physician's preference and particular practice needs.

TELEPHONE HARDWARE AND SOFTWARE SYSTEMS

Medical assistants should become familiar with, and continually update, their knowledge of the various telephone systems available. The most logical source of information regarding these systems is the local telephone utility. Most telephone companies maintain a customer service representative whose job is to visit clients, propose systems which would facilitate the needs of a particular office, and train office personnel in the effective use of phone equipment. Since this service is almost universally provided at no cost, medical assistants should contact the local telephone company on a periodic basis so that they can learn about the latest developments in equipment and services.

Hardware

The most obvious part of a telephone system is the phone itself. Available hardware systems range from the simple single telephone which sits on the receptionist's desk to the more complex multi-function units which include numerous extensions.

If the office is a one physician practice, and the doctor prefers not to move toward more intricate systems, an ordinary receiver may be adequate, although the receptionist must move through the office to notify each person receiving a call. Most offices find, however, that a multiple extension system provides needed efficiency at a reasonable price. With the multiple extension system it is possible to have a centrally located individual answer all calls. If a particular call must be transferred to a person in another location, the system can be augmented by a buzzer-signal device. Thus a call for the clinical medical assistant can be transferred to a particular station by means of an electronic signal. The telephone manager can then switch to another line and make additional calls if desired. Another advantage to this approach is that the physician may use any of the extension phones to place a call. There is no need to go to a central location or wait until the phone is free.

Some physicians prefer the convenience and efficiency of an electronic intercom system used in series with the telephone extensions. Such a system makes it possible to speak to persons in any area of the clinic or office, to amplify phone calls, or to have conference calls connected to several areas of the office simultaneously.

If medical assistants are employed in very large offices or clinics which service a large number of physicians, they may find themselves operating a small electronic switchboard. Each type of switchboard has its own unique advantages and operations.

Software

The general category of telephone software refers to items such as telephone number files, procedures manuals, or auxiliary telephone accessories which are purchased or designed by a particular office staff member to enhance the basic instruments provided by telephone companies.

The most essential software accessory which is utilized by the medical assistant is a system for storing and accessing commonly used telephone numbers. It is not necessary to develop or maintain an enormously complex system, but it is wise to arrange commonly used numbers, such as laboratories, pharmacies, hospitals, and consulting specialists, in a central file for quick reference. This will save the medical assistant the time required to repeatedly obtain these numbers from the directory. A large number of commercial telephone filing systems are currently available. Many of these, however, are not appropriate for medical office use.

In the absence of a commercial system which will allow for continuous updating of numbers listed, a file box which holds 3 × 5 index cards is preferable. The cards can be arranged in alphabetic order and separated by index tabs, permitting ease when number changes or withdrawals are required. A rolladex file system can serve the same purpose.

The creative medical assistant should search for other kinds of software approaches to making telephone communications management more efficient. If the MA strikes upon an idea, it should be discussed with the physician before major or expensive innovations are introduced.

THE ANSWERING SERVICE

There are several different types of answering services. All of these fall within the general category of software systems. Each provides a particular set of advantages and disadvantages. In some offices it will be most economical and efficient for the office staff to purchase or lease their own equipment. Generally, phone answering devices are activated by an on-off switch. When an office staff member is not on duty, a prerecorded message informs the caller that the office is closed and directs the caller to leave a message on the recording. When the medical assistant returns to the office, the recorded messages are played back.

The type of answering service most often used by physicians is the operator-answering system. When calls are received after office hours, the answering service can contact the physician directly. The physician will periodically check with the service for messages. Professional answering services are available around the clock. Only the emergencies are immediately relayed to the physician. Other messages are called into the office and the receptionist, at the beginning of office hours, will assemble the list of calls received the previous evening or during other times when calls could not be personally handled.

If the physician subscribes to such a service, it will be the medical assistant's responsibility to coordinate the use of the service with the office answering system.

PERSONAL PAGING DEVICES

Most regional phone utilities make available a small radio-controlled pocket device for personal paging. Upon leaving the office, the physician activates the electronic pocket device so that when an emergency arises, the medical assistant dials a predetermined phone number which alerts the physician by an audible beeping signal from the device. The physician may then go to any available telephone and call the office. These paging devices are inconspicuous and can be comfortably carried.

PLACING LONG-DISTANCE TELEPHONE CALLS

There will be various occasions on which the physician will need to speak to an individual in another city or state. The medical assistant will usually place the long-distance call and will summon the physician when contact has been achieved. Patients, suppliers, or other doctors, although hundreds or thousands of miles away, may need to exchange important, sometimes crucial, information. All of the rules of telephone answering and identification procedures apply to a long-distance call. You are still making an effort to communicate information to persons whom you cannot see. Thus the basic nonverbal problems will persist.

To avoid unnecessary charges, the medical assistant must become familiar with long-distance rates during different times of the day. Person-to-person calls are usually more economical than station-to-station calls. Knowledge concerning the various time zones is also essential when placing long-distance calls.

A stepwise approach to placing local and long-distance calls is given below.

Local:

1. State your name and identify the office.
2. State the purpose of the call.
3. Record the response and the speaking name when appropriate.
4. Repeat information for clarification when appropriate.
5. Close the conversation cordially.

Long-Distance:

1. Before placing the call, check the name and number for accuracy.
2. Identify the time difference if applicable.
3. Select the method of call placement—direct dial, station-to-station, or person-to-person.
4. Prepare any materials that will be used for reference by the physician and place these in a spot convenient to the telephone.
5. Place the call.
6. Follow the steps described in placing a local call.

TELEPHONE HANDLING PROCEDURES

Procedure	Principle
1. Answer the telephone promptly.	1. Allowing the telephone to ring several times causes further disruption to the office staff and annoyance to the caller.
2. Extend greeting, and identify the office and the speaker.	2. This is an expected professional courtesy, and directs the caller to identify himself. This orientation provides the caller with the information required to proceed with the conversation.
3. Focus on the purpose of the call, and record the information received.	3. Concentrating on what is being said and determining the main idea will facilitate the avoidance of repetitious conversation. Recording ensures accurate message interpretation.
4. Ask pertinent questions when necessary.	4. Questions facilitate classification and direct the caller to provide the required information.
5. Close with a cordial expression.	5. A friendly closing leaves the caller with the feeling that he was well received and further aids in establishing a positive interaction.
6. Proceed with appropriate followup.	6. This ensures that the caller's message will be properly managed and not forgotten or misplaced.

SUMMARY

The management of telephone communication is a major responsibility of the administrative medical assistant. Handled effectively the telephone is the major resource available for establishing positive rapport with patients and others contacting the office. Ones telephone voice and manner are reflective of the general office environment and will set the tone for all interactions which follow.

This chapter has focused on the techniques which facilitate effective telephone usage. Application of these techniques ensures that each call will be managed appropriately and that the messages received will be accurately processed.

APPLICATION EXERCISES

To participate in the following class exercise each student will need to have several pieces of paper and a pen or pencil.

1. Divide the class into groups of four or five.

2. Select two persons and have them sit back to back so that they cannot see each other. Choose one person to be the caller and another the listener. The remaining students will observe.

3. The caller will draw a group of five squares such as the one shown on page 182. The squares must be touching each other and of roughly similar size.

4. The caller will then attempt to describe to the listener what the diagram looks like and have the listener duplicate the description on paper.

5. Repeat the exercise so that each group member has participated.

6. Discuss the problems encountered in the execution of this assignment. What were the approaches of the more successful caller-listener combinations?

7. One representative from the group should share the group's findings with the class. Try to identify the similarities in the reports.

Record the following two calls using the telephone message blanks on page 183 as guides. Describe any other followup that might be indicated.

1. Mrs. Coffey calls and states that she is still getting headaches even though she has been taking her blood pressure medicine. She asks if she should continue to take it of if she needs a change in medication. Her telephone number is 871-4326.

2. Mr. Balczon calls and states that there is still some redness around his puncture wound. He finished taking his medication yesterday. He asks if this is normal or if he needs another dose of antibiotic. His telephone number is 554-6210.

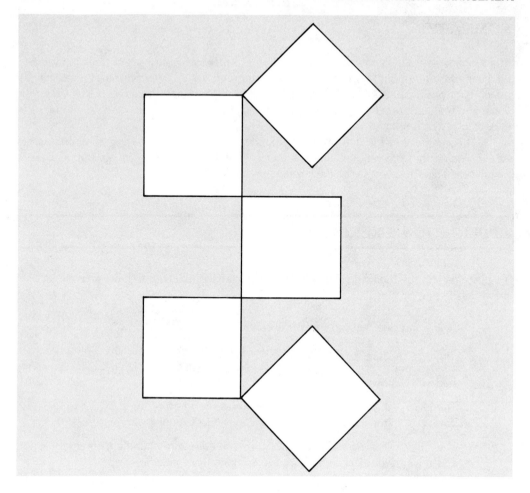

Screen the following patients to determine the urgency of the visit requested and the proper management of the call.

1. Mrs. Jones begins: "I would like to speak to the doctor. I was in last week with this sore throat and it's not any better."

2. Mr. Collins begins: "I would like to be seen today. I've been sick for the past 4 days."

3. Mrs. Stevens begins: "I would like to speak to the doctor. My husband is having terrible chest pains and he's very upset."

This exercise requires the students to role-play the parts of the medical assistant and the patient in the following situations. Begin with the ring of the telephone and identify the office. Continue the conversation to its logical end.

TELEPHONE RECORD

To _____

Date _____ Time _____

Caller _____

Phone No. _____

Message _____

_____

_____

_____

Action Required _____

_____

_____

Received by _____

TELEPHONE RECORD

To _____

Date _____ Time _____

Caller _____

Phone No. _____

Message _____

_____

_____

_____

Action Required _____

_____

_____

Received by _____

1. A patient calls and complains that the bill you sent was incorrect. She appears angry.

2. A patient calls, will not identify himself, and persists in asking to speak to the doctor.

3. A patient calls and requests the results of her laboratory tests.

4. A patient calls and requests a prescription refill.

5. A patient calls and complains that the doctor's prescribed treatment is not helping her.

6. A patient's mother calls and asks if her daughter's pregnancy test was positive.

7. An individual calls and asks for a contribution to a local service organization.

8. A physician calls and asks to speak to the doctor.

9. A friend calls and wants to discuss last weekend's happenings.

10. The hospital calls to tell the doctor that the patient's condition is unchanged.

COMPLETING THE LEARNING LOOP

As a prospective medical assistant, you can begin to develop your telephone skills while still in the training process. Begin to view each use of the telephone as a learning experience. Try to utilize the concepts which have been presented in this chapter in an effort to become a better telephone communicator now. You have also learned some valuable lessons regarding communication that can be applied to subsequent procedures and to all kinds of interactions.

As the chapters proceed, you will begin to realize how each task is related to the others, particularly in the area of attitude development.

BIBLIOGRAPHY

Blankenship, A. B.: *Professional Telephone Surveys.* McGraw-Hill, New York, 1977.
Collier, L.: *Telephone Tactics That Make You A Winner.* Rawson, Wade, New York, 1981.
de Sola Pool, I.: *Social Impact of the Telephone.* MIT Press, Cambridge, Mass., 1977.
Sunier, J. H.: *The Handbook of Telephones and Accessories.* TAB Books, Blue Ridge Summit, Pa., 1978.

CHAPTER 10

LETTER WRITING
AND MAIL HANDLING

SPECIFIC OBJECTIVES

Upon completion of this chapter you will be able to:

1. Communicate effectively through correspondence.
2. Design and process original written communications including memos and letters.
3. Manage incoming and outgoing mail efficiently.

INTRODUCTION

In the previous chapter the problems associated with telephone communication were discussed. The major difficulty in telephone conversations was found to revolve about the concept, that the communicaters could not visualize one another. Thus facial expressions and other nonverbal means of communicating were unavailable. Letter writing and other forms of written communication also possess this shortcoming. Not only are the nonverbal tools missing, but the letter writer has no quick way to test for reactions or for message effectiveness. The phone caller has the opportunity to repeat or rephrase a question, which is not true in the case of the letter writer.

In another sense, a letter is a long-term reflection on its writer. Unlike a conversation which lasts for a short time and then is slowly lost to memory, a letter can be read several times, filed, passed from person to person, or pinned on a bulletin board. It is essential that the medical assistant make each letter an effective, attractive, and accurate projection of the doctor's office.

ESTABLISHING OFFICE ROUTINE

The new medical assistant will probably be introduced to a preferred system for letter writing and sending. It is advisable that before an existing process is disassembled, the MA take time to learn how it functions. It is possible that an existing process was carefully designed by the physician, but it is more likely that the overall approach, or at least some aspects of the existing procedures, simply evolved by accident. Thus it is imperative that the MA introduce new ideas or suggestions carefully and tactfully to the physician to be sure that the physician agrees with prospective changes prior to their initiation.

Equipment Needs

The key to an effective written communications system is a typewriter in excellent condition which meets the needs of the office and is properly situated. A special typing area should be provided, including a table or desk which is the proper height for working. In addition the MA should ensure that the typewriter itself receives the best possible care, which includes covering the machine in the evening and cleaning it at regular intervals. Local service representatives are often available for advice regarding cleaning and repair. Most manufacturers provide this assistance at no charge.

A typewriter can often be purchased with a service contract. This is an agreement between the customer and a service agency to provide regular care and maintenance. Many service contracts include a number of emergency repair visits as well.

All of the auxiliary equipment required to operate and maintain a typing system should be placed within easy reach of the typewriter in a drawer or cabinet.

Stationery

Most physicians choose a letterhead containing their name and address. The selection of an appropriate letterhead coupled with the quality of the paper constitutes a projection of the office image which can be substantially more powerful than the message itself. Various styles of letterheads and paper quality can be requested and purchased. Many organizations are moving toward logos or graphics which help to project the image of the office more dynamically. While physicians will probably wish to be consulted concerning design, changes, and subsequent purchases, they are more concerned with their medical practice than with office procedures, and the medical assistant's initiative and suggestions are generally welcomed.

APPROACHES TO LETTER WRITING

Many office assistants take a rather negative approach to letter writing. They seem to feel that their job consists simply of transferring the physician's ideas or written words onto a piece of business stationery without spelling or punctuation errors. While it is clear that the skills of an accurate and proficient typist are undeniably important, the MA should also provide expertise in composing many types of medical correspondence, including subscription renewals, equipment orders, travel arrangements, and payment requests.

The role of the medical assistant is clearly that of innovator, information gatherer, and facilitator. The more responsibility he or she is able to successfully assume for the business management of the practice, the closer physicians can come to the realization of their goals for patient care.

Since medical assistants are knowledgeable in both the clinical and administrative aspects of medical office managment, they should encourage the physician to utilize their expertise in the construction of letters. For example, the physician should be able to say, "Send a letter to the Rotary Club and tell them that I will speak at the luncheon meeting on July 12 at noon on 'Current Developments in Cardiology.' " The MA should respond by making notes of the major points (date, time, subject), then constructing a letter for the physician's approval and signature.

This approach results in valuable time-saving for physicians as they can depend on the creative skills of the medical assistant to relieve them of routine and burdensome letter-writing duties. The physician need do no more than review the work and sign the letters.

TECHNIQUES OF LETTER WRITING

In order to perform the task of letter writing competently, it is essential that the medical assistant understand the basic aspects of composing correspondence. Since several styles and techniques for writing are available, the MA should be aware of alternatives and assist physicians in selecting those which most appropriately reflect their needs.

The Form

The physical presentation of a business letter is as important as the message itself. The overall format and presentation provide a projection of the office and either add to or detract from the written message. The are five basic forms of business letters:

1. block
2. semiblock
3. full block
4. hanging identification
5. simplified

Each of these forms is illustrated in Figures 10-1 through 10-5.

The block and semiblock forms are used most frequently. These forms are conventional and project a "traditional" or "conservative" image. The full block form is a newer "hybrid" form which is generally favored by secretaries because of its margin consistency. The hanging identification form has achieved great popularity with sales and purchasing firms, and, although rarely adopted by physicians, the medical assistant is likely to encounter its use on many incoming letters. The simplified form is enjoying a steadily increas-

```
                        S. R. SELLARO, D.O., INC.
                           GENERAL PRACTICE
                            ANESTHESIOLOGY
                       306 WEST ELEVENTH STREET
                           ERIE, PA. 16501
                              ———
                       TELEPHONE 814 - 455-1311


                                             January 17, 1980




   Mr. P. J. Browning
   214 West Elm Street
   Erie, Pennsylvania 16513

   Dear Mr. Browning:

   Thank you very much for the invitation to speak with the Rotary Club of Erie.
   I have been affiliated with Rotary Clubs for several years, and I am honored
   that you would ask me.

   My choice of a topic for your gathering would be, "Sports Medicine."  I have
   been interested in this area for several years, and believe that some of the
   most recent developments could be of use to many of your members.

   I understand that the meeting will be held at the Chambers Restaurant, at
   12:00 noon on the 13th of March.

                            Sincerely yours,




                            S. R. Sellaro, D.O.

   SRS:mk
```

FIGURE 10-1. Block form.

ing use. It conveys a feeling of warmth and efficiency (replacing needless rules and procedures), and typically expresses a sense of informality. Most physicians who use the simplified form do so because of the added advantages of brevity and clarity.

The Message

To the letter writer, selection of words is as imporant as the use of color is to the artist. Carefully composed, the letter reflects a multi-level message combining feeling, information, and visual appeal.

The following seven rules may be applied to the overall art of letter construction. Each is a powerful aid to the prospective letter writer.

S. R. SELLARO, D.O., INC.
GENERAL PRACTICE
ANESTHESIOLOGY
306 WEST ELEVENTH STREET
ERIE, PA. 16501

TELEPHONE 814 - 455-1311

January 17, 1980

Mr. P. J. Browning
214 West Elm Street
Erie, Pennsylvania 16513

Dear Mr. Browning:

Thank you very much for the invitation to speak with the Rotary Club of Erie. I have been affiliated with Rotary Clubs for several years, and I am honored that you would ask me.

My choice of a topic for your gathering would be, "Sports Medicine." I have been interested in this area for several years, and believe that some of the most recent developments could be of use to many of your members.

I understand that the meeting will be held at the Chambers Restaurant, at 12:00 noon on the 13th of March.

Sincerely yours,

S. R. Sellaro, D.O.

SRS:mk

FIGURE 10-2. Semiblock form.

1. *Utilize cue notes.* Cue notes refer to note taking *prior* to letter writing to identify the major points to be expressed in the letter. For example, the physician may request that the medical assistant write a letter to Dr. Jones thanking him for the patient referral and notifying him that the results of the consultation will be sent to him by the end of the month.

   Notes: To: Dr. Jones
           Re: Thank you—referral. Mrs. J. Albertes will receive results by end of the month.

   Cue notes assist in letter organization and clarity.

S. R. SELLARO, D.O., INC.
GENERAL PRACTICE
ANESTHESIOLOGY
306 WEST ELEVENTH STREET
ERIE, PA. 16501
—
TELEPHONE 814 - 455-1311

January 17, 1980

Mr. P. J. Browning
214 West Elm Street
Erie, Pennsylvania 16513

Dear Mr. Browning:

Thank you very much for the invitation to speak with the Rotary Club of
Erie. I have been affiliated with Rotary Clubs for several years, and
I am honored that you would ask me.

My choice of a topic for your gathering would be, "Sports Medicine." I
have been interested in this area for several years, and believe that
some of the most recent developments could be of use to many of your
members.

I understand that the meeting will be held at the Chambers Restaurant,
at 12:00 noon on the 13th of March.

Sincerely yours,

S. R. Sellaro, D.O.

SRS:mk

FIGURE 10-3. Full block form.

2. *Establish an effective beginning.* The most common error in letter writing is failure
to adequately introduce the topic in the first paragraph. The quality of the letter
often increases as the writing progresses. A corrective technique is to rewrite the
first paragraph after the entire letter is completed. Since the purpose of the first
paragraph is to gain the reader's attention, introduction of the topic should appear
in the first four sentences.

3. *Be brief and precise.* Unnecessary length should be avoided without jeopardizing
content. The medical assistant should attempt to convey the message with precision. Wordiness clouds the message, forcing the reader to sort through the verbiage for the main idea. A rough draft should be written from the cue notes and
should be rechecked for wordiness prior to acceptance of the final draft.

S. R. SELLARO, D.O., INC.
GENERAL PRACTICE
ANESTHESIOLOGY
306 WEST ELEVENTH STREET
ERIE, PA. 16501
—
TELEPHONE 814 - 455-1311

January 17, 1980

Mr. P. J. Browning
214 West Elm Street
Erie, Pennsylvania 16513

Thank you very much for the invitation to speak with the Rotary Club of
Erie. I have been affiliated with Rotary Clubs for several years,
and I am honored that you would ask me.

My choice of a topic for your gathering would be, "Sports Medicine." I
have been interested in this area for several years, and believe
that some of the most recent developments could be of use to many
of your members.

I understand that the meeting will be held at the Chambers Restaurant,
at 12:00 noon on the 13th of March.

Sincerely yours

S. R. Sellaro, D.O.

SRS:mk

FIGURE 10-4. Hanging identification form.

4. *Avoid use of the first or second person.* Although there are circumstances in which
the first or second person may be used in a personal letter, it is usually preferable
to write in the third person. Avoiding the use of "I," "We," or "You," whenever
possible, adds a sense of objectivity and professionalism to whatever is written.
For example, it is better to say "It has been determined . . ." than to say "I (or We)
have determined . . . ."

5. *Use proper grammar and punctuation.* Errors in grammar and punctuation serve
as a negative public relations factor. Spelling errors, sentence fragments, and
misuse of words and punctuation suggest incompetence in all aspects of the medical practice. Although inaccurate, this perception is easily acquired, especially
when the letter is an initial contact. A dictionary and a comprehensive guide to

S. R. SELLARO, D.O., INC.
GENERAL PRACTICE
ANESTHESIOLOGY
306 WEST ELEVENTH STREET
ERIE, PA. 16501

TELEPHONE 814 - 455-1311

January 17, 1980

Mr. P. J. Browning
214 West Elm Street
Erie, Pennsylvania 16513

Dear Mr. Browning:

Thank you very much for the invitation to speak with the Rotary Club of
Erie. I have been affiliated with Rotary Clubs for several years, and
I am honored that you would ask me.

My choice of a topic for your gathering would be, "Sports Medicine." I
have been interested in this area for several years, and believe that
some of the most recent developments could be of use to many of your members.

I understand that the meeting will be held at the Chambers Restaurant, at
12:00 noon on the 13th of March.

S. R. Sellaro, D.O.

FIGURE 10-5. Simplified form.

grammar should be kept in the work area for ready reference. Proofreading the
rough draft for errors of all kinds is imperative. Unfortunately, the medical assistant may never receive credit for hundreds of perfect letters, and instead receive
criticism for one letter containing errors. (It may be helpful to consult Punctuation
Patterns in Medical Correspondence, found in the Appendix.)

6. *Use professional terminology but write clearly.* Medical terminology must be used
   where appropriate, but the use of uncommon vocabulary throughout a letter
   should be avoided. Clarity is very much related to word choice. The letter should
   be professional in tone but not deliberately complex. The reader should not need
   a dictionary to interpret the message.

7. *Close with a paragraph which suggests action.* The purpose of the final paragraph should be to motivate the reader to act when a response is needed. The urgency of the response and the form it should take (a return call, a visit, a return letter) should always be clearly indicated.

Letter Mechanics

Since the quality of their work reflects upon the office image, it is essential that medical assistants ensure that each outgoing letter is mechanically perfect. The top and bottom margins should be well planned so that the letter is centered on the paper. Each line should be within the proper right-hand margin.

There are variations in preference for spacing and margin designs. The following guidelines are in common use:

Margins: A minimum of one inch is needed on either side of the body (10 spaces for pica, 12 spaces for elite). At least two inches of block space are needed at the top of the paper, and a minimum of one inch at the bottom.

Spacing: Depending on the form used, if indentation is required, an indent of five spaces before the beginning of each paragraph is universally accepted. Letters are usually single-spaced between lines and double-spaced between paragraphs.

Typing and spacing errors should be double-checked before the letter is removed from the typewriter. All corrections should be made neatly, and "strike-overs" should never appear on the finished copy.

COMPOSING AN ORIGINAL LETTER

Integration of all the aspects of letter writing discussed in the foregoing sections is essential to the composition of an original letter. The steps outlined below can be followed in the preparation of most letters that are routinely encountered in medical office practice.

Procedure	*Principle*
1. Assemble materials: stationery, references, typing accessories, and cue notes.	1. An adequate work area and availability of necessary materials result in efficient use of time and resources.
2. Begin to draft the letter, using pencil. Use the cue notes for the planning and organizing of main ideas.	2. A rough draft promotes good writing because sufficient thought and planning have been exercised. This serves to reduce the incidence of error.

3. Identify the person to whom the letter is being sent. Include name and address. Place on left-hand side of letter (refer to Figs. 10-1 through 10-5).

3. Called the "inside address," this information serves to reference the letter, and adheres to traditional form.

4. Date the letter. Place on right-hand side of letter, depending on style (refer to figures).

4. Dating the letter is extremely important as the letter, once written, is an historical document often needed for legal and other reference.

5. Two spaces below the inside address place the salutation (Dear Mr., Mrs., Ms., Dr. ——:).

5. A salutation is necessary to adhere to proper form and personally address the receiver.

6. The body of the letter is now composed. The body contains the content of the letter—why the letter is being written and what response, if any, is required of the recipient. Wordiness and grammatical errors must be avoided.

6. The body consists of an introduction, a message, and a closing. Word choice and clarity are important assets to the reader's understanding of the content. An awareness of the nature of the message and the identity of the recipient are integral components of successful composition.

7. Choose an appropriate closing (Sincerely, Yours truly, Cordially, etc.).

7. The closing should convey the feelings of the writer. Usually the medical assistant will compose the letter as though the physician were the writer, and the closing should thus be acceptable to the physician.

8. Proofread the draft and type the letter.

8. Checking for errors in spelling, punctuation, word choice, and sentence structure assures a satisfactory projection of the office image.

9. While the letter is still in the typewriter, check for typing errors.

9. It is much easier to make corrections while the paper is in the typewriter and spacing is predetermined.

10. Obtain the physician's signature.

10. The physician's signature should be affixed in ink to ensure his approval and to personalize the letter.

11. Make a carbon or photocopy of the letter and file it.

11. An outgoing correspondence file is a valuable reference and source of proof.

FORM LETTERS

In office practice, certain types of letters are used repeatedly. Most physicians employ a form letter to meet routine needs. The advantage of the form letter is that it is a time-saving device that can be readily applied to uniform situations. The disadvantage is that most form letters can immediately be recognized as such, and the recipient may feel that he has been treated impersonally.

The decision concerning which form letter to use and when this use is acceptable should be made in consultation with the physician. To a large extent this decision may be dictated by the office workload. If it is generally difficult to complete all of the office paperwork, a series of form letters may be required to resolve the difficulties in time management.

Form letters can be adopted for correspondence related to letters of collection, information regarding professional fees, request letters (such as for drug samples or reprints), and some referrals.

"Fill-In" Form Letters

For letter-writing problems which are repeated and predictable, the "fill-in" form may be the best solution. A common usage occurs in instances such as notifying the patient of test results and scheduling appointments. Figure 10-6 is an illustration of this method. The medical assistant should develop a series of these "fill-in" letters so that the items can be completed and mailed as needed. There are several logical uses for these kinds of form letters, but when used exclusively and nonselectively they can fail to project the desired image or obtain results when action is necessary. The office practice needs and ultimately the physician's preference will dictate which particular situations warrant this approach.

```
                                        Robert P. Green, M.D.
                                        843 Cherry Street
                                        Erie, Pa.  16503

                                        Telephone 456-1212




        To:


        The following patient is currently under treatment:

            Name:

            Address:

            Birthdate:

        Please forward the information requested below.




        Your earliest reply will be appreciated.


                              Sincerely,



                              R. P. Green, M.D.
```

FIGURE 10-6.   A "fill-in" form letter.

Semi-Form Letters

A modified approach to form letter writing is useful for those letters which are repeated but not in their exact form. This approach employs the "semi-form letter." Once the medical assistant has prepared a letter of promising utility, a copy should be made and filed as a model for future letters of similar intent. A recommended approach to developing such a file is to use a subject-divided notebook. The subject file might include letters of recommendation, inquiry, acceptance, and other common types of correspondence. After the MA has developed a series of each of the basic types of letters, one or more of each type may be used as a guide to the construction of new letters as they are assigned.

While the semi-form approach is neither as fast nor as efficient as the basic form letter, it retains some of the warmth of an original letter while saving substantial time.

LETTER PROCESSING

Letter processing refers to the handling of both incoming and outgoing mail. In the medical office much mail is sent and received daily. This necessitates efficient methods of handling.

Incoming Mail

The first concern in handling incoming mail is sorting. The medical assistant assumes this responsibility as well as that of opening the mail and directing it to the addressee. Usually the MA will open all mail unless it is addressed to the physician and marked "personal."

Before beginning the implementation of any mail processing system, the MA's ideas should be shared and discussed with the physician. The doctor's preferences will determine the mail handling process. Sorting can be categorized according to the action required:

1. *Mail the medical assistant can handle.*

   This category refers to mail which is addressed to the MA directly or sent to the physician, such as advertisements for office supplies, payments for office visits, etc. Complete mail handling by the medical assistant consists of opening, reading, and following through appropriately. Once mail is identified as that which can be handled by the MA, the action taken should be recorded on the letter itself in the form of a notation above the date.

2. *Mail the physician handles.*

   Mail which cannot be handled by the medical assistant must be sorted and annotated for the physician. Annotation is the term applied to the identification and isolation of important points in the letter. It is an effective means of saving time for the physician as well as preventing valuable information from being overlooked. Annotation is accomplished by underlining important words or phrases and writing notes in the margin.

Figures 10-7 and 10-8 represent a letter which was received and the corresponding annotation which was carried out by an MA, using the procedures that follow.

January 20, 19__

Adam Williams, M.D.
110 Perry Square
Townsville, PA 14502

Dear Dr. Williams:

As you know, the AMA is preparing for its next convention.
We are recruiting guest lecturers and workshop facilitators.
You were referred to our office by Dr. Paul Brown as an expert
in the field of gerontological medicine. We invite you to
submit a proposal for a workshop. Please send an outline
and other materials that would assist the committee in their
determination of the compatibility of your work with our intent.
Enclosed please find information describing the workshop sessions.
Contact our office if we can be of further assistance. We look
forward with great anticipation to your response and are hopeful
that you will join us as a workshop facilitator.

Sincerely,

John Adams, M.D.
Director of Continuing Education
American Medical Association

JA/mf
Enclosure

FIGURE 10-7. A sample invitation letter.

PROCEDURE FOR ANNOTATING INCOMING MAIL

Procedure	*Principle*
1. Place the date received in the top margin. *Example:* Rec. 1/19/80	1. The identification of the date received is helpful in future referencing. The dateline typed on the letter may inaccurately reflect the time that the letter was actually sent.

Rec. Jan 29th
January 20, 19__

*Note: dates on brochure
conflict with your
scheduled vacation time.*

Adam Williams, M.D.
110 Perry Square
Townsville, PA 14502

Dear Dr. Williams:

Re: As you know, the <u>AMA</u> is preparing for its next <u>convention.</u>
We are recruiting guest lecturers and workshop facilitators.
You were referred to our office by Dr. Paul Brown as an expert
in the field of gerontological medicine. <u>We invite you to</u>
<u>submit a proposal for a workshop.</u> Please <u>send</u> an <u>outline</u>
<u>and other materials</u> that would assist the committee in their
determination of the compatibility of your work with our intent.
<u>Enclosed</u> please find <u>information describing the workshop sessions.</u>
Contact our office if we can be of further assistance. We look
forward with great anticipation to your response and are hopeful
that you will join us as a workshop facilitator.

                         Sincerely,

                         John Adams, M.D.
                         Director of Continuing Education
                         American Medical Association

JA/mf
Enclosure

FIGURE 10-8.   The letter shown in Figure 10-7 with annotations added by the medical assistant.

Procedure	*Principle*
2. Read the letter and underline or bracket important points. *Example:* Thank you for the Re: *consultation referral on Mrs. Nancy Jones.* I have placed Mrs. Jones on a regimen of *Indovin tablets* and a *low purine diet.*	2. Since the objective is to highlight important information for the physician, the format used should be consistent. In the example "Re" denotes the main topic. The physician's attention will immediately be drawn to the underlined words, thus eliminating the need for rereading the letter.
3. Note any action to be taken in the upper margin; if not, explain and underline in the body of the letter. *Example:* Reply necessary.	3. Notes regarding action assist the physician in the organization of work activities. The note will immediately acquaint the physician with the nature of the letter.

4. Attach supplemental material or patient's file where appropriate.

   Example: With a letter relating to test findings on a patient, the patient's complete file should be attached.

4. The physician may be better able to interpret the content of the letter when pertinent materials are attached.

ESTABLISHING PRIORITIES FOR INCOMING MAIL

Proper handling of incoming mail necessitates decision-making as to the order of informational importance and the immediate form of action required:

1. *Most important.* This mail should be brought to the physician's attention daily and should be placed on the top of the stack. Personal letters, of course, would take precedence.

   Examples: Results of laboratory tests.
   A problematic insurance claim.

2. *Potentially important.* Some correspondence which is addressed to the physician may be of potential usefulness but not of immediate concern. Journals and notifications of meetings can be delivered to the physician less frequently or stacked below the items of most importance.

3. *Unimportant.* Mail such as supply catalogues, descriptions of new products, and other miscellaneous items can be disposed of, or, if potential use is anticipated, placed in a designated area for future reference.

Incoming mail can be handled effectively and efficiently when an organizational system such as the one described in this section has been developed.

Outgoing Mail

Outgoing letters sent by the physician can also be successfully organized to facilitate expediency. The decision as to which class to assign to the letter is related to the importance of the content and possible deadline restrictions.

1. *First Class*

   Most letters are sent first class. The envelope is sealed and the correct first class postage is affixed. Typewritten reports are considered first class. Other examples include postcards and handwritten letters and materials. Mimeographed or printed materials are exceptions.

2. *Second Class*

   Newspapers, magazines, and journals registered at the Post Office are considered second-class mail. Special rates are charged for these items, and journals and magazines sent by the office are more expensive than those mailed by the publisher.

3. *Third Class*

This classification includes books and catalogs of 24 or more bound pages, manuscript copy, identification cards, circulars and other printed materials, and all other matter weighing less than 8 ounces, not included in first- or second-class mail. Special rates are applicable to bulk mailing, and the Post Office should be consulted.

4. *Fourth Class*

This classification is reserved for all other merchandise and materials not included in the other classifications, such as films and books of more than 24 pages. Since postal regulations will vary, the Post Office should be consulted when questions arise. Handbooks that explain mailing procedures and list current rates are service publications obtainable from the Post Office on request.

5. *Special Designations*

a. *Priority Mail.* Any package or letter stamped as priority mail will be sent using the quickest available transportation.

b. *Special Delivery.* Mail which is delivered immediately upon receipt at the Post Office of destination is termed special delivery. This designation, although more expensive, ensures that the letter or package will not be delayed by routine sorting and handling.

6. *Protective Designations*

There are certain protective designations for use when money or important papers must be mailed.

a. *Registered Mail.* This refers to mail for which a receipt of delivery is provided. The mail carrier obtains the signature of the receiver at the address specified. The sender then receives a copy of the receipt, thus providing proof of delivery.

b. *Certified Mail.* This is a mailing system which provides a record that documents were mailed. A receipt is given to the sender.

7. *Mailing Currency*

a. *Cash on Delivery.* COD is one method of utilizing the mail service as a collection intermediary. The receiver pays the amount due the sender upon delivery of the mailing. The Postal Service then returns the payment to the sender by postal money order.

b. *Money Orders.* These are negotiable certificates of currency transfer. The Post Office collects from the sender the amount of money required by the receiver, sends the certificate to the receiver, and the receiver goes to the Post Office to convert the certificate back into cash. This service functions in a manner similar to a bank checking system, except that a money order does not need to be cleared.

These postal classes and categorizations should serve as an informational guide. However, postal categories and regulations are changeable. Consult the local Post Office for the latest regulations. In the office, current literature supplied by the Post Office describing its procedures, rules, and regulations should be included in the procedures manual for ready reference.

SUMMARY

Letter writing and mail handling are important skills that medical assistants must possess if they are to alleviate the demands placed upon the physician. These tasks are well within the boundaries of medical assisting functions. The physician will come to depend on the MA for the performance of these vital functions.

Original letter writing skills will be an extremely valuable asset in the employability of the medical assistant. The more varied and numerous the skills of the MA, the more essential she or he is to the successful operation of the medical office.

APPLICATION EXERCISES

1. Compose and type the following letters:

   a. Cancel a subscription to *Pediatric Monthly*.
   b. Order a filing cabinet.
   c. Accept an invitation for the doctor to speak at a conference.

   Letter particulars may be contrived or developed as the instructor specifies.

2. The instructor will give you samples of the mail received in the physician's office. Sort accordingly with restrictions and guidelines outlined by the instructor. Discuss results.

3. Annotate the five practice letters on the following pages.

4. Proofread the final practice letter. Discuss results. (Note: only the body of the letter is provided.)

5. Discuss how the following examples of mail would be handled:

   a. Medication samples.
   b. A letter to the doctor requesting a donation for an organization (office policy is no donations).
   c. A letter from the hospital stating that they have not yet received x-rays that were to have been sent.
   d. A letter requesting personal information on a patient for an insurance application.
   e. A letter not marked personal but obviously of a personal nature.

March 10, 19__

Warren Bennet, D.O.
207 Sun Dr.
Townsville, PA 12075

Dear Dr. Bennet,

        I am writing to thank you for referring Mr. John Frese to
me. I found that Mr. Frese's facial dermatitis to be linked
to a shaving cream he was using. Mr. Frese has been instructed
to use a natural-base preparation. His rash is clearing and
I I am returning him to you for follow-up. Attached are copies
of treatment sheets. Thanks again.

                                Sincerely,

                                John Wright, M.D.

    JW:mf

March 10, 19__

Warren Bennet, D.O.
207 Sun Dr.
Townville, Penna. 12075

Dear Dr. Bennet,

    We are unable to process your order for VIX05 Electrocardiogram
Unit. We have discontinued this model. Enclosed please find
literature which explains and illustrates the alternative models
available.

    We apologize for the inconvenience this may have caused
you and look forward to meeting your future orders successfully.

                                Sincerely,

                                Ronald Rose
                                Sales Representative

    RR/mf

March 10th 19__

Warren Bennet, M.D.
207 Sun Dr.
Townsville, Penna. 12078

Dear Dr. Bennet,

We received your letter concerning the potential for placement of your patient in Lakeview Convalescent Home. We will
have a vacancy beginning June 10th. This is a single room and
the charge is $210 weekly. Of course, medication and treatment
charges will be additional. Contact us by April 1st, to reserve
the room. As you know, there is quite a long waiting list and
we will not hold the room after the 1st. The patient should
contact us prior to April 1st so that we may answer questions
and describe our services. A deposit would also be expected
at that time.

Thank you for considering Lakeview Convalescent.

Sincerely,

Michael Levinson
Director

ML/mf

Thank you for referring Mrs. Marks to me. As you indicated

this is a complex case. Initial examination uncovered a bile

duct blockage. I am recomending surgical asperation of the

Blockage. Attached are the findings for your records. Mrs.

Mark's will be contacting you for continuation of treatment

of her bladder infection which must be cleared prior to the

scheduling surgery. At this time Mrs. Marks can contact the

office for an appointment. Please forward her copy of her file

after her treatment has been completed.

> I am informing you of my disatisfaction with your sales
> repesentative. He is pushy and rude and Ive instructed my
> assistants to refrain from making an appointment for him to
> meet with me. While I regret terminating of my relationship with
> your company I will not resume the association until I have been
> asured, that a sales representative with a sense of profession-
> alism will be calling on me.

COMPLETING THE LEARNING LOOP

As a student, the prospective medical assistant will have the opportunity to begin to develop letter-writing skills which can later be employed in a professional career. The student should seize every opportunity to improve upon writing skills. Courses in business and professional writing or in creative writing can be of great help, but practice is the key to the development of medical letter-writing proficiency.

Another area of communication for which the medical assistant is responsible is patient teaching. The development of patient-teaching skills is the primary focus of the next chapter.

BIBLIOGRAPHY

Brown, L.: *Communicating Facts and Ideas in Business.* Prentice-Hall, Englewood Cliffs, N.J., 1970.
Effenbein, J.: *Handbook of Business Form Letters and Forms.* Simon & Schuster, New York, 1972.
Ewing, D.: *Writing for Results.* John Wiley & Sons, New York, 1974.
Newman, L.: *Ten Letter Writers.* Books for Libraries Press, Freeport, N.Y., 1968.

11

PATIENT TEACHING

SPECIFIC OBJECTIVES

Upon completion of this chapter you will be able to:

1. List the basic teaching techniques and explain their uses.

2. Apply these techniques to simulated situations.

3. Describe the role of the medical assistant in patient teaching.

4. Describe the importance of patient education in the practice of medicine.

INTRODUCTION

From the patient perspective, the attainment of an accurate clinical diagnosis and the receipt of satisfactory treatment for the existing condition is not always a sufficient return for the cost of medical care. The physician's practice of medicine is experiencing dynamic shifts in patient care objectives. Medical management is a current term used to describe the multifaceted aspects of patient care.

In addition to a desire for diagnostic expertise and quality treatment, many patients are now expressing interest in the teaching of illness-prevention, clues to achieving optimum states of wellness, and a counseling-conscious approach to total health care.

While the physician is being required to assume these responsibilities in an expanded way, the medical assistant is also becoming involved in this holistic health care concept. *Holistic medicine* is the term used in reference to health care which is sensitive to the needs of the whole person through consideration of his psychologic and physiologic condition as well as the intellectual and spiritual dimensions of his being.[1]

The doctor-patient relationship is changing. Because the relationship of the patient with various allied health professionals flows from the doctor-patient relationship, all members of the health team are facing new expectations imposed by the patient.

While patient education has always existed, its scope is rapidly expanding. The medical assistant should have an awareness of the role patient education plays in holistic medicine and possess the ability to apply teaching behaviors successfully. The MA with teaching skills becomes an ever more valuable asset to the office structure. A better qualified staff affords the physician greater autonomy in providing comprehensive health care services to the patient.

CHANGING DIMENSIONS OF HEALTH CARE

The British Parliament recently ruled the controversial "heart transplant" operation to be illegal. In carrying out this symbolic act the British government was reflecting a worldwide shift in emphasis away from mechanical, "fix the symptoms" health care and toward a broader, holistic approach. The basic idea behind the Parliament's ruling was that if the monies which were allocated to a few enormously expensive heart operations could be diverted to overall health education, a much greater social good would be effected. In the long run fewer persons would need expensive heart surgery or, for that matter, many other high-technology medical procedures.

The proponents of open heart surgery argue that the knowledge which is gained by the persons who pursue such complex and difficult procedures provides a very positive gain for persons who function in related areas of medicine. The family physician, for example, will ultimately gain in his understanding of the cardiovascular system from the struggles of the few pioneering heart surgeons specializing in such rare procedures. And for the moment it is quite impossible to completely discount this argument. In fact it is such a strong and logical case that the most prudent position at this juncture is to accept it.

The purpose here, however, is not to rationalize a particular approach to medicine, but rather to introduce the MA to the fact that issues such as the holistic medicine controversy do exist, and that they will continue within all of the known medical specialties.

Identifying the Physician's Philosophy

Before practicing medical assistants become involved in the implementation or design of a patient teaching program, they should attempt to determine the basic philosophy of the physician by whom they are employed. Some doctors prefer to take a relatively narrow or specialized view of their services. Particularly if a physician is a specialist, he or she may be concerned only with the mechanical problems at hand, dealing exclusively with the patient processes which relate to the primary problem. Naturally, physicians who prefer to limit their attention to the symptomatology and treatment which is connected with a short-term set of problems will create an educational system for patients which is quite different from that of more "holistic" doctors. It should again be emphasized that there is nothing wrong with this approach. It may lead, in fact, to a greater level of attention to detail.

If the physician indicates an interest in exploring the broader context of each patient, then he or she is probably a proponent of holistic medicine: one who seeks an understanding of the relationship between lifestyle and illness. In this case the program of health care education might extend well beyond the basic mechanics of medical practice.

Some dentists, for example, attempt to educate patients about diet and hygiene, linking these lifestyle variables to a program of overall dental health. The holistically oriented dentist might be interested in delivering nutritional information or reports on toothbrush quality. The more mechanistic dentist might be more concerned with simply supplying information directly related to dental procedures, such as instructing a patient not to chew on a new filling for 12 hours.

Lifestyle-Disease Syndromes

Holistic physicians are continually attempting to link illness with lifestyle and then to provide education which attempts to promote fundamental changes in lifestyle. The argument from this perspective holds that to treat symptoms without attacking root causes which are based in the lifestyle is not only an inefficient use of the physician's time and energy, but also a disservice to the patient.

To perform open heart surgery on a patient who has a high fat diet, smokes, and leads a sedentary life may temporarily relieve some symptoms of disease, but does such a procedure have a long-term impact upon the progress of the disease? Many holistic physicians suggest that it does not. Perhaps, in addition to the operation (or, even better, before the operation becomes a necessity), the physician should attempt to bring about a change in the basic lifestyle variables (diet, smoking, and exercise) which quite probably are contributing to the disease.

The family physician who is holistically oriented might look for a medical history which is indicative of a certain group of problems, such as heart disease, then immediately begin an educational process which attempts to bring about positive changes in the lifestyles of patients. The orthopedic specialist who is working on a specific problem such as "tennis elbow" might recognize the importance of exercise to a particular patient and suggest substitute sports which would not compound the affected joints.

Self-Destructive Tendencies

A real puzzle in the holistic approach to medicine, and perhaps in logical arguments against it, is the apparent zeal with which many persons abuse themselves. Even in an evolving era of public information which links such practices as smoking, drinking, and overeating to health dysfunctions and disease, large numbers of people seem to persist enthusiastically in these obviously bad habits.

In several recent large-scale literature reviews on the subject of health and nutrition, the one conclusion universally reached was that the most powerful predictor of good health is understanding.[2] Nevertheless, an estimated 60 million persons in the United States are clinically overweight. Even though every package of cigarettes sold contains a clear health warning, approximately 50 million Americans continue to smoke at an estimated cost of 12 billion dollars in health care for treating primary smoking-related disorders.[3] There are at least 10 million alcohol abusers in the United States who apparently insist upon doing systematic damage to their livers, kidneys, and other vital organs.

Thus the perplexing problem of health education is not only one of identifying the relationships between disease symptoms and lifestyle, but also of bringing about real changes in lifestyles once the problem has been isolated.

DESIGNING AN INFORMATION SYSTEM

For a health care education system to be effective there must be a concerted team effort to educate. The design of a patient education system must logically be connected to the philosophy of the physician who directs the office staff, but regardless of basic approach or specialization, some common educational objectives can be identified.

Basic Office Mechanics

No matter how patient and thoughtful the medical staff may be, patients are quite often propelled into such a high state of anxiety that they may be oblivious to many of the most obvious mechanical functions of the office. For this reason it is usually a good idea to provide a brochure or pamphlet which describes the basic functions of the office. Typical inclusions would be as follows:

1. *The physician's specialty.* In addition to the general title, this area of the pamphlet should contain a description of the specialty and explain the scope of services in language which any patient can easily comprehend.

2. *A statement of philosophy.* The physician should dictate a brief summary of his most important policies or approaches, including how he feels about second opinions, his preference in patients (by age or other criterion), and other pertinent information.

3. *Office hours.* A list of the hours during which the office is normally open should be included, as well as the procedure by which patients may make appointments.

4. *Payment policies.* The preferred methods of payment and other information pertinent to insurance or fees should be outlined.

5. *Medical questions.* A procedure should be given which the patient can follow if he has questions, needs general assistance, or is seeking additional information about his medical care.

6. *Emergency procedures.* The proper procedures to follow in an emergency should be included.

7. *Coverage systems.* This information should include what to do if the patient needs to contact the physician before or after office hours, on weekends or during vacations.

8. *Other staff members.* The names and functions of other regular staff members should be included in the brochure.

Figure 11-1 provides an illustration of a typical information sheet containing answers to basic questions about a medical office.

Treatment Procedures

Another area of the medical practice which calls for a patient teaching program is that of common treatment procedures. Many physicians make a fundamental error in assuming that persons understand and will follow their orders. However, in a recent study of patients with high blood pressure, it was found that almost 40 percent of the individuals who were under treatment were suffering from hypertension because they were not taking their medication properly.[4] In similar studies by researchers who have been interested in finding out whether patients would take the entire prescribed dosage of a medication, it has generally been found that a full 50 percent of individuals will terminate their medication at a premature date.[5,6]

It can logically be concluded from studies such as these that patients are likely to misunderstand or fail to follow even the simplest of instructions. Perhaps this happens because

---

Some Answers To Common Questions About Dr. White's Office

1. What is Dr. White's Specialty?

   Answer: Dr. George White is an orthopedic specialist who has developed a sub-specialty in sports medicine. This means that he is particularly interested in the kinds of orthopedic problems which have resulted from or contribute to the inability to participate in sports.

2. Do I have to be a professional athlete to see Dr. White?

   Answer: No! Dr. White is convinced that all of us would be happier and healthier if we would maintain an active participation in lifelong sports activities. He is as interested in a grandmother who can't jog because of a sore foot as he would be in treating a professional football player.

3. Is Dr. White's service expensive?

   Answer: We will be pleased to discuss our professional fee structure with you before you begin treatment. In the long run most persons would consider this kind of treatment to be less expensive than the surgery which might result from an undiagnosed problem.

4. How should I pay the Doctor?

   Answer: Normally, patients should pay for services at the time of the office visit. If there are

extenuating services we will be happy to discuss them with you.

5. What are the office hours and how can I make an appointment?

   Answer: Except for emergency cases all office visits are by appointment. The office is open Tuesday, Thursday and Saturday from 10:00 A. M. to 7:00 P.M.

6. What if I have questions?

   Answer: We welcome you to call us at 412–3768 during regular office hours. We will either get an answer to your question or arrange an appointment.

7. What about emergencies or questions during non-office hours?

   Answer: If the question can wait until regular hours we would appreciate your not calling until then, but in the event that an emergency occurs you may reach Dr. White any time by calling 412–3768 and reaching his answering service.

FIGURE 11-1. A typical office mechanics brochure.

the kinds of procedures which seem commonplace to the office medical staff (because they are practiced hundreds of times per week) can be a great mystery to the average patient.

It is quite useful, then, to provide resource materials for patients who are being asked to follow even the most basic procedures. In fact, the more common and repetitive the problem, the more it makes sense to provide helpful materials such as pamphlets or mimeographed instruction sheets which explain the details. Such resource material is not designed to replace the practice of medicine or the ordinary instructional processes of a medical office. Rather its purpose is to reinforce doctor's instructions.

Depending upon the kind of medical office, materials could be prepared for patients who

1. have an infection;
2. are experiencing tension and anxiety;
3. are troubled by lower back pain;
4. have a cast for the first time;
5. need to learn how to use crutches;
6. are following a special diet.

Usually these materials can be gathered, free of charge, from local organizations (The American Cancer Society will provide literature on how to stop smoking, and the Heart Association will provide information on low-fat diets.) Materials relating to a particular office practice may need to be originally designed and duplicated.

Patient education is as much a part of the practice of medicine as are diagnosis and treatment. How valuable are proper diagnosis and skillful treatment design if the patient fails to follow instructions?

Lifestyle Suggestions

For physicians who prefer a more holistic approach to their patients, the office information systems may be extended into the generalized areas of lifestyle, thus dealing with such overall issues as nutrition, exercise, diet, and coping with stress. Some physicians are interested in providing information in the form of articles and pamphlets for their patients. The implied purpose is to stimulate good health habits, thus preventing sickness rather than treating symptoms at a later date.

A number of strategies are available for physicians who wish to carry out a basic health education program with their patients. Some physicians may feel that once they have identified lifestyle problems such as smoking or overeating, their role is to direct a basic set of materials to the patient. If this is the prevailing approach of a particular physician, it may be sufficient to maintain a supply of articles or brochures of a rather general nature which can be given to individual patients.

Other physicians will prefer to encourage their patients to take a more active role in health care by suggesting reading materials such as books and magazines containing useful guidelines and recommendations. If this is the case, the doctor may wish to keep samples of these materials in the office to show to patients.

The Role of the Medical Assistant

The medical assistant will be responsible for maintaining and managing an inventory of the kinds of materials which could be of use to patients. Before beginning an information system or altering an existing one, the MA should discuss this entire area with the physician. Having determined the physician's general philosophy relative to the medical practice and the desired approach to the problem of written information, the medical assistant will be able to act as an efficient information director. In this capacity MAs may find themselves searching for information such as pamphlets, brochures, and articles, or even writing their own information sheets.

SEEKING PATIENT INVOLVEMENT

Patient-Assisted Diagnosis

Patients must learn that they play a critical role in the diagnostic process. They must be absolutely objective and honest with the physician and staff if they are to receive a proper assessment. If patients take a challenging attitude—"OK, let's see if you can figure out what I've got"—the task of the physician-diagnostician is made substantially more difficult. If patients are in a state of great anxiety or attempt to hide information from the physician, there is little chance that they will receive a quality diagnosis.

Beginning with patient history questions such as the number of cigarettes smoked per day (one of many questions which might tempt the patient to provide an overly optimistic answer), patients must be convinced that their input is vital to proper medical care. Patients must also understand that they need to be objective reporters. If they are upset or prone to exaggeration, the information which they provide could lead to an incorrect diagnosis.

Patient-Assisted Treatment

If the patient is encouraged to take an active role in treatments, the classic "I'll bet you can't cure me" stance is changed to a "let's work together to make me feel better" perspective. Patients who feel that they are essentially responsible for their own cure (and that the physician is a resource person) are more likely to listen to instructions, ask for brochures and other information relative to their problems, and otherwise move successfully through the process of treatment. Thus a cynically resistant attitude—"I only took half of my medicine but I'll get better"—gives way to a more positive assessment of treatment—"the physician said to take four pills per day for ten days, so I will!"

The traditional passive patient is the most likely to misunderstand or ignore procedures. The active patient is likely to ask questions, to seek additional information, and to follow orders quite explicitly.

Educational System Design

It is clear that a sound patient education system must go well beyond the development of a series of printed materials and brochures. The delivery of patient education requires the active involvement of patients from their very first office visit. They must be encouraged to ask questions and to seek information. Naturally, this places a greater burden upon the staff. Rather than accepting the role of "automatons" who are herded from step to step, charged a fee and then sent home, actively involved patients will probably be assertive. They will want answers at times when staff members may be preoccupied or when answers are not readily available, but the outcome in terms of quality medical care is well worth the trouble.

IMPLEMENTING A PATIENT EDUCATION SYSTEM

Once the medical assistant has discussed the program of patient education with the physician and determined both the physician's basic educational philosophy and the optimum set of educational materials, the basic responsibility will be to administrate this process. The MA acts as a liaison or resource person, connecting the patient with the medical office and the physician.

The Medical Assistant as an Educational Resource Person

Many patients feel that physicians and nurses are in such a rush to provide critically needed services for other patients that they are too busy to answer questions. In addition, the actual treatment or diagnosis seems to move so quickly that before the patient realizes what has happened, he is by himself, putting his clothing on and wondering whether the doctor said to soak the sprained ankle in hot or cold water.

Much of the typical failure of patients to follow instructions comes as a result of their being confused or simply reluctant to persistently ask questions. Sometimes the most important questions don't even come to mind until the patient has left the office and gone home. Then the patient may be even more reluctant to ask questions since he feels that he may be asked to return for a second appointment or even charged for the advice.

The medical assistant should help patients to feel at ease and display a willingness to obtain answers to any questions. Before the patient leaves the office, the MA should ask the patient if there are any questions, and then respond clearly and precisely.

Patient: Goodbye Miss Green, I'll be seeing you again in a few weeks.

MA: How are you feeling, Mrs. Smith?

Patient: Much better, thank you, and the doctor gave me a new prescription.

MA: Are you going to finish your old prescription before you begin the new one or start the new medication immediately?

Patient: I don't remember. What do you think I should do?

MA: Just a moment and I'll ask the doctor for you. . . .

MA: Dr. White feels that you should begin the new medication as soon as possible. Do you have any other questions?

Patient: I was wondering which foods to avoid with an allergy like this one.

MA: We have a pamphlet here which describes a proper diet for persons who are allergic to chocolate. Why don't you take it home, read it and call me at the office if you have any questions.

Note that the MA has intervened in the process above and has changed a passive and confused patient into one who is

1. relatively sure of the procedure which she should follow;
2. actively involved in studying and participating in her own treatment;
3. aware of the MA as a potential resource for answers to questions.

Offering oneself as a resource person requires more than simply expressing a willingness to answer questions. MAs must use all of their interpersonal skills to determine ways in which they can help patients to be trusting and at ease. With some individuals the MA will have to be very patient and nondirective. Others will easily adapt themselves to a straightforward approach—"Do you have any questions?" Anticipation of the types of questions that patients have and a general empathetic sensitivity to patient needs will facilitate this process.

Using Prudent Judgment

Medical assistants must guard against setting up an alternative diagnostic or treatment center in the office. They must not divert persons from the physician's judgments. Rather they should provide a support system to assist patients in asking and interpreting the physician's advice.

Sometimes a patient will ask a question which clearly falls within the training and expertise of the medical assistant. In this case the MA should offer the assistance that she or he feels is necessary. With questions which relate to the practice of medicine, however, the MA should serve as an information resource only. Patients should be told that the doctor's advice will be sought and that they will have an answer as soon as possible. If there will be an unexpected delay in returning information to a patient, it is a good practice to call and explain the situation.

MAs should keep a log of telephone calls and the advice which they have given to patients so that they can periodically report activities to the physician. Even relatively trivial occurrences should be reported so that the physician will be aware of the total situation.

Maintaining a Patient Information Library

Medical assistants should act as administrators of the patient information library. In this capacity they must organize the brochures and other free literature so that they know where each piece of material is located and when a particular piece is in short supply.

The MA should also be resourceful and always on the lookout for materials which might augment the office information system. When a new pamphlet or article is located which might be of use, the MA should call it to the attention of the physician and offer to order it if the doctor feels that it would be a good addition.

THE PATIENT EDUCATOR

In many medical offices at least one staff member is accorded the role of patient educator. Generally the staff member who is charged with patient education will perform all of the administrative duties which were previously mentioned, as well as getting involved in both formal and informal programs.

The patient educator may be asked to design and run special workshops for the physician's clients. During these sessions the educator may try to acquaint groups of patients with new information which is relevant to the particular problems which they are experiencing.

Most patient educators are expected to keep abreast of the patient's diagnostic and treatment process so that proper feedback channels can be established. The patient educator should make a concerted effort to

1. ask "appropriate" questions which allow patients, in a nonthreatening environment, to freely discuss problems or concerns;

2. gently lead patients toward the answers so that when they arrive at the solutions to their problems they feel that they have taken an active role;

3. provide positive reinforcement for patients, thus helping to shape new behaviors which will allow the treatment to progress.

Because of their training and their basic role in the medical office, medical assistants are the obvious choice to be patient educators.

GUIDELINES TO EFFECTIVE PATIENT TEACHING

Procedure	*Principle*
1. Develop a brochure which lists the common office mechanics such as hours and payment methods.	1. Most patients need to be oriented to basic office processes. Since the staff is in the office on a full-time basis, they can easily lose touch with these simple questions.
2. Presume that the patient has questions and help him articulate these.	2. Many patients are too nervous or confused to develop clear questions about matters of concern.
3. Act as a liaison or resource person for patients.	3. If patients feel that the MA is at their service, they are more likely to seek the answers to important questions relating to their condition and treatment.
4. Make the patient feel that he is an active participant in his health care.	4. Patients who take an active role in the treatment process recover faster and experience more satisfaction.
5. Make an attempt to learn the physician's philosophy.	5. MAs can support the physician's approach effectively only if they understand it.
6. Stock a comprehensive variety of literature for patients.	6. Informational materials facilitate the involvement of patients in their own health care.

SUMMARY

Trends in the practice of medicine indicate that the overall mission of the typical medical office is changing dramatically. Increasingly, physicians are being asked to act as facilitators of health and teachers who cooperate with patients in designing a healthful life rather than approaching the human body mechanistically.

Since a major portion of their training, as well as a large share of their attention, is clearly devoted to the diagnosis and treatment of specific disorders, and since they are usually overworked and enormously busy, physicians generally find a holistic approach to be quite difficult.

Physicians cannot be expected to carry out holistic medicine alone, but they should be able to rely on the support of a staff that is knowledgeable and aware of the holistic perspective. Without challenging the physician's philosophical approaches, medical assistants should provide the catalyst for patient education. Understandably, this would be the responsibility of advanced medical assistants with extensive experience and specialized training. They would then serve as office informational resources, anticipating questions, providing answers, intervening and interpreting when necessary, and changing patient orientations from negative and passive to positive and active.

APPLICATION EXERCISES

To prepare for the classroom exercise, the MA student should complete the following assignment at home. On paper jot down two or three events which took place during your personal experience as a patient. (If you would rather, you may use the experiences of a friend or relative.)

The classroom exercise should proceed as follows:

1. Organize the class into several groups of four or five students.

2. Appoint one student to be the group secretary and as each student shares her experiences with the group, make a brief master list of common problems.

3. Use the list as a guide and develop a second master list containing positive strategies which an MA might utilize to avoid the problems.

4. The groups will reconvene with the overall class to share their strategies. The classroom instructor will serve as a leader and list all of the strategies on the blackboard.

5. Discuss ways in which the approaches outlined in this chapter might have alleviated the problems which were identified in the groups.

COMPLETING THE LEARNING LOOP

As an MA student you should begin to cultivate an interest in the field of medicine and its recent developments. It would be advisable for each person in an MA curriculum to visit the library on a regular basis and become familiar with some of the multitude of medical and health care journals, including the *Professional Medical Assistant*. In this way MA graduates will bring a broader understanding of medical practices and trends to their first position, thus ensuring their role as a valued member of the health care team.

The following chapter will aid the medical assistant in acquiring skill in the reading and abstracting of professional journals.

REFERENCES

1. Parsons, T.: Definitions of Health and Illness in Light of Social Structure. *Journal of Social Issues,* No. 4, 1952, pp. 2-44.
2. Stuart, R. B., and Davis, B.: *Slim Chance in a Fat World.* Research Press, Champaign, Ill., 1972.
3. Somers, A. R.: *Promoting Health.* Aspen Systems, Germantown, Pa., 1976.
4. Wilber, J., and Barrow, J.: Hypertension: A Community Problem. *American Journal of Medicine,* May 1972, pp. 653-663.
5. Charney, E., et al.: How Well Do Patients Take Oral Penicillin? *Pediatrics,* August 1967, pp. 188-195.
6. McKenney, J., et al.: The Effect of Clinical Pharmacy Services on Patients with Essential Hypertension. *Circulation,* November 1973, pp. 1104-1111.

12

LIBRARY AND RESEARCH RESPONSIBILITIES

SPECIFIC OBJECTIVES

Upon completion of this chapter you will be able to:

1. Organize the physician's personal and office library in a logical and effective manner.

2. Utilize the office library to locate resource materials for the physician.

3. Gather information for the physician at the local public, university, or hospital library.

4. Assist the physician in the preparation of papers, manuscripts, and abstracts.

INTRODUCTION

Most individuals who would attempt to name the aspect of modern physicians' careers that is the most important to them would be incorrect in their guess. They would probably suggest that physicians are only concerned with the obvious aspects of their practice such as surgical skills, making the office more efficient, or constructing a new medical building. But the reality of the typical physician's practice would tend to indicate something quite different.

Because of the dynamic nature of the field of medicine, most physicians find that the hardest aspect of their career is keeping up with the latest research. Unlike many other fields, medicine depends upon its practitioners to contribute their learning experiences to the ongoing literature.

For the medical assistant this means that most physicians will constantly be gathering information which is relevant to their fields. Physicians may also feel that they should contribute, from time to time, by preparing papers or manuscripts which contain information gained through their own practice or research. Since the physician typically perceives this to be an extraordinarily important function, the MA must internalize this imperative and be prepared to assist the physician by possessing appropriate library and manuscript skills.

THE OFFICE LIBRARY

Physicians will usually attempt to build and maintain an office library of the particular resource material most relevant to their interests and medical specialties. This library will contain books, journals, and other reference material. The MA should be able to develop a logical system for organizing these materials.

Physical Management

The first step in organizing the reference materials is to determine the proper area of the office in which to set up the library. Naturally the physical area should be of adequate size to contain the current materials and allow for future expansion. The area must include several sturdy bookshelves with adjustable dividers. It is also advisable that the library area be in a quiet corner of the office which contains a reading table and a lamp. Many times this will be within the physician's private office.

The professional library should not be in an area of heavy staff activity because of the distractions which might occur, nor should it be easily accessible to patients who might disturb the logical order of the resources or read and misinterpret technical information.

Organization

Before medical assistants can begin an organizational system or rearrangement, they must become aware of the function of an office library. The sole purpose of the office library is to provide the physician and staff with needed reference materials which are readily accessible. Thus it is imperative that the MA discuss the sequencing of books with the physician. Once the preferences of the physician are understood, a logical arrangement by speciality, subject, or author can be initiated.

It is generally helpful to place appropriate labels on the shelves. This will assist the MA in utilizing shelf space effectively, and it will assist the physician in scanning the library to locate the desired text.

The typical office library includes separate areas for books and journals. Within these separations the journals are usually arranged alphabetically. Books are most often arranged in alphabetical order by the author's last name. Some physicians may prefer to organize their books according to subject matter, with sections devoted to diagnostic procedures, general medicine, and specialties.

Each book should be clearly inscribed with the physician's name and office address. If he has not previously used one, the MA might suggest a rubber stamp for this purpose.

Journals

Often the most up-to-date and essential information will be contained in medical journals rather than in books. For this reason most of the MA's attention is likely to be devoted to the organization and management of the office journal collection. There are literally thousands of different journals in the field of medicine. Of these the physician will probably select a few which are most closely related to his specialization or interests.

Since journals are published on a periodic basis (monthly, bimonthly, or quarterly in most cases), the first concern in handling journals is to collect similar periodicals in a central location. There are several satisfactory approaches to this task. One is to obtain file boxes which will adequately hold one year of issues of a particular journal. The issues are then placed in the box and labeled accordingly. Another logical approach is to designate a horizontal area on the shelves for recent issues that are stacked for ready access until the current year has ended.

When journals have accumulated for a year, the MA may elect to have the complete volume bound at a commercial bindery or to place the box containing the journals in the appropriate space on the shelves. For a small fee, many journals will provide a specially designed container to hold a year of issues. With binding, however, there are no lost issues and storage is facilitated.

Special Interest Files

Most physicians develop at least one special interest. As a result they may begin to search systematically through journals, books, and reprints for information relative to these interests. To facilitate this activity the MA should obtain a large loose-leaf notebook and help the physician to find and reproduce such materials and to arrange them in some logical order. A label indicating the subject can be attached to the notebook and the notebook itself can then be housed in the library. New additions can be hole-punched and inserted for future reference. The skills required to locate research materials in other libraries will be discussed in a later section.

Cataloging

In most office libraries the creation of a card file is unnecessary. Unless the physician makes a regular practice of lending or has a problem with materials disappearing, the MA should simply concentrate on keeping the shelves in order. Most of the doctor's specialized materials can be handled by placing reproductions of important articles or sections of books in the "special interest" notebooks, instead of maintaining a complex filing system.

If the MA becomes the custodian of a very large library, perhaps one which is associated with a group practice or a clinic, then a catalog system might prove useful. Such a system is best accomplished with two basic approaches:

1. A card file which includes an alphabetized series of 3×5 index cards can be maintained in the library area. Each book should be cross-referenced on three or more cards according to title, author, and subject matter. The index cards can be housed in plastic containers which are available at most stationery stores.

2. A master list of journals can be developed, including the volume numbers, issue numbers, and dates of those contained in the library. If the doctor is in the habit of loaning books from his or her professional collection to friends or colleagues, the MA should attempt to keep a record of which books are "out" and who has them.

COORDINATING LOCAL LIBRARY FACILITIES

The medical assistant should attempt to become familiar with all of the libraries in the local area which might have journals or books which could be of value to the physician. In addition to the local public library there are probably nearby hospitals and universities which have medical resource materials.

For a nominal fee, many libraries will make available a list of their current journals. A master list of the journals maintained at all of the local libraries could prove to be a valuable source of information for the physician.

Most college and university libraries participate in the Inter-Library Loan Program, which can furnish photocopies of virtually any journal article by means of its worldwide cooperative network. There is usually a small fee for this service, but the potential for gathering broad volumes of information is limitless.

THE RESEARCH ABSTRACT

The medical assistant may be asked to assist the physician in gathering information or doing library research. One of the most important tools in fulfilling this function is the research abstract, an aid which is largely unfamiliar to many students.

Journals versus Magazines

Many of us have a broad variety of interests which can lead to the faithful reading of periodicals. There are publications for general audiences and for hobbyists of all kinds, but none of these is a journal in the true sense of the word. Journals are publications which are written by and for professionals and which contain primary research data. Just as the sports enthusiast reads sports magazines to get the "latest" information relative to his particular interest, the physician will constantly strive to keep up with medical advances by reading journals.

Journal reading, however, tends to be more difficult than magazine reading. For one thing there are thousands of different journals from which to choose, and for another, the time and energy required to wade through a complex technical article are substantial compared to the reading of a light magazine piece on bowling or archery.

What Is an Abstract?

Most journals include a brief summary of each article as a service to readers. The length or style of an abstract may vary according to the journal, but essentially it is a condensation of the entire article, describing the purpose of the research, the methods used, and the conclusions reached.

The basic purpose of the research abstract is to give readers the general sense of an article so that they can decide whether a full reading would be useful. Often the information contained in an abstract spares the reader the time-consuming process of perusing an article only to find that its information does not really apply to his needs.

The examples given below are abstracts reprinted from two well-known journals. The first, taken from the *Journal of the American Medical Association*, outlines a study of a treatment approach for patients with pulmonary complications. The second, from the *American Journal of Orthopsychiatry*, describes a sociological study of family therapy.

Article title:

"Pulmonary Dysfunction Following Traumatic Quadriplegia: Recognition, Prevention, and Treatment"

Abstract:

A prospective study of the pulmonary complications occurring in 22 consecutive patients admitted to hospital within 24 hours after acute traumatic quadriplegia was compared with the findings of a retrospective survey of 22 comparable patients. Patients in the prospective group received therapy designed to prevent or reverse secretion retention. All patients in this group survived. In the retrospective group there were nine deaths; pulmonary complications and the need for tracheal intubation and mechanical ventilation were three times more frequent. Serial pulmonary function testing in the prospective group demonstrated a greater compromise of expiration than inspiration and progressive improvement in diaphragm function with time. It is concluded that vigorous pulmonary therapy in the prospective group was associated with increased survival, a decreased incidence of pulmonary complications, and a decreased need for ventilatory support.

Article title:

"Family Therapy: The Making of a Mental Health Movement"

Abstract:

Family therapy, unlike many fleeting therapeutic fads, has flourished in established mental health circles for the past 25 years. This paper examines the socio-historical sources of family therapy's popularity, and considers the growth and development of this contemporary American therapeutic phenomenon from a sociological perspective.

In both of these examples it may be noted that there is sufficient information to inform the reader of the general nature of the articles to follow. If, for example, the physician was looking for information about how to practice family therapy, the second abstract indicates that he would not find such information within the article in question.

Sources of Research Abstracts

In addition to the fact that research abstracts accompany most articles in the majority of professional journals, physicians may consult *Excerpta Medica*, a general compilation of medical research abstracts, which is available in all hospital and medical center libraries.

Excerpta Medica is organized by specialty so that the researcher looking for articles which deal with a particular aspect of medicine, such as anesthesiology or internal medicine, can find abstracts indexed by topic within a specific section entirely devoted to that subject.

The physician searching for information relative to a certain aspect of medicine may consult *Excerpta Medica*, read the pertinent abstracts to see if the articles to which they refer are of use, and then attempt to obtain the articles themselves. This would be the ideal time to consult a master list of journals which are available in area libraries or to check with Inter-Library Loan.

ASSISTING THE PHYSICIAN WITH RESEARCH

Many times in the course of a medical practice a problem will emerge which the physician cannot immediately answer. Sometimes sources of information will be readily available to the doctor, and she will need to go no farther than her personal library. At other times physicians will have to begin a systematic search of books and journals to find the needed information.

When an extensive search is necessary, a skilled MA can provide valuable assistance. If the physician is able to explain his needs to the medical assistant, the MA can search the appropriate journals for preliminary information, thus relieving the physician of the mechanical aspects of a literature review.

In most cases MAs should not attempt to make judgments relative to the potential value of articles. Their task is to find articles which deal with the kinds of problems in which the physician is interested. They should ask the doctor which strategy is preferred:

1. making a list of articles relating to a particular problem;
2. making reproductions of the abstracts of those articles;
3. making reproductions of entire articles; or
4. sending for reprints.

If a large number of articles is available, strategy 1 or 2 would probably be the practical choice. The physician could then select the articles which are most promising, and the MA could in turn have reproductions made.

If the MA is working from *Excerpta Medica*, the abstracts may be far easier to find than the journals from which they were taken. If the physician has time to wait, the articles may be ordered from a local library which participates in an inter-library loan system. Before ordering an article, the MA should check to be sure that the journal in question is not available at a local library.

Many institutions of higher education, especially state-affiliated schools, make available a literature review service. Many of these services are computerized and draw resources from an enormous body of materials. Generally these services are offered at a very modest cost. Even if the physician is not located in close proximity to such an institution, a simple long-distance phone call or a visit to a branch campus might point the way to a valuable research asset at a very reasonable cost. The typical computer-assisted literature search might reveal a hundred or more contemporary titles at an approximate cost of $20 to $50. If the total expenses of sending a person to do a library search are considered, this fee will seem quite attractive.

MANUSCRIPT PREPARATION

Perhaps to a greater extent than other professionals, physicians are charged with the responsibility of sharing their learning experiences with their colleagues. Since advances in the art and science of medicine can be of vital importance to the continued development of the field, many physicians will regularly prepare papers which they might offer either for publication in one of the many journals, or for discussion at a professional meeting.

Medical assistants should be prepared to aid physicians in the preparation of these manuscripts. This will be especially true if the MA has assisted the physician in gathering research materials for the project. In addition to the mechanical assistance which MAs can provide by typing papers and checking for spelling and punctuation, they should also be prepared to provide both editorial and stylistic support.

Scientific Writing Styles

The kind of writing which is done in a scientific manuscript is quite different from that which might be used in a textbook or magazine article. If medical assistants are asked to edit a physician's paper, they should be aware of the important differences. Scientific inquiry is supposed to be carried out from a position of curiosity. Thus a research paper should be free of dogmatic language. A scientific paper, for example, should not contain a statement such as the following:

> . . . the results of the experiment definitely proved that the medication cured all of the patients.

A better wording would be:

> . . . the results of the experiment supported the hypothesis that the medication was useful in treating many patients.

The first editorial task of the medical assistant is to carefully exclude all of the dogmatic assertions which are contained in the paper.

A second and connected task is to be sure that the paper is written in the third rather than the first or second person (I, we, and you). It is a basic convention of scientific research that all papers be written in the third person. Thus a statement such as:

> . . . I administered the treatment to the patients, we measured the results and then I concluded . . .

would be replaced with one such as:

> . . . the treatment was administered to the patients, and the results were measured. It was concluded that . . . .

Writing in the third person adds an aura of credibility and objectivity to a research report.

Professional Style Guides

In addition to providing editorial assistance, the MA should ascertain the stylistic requirements of the particular journal or professional society for which the manuscript is intended. The most logical way to learn about these requirements is to write to the association or journal in question and request a style guide for potential contributors. Generally these guides will list mechanical requirements such as paper length, margin sizes, style of type, abstract size, referencing, and footnotes. If a style guide is not available, the MA may be able to determine the required style by referring to other articles which have been published by the particular source which is to receive the manuscript.

General Editing

Medical assistants should devote as much energy as they can to the task of editing manuscripts. It is evident that the credibility of a research paper or report would be suspect if the writing quality, spelling, or punctuation were in any way deficient. Thus the MA should carefully examine the paper for editorial integrity. Try to remember as you carry out this procedure that an error will be a published testimonial to your incompetence.

The Appendix to this book provides useful information on proofreading, medical terminology, and the use of abbreviations, numerals, and symbols.

SUMMARY

Being a research assistant is a little like "playing" detective. It can be fun, challenging, and exciting if it is approached correctly, or it can be a complete drudge. The secret is in the attitude! To be successful the library "detective" must presume that she or he is doing an important and useful job. If the MA trudges off to the library thinking that "the doctor should do this himself" or that "I'll never find anything," she will be a failure. Not only will she fail to find anything, but she will allow her mood to rule out an opportunity to be a valuable support to the physician.

The approach needs to be one of enthusiastic optimism. "I know that there is information on exercise therapy for patients with tendinitis of the knee, and I am going to find it!" Naturally, the first few times that MAs venture into the world of research journals, they will be awestruck by the information overload, and confused and concerned about their capacity to do a good job. But to be an effective MA you must get over this hurdle and develop confidence in yourself. To a large extent this is simply a matter of experience.

GUIDELINES FOR EFFECTIVE LIBRARY AND RESEARCH ASSISTING

1. Attempt to understand the research interests of the physician, including the kinds of articles and books with which he or she is most concerned.

2. Attempt to organize and maintain the physician's office library in a way which is readily useful.

3. Learn the locations and contents of other library facilities in the immediate area.

4. Spend some time reading a few of the journals which relate to the particular interests of the physician.

5. Let the physician know that you are willing to help with these responsibilities.

6. Do a perfect job of proofreading and editing materials. Be slow and demanding rather than fast and sloppy.

APPLICATION EXERCISES

To prepare for this exercise each MA student should perform the following assignment before class. Using no more than 150 words, write an abstract of this chapter. Bring the abstract to class.

The class should divide itself into groups of four or five students. Within each group students are to perform the following tasks:

1. Take turns reading each abstract.

2. As a group, critically evaluate each abstract. What are its strong points? Has important information been omitted? What are its weaknesses?

3. Working as a group, develop one good abstract.

4. A representative of each group will read the group's abstract to the overall class.

5. The instructor will lead a discussion in which the characteristics of a good abstract are highlighted.

COMPLETING THE LEARNING LOOP

More than any other single factor, the thing which will enable a medical assistant to be effective as a library and research aide is a good attitude. If MAs understand that research is a vital link between the developing theories of medicine and their physician's capacity to practice good medicine, and if they see their role as one of assisting the doctor in every way possible, then they will have the capacity to be a valuable asset to the office.

The MA needs to appreciate the fact that keeping the journals in order, organizing an office library, and proofreading a paper are every bit as important as the clinical aspects of assisting, such as giving shots and taking blood pressures. If she can help the physician through her library and research skills, she will have established her value as a medical assistant.

Naturally, this is easier said than done. It is ever so tempting, when one is already busy with accounting ledgers and recordkeeping, to make excuses when it comes to library duties. Nevertheless, MAs who wish to establish their value as an office resource must constantly remind the physician of their willingness to take on research responsibilities.

BIBLIOGRAPHY

Cushieri, A., and Baker, P. R.: *Introduction to Research in Medical Sciences.* Churchill Livingstone, New York, 1977.

Day, R.: *How to Write and Publish a Scientific Paper.* ISI Press, Philadelphia, 1979.

Hauer, M., et al.: *Books, Libraries, and Research.* Kendall/Hunt, Dubuque, Iowa, 1978.

Hook, L.: *The Research Paper: Gathering Library Material.* Prentice-Hall, Englewood Cliffs, N.J., 1962.

Nolting, K. B.: *The Art of Research.* Elsevier, New York, 1965.

Payton, O. D.: *Research: Validation of Clinical Practice.* F. A. Davis, Philadelphia, 1979.

Strawn, R. R.: *Topics, Terms, and Research Techniques: Self-Instruction in Using Library Catalogs.* Scarecrow Press, Metuchen, N.J., 1980.

4

MEDICAL LAW
AND ETHICS

The growing sophistication of the health professions and the developing legal consciousness of the public have given new prominence to the fields of law and ethics as they relate to the delivery of medical services. As members of the health care team, medical assistants must acquaint themselves with the nature and implications of these closely related concerns both to assure the quality of their performance and to protect themselves from compromising or injurious situations. Both law and ethics derive largely from social custom, but the difference between them is crucial. Ethics involves the making of moral choices and the transformation of those choices, or values, into "rules" of conduct. Law, although deriving from accepted values, has the additional characteristic of being interpreted by a system of courts and enforced by the power of the state. The two chapters contained in this unit should help medical assistants to function knowledgeably when confronted with the legal and ethical aspects of their work.

UNIT OBJECTIVES

Upon completion of this unit you will be prepared to:

1. Explain the legal responsibilities of working in a medical office.

2. Distinguish between the liability of the physician and that of his staff members.

3. Discuss the relationship of medical care and professional integrity.

4. Explain the meaning of social responsibility in the delivery of health care services.

13

EVOLVING ISSUES IN MEDICAL LAW

SPECIFIC OBJECTIVES

Upon completion of this chapter you will:

1. Possess a reasonable understanding of contract law.

2. Be prepared to act responsibly as the physician's legal agent in a medical office setting.

3. Understand the legal ramifications of practicing as a medical assistant.

4. Be able to assist the doctor in the proper management of narcotics.

5. Be aware of how to deal effectively with patients without subjecting the office to potential suits.

6. Realize the most common sources of potential lawsuits and understand how to avoid these.

INTRODUCTION

Today's physician has become a major target of potential lawsuits. Because of the sensitive nature of medical practice and the apparent assumption that doctors are an "easy mark," recent years have witnessed an alarming increase in the number of patients who are suing physicians. These lawsuits cover a wide spectrum of claims ranging from lost time and inconvenience due to waiting in the office to errors of diagnosis or treatment and gross negligence. While the vast majority of physicians carry insurance which protects them against personal loss resulting from these claims, the optimum approach to this problem is one which will minimize the potential of a lawsuit.

The role of the medical assistant in this regard is quite clear. The MA must coordinate the efforts of the office team to protect the physician from needless harassment by lawsuits. To effectively play this role, the medical assistant must understand the basics of medical law. It may be helpful to consult the glossary of medical-legal terms found in the Appendix to this book.

AVOIDING THE LAWSUIT MENTALITY

Once a person has been sued, whether or not he wins the case, there is a great danger that a kind of brutal skepticism will set in. While most MA students will probably not be able to relate directly to these feelings, imagine how a physician must feel, after devoting years to learning the practice of medicine, struggling to keep up with the field and working diligently to provide quality care for patients, when a disgruntled person makes an accusation of malpractice. To many physicians the first suit is a crushing and highly emotional experience.

To make matters worse the typical lawsuit drags on for months and constantly reminds the physician that his competence is in question. Even though in some situations the patient is simply seeking financial compensation and bears no real malice, the suit will cause needless anxiety, self-questioning, and introspection on the doctor's part.

There is a danger that the anxiety generated by a suit will infect an entire office staff and cause a dehumanization of services. The medical assistant may begin to view each new patient as a potential enemy; a "lawsuit mentality" can easily set in.

The prudent approach is simply to accept the statistical probability of a lawsuit but to carry on office business in such a way as to minimize its potential. The medical assistant must never approach patients as potential lawsuit claimants.

CONTRACT LAW

The relationship between the physician and the patient is covered by the Law of Contracts. A contract is an agreement between two persons. The agreement does not necessarily have to be a written one. In the case of a professional who offers a commonly understood service, many of the aspects of the contract are generally understood or implied.

To be valid a contract must have four characteristics:

1. *Manifestation of assent.* There must be both an offer and an acceptance.

2. *Legal subject matter.* The contractual issues must be valid legal matters.

3. *Parties having legal capacity.* Both parties must legally be capable of entering an agreement.

4. *Consideration.* Both parties must understand the agreement.

The party who makes a contractual offer is known as the *offerer,* and the party to whom the offer is made is called the *offeree.*

The physician who begins a medical practice is, in legal terms, "inviting an offer." The patient who comes to the physician for treatment is then the *offerer,* the physician who begins treatment is the *offeree.* Generally, the process of contractual law between the patient and physician begins at this point and falls within the implied logic of contracts. This suggests that the patient has agreed to pay the physician's fees, and the physician has agreed to execute treatment using reasonable care and judgment. The physician further attests that he possesses at least a reasonable level of training, skill, and knowledge relative to all other similar physicians who are practicing within his geographic area.

Even though no formal contract is signed by patient and physician, all of these components of the implied agreement are assumed within contract law. If, for example, the physician attempted a procedure which was out of his area of expertise, he would be in violation of the law unless:

1. The procedure was an emergency.

2. There was no specifically qualified physician within the geographic area, and no possibility of getting the patient to a specialist in another area.

Promise of a Cure

If at some particular time during the diagnosis or treatment the physician or an authorized representative (possibly the medical assistant) was to promise a cure, this would become a part of the contract. This fact of law should make it clear to the MA that no one in a medical office, including the doctor, should ever promise that the patient will be cured. If, in a particular instance, complications occur and the patient is not fully cured, then a lawsuit may result. Discussions with patients need to be based upon logical diagnosis, treatment explanations, and probable outcomes. The medical assistant should never make such statements as, "Of course the doctor can fix your broken finger; he is an excellent physician and ten weeks from now it will be as good as new." Instead she might say, "Dr. Smith has treated several cases just like yours and almost everyone has acquired full use of their finger after ten weeks."

Third Party Contracts

One of the more common contractual problems for the physician is the treatment of a third party who is not legally responsible. Mr. Jones, who is a regular patient, brings in his next door neighbor, Jack, and explains that Jack hurt his back helping to push his car out of a snow drift; therefore Mr. Jones is going to pay the doctor bill.

On the surface a situation like this may seem quite innocent, but sometimes these matters can become quite complicated. For example, the doctor may find that an extensive treatment will be required which will cost several thousand dollars. Meanwhile, Mr. Jones learns that Jack has had a bad back since he was injured ten years before playing shuffleboard. Jones tells Jack that he won't pay; Jack tells the doctor that he will have to get his money from Jones, and the physician may find it impossible to collect his normal fee.

This example illustrates the fact that unless a person asks for treatment for himself or for a dependent (wife or child), the physician must obtain a written agreement which is signed and witnessed. If physicians do not secure a written agreement, they will subsequently find that they have no legal right to payment.

Terminating a Contract

Having entered into a verbal contract with a patient, the physician is legally obliged to continue caring for the patient. If this relationship is to end, the physician must protect himself by writing a letter of termination of services, sending the letter by certified mail, and filing both a carbon or photocopy of the letter and the mailing receipt. There are three general instances in which the physician may withdraw from a case:

1. If the patient fails to uphold his part of the contract either through refusal to make reasonable payment or through not following doctor's orders.

2. If the patient leaves the hospital without the permission of the physician.

3. If the patient requests that the doctor not continue services.

In all of these cases a letter, which may later serve as legal protection, should be sent to the patient, and a copy should be filed by the physician.

"Good Samaritan" Acts

In an emergency, such as an automobile accident or an injury at a basketball game, physicians, nurses, or other allied health professionals may be called upon to render immediate care. To protect such persons from later suits by patients or their families, most states have passed "Good Samaritan" acts. While the exact areas of applicability vary from state to state, the general purpose of these acts is to ensure that the physician or other person who gave care in good faith and used reasonable concern, given the circumstances, is protected from civil liability.

The medical assistant should check the "Good Samaritan" laws of her state to see if they apply to her, and if they do not she should discuss this potential problem with the physician.

TYPES OF MEDICAL LIABILITY

If a physician is sued, the basis of the litigation will either be malpractice, negligence, or breach of contract.

Malpractice is at issue when a patient claims to have been detrimentally affected by treatment. There are three basic types of malpractice:

1. *malfeasance,* a claim that an incorrect treatment was performed;

2. *misfeasance,* a claim that the treatment was incorrectly performed;

3. *nonfeasance,* a claim that proper treatment was delayed for no apparent reason.

Negligence is at issue when a patient claims that a physician (or someone acting on his instructions) accidentally carried out an action which harmed the patient, and that this action is one which is not normally done, such as when an instrument or sponge is accidentally left inside a patient following surgery.

Breach of contract is at issue when a patient claims that a physician did not live up to his part of the implied doctor-patient contract. Violation of confidentiality and failure to perform prescribed services would fall within this category.

Medical assistants must protect both themselves and the physician from litigation by:

1. Making copies of all important documents, such as letters of withdrawal, and filing these copies accurately.

2. Never admitting fault unless it is with the advice of the physician's attorney or insurance agent.

3. Not making contractual promises to patients, such as promises of cure or commitments of the physician's time.

MEDICAL LICENSURE

The individual states have historically developed procedures for licensing persons who practice the healing arts. The original purpose of these Medical Practice Acts was to protect the citizens of the state from "quackery."

Although the process of licensure may differ from state to state, the following basic requirements may be cited. The physician must

1. have graduated from an accredited medical school;
2. have completed an internship approved by the state board of medical examiners;
3. be at least 21 years of age and a U.S. citizen;
4. be a state resident of good moral character;
5. satisfactorily complete the state board examinations.

There has been an organized effort to standardize these requirements by the American Medical Association. To this end the National Board of Medical Examiners has been charged with the responsibility of administering a "National Level Board Test." Most states now recognize these scores in lieu of state board scores.

Each practicing physician has a legal responsibility to obtain a license to practice medicine, to display that license in his office, and to renew the license periodically. Physicians who dispense drugs must also obtain a narcotics license from the federal government. The license number must appear on each prescription for a narcotic substance.

SPECIAL LEGAL PROBLEMS OF DRUGS

Due to the growing problem of drug abuse, a government agency—the Drug Enforcement Administration (DEA)—was established under the Controlled Substances Act of 1978. One of the primary responsibilities of the DEA is to control and regulate the physician's dispensation of narcotics. Because of the paperwork involved in these procedures, the medical assistant will probably become involved in the physician's dealings with the DEA.

Each physician must register with the DEA. If a doctor has more than one office in which he maintains a supply of drugs, administers drugs, or dispenses drugs, he must register each of these offices individually.

There are several categories, or schedules, of drugs covered by the Controlled Substances Act:

Schedule I:
a. The drug or other substance has a high potential for abuse.
b. The drug or other substance has no currently accepted medical use in treatment in the United States.
c. There is a lack of accepted safety for use of the drug or other substance under medical supervision.

Schedule II:
a. The drug or other substance has a high potential for abuse.
b. The drug or other substance has a currently accepted medical use in treatment in the United States or a currently accepted medical use with severe restrictions.
c. Abuse of the drug or other substances may lead to severe psychological or physical dependence.

Schedule III:
a. The drug or other substance has a potential for abuse less than the drugs or other substances in schedules I and II.
b. The drug or other substance has a currently accepted medical use in treatment in the United States.
c. Abuse of the drug or other substance may lead to moderate or low physical dependence or high psychological dependence.

Schedule IV:
a. The drug or other substance has a low potential for abuse relative to the drugs or other substances in schedule III.
b. The drug or other substance has a currently accepted medical use in treatment in the United States.
c. Abuse of the drug or other substance may lead to limited physical dependence or psychological dependence relative to the drugs or other substances in schedule III.

Schedule V:
a. The drug or other substance has a low potential for abuse relative to the drugs or other substances in schedule IV.
b. The drug or other substance has a currently accepted medical use in treatment in the United States.
c. Abuse of the drug or other substance may lead to limited physical dependence or psychological dependence relative to the drugs or other substances in schedule IV.

Narcotic and Non-Narcotic Drugs

Under DEA regulations, substances may be divided into two distinct generic categories: narcotic and non-narcotic. While the primary concern of the agency is with narcotic drugs, physicians who dispense non-narcotic drugs on a regular basis must inventory these substances and keep an updated record of all transactions for two years. Agents of the DEA may ask to review these records at any time, and the physician is required by federal law to provide them.

Many physicians do not regularly dispense dangerous non-narcotic drugs, but they do accumulate moderate supplies of samples which they may pass along to patients on a random basis. For example, a "needy" college student requires a decongestant, and the physician, remembering how difficult it was to work his way through college, may simply give the patient a bottle from the sample shelf. This basic approach is not considered a regular process of dispensing and thus does not require a records system.

Narcotic Inventory Control

With substances which are defined as narcotics by the DEA, both physicians and their staffs are required to practice several routine precautionary procedures. First, and perhaps most important, is the requirement that all narcotics be stored in a locked cabinet or safe and that access to keys to that container be carefully controlled. Theft or other loss of substances from the locked area must be reported to the regional DEA office as soon as the loss is discovered. Local law enforcement agencies should also be informed.

All narcotic drugs should be ordered on DEA triplicate order forms so that the agency can keep track of these substances using the third part of the form. Physicians must also maintain two years of inventory records for their supplies of narcotic drugs.

PATIENT CONSENT FORMS

There are times when the physician should secure a signed consent form such as the one shown in Figure 13-1. The American Medical Association suggests that this procedure be followed in the event that a particular medical treatment presents either a recognized risk or involves hospitalization. To sign such a form the patient must be of legal age (which varies from state to state) or be an emancipated minor (a technical minor who has been declared to be of legal age by the state). In the event that the patient is in grave danger and at the same time unconcious or otherwise unable to respond, the physician may proceed without signed consent forms.

Another procedure which requires that the prudent physician obtain release forms is voluntary sterilization. In this case it is further required that the physician obtain both the signature of the patient and that of his or her spouse. A sample form is shown in Figure 13-2.

Informed Consent

For a consent form to be valid, the patient must fully understand not only the procedure which he or she is about to undergo, but also the risks which are involved and all of the

AUTHORIZATION FOR MEDICAL AND/OR SURGICAL TREATMENT

I, the undersigned, a patient in this hospital, hereby
authorize Dr._____(and whomever he may
designate as his assistants) to administer such treatment as is
necessary, and to perform the following operation_____
_____and such additional operations or procedures
as are considered therapeutically necessary on the basis of
findings during the course of said operation. I also consent
to the administration of such anesthetics as are necessary, by
Dr._____and associates. Any tissues or parts surgically
removed may be disposed of by the hospital in accordance with
accustomed practice.
I, hereby, certify that I have read and fully understand the above
Authorization for Medical and/or Surgical Treatment, the reasons
why the above named surgery is considered necessary, its
advantages and possible complications, if any, as well as
possible alternative modes of treatment, which were explained
to me by Dr._____. I also
certify that no guarantee or assurance has been made as to the
results that may be obtained.

Date_____ Signed _____
                                                        PATIENT

Witness_____ or _____
                                                NEAREST RELATIVE

                            Relationship to patient_____

(Authorization must be signed by the patient, or by the nearest
relative in the case of a minor or when patient is physically
or mentally incompetent.)

14-99 (R/1/73)

FIGURE 13-1. Sample authorization form for medical or surgical treatment.

generally accepted alternatives to the treatment along with their associated risks. All of this information must be made available to the patient in simple, nontechnical language.

PATIENTS WHO FAIL TO FOLLOW ADVICE

The physician will sometimes encounter a patient who terminates treatment at a premature date or otherwise refuses to follow the physician's advice. There are at least two reasons for attempting to contact these individuals to inform them of the dangers in their reluctance to continue with treatment. The first is an ethical consideration. Instead of feeling irritated with or insulted by these persons, the physician and staff should presume that the patient is sim-

---

STERILIZATION PERMIT

Date _____ Hour _____ .M.

I hereby authorize and direct Doctor _____ and assistants of his choice to perform the following operation upon me at the above named hospital _____ _____ and to do any other procedure that his (their) judgment may dictate during the above operation. It has been explained to me that I may (or will probably) be sterile as a result of this operation but no such result has been warranted. I understand that the word "sterility" means that I may be unable to conceive or bear children and in giving my consent to the operation have in mind the possibility (probability) of such a result. I absolve said doctor, his assistants and the hospital from all responsibility for my present condition or any condition that may result from said operation.

Signed _____

Signature Witnessed:

By _____

By _____

I join in authorizing the performance upon my wife (husband) of the surgery consented to above. It has been explained to me that as a result of the operation my wife (husband) may be sterile.

Signed _____

Signature Witnessed:

By _____

By _____

FIGURE 13-2. Sample sterilization consent form.

ply using bad judgment because of his illness and its associated trauma. In this case a gentle but firm letter, such as the one shown in Figure 13-3, may convince patients or their families to seek help. A second, legal, consideration is that a patient file which contains a formal record of the patient's failure to complete a treatment procedure may protect the physician from suit at a later date.

THE LEGAL RESPONSIBILITY OF THE MEDICAL ASSISTANT

As licensed and trained members of the allied health care professions, and as duly authorized representatives of a physician, medical assistants are in a position to bring suit either

---

Dear Mrs. Green,

When I examined your injured hand yesterday, I suggested
that it might be broken and that we should meet at the hospital
for an x-ray examination. Your failure to meet me for this
procedure may result in serious consequences if a fracture does
exist.

I would urge you to contact either me or another physician
of your choice to have this problem diagnosed as soon as possible.

FIGURE 13-3.   Sample letter to a patient who has failed to follow advice.

upon themselves or the physician they represent if they act in an inappropriate manner. MAs who are negligent in the execution of their job may be sued, but in most cases patients will sue the physician, owing to the fact that the employing physician is generally held liable for the actions of employees.

A major concern of the medical assistant relative to potential litigation must be the protection of the physician. The two most common areas of concern for potential litigation of this sort are (1) misinstructing patients and (2) emergency care in the doctor's absence.

Misinstructing Patients

As an authorized agent of a physician, what the medical assistant says to a patient is legally presumed to be at the physician's instruction. Extreme care must therefore be taken in explaining treatments and other procedures. The MA must be sure that patients fully understand any instructions which they have been given.

Medical assistants also must be prudent in their choice of language with regard to appointments, diagnoses, treatments, and outcomes. If, for example, a medical assistant tells a patient that the doctor will meet him at the emergency room in 30 minutes, the MA has legally bound the doctor to an agreement or contract. If the physician is an hour late due to an emergency, he may be subject to suit. Thus the medical assistant must learn to use nonspecific language:

> *Nonspecific:*
> "Please be at the emergency room at 9:00 a.m. The physician will see you as soon as he has completed his rounds."
> *Specific:*
> "Dr. Jones will meet you in the emergency room at 9:00 a.m."

> *Nonspecific:*
> "Most patients find that this medication does not make them nauseated."

Specific:
"Don't worry, you won't get sick as a result of this drug."

Nonspecific:
"Several of our patients have gotten over the flu in three or four days when they followed these instructions."
Specific:
"Take your prescription, drink plenty of fluids, and you will be better by next Friday."

Although the physician is legally responsible for the actions of a representative who does not have the required professional skills or who follows physician's instructions which prove to be improper, he is not responsible for negligence or a failure to follow instructions. Thus it is imperative that the medial assistant, acting as agent for the physician, clearly understands and accurately follows all instructions.

Emergency Care in the Office

There is a reasonable chance that the medical assitant will confront a medical emergency in the physician's office while other professionals are not available. For example, the MA may be handling the switchboard during lunchtime when a waiting room patient collapses or falls and hurts himself. The general rule of thumb in such a situation is that the medical assistant, or any person present for that matter, may carry out whatever emergency procedure is clearly called for as long as the individual works within the limits of his or her skill and training, and consistent with routine first aid procedures. The MA should discuss this eventuality with the physician and ask for advice regarding these situations.

SUMMARY

The medical assistant must walk a narrow line between protecting the physician from litigation and acting in an inhumane and bureaucratic manner. On the one hand, MAs must continually guard against making imprudent statements or commitments on behalf of the physician, and on the other, they must not forget their important role as human relations facilitators for patients. It takes a great deal of experience to attain this balance and substantial skill to maintain it.

GUIDELINES FOR EFFECTIVE MEDICAL-LEGAL ASSISTING

Procedure	Principle
1. Do not approach patients as if they were potential troublemakers or litigators.	1. Such an approach does not lead to prudent caution; it creates a mechanistic atmosphere of bureaucracy.
2. Never promise a cure.	2. The promise of a cure creates for the physician a legal responsibility to deliver a cure.

3. Maintain an accurate record of all narcotics.

3. Physicians are as legally responsible for narcotic records management as they are for the narcotics themselves.

4. Secure signed consent forms for all hospitalizations, sterilizations, and other reasonably risky procedures, and file them properly.

4. The signed consent form serves as an insurance against later litigations.

5. Send letters of advisement to all patients who explicitly fail to follow advice.

5. The letter of warning ensures physicians that they have done all within their power to secure proper care.

6. Don't make specific patient scheduling commitments for the physician.

6. A promise of an appointment time constitutes a contract between the physician and the patient.

APPLICATION EXERCISES

The following classroom exercise requires the use of a pen or pencil. The class should divide itself into groups of four or five students and then spread itself throughout the classroom to avoid noise congestion.

1. Within each group the students should select one individual to take the role of the medical assistant, another to take the role of the patient, and two or three remaining students to act as observers.

2. The medical assistant and the patient should face each other and spend approximately five minutes working through the patient roles which follow:

   The medical assistant should attempt to deal with the patient in a humane but responsible manner.

   The observers should keep track of the time, and use the guide which follows to evaluate the dialogue.

Evaluation Guide

Procedure: List measures taken by the medical assistant which seemed to reassure or calm the patient, and those which seemed to irritate or activate the patient.

Positive Strategies	Negative Strategies
1.	1.
2.	2.
3.	3.
4.	4.
5.	5.

3. The patient should select one of the following roles:

   a. *Mrs. Brown:*
   You are about to leave the office to meet the physician at the hospital for tests. You have been having chest pains and you are very worried.

   b. *Mrs. Black:*
   Your child has the flu. He is also the star of his grade school soccer team which has a playoff game in six days. You want him to be well for the contest. You are a typical "little league" parent.

   c. *Mrs. Green:*
   You are an avid tennis player, but you have tennis elbow. You want to know how soon you can return to the courts. You are anxious.

   d. *Mrs. White:*
   Your husband fell and hurt his leg. The doctor has asked that he go for x-ray examination, but you heard that x-rays cause cancer. You don't want unnecessary x-ray treatment for your husband. You are hostile.

   e. *Mrs. Purple:*
   You have had a persistent respiratory infection for three weeks. Your friends who had the same "cold" went to another physician and recovered in a few days. You are angry.

4. As the patient and medical assistant discuss the problem, the observers should record positive and negative responses by the medical assistant. They should pay particular attention to the MA's capacity to avoid getting upset.

5. Each student should take a turn as the medical assistant and the patient.

6. After the group has completed its role-playing rounds, the students should discuss their observations.

7. The instructor will lead a classroom discussion in which the positive and negative strategies of the medical assistants can be identified.

COMPLETING THE LEARNING LOOP

It will take years of experience for the medical assistant to develop the skills required to become a humane and warm listener who is concerned for the problems and needs of the patient without inadvertently making irresponsible promises or statements which cannot be supported by the physician. As you spend the next few years at college, you should begin to identify persons with whom you come in contact as being either skilled in this regard or prone to error. In your dealings with the college or university that you are attending as well as with other professional offices, you should pay close attention to office secretaries and other assistants.

Do these individuals make the error of taking an overly rigid, alienating posture of protecting the "status quo" without regard to the persons that they represent? Do they seem to side with the client and agree to all kinds of promises? Or do they find a balanced position?

The competent and valuable medical assistant is one who learns to find that equilibrium point.

BIBLIOGRAPHY

Curran, W., and Shapiro, E.: *Law, Medicine and Forensic Science.* Little, Brown, Boston, 1970.
Lander, L.: *Defective Medicine: Risk, Anger, and the Malpractice Crisis.* Farrar, Straus & Giroux, New York, 1978.
Medicolegal Forms with Legal Analysis. American Medical Association, Chicago, 1973.
Moritz, A., and Morris, R.: *Handbook of Legal Medicine.* C. V. Mosby, St. Louis, 1975.
Morris, R., and Moritz, A.: *Doctor and Patient and the Law.* C. V. Mosby, St. Louis, 1971.
Practitioner's Information Outline of the Controlled Substances Act of 1970. Bureau of Narcotics and Dangerous Drugs, U.S. Department of Justice, Washington, D.C., 1972.

CHAPTER 14

PROFESSIONAL ETHICS FOR HEALTH CARE

SPECIFIC OBJECTIVES

Upon completion of this chapter you will be able to:

1. List the ten principles of medical ethics as outlined by the American Medical Association.

2. Explain the importance of the principles of medical ethics to the medical assisting profession.

3. Apply the principles of medical ethics to medical office situations.

INTRODUCTION

Every profession adheres both to the legal regulations imposed upon its practice and to an expected code of behavior for its practitioners. In this chapter the code of behavior for the medical professions is explored. This code, based on certain defined principles, is the subject of medical ethics.

The medical assistant, assuming the role of a valued member of the health team, must internalize the principles of medical ethics and acquire an understanding of the relationship of an ethical code to the law. The Appendix to this book provides a practical list of terms having direct application to the field of medical ethics.

ASPECTS OF MEDICAL ETHICS

The term medical ethics refers to the principles that reflect a code of behavior based on moral standards of medical practice. According to the American Medical Association, medical ethics provides standards which transcend that which is required by law. Another dimension of medical ethics is bioethics, a new term coined to denote the study of moral issues as they relate to medical research and its applications. Bioethics combines the fields of medicine and philosophy in a quest for moral responsibility and judgment in critical questions posed by medical technology.

Medical ethics is based upon historical custom in general and upon the Hippocratic Oath in particular. The oath which Hippocrates required of his students in the fourth century B.C. is still in use today:

> I swear by Apollo the physician, and Aesculapius, and Health, and Allheal, and all the gods and goddesses, that, according to my ability and judgment, I will keep this oath and stipulation, to reckon him who taught me this art equally dear to me as my parents, to share my substance with him and relieve his necessities if required; to regard his offspring as on the same footing with my own brothers, and to teach them this art if they should wish to learn it, without fee or stipulation, and that by precept, lecture and every other mode of instruction, I will impart a knowledge of the art to my own sons and to those of my teachers, and to disciples bound by a stipulation and oath, according to the law of medicine, but to none other.
>
> I will follow that method of treatment which, according to my ability and judgment, I consider for the benefit of my patients, and abstain from whatever is deleterious and mischievous. I will give no deadly medicine to anyone if asked, nor suggest any such counsel; furthermore, I will not give to a woman an instrument to produce abortion.
>
> With purity and holiness I will pass my life and practice my art. I will not cut a person who is suffering with a stone, but will leave this to be done by practitioners of this work. Into whatever houses I enter I will go into them for the benefit of the sick and will abstain from every voluntary act of mischief and corruption; and further from the seduction of females or males, bond or free.
>
> Whatever, in connection with my professional practice, or not in connection with it, I may see or hear in the lives of men which ought not to be spoken abroad, I will not divulge, as reckoning that all such should be kept secret.
>
> While I continue to keep this oath unviolated, may it be granted to me to enjoy life and the practice of the art, respected by all men at all times, but should I trespass and violate this oath, may the reverse be my lot.

A modern treatment of the code composed by Hippocrates is found in the ten principles of medical ethics adopted by the American Medical Association:

> 1. The principal objective of the medical profession is to render service to humanity with full respect for the dignity of man. Physicians should merit the confidence of

patients entrusted to their care, rendering to each a full measure of service and devotion.

2. Physicians should strive continually to improve medical knowledge and skill, and should make available to their patients and colleagues the benefits of their professional attainments.

3. A physician should practice a method of healing founded on a scientific basis, and he should not voluntarily associate professionally with anyone who violates this principle.

4. The medical profession should safeguard the public and itself against physicians deficient in moral character or professional competence. Physicians should observe all laws, uphold the dignity and honor of the profession and accept its self-imposed disciplines. They should expose, without hesitation, illegal or unethical conduct of fellow members of the profession.

5. A physician may choose whom he will serve. In an emergency, however, he should render service to the best of his ability. Having undertaken the care of a patient, he may not neglect him; and unless he has been discharged, he may discontinue his services only after giving adequate notice. He should not solicit patients.

6. A physician should not dispose of his services under terms or conditions which tend to interfere with or impair the free and complete exercise of his medical judgment and skill or tend to cause a deterioration of the quality of medical care.

7. In the practice of medicine a physician should limit the source of his professional income to medical services actually rendered by him, or under his supervision, to his patients. His fee should be commensurate with the services rendered and the patient's ability to pay. He should neither pay nor receive a commission for referral of patients. Drugs, remedies or appliances may be dispensed or supplied by the physician provided it is in the best interests of the patient.

8. A physician should seek consultation upon request, in doubtful or difficult cases, or whenever it appears that the quality of medical service may be enhanced thereby.

9. A physician may not reveal the confidences entrusted to him in the course of medical attendance, or the deficiencies he may observe in the character of patients, unless he is required to do so by law or unless it becomes necessary in order to protect the welfare of the individual or of the community.

10. The honored ideals of the medical profession imply that the responsibilities of the physician extend not only to the individual, but also to society where these responsibilities deserve his interest and participation in activities which have the purpose of improving both the health and the well-being of the individual and the community.

The sections to follow will serve to explain and develop these ten general principles.

Service to Humanity

The purpose of the medical profession is to "render service to humanity with full respect to the dignity of man." Thus the role of each physician and supporting staff is to provide health care to the best of their combined abilities and, in so doing, to treat and regard the patient humanely. This statement rejects the notion of treating the patient as a disease entity or body part rather than as a human being with a complex scope of sensibilities.

Physicians and their staffs are thus called upon to practice holistic medicine—to treat the patient in his totality. Administering to the patient in this sense implies that a respect for and attention to the patient's intellectual, emotional, spiritual, psychological, and physiological states are required in fulfilling the ethical goals of the medical profession.

Continued Pursuit of Excellence

The physician's training and education do not end with formal schooling. He or she is charged with the lifelong task of maintaining skills and increasing knowledge. While this process applies to all professionals, it may be argued that since the ramifications of a physician practicing dated medicine are more serious than those of, say, a tax accountant who missed some recent adjustment in the tax laws, this particular ethical principle is indeed critical for the physician.

Physicians usually commit themselves to the reading of journals and current medical textbooks, to attendance of conferences, and to accommodation of continuing education units. To a great extent, the physician assumes this responsibility at the expense of interrupting the practice of medicine. Thus the pursuit of this principle may carry a corresponding loss of income. This principle implies that while the patient has the right to expect reasonably current modes of medical practice, the physician has the obligation to provide up-to-date, well-informed care for as long as he intends to function as a medical practitioner.

Scientific Methods of Healing

Physicians practice the art of healing which is based upon a scientifically verifiable model of medicine. As such their professional responsibilities require that they practice within the confines of their understanding of medical practices, and that they assist, if possible, in the dynamic evolution of that model by contributing their own learning experiences to the shared body of knowledge.

It would be unethical for physicians to extend their diagnosis to areas which had no basis in scientific prediction or to adopt methods with a nonscientific basis. This principle further calls upon the physician to reject any professional association with individuals professing the use of nonscientific methods. This ethical code of behavior serves to protect the physician, the patient, and the integrity of the medical profession.

Upholding the Profession

The physician assumes the responsibility of maintaining the "dignity and honor of the profession." Operationally, the ethical behavior implied is two-dimensional. On the one hand, the physician must demonstrate the utmost confidence in and respect for colleagues, and must never indiscriminately criticize the approaches or methodologies of another physician in public. On the other hand, he must do everything that is within his power to expose any illegal or unethical behavior by fellow physicians.

Since the practice of medicine is so technically complex, and at the same time held in high esteem by the general public, physicians themselves are charged with the heavy burden of monitoring and maintaining the competent and ethical practice of their own profession. In this way the public is protected from negligent or harmful medical practice, and society's faith in the profession remains intact.

Responsibility to a Patient

Under normal circumstances, physicians are free to choose their patients. By virtue of office location, specialty, or the determination of optimal practice size, physicians may effectively refuse to undertake the care of persons requesting their services. It is also acceptable for a physician to suggest to a regular patient that he would be better served by a different physician. Withdrawal from the rendering of services necessitates that the patient be duly informed of the decision. This is both an ethical and a legal responsibility. In emergencies, however, the physician should care for the patient to the best of his or her ability until other adequate medical care becomes available.

Physicians cannot neglect patients entrusted to their care. They can discontinue service upon notifying the patient, as indicated earlier, but the code of ethical behavior reminds physicians that they may not delay or abandon patient care according to their own preferences. Moreover, this principle states that solicitation of patients is unethical. Therefore, advertisements or other urgings are not acceptable.

Appropriate Terms and Conditions

Physicians must constantly strive to ensure that they are practicing within an environment which supports both the practice of quality medical care and the continuation of ethical behavior.

In practical terms this principle implies that physicians should not associate with an organization (hospital or other) which places pressures upon them to practice medicine of inferior quality or to compromise their own moral code. Nor should the physician enter into a contract with a patient which would result in the same outcome.

Physicians must avoid all situations which dictate that their medical practices be any other than those which they would consider to be fully competent and morally acceptable.

Income for Direct Services

The physician's income should be earned in exchange for direct medical services rendered either by him or by an individual in his employ and under supervision. Fees should be based upon the general market value of the particular services and upon the patient's ability to pay. With third party intervention, such as insurance, the patient's ability to pay has become an obscured consideration. Insurance fee schedules influence physician charges.

Physicians should not compensate each other for referrals or consultations, thereby supplementing their income for favors bestowed or received. Nor should the physician enter the general business of supplying drugs or appliances unless dispensing these items provides a necessary service to the patient.

This principle emphasizes that the physician's fees should be compatible with the services provided and implies that fee-splitting or kickback is unethical. Fee-splitting is another term for the sharing of fees when one physician refers a patient to another doctor and then receives a portion of the patient's fee.

Consulting with Fellow Physicians

This principle sets forth a code of ethical behavior governing consultation. Whenever a physician encounters diagnostic or treatment difficulties that appear beyond the scope of his or her experience or knowledge, or when a reasonable doubt arises and a second opinion is desired, the physician should willingly consult with colleagues or specialists known to be knowledgeable and skillful in the particular area in question.

In the event that a patient requests a second opinion, physicians should also pursue a consulting relationship regardless of their own feelings concerning the necessity of the consultation. Physicians must never allow the fact that a patient requested a second opinion to influence their opinion of the patient or their approach to the case. The patient retains the right to acquire a consensus in treatment or diagnostic methodology.

The physician who encourages patients to seek a second opinion in cases where diagnosis or treatment poses severe consequences is generally regarded as showing integrity and high moral character.

Confidentiality

Often the information gained by a physician in the diagnosis or treatment of a case could be deleterious to the patient. Character flaws, personality problems, drug and alcohol addiction, and other potentially volatile information are often divulged in the physician's office. The ethical code dictates confidentiality in all patient-doctor exchanges.

Unless they are required by law or believe that the process of sharing the information obtained would protect society or the patient from serious harm, physicians may not reveal the content of private conversations.

Social Responsibility

While the ethical practitioner of medicine has a series of responsibilities to individual patients, these responsibilities also apply to society at large. This principle of social responsibility implies that physicians of moral character will contribute to the general welfare of their communities. If physicians can benefit society by the prudent application of their professional knowledge, it is their obligation to do so.

The code of ethical behavior here described contains the expectation that physicians will actively participate in community activities and that their involvement will reflect the ideals and ethics esteemed by the profession.

A CODE OF ETHICS FOR THE MEDICAL ASSISTANT

Just as the AMA has adopted a code of ethics for physicians, the American Association of Medical Assistants has recently composed a set of principles for MAs.

1. The medical assistant must render service to humanity with full respect for the dignity of the person.

   MAs should approach each individual with a positive and humanitarian attitude which demonstrates a high regard for his or her uniqueness.

2. The medical assistant must respect confidential information gained through employment unless legally authorized or required by responsible performance of duty to divulge such information.

   Confidentiality is perhaps the most easily and most often breached principle. Yet this is the single most observable aspect of respect for human dignity. The patient's right to privacy must be guarded by the physician, the staff, and the MA.

3. The medical assistant must uphold the honor and high principles of the profession and accept its disciplines.

   MAs should continually act to foster respect for the medical profession. Self-control is mandated by the nature of the profession.

4. The medical assistant must seek to continually improve the knowledge and skills of medical assisting for the benefit of patients and professional colleagues.

   Membership at the national, state, and local levels of the profession reflects the MA's pursuit of excellence. Advanced training, coursework, and the earning of continuing education credits are important aspects of an ongoing effort to build skills.

5. The medical assistant must participate in additional service activities which aim toward improving the health and well-being of the community.

   MAs have a responsibility to aid in the advancement of their communities. To this end they should involve themselves in voluntary work which serves to promote the ideals of the profession.

In addition to upholding the ethical principles of the physician, medical assistants must strive to understand and practice the principles of their profession.

PRACTICAL CONSIDERATIONS FOR THE MEDICAL ASSISTANT

The reader is about to leave the study of administrative considerations and move into the clinical half of this book, the area that many MAs consider more interesting. There is a great danger, however, in overlooking a vitally important aspect of being a good medical assistant—that of upholding medical ethics in practice.

It is quite natural to imagine the skilled MA as a person who researches the literature in a medical library, or comforts a young child, or takes a blood pressure accurately. But it is equally important, in a practical sense, that the skilled MA understand the ethical considerations involved in being a member of the medical team.

Suppose, for example, that you learn at the office that a patient, Mrs. Smith, has been drinking too much and that the doctor is treating this problem. How will you react the following week when you are at a party with your friends and one of them mentions that Mrs. Smith is her next door neighbor? Will you say something about her "drinking problem"? You might rationalize this behavior by concluding that you only told one person and that the person is a close and trusted friend. But no matter how you explain your behavior, you will have been unethical.

Being a supporter of the physician's ethics is at times problematic. MAs must struggle to understand and accurately interpret the basics of medical ethics. Then they must constantly guard against the many temptations to act improperly. In the real world these theoretical issues quickly become difficult practical problems.

CONTEMPORARY ISSUES

Because of the dynamic nature of society and of the field of medicine itself, new moral-medical issues of a problematic nature are constantly arising. Typical contemporary examples include abortion on demand, genetic engineering, euthanasia, and behavior control.

Perhaps the greatest problem in dealing with these kinds of issues is that they may seem to be immoral when viewed from the perspective of particular religious beliefs. Taken in light of the fact that many MAs and other allied medical personnel are trained in colleges and universities which are religiously affiliated, the difficulty in dealing with issues which challenge both personal and institutional value systems grows enormously. How is an MA who believes that abortion is morally wrong to cope with the process of abortion during her medical career? And even more important, how will the MA who believes that abortion is morally right deal with abortion?

It is not possible to present specific moral precepts within the context of this discussion. Even if they could be fully presented, such precepts would offer no conclusive answers to complex moral-medical questions. There is, however, a logical guide to the preservation of ones unique system of ethics:

1. MAs should not be forced to change their moral convictions because of their professional training. Even if there is controversy regarding the "rightness" of an issue, MAs should hold to their convictions.

2. MAs should not attempt to force their beliefs upon other individuals. If there is a moral controversy regarding an issue, they must allow for persons with opposing beliefs.

3. MAs should attempt to find employment in an environment which does not continually challenge their moral positions. This is perhaps the key to job satisfaction for professionals.

In issues of morality there are no clear lines. Most of the controversies arise out of difficult interpretations. It is relatively easy to deal with the more obvious cases, such as "should the Roman Catholic MA work in an abortion clinic?" Clearly this would challenge her moral position. But how should the MA react to a patient who is unconscious, critically needing a blood transfusion, but of a religious conviction which doesn't allow blood transfusions? Would you save the patient by violating his or her beliefs? In issues such as this one the answers are not all clear. They are difficult issues which mix law and morality with the practice of medicine.

As an MA you will find these issues within medicine to be both dynamic and challenging. The question of ethics relative to the contemporary issues of medicine will never be settled. There will, however, be a continuous evolution of thinking about appropriate ethical and moral solutions to various issues. The ongoing task for the MA will be one of participation in an active role as problem solver, thinker, and evaluator.

SUMMARY

The most difficult practical aspect of ethics is that no one seems to notice or reward ethical behavior. An accurate temperature reading or a well-composed letter is a monument to the MA. Ethical behavior, however, is simply expected.

For the MA who hopes to provide quality assistance in the practice of medicine and become a valued member of the office medical team professional ethics is a prerequisite.

APPLICATION EXERCISES

To participate in the following classroom exercise, each student should have several sheets of paper and a pen.

1. The class should be divided into groups of four or five students.

2. Working in groups, each student should participate in a discussion which leads to an example of how an MA could contribute to one of the principles of medical ethics. (Your instructor will divide up the ten principles of medical ethics among the classroom groups.)

3. When each group is confident that it has identified a good example of practicing a particular principle, the members should prepare a short (3- to 5-minute) presentation.

4. One member of each group should be appointed to share the group's example with the entire class.

5. Using the same group format, each group should choose one of the following moral-medical issues:

   a. genetic engineering
   b. abortion

c. behavior control/behavior modification

d. euthanasia

e. artificial maintenance of life (use of life support devices)

6. Group members should discuss their chosen issue and present a brief (3- to 5-minute) synopsis to the class.

7. Your instructor will lead a class discussion and attempt to answer questions.

COMPLETING THE LEARNING LOOP

Students of medical assisting do not have to wait until they begin to function as office assistants to become ethical professionals. Medical ethics asks that the physician choose a standard of behavior which is well above that which is expected or required by law. Perhaps the MA could best prepare for a career in the physician's office by attempting to set standards of personal behavior which are higher than those which are expected of a student. This is a difficult task because you will be seeing other students, either in training as MAs or for other professions, whose behavior is clearly not ethical. But if you want to separate yourself from the crowd—to become the best MA you can become—the task is well worth the effort.

BIBLIOGRAPHY

Brody, H.: *Ethical Decisions in Medicine.* Little, Brown, Boston, 1976.
Campbell, A. V.: *Moral Dilemmas in Medicine.* Churchill Livingstone, New York, 1972.
Fromer, M. J.: *Ethical Issues in Health Care.* C. V. Mosby, St. Louis, 1981.
Hiller, M. D.: *Medical Ethics and the Law.* Ballinger, Cambridge, Mass., 1980.
Hunt, R., and Arras, J.: *Ethical Issues in Modern Medicine.* Mayfield, Palo Alto, Cal., 1977.
McFadden, C. J.: *Medical Ethics,* ed. 6. F. A. Davis, Philadelphia. 1967.
Ramsey, P.: *The Patient as a Person.* Yale University Press, New Haven, Conn., 1970.
Walters, L. (ed.): *Bibliography of Bioethics.* Gale, Detroit, 1975.

THE CLINICAL MEDICAL ASSISTANT: THEORY AND PRACTICE

5

PREPARING FOR THE PHYSICAL EXAMINATION

The physical examination is the cornerstone of office medicine. Like most other activities, a physical examination will be most effective when it is properly planned. The medical assistant should be prepared to aid both the physician and the patient by understanding the procedures involved and by readying the patient and all needed office equipment for the examination.

UNIT OBJECTIVES

Upon completion of this unit you will be able to:

1. Assist the physician in the preliminary interview and history.

2. List the skills required of an interviewer.

3. List, explain, and measure the vital signs, height, and weight.

4. Prepare the patient for the physical examination.

CHAPTER 15

THE PATIENT INTERVIEW AND HISTORY

SPECIFIC OBJECTIVES

Upon completion of this chapter you will be prepared to:

1. Assist the physician in the patient interview and history.
2. Provide resource materials for patients.
3. Interview patients, thus providing a screening process for the physician.
4. Take a patient history.
5. Build and maintain the patient file.

INTRODUCTION

In the generic sense, the first and most fundamentally important step in the clinical process is the patient history and interview. Essentially these can be thought of as two different kinds of procedures.

The *history* is a systematic and thorough discussion and record of all relevant past medical data which may affect the diagnosis or treatment of a particular patient. Generally, the history is taken only one time, but is then filed and updated during subsequent visits and treatments.

The *interview* is the preliminary screening which takes place at the beginning of each office visit. It is during the interview that the patient will be asked to relate specific complaints, concerns, or the particular reason for the visit. If the office visit is one of an outgoing system of visits, the interview can be used to process information concerning progress since the last such visit.

The purpose of this chapter is to introduce the medical assistant to both the concepts and techniques of the interview and history.

THE ROLE OF THE MEDICAL ASSISTANT

Throughout this chapter the approach will be to present the mechanics of patient interviewing and history-taking as they might essentially be viewed by the physician. This is not because medical assistants are expected to take the role of the physician in the interviewing or history-taking process, but it is much easier for MAs to take on a partial responsibility when they understand the entire system. In actual practice the medical assistant will have to understand and conform to the wishes of the doctor. This approach will be to teach interviewing and history-taking as an overall process.

Physicians basically fall into three categories relative to actual practice mechanics. Each of these approaches is discussed below.

The Physician-Only Approach

Some doctors prefer to carry out all interviewing and history-taking themselves. They feel that the patient should provide information only once, and that this information should be directed to the physician. Many specialists take this approach because they feel that the diagnostic power of the physician must be utilized in order to make the proper use of patient information. Some physicians may feel that when a patient divulges information to two different individuals he may forget exactly to whom he told what, and then leave out important bits of information.

If medical assistants work for physicians whose preference is for this kind of approach, they need to respect his or her wishes and discourage patients from communicating information which would be important to the diagnostic interview or history. This needs to be done in a gentle but firm way which doesn't lead the patient to feel that the MA is not interested. The medical assistant should suggest that patients collect their thoughts so that these might later be shared with the physician. The MA might offer to discuss any questions or concerns with the patient after the physician has reviewed the case. This will help to establish effective lines of communication between the patient and medical assistant, while respecting the philosophy of the physician.

The Physician-Medical Team Approach

Some physicians feel that "two heads are better than one" in the sense that a history given twice (to two separate individuals), or an interview done twice, is more likely to divulge important data. This does not suggest that the medical assistant will be taking over the responsibility for this aspect of medical care; rather the MA will be cooperating with the doctor in gathering information.

Generally, physicians will ask the medical assistant to precede them in the process. The advantages to this approach are quite clear. First, the patient has the opportunity to "practice" giving his information to the medical assistant. This may help the patient to become more comfortable and skillful at relating pertinent data. The MA can assist in this process by helping the patient to focus upon critical issues. Then when the physician does conduct an interview with the patient, he will benefit by the learning/practicing process which has already taken place.

Physicians who prefer to take a team approach will generally spend substantial time training their assistants in interviewing methods and procedures. Medical assistants who work for such a physician must make every effort to understand the physician's preferences and must pattern their approaches to facilitate the doctor's needs. Team-oriented physicians will probably want to have a conference with the medical assistant before they see the patient so that they can learn what insights the MA has gained and refer to notes or forms which have been completed.

The Patient-Directed Approach

A technique which has grown in popularity, especially in the process of history-taking, is the patient-directed approach. Here the patient is given a form to complete containing the critical aspects of his own history. Several different standardized forms are available, or the doctor may prefer to design one.

If medical assistants function within this framework, they should serve as patient facilitators and resource persons, providing whatever assistance is needed for the patient to complete the particular format which is required.

MEDICAL INTERVIEWING SKILLS

Before dealing with the nature of the specific materials or information which is to be exchanged during an interview or history, it is essential that the basic skills required by the interviewer be discussed.

The Psychophysical Presence

Before beginning an interview it is a good practice to stop for a few seconds outside the interview room and collect ones thoughts carefully. The object is to shed all previous concerns and anxieties in order to devote full attention to the current patient.

The interviewer should appear to be physically as well as psychologically fresh. The attitude of the interviewer should be professional and not suggestive of tiredness or disinterest. The clothing and grooming must be innocuous, permitting patients to focus upon their own needs rather than on the unusual appearance of the interviewer.

Observational Skills

Medical assistants should strive to use all of their senses during the interview process. Adding visual and contact senses to the traditional listening mode can add a great deal to the forthcoming information value. Does the patient appear to be at ease? Is the patient visibly ill or otherwise distressed? Observation of posture, grooming, clarity of expression, and other attributes may assist in the diagnosis. All of these bits of information should be summarized and compiled before making a final report to the physician.

Verbal Tactics

Naturally the common medium for interviewing is verbal. Patients discuss their problems, while interviewers probe with questions. A series of six interviewing guidelines designed to assist in the medical context is given below.

1. *The interviewer must be nonjudgmental.*

   There is no quicker way to destroy the continuity of a conversation between a medical assistant and a patient than for the MA to offer judgments. Whether positive or negative, judgments by the interviewer interfere with the objectivity of the information transfer process. Negative feedback tends to stifle the patient. Positive feedback sends the patient onto meaningless tangents. The medical assistant/interviewer needs to *listen, ask probing questions,* and *record answers when appropriate.* But she should *never pass judgment.*

   Patient: "Whenever I'm hungry at night I have a bowl of ice cream with chocolate syrup."

   Incorrect response: "Well, you know that you'll never lose weight like that."

   Correct response: "What size serving do you usually eat, Mrs. Smith?"

2. *Interrupt long statements with probing questions.*

   Many times patients begin a dialogue or description which becomes dysfunctionally long. After a few minutes they will need some structure as well as a positive indication that the medical assistant is really listening. When the patient has reached such a point, he will generally begin to drift from the main theme. This is the appropriate time for the interviewer to interrupt with a probe.

3. *Use short, probing questions.*

   When the medical assistant does interrupt to provide a transitional place in dialogue, she should guard against adding to the patient's confusion by drifting off onto a new tangent. The best approach is to use brief probing questions such as:

    a. "Could you clarify that?"
    b. "Please describe that more specifically?"
    c. "How often did it happen?"
    d. "How did you feel about it?"

These probes serve to provide a needed structure in the dialogue. They help the interviewer to clarify important points and slow the process at critical events so that the interviewer can absorb them. In addition they provide a kind of verbal feedback which assures the patient that the interviewer is really listening.

4. *Respond with interest.*

During the process of probing it is important for the medical assistant to demonstrate interest in the patient. Much of the training of MA/interviewers would lead them to suspect that they should not get emotionally involved with the patient. MAs should take a scientific and rational approach, guarding against making uneducated guesses or offering too much information. But there is a clear danger that by taking this approach the medical assistant might suggest a lack of interest, thus "turning the patient off."

Medical assistants should use their probes to demonstrate attentiveness and interest to the patient. This can be accomplished by adding phases such as "That's very interesting" or "I'm not sure that I understood" to the probes which were previously discussed.

5. *Use basic questions which the patient will understand.*

The medical assistant should attempt to remember that the patient is relatively untrained in medical terminology and office procedures. All questions should be developed in language and structure which the patient can easily understand and deal with.

6. *"Mirror" the patient's important statements.*

In addition to interrupting the patient with an occasional probing question, the medical assistant/interviewer should make a practice of looking for and "mirroring" critical statements. During the course of discussion the patient will ultimately come to two or three critical events. These are, in the judgment of the medical assistant, the most important aspects of the description—the particular bits of information which must be recorded and transmitted to the physician.

    To ensure that the quality of this information is maximized, the medical assistant should attempt to "mirror" the patient's statements by stopping the conversation and repeating the information for the patient to listen to.

Patient: "... and every time that I ate red meat during a meal I would wake up during the evening with a severe stomach ache."

MA: "Just a moment, let me see if I understand you. Each time you eat red meat you are awakened during the evening because of stomach pain?"

Pinpointing

Both diagnostic and therapeutic procedures require the gathering of accurate data during patient interviewing. To facilitate the usefulness of such information, the medical assistant should develop skills which lead to the "pinpointing" of specific symptoms or other medical clues. Pinpointing is the process of moving language from the general to the specific. A pinpointed statement is one which is clear, observable, and accountable.

Below is an example of a patient description which is changed from a vague or general state to a more precise and useful "pinpointed" perspective:

Vague: "It seems that I always have this stupid headache. I must use a ton of aspirin every year. Even my kids have noticed that I'm not myself."

Pinpointed: "I have been bothered by headaches lately. During the past two weeks I have had six headaches. Three of these were so severe that I had to take aspirin; and even my children noticed that I was ill."

Converting a patient's vague and generalized statements into pinpointed and qualified descriptions will assist the physician in understanding both the nature and severity of a particular problem. Thus the role of the medical assistant during patient interaction is to gently move the patient toward more specific language. In most cases, once patients begin to grasp the nature of the pinpointing process, they will automatically begin to do their own pinpointing, thus making the MA's task easier.

The medical assistant should attempt to use probes whenever the interviewee begins to describe an important symptom or a related event. The object is to slow the patient down at the critical places so that he is forced to focus upon these. Once the critical events have been clearly described, the MA should attempt to help the patient count the frequency of these issues. If the patient is not able to remember accurately, the medical assistant should involve the patient in keeping a record of such events in the future. An additional but important aspect of pinpointing is the elimination of meaningless or emotional expletives and the control of exaggeration.

Incorrect: "I think that I have had this miserable cold for a year!"

Correct: "I have had a throat and nasal congestion for the past eight days."

For the medical assistant, the pinpointing process is very clearly an interpersonal interviewing skill. She must very gently but persistently guide the patient-interviewee toward specific, accurate, and quantified descriptions.

THE PATIENT INTERVIEW

Each time the patient visits the office, an interview will take place, usually before the diagnostic or treatment procedure.

The content and process of the interview itself are just as important as the skills which are utilized by the interviewer. Perhaps the most critical aspects of the interview are related to patient confidentiality and privacy. Many patients have concerns or reservations about revealing the details of their illness. Thus the interview should be conducted in a private area which is removed from office traffic. The approach should be time-efficient without giving the patient an impression that there is a "rush" to get finished.

During the interview the following structure should be followed: *

1. *What is the chief complaint?*

   Patients should be encouraged to begin the interview by relating the chief complaint in their own words. The complaints should be articulated with the use of pinpointed symptoms.

2. *What is the history of this illness?*

   Patients should be allowed to develop a narrative of how the chief complaint became a particular problem and the events or symptoms which seem to be associated with it.

3. *How long has the complaint been present?*

   The duration of the illness should be expressed in accurate terms.

4. *In what physical area is the problem localized?*

   Patients should accurately describe the specific location which is affected. If more than one area is involved, how are these interacting?

5. *How are the symptoms progressing?*

   Are the symptoms moving throughout the body? Did the trouble develop suddenly or slowly?

6. *What is the character of the symptoms?*

   Is the complaint best described as a discomfort, a dull ache, or a severe pain? Do these symptoms come and go suddenly or slowly?

7. *How is the complaint related to activity?*

   Can the patient's problems be linked with a particular activity such as sleeping, eating, or walking?

Once these seven major steps have been completed, the interviewer should conclude by discussing two general issues. First she or he should try to determine what, if any, treatment has been attempted in the past, either by other physicians or by the patient. Second, an attempt should be made to learn the general effects of the problem—physical, psychological, and social. The interviewer should inquire about the patient's general physical condition, including weight, sleep habits, energy level, and state of mind, and about the patient's family and work life.

All of this information should be recorded for further study by the physician and subsequent inclusion in the patient's file. Some physicians prefer to use a standardized interview

---

* Suggested by Delp and Manning: *Major's Physical Diagnosis*. W. B. Saunders, Philadelphia, 1968.

form such as the one shown in Figure 15-1. Others may record interview data on a form of their own design or on plain paper.

THE PATIENT HISTORY

The general history is taken during the patient's first office visit. The basic steps discussed below comprise the typical format or structure for taking the history.

The Patient Description and Narrative

The first step in the recorded history should be to accumulate a brief package of information which generally describes the patient. The intent here should not be to list symptoms or elaborate upon specific disorders, but rather to describe the "whole person" including his

Patient _____   Date _____

                                               Interviewer _____

1. Chief Complaint:

2. History:

3. Length of Complaint:

4. Physical Area Affected:

5. Progress of Symptoms:

6. Character of Symptoms:

7. Problems with Basic Activities:

8. Miscellaneous:

FIGURE 15-1. A standardized interview form.

personality, his general appearance, and his mental status. This is accomplished with two basic steps: the relevant demographic data and a brief descriptive abstract. A typical example appears below.

Demographic Data:

Name: George Adams
Birth Date: March 12, 1941
Marital Status: Married
Children: Darlene (16), Harry (12), Albert (6)
Occupation: High School Teacher—Math.
Educational Level: Master's degree

Descriptive Abstract:

Teaches math at Central High, and appears to enjoy his work. In addition he is the school's head baseball coach. During the summer George paints houses for extra income. His total annual earnings are $21,000, and his wife works part-time as a substitute teacher. The entire family engages in his favorite hobbies of camping and fishing. George was raised a Baptist. His father was a factory worker, his mother a housewife.

In most cases the interviewer will take the demographic information at the beginning of the interview but will wait until the end of the process to sit down and formulate the narrative. During subsequent visits the physician may wish to refer to the narrative. Often a sudden change in emotional status or lifestyle will be made apparent from the information contained in this narrative. Such data may help the physician to "key in" on the important aspects of a patient's life as these may contribute to the patient's condition.

Basic Habits

The history procedure should attempt to identify personal habits. The purpose is to gain insights into the mode of living of the patient so that subsequent connections can be drawn between medical problems and the patient's lifestyle. The interviewer should cover the following aspects:

1. *Diet and Nutrition.* What kinds of foods are eaten and in what volume: how much meat, processed food, "junk" food?

2. *Patterns of Weight.* Is the weight satisfactory to the patient. Is it stable? If it fluctuates over the years, by how much?

3. *Exercise.* Does the patient engage in regular exercise? How much, what type, how often?

4. *Smoking.* If the patient smokes, how much and what type of materials (pipes, cigars, cigarettes)?

5. *Drinking.* What kind of alcoholic beverages are used, and in what quantity?

6. *Sleeping.* Does the patient have regular sleep habits? If so, how many hours per day does he sleep?

7. *Drugs.* Which legal or illegal drugs are used on a regular basis (include vitamins, aspirin, etc.)?

Family History

Since many diseases seem to follow particular families, it is important to trace the family history as a part of the patient history. The point here is not to establish the genetic as opposed to the social influences of particular diseases such as diabetes or cancer, but rather to establish existing familial patterns.

The patient should be asked to describe both parents in a general manner. The patient should attempt to focus upon their general health and conclude with their age at the time of death and its cause (if appropriate). If the father ultimately died of heart failure, for example, it would be useful to know if he was overweight and if he smoked or exercised on a regular basis. Once the health patterns of both parents have been established, the patient should be asked to describe his maternal and paternal grandparents, as well as any brothers and sisters.

Past Illnesses

The patient should be asked to provide a record of all past illnesses, including injuries. There is no need to detail common colds or minor flu viruses, but a note as to the patient's basic tendencies would be in order. For example, a patient may report that he gets an average of two minor colds per year.

The list should include infant and childhood diseases (with approximate dates), incidence of pneumonia, hospitalization, operations, chronic conditions such as arthritis, pregnancies, hayfever, allergies, and drug sensitivities.

Self-Perception

To put the entire history in perspective, it is generally useful to ask the patient a leading question such as, "How would you describe your general health at this time?" and then record the answer. This procedure will give the physician an excellent insight into the patient's self-perception. Such a perspective may be important in designing a treatment or diagnosing a problem.

The patient who puts on a "tough-guy" image might be expected to overlook or negate symptoms of pain or discomfort. Another patient with a more fragile self-concept may overstate similar problems.

Basic Systems

The final step in the history-taking procedure is the assessment of each of the major body systems and the symptoms which may be associated with them. These include:

1. *Head:* headaches, pains, tension.

2. *Eyes:* visual problems, strain, infections.

3. *Ears, nose and throat:* hearing problems, infections, roughness, congestion, sinus.

4. *Mouth:* dental and/or gum disease, sores, bleeding.

5. *Cardiovascular system:* palpitations, dizziness, exhaustion, pain, high or low blood pressure.

6. *Respiratory system:* shortness of breath, breathing irregularities, asthma, discharge or expectorant.

7. *Urinary system:* voiding habits, discharges, frequency, strongness of urine, sexual habits.

8. *Gastrointestinal system:* dietary habits, weight changes, stomach disorders, indigestion, hunger pains, nausea, types of stools, bowel movements, hemorrhoids.

9. *Menstrual cycle:* interval, regularity, discharge.

10. *Neurological system:* dizziness, weakness, sporadic loss of coordination, loss of memory or difficulty in concentrating.

11. *Psychological assessment:* state of mental health, nervousness, symptoms of distress.

With each subsystem the medical assistant/interviewer should direct the patient's attention to that particular area and inquire as to the history, evolution, and present condition of symptoms which are connected.

Interviewer: "Now that we have some information about your urinary system, what can you tell me about your stomach and bowel habits? Why don't you begin by discussing your day-to-day eating habits and how your stomach reacts to various foods."

Patient: "Well, I used to eat quite a lot, but lately I've had to cut down because I'm watching my weight. I can eat just about anything I want with the exception of fried foods which seem to give me indigestion."

Interviewer: "Exactly which foods do this to you?"

Patient: "Well, I've noticed that fried potatoes and meats, especially hamburgers, cause quite a bit of stomach pain."

Interviewer: "Does this happen every single time you eat fried food?"

Patient: "I would say about 80 percent of the time."

Interviewer: "How about your bowel habits?"

Patient: "Well, I seem to be quite regular with normal stools. I rarely have trouble with diarrhea or constipation."

Interviewer: "Do you ever experience nausea? Have you had any trouble with hemorrhoids? Do you have problems with indigestion?"

When the medical assistant strikes upon a particular dysfunction, the topic should be pursued, as in the interview above, in an attempt to gain as many insights as possible.

RECORDING THE HISTORY

While the basic framework for taking the history may be a scientifically designed process which is generally found to contain the important or critical parameters of health, the recording of data is an art. The most obvious problem is that of condensing the patient's conversation into a brief and useful record. All of this must take place while the medical assistant is talking and listening.

The key to developing this skill is practice. The MA must learn to listen for key words and concepts, write these down during the interaction with the patient, and then return to the history at a later time to "fill in the blanks." It is essential that the interviewer not wait too long before returning to the history, or important information may escape the process.

The physical record itself should be neat, easy to read, and well-organized. Generally this means that the approach to history-taking should be consistent. A good history facilitates the continued efficient use of the history portion of the file, thus enhancing medical care.

There are a number of different approaches to the format itself. Some physicians prefer to use either a "plain paper" approach or a simple framework such as the one shown in Figure 15-2, whose purpose is to keep the interviewer on track and make sure that nothing is omitted. It is likely that a particular physician may design a format which is pleasing to him and then continue using it. Other physicians prefer a standardized form. Whatever the physician's preference, medical assistants must make an effort to adapt themselves and their approaches to the doctor's needs.

THE NEEDS OF SPECIALISTS

If medical assistants find themselves working for a specialist rather than a family practice physician or internist, they will probably discover that the particular focus of specialized medical care requires some rather substantial deviations from the history-taking approach which has been discussed here. Cardiologists or orthopedists, for example, will probably be interested in a more specific set of symptoms than the family practitioner, and, in fact, they will generally not want to spend time dealing with the broad categories which were previously developed. It is quite likely that medical assistants who aid these specialists will *not* be directly involved in interviewing and history-taking per se.

```
┌──────────────────────────────────────────────────────────┐
│                                                          │
│                   INTERVIEWER'S GUIDE                    │
│                                                          │
│                                                          │
│      1. Patient Description and Narrative                │
│      2. Basic Habits                                     │
│           a. diet                                        │
│           b. exercise                                    │
│           c. smoking, drinking                           │
│           d. sleep                                       │
│           e. drugs                                       │
│      3. Family History                                   │
│      4. Past Illnesses                                   │
│      5. Self-Perception                                  │
│      6. Basic Systems                                    │
│           a. eyes, ears, nose, throat, mouth             │
│           b. cardiovascular                              │
│           c. respiratory                                 │
│           d. urinary                                     │
│           e. gastrointestinal                            │
│           f. menstrual cycle                             │
│           g. neurologic                                  │
│           h. psychological assessment                    │
│                                                          │
└──────────────────────────────────────────────────────────┘
```

FIGURE 15-2. A history recording framework.

BUILDING THE MEDICAL FILE

The patient history and subsequent interviews comprise the essence of a medical file. The history is placed in the patient's folder so that each time he or she is seen, the physician may take a moment to refresh his memory as to the particular medical history. To be effective, however, the patient file must be dynamic. It should represent not only the past history of a patient, but also the progress of that patient while under the physician's care.

During each office visit an interview should be carried out, recorded, and added to the file data. This record of interviews will provide a future history of each patient's medical care, including overall observations, measurements which are carried out during a typical office visit, and any treatments which are prescribed. It is the role of the medical assistant to support the physician in the continued performance of this duty.

SUMMARY

As a medical assistant, you may be expected to serve as the preliminary or screening person during patient interviews. You may also be asked to assist in the taking of medical histories. Medical assistant/interviewers play a vital role in the delivery of health services. They act as a sounding board and confidante to patients. Moreover, they help patients communicate their problems and concerns to the physician.

APPLICATION EXERCISES

To prepare for this classroom exercise each student will be required to have a pen and several sheets of paper.

1. The class will be divided into groups of three students.

2. Within each group of three, students will take turns playing the role of interviewer, patient, and observer.

3. During each of three rounds, the interviewers will take complete case histories of the patients, while the observer watches carefully, noting the strong and weak points of the interviewer on the form provided below. The interviewer should use the suggested framework shown in Figure 15-2, and record the history on plain paper.

4. After the exercise the instructor will lead a discussion in which the whole class will attempt to summarize the important notes made by the observers.

Observer Rating Form: Patient History

Procedure: Using the space below, record interviewer strategies which were effective in gaining information, and those which were ineffective and tended to obscure information.

Effective Strategies	*Ineffective Strategies*
1.	1.
2.	2.
3.	3.
4.	4.
5.	5.

COMPLETING THE LEARNING LOOP

As a student you can begin to practice your newly acquired interviewing skills. When you talk to or counsel your friends or are involved in discussions with your teachers, try to apply the communications skills which have been suggested throughout the chapter. If you begin now to work through this important learning process, you will bring a higher level of professional skill to your first position as a medical assistant.

BIBLIOGRAPHY

Berne, E.: *Principles of Group Treatment.* Grove Press, New York, 1966.

DeGowin, E. L., and DeGowin, R. L.: *Bedside Diagnostic Examination,* ed. 3. Macmillan, New York, 1976.

Delp, M. H., and Manning, R. T.: *Major's Physical Diagnosis.* W. B. Saunders, Philadelphia, 1968.

Neelan, F. A., and Ellis, G. J.: *A Syllabus of Problem Oriented Patient Care.* Little, Brown, Boston, 1974.

Thompson, D.: *Managing People by Influencing Behavior.* C. V. Mosby, St. Louis, 1978.

16

THE VITAL SIGNS, HEIGHT, AND WEIGHT

SPECIFIC OBJECTIVES

Upon completion of this chapter you will be able to:

1. List and explain the vital signs.
2. Perform the vital signs.
3. Measure height and weight.
4. Care for the equipment used.
5. Define all relevant terms.

INTRODUCTION

A thorough understanding of both the physiologic and measurement aspects of the vital signs, height, and weight is the foundation of clinical medical assisting. The purpose of this chapter is to introduce these concepts to the student medical assistant. The discussion is divided into five distinct sections: (1) body temperature; (2) pulse; (3) respiration; (4) blood pressure; (5) height and weight. Each section will contain a separate statement of specific skills objectives.

The vital signs, also known as cardinal signs, are measurements which indicate the state of health of the human body. "Vital" comes from the Latin *vita* meaning life. The vital signs are indications of the condition of life. In a state of well-being all the vital signs—body temperature, pulse rate, respiratory rate (TPR), and blood pressure (BP)—will fall within an average range. In a state of ill health these same signs will vary, depending on the cause, and fall below or above the average range. Factors other than disease can sometimes cause fluctuations of these signs. Environmental changes, activity, and emotional state greatly influence the vital signs. The determination of these signs is an important diagnostic aid providing the physician with necessary information. Together with results of laboratory and other clinical tests and the physical examination, vital signs enable the physician to reach a diagnosis. The measuring and recording of vital signs is often a major responsibility of the medical assistant.

BODY TEMPERATURE

Skills Objectives

Upon completion of this section you will be able to:

1. Define body temperature and explain the physiology.

2. Demonstrate the proper procedure for taking oral, rectal, and axillary temperatures.

3. Explain why a particular site is chosen.

4. List and explain the factors taken into consideration when evaluating body temperature.

5. Explain the principles corresponding to each step in oral, rectal, and axillary temperature procedures.

6. Demonstrate the proper method for cleaning thermometers.

Physiology of Body Temperature

Body temperature represents the balance maintained by the body between heat lost and heat produced. Body heat is described in terms of heat units called degrees which are measurable through use of a thermometer.

Heat is produced in the body, and body temperature is derived from a process called metabolism which involves *all* the chemical and physical changes taking place in the body, such as digestion of food, respiration, and muscle activity. External conditions, such as environment and emotion, are other factors that sometimes affect heat production. Therefore, a heathy person's temperature will vary during the day depending on the internal and external state of the body.

In the unhealthy individual, illness upsets the metabolic process and disturbs the amount of heat being produced. In most disease processes, the metabolic activity is increased, thus increasing body temperature. There are, however, conditions and illnesses which decrease body temperature, such as fainting, fasting, dehydration, and injury to the central nervous system.

Any other factors influencing the metabolic rate will thereby influence body temperature as well. Metabolism in infants and children differs from adults due to the great expenditure of energy required for early growth and development. In addition there is a general immaturity of the heat-regulating system and their young bodies are more responsive to chemical and physical changes.

The heat-regulatory system consists of receptors in the skin and in the hypothalamus of the brain. These receptors monitor the balance between heat produced (as in digestion, physical activity and fever) and heat lost (as in perspiration, urination, and defecation).

Since heat is produced continuously during life, it must also be lost continuously. The mechanisms of heat regulation are extremely effective in maintaining temperature balance. When the body overheats there is a contrasting cooling system called perspiration. Perspiration is the excretion of moisture through the pores of the skin.

Heat is also lost through urine, fever, and water vapor in the lungs during expiration. When moisture from these sources (including perspiration) evaporates, heat is released, and the body is cooled.

Other causes of heat loss are external. Environmental changes such as those occurring from a cold breeze increase heat loss.

When more heat is produced than is lost, the body temperature is above normal, or elevated. Conversely, when more heat is lost than produced, the body temperature will drop below normal.

Normal Body Temperature

The average normal *oral* temperature for adults is considered to be 98.6°F (37.0°C). The average normal *rectal* temperature is 100°F (37.8°C), and the average normal *axillary* temperature is 98°F (36.6°C). Oral temperature refers to temperature in the mouth; rectal refers to temperatures in the anal canal; and axillary refers to temperature in the axilla, or armpit area.

Variations in temperature do occur. The average temperature range usually considered to be within normal limits is 0.5° to 1.0°F (0.3° to 0.6°C). Because of metabolic, environmental, and emotional changes previously discussed, body temperature is usually lowest in the morning prior to the initiation of daily routines. It then follows that body temperature is highest in the late afternoon or evening.

Elevated Body Temperature

An abnormally high body temperature is called *fever*, hyperthermia, or pyrexia; the patient is said to be febrile. A temperature of 105.8°F (41°C) is life-threatening in that brain functioning is impaired.

Fever is further categorized by descriptive terms which refer to the phase of the fever. The onset, or *invasion*, is the period when fever begins. Fever may occur suddenly or have a gradual onset. When temperature fluctuates between periods of normal or subnormal and periods of fever it is termed *intermittent*. A *continuous* temperature remains constantly elevated. *Remittent* temperature fluctuates several degrees above normal but does not reach normal between these periods of fluctuation. *Subsiding* fever is a stage which occurs when the temperature returns to normal. A *crisis* occurs when fever ends suddenly; *lysis* occurs when it ends gradually. The stage of crisis is usually accompanied by *diaphoresis* or profuse sweating (Fig. 16-1).

Another term for subnormal temperature is *hypothermia*.

Equipment for Measuring Body Temperature

A clinical thermometer is used to measure body temperature, and is calibrated in either Fahrenheit or Celsius (centigrade) degrees. Oral thermometers have a long, slender mercury bulb which gives the largest surface contact with tissues under the tongue or in the axilla. A shorter, blunter bulb thermometer is used to obtain the rectal temperature as the shape helps to prevent injury when inserted into the anal canal and can be securely held by

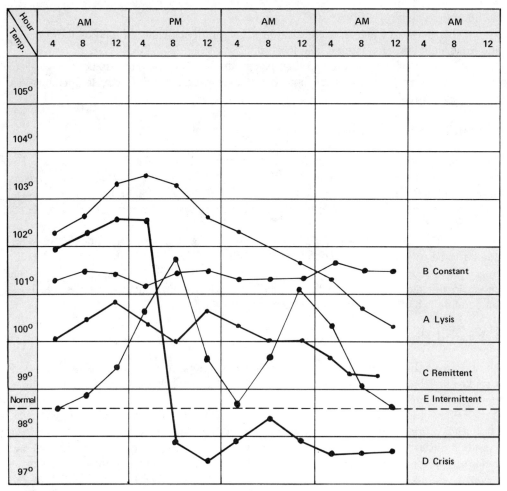

FIGURE 16-1. Fever categories.

rectal tissue. The end tips of rectal and oral thermometers are color-coded for ease in identification: blue (rectal) and red (oral). A security bulb thermometer has a special encasement
to prevent breakage and is sometimes used for the disoriented patient (Fig. 16-2).

Electronic thermometers are also available. These are equipped with disposable
covers, are color-coded, and are used for both oral and rectal temperatures. A reading can
be obtained in 5 seconds with ±0.2° accuracy. While becoming widely used in hospitals,
most physician's offices utilize glass thermometers.

Upon contact with warm human tissue, the mercury in the bulb of the glass thermometer will rise. After a designated period of time, usually 3 to 5 minutes, the temperature
will register and will not increase. The temperature reading is obtained by referring to the
calibration scale on the thermometer and noting the point reached by the mercury.

On both the Fahrenheit and Celsius scales, the long lines on the thermometer represent 1° of temperature. However, on the Fahrenheit scale, the shorter lines represent 0.2°,
while on the Celsius scale they are read as 0.1° (Fig. 16-3).

Procedure for Obtaining Body Temperature

The procedure for obtaining body temperature varies with the site utilized. Oral temperature
readings are taken on most individuals. A rectal temperature reading is taken on infants and

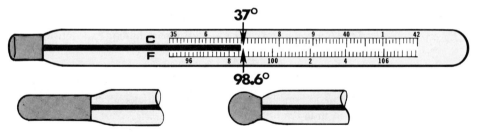

FIGURE 16-2. Types of thermometers. (Reproduced from Saperstein, A. B., and Frazier, M. A.:
Introduction to Nursing Practice. F. A. Davis, Philadelphia, 1980.)

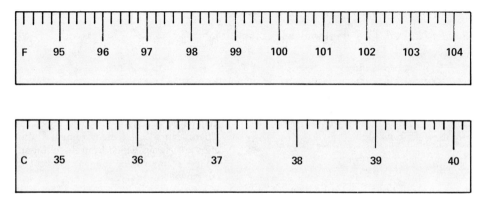

FIGURE 16-3. Comparison of Fahrenheit and Celsius scales.

young children or adults who cannot hold a glass thermometer securely in the mouth. An axillary temperature is taken in special circumstances when neither oral nor rectal temperature readings can be obtained. A procedure guide for each method is described in the sections to follow.

EQUIPMENT CARE

Since the thermometers are constructed from glass, care must be taken to avoid breakage. If breakage should occur, all pieces must be carefully disposed of to prevent injury to the office staff and the patient. Escaping beads of mercury should be brushed onto a piece of paper, wrapped in the paper without touching the skin, and disposed.

The following procedure is used to clean and disinfect glass thermometers:

1. Wash in cool, sudsy water to remove surface soil. (Hot water cannot be used because it will cause the mercury to expand too far up the sealed column and break the glass.)

2. Rinse in cool running water.

3. Dry thoroughly. If still wet when immersed in a chemical solution for disinfecting, the solution strength will be decreased.

4. Place the thermometer in a disinfectant solution such as isopropyl alcohol or zephiran chloride. A minimum of 20 minutes is recommended to ensure proper disinfection.

5. Rinse under cool water to remove residual disinfectant.

6. Place in proper storage container, usually a sterile metal receptacle, or retain in disinfectant solution until ready for use.

TAKING ORAL TEMPERATURE

Purpose: To gain important reliable knowledge of the patient's general condition or to detect any change in condition.

Equipment Needed: Oral thermometer, cotton ball.

Procedure	Principle
1. Select a thermometer. If the thermometer has been stored in a chemical solution, rinse with cool water and wipe dry with a cotton ball from the bulb to the tip.	1. Chemicals may irritate the mucosa of the mouth and may be foul-tasting. Hot water may cause the thermometer to break and interfere with accurate measurement Thermometers are always wiped from the clean surface to the contaminated one to prevent cross-contamination.
2. Check the level of mercury by holding the thermometer with calibration toward you and at eye level.	2. If the level of mercury is above 96°F, it will have to be shaken down in order to obtain an accurate reading. The thermometer is shaken

3. Identify the patient and explain the procedure. Have the patient in a sitting or lying position.

4. Position the thermometer under the patient's tongue and leave in place 2 to 3 minutes. Instruct patient to close mouth.

5. Remove the thermometer and wipe with cotton ball, *once* from the end of the stem down to the bulb, using a firm, twisting motion. Discard cotton ball.

6. Read the thermometer. Once temperature reading is obtained, shake mercury to 94°F. Place in proper container.

7. Record the reading on the designated form or chart. Patient's name, date, time, and reading are included. Abbreviation for temperature is T.

8. Wash hands.

down by holding the thermometer firmly between the thumb and forefinger and shaking downward with a snapping wrist action.

3. It is necessary to ask patients *if they have consumed a hot or cold drink* prior to taking the temperature. If so, *wait 30 minutes*. Patients will be better prepared for the procedure if they understand what is occurring and why.

4. When the bulb rests against the superficial blood vessels in the pocket on either side of tongue and the mouth is closed, a reliable measurement is obtained.

5. The removal of mucus will allow an accurate reading and carry microorganisms away from the medical assistant's fingers. Friction helps loosen foreign material from a glass surface.

6. The temperature is read where the mercury level ends. Hold the thermometer between the thumb and index finger at the tip end, away from the bulb. Rotate the thermometer until the silver mercury line can be identified; follow the line until it becomes opaque. The mercury has risen in the column as a direct result of body temperature radiated. Used thermometers are placed in the proper container to prevent contamination of clean thermometers and utensils. Oral thermometers are kept separate from rectal thermometers.

7. Patient data must be immediately and properly recorded to prevent error in the diagnosis.

8. Washing hands between patients and procedures is imperative to prevent the transfer of microorganisms to other patients and to the medical assistant.

TAKING RECTAL TEMPERATURE

Purpose: To obtain temperatures for infants and children, unconscious and irrational patients, and other patients when indicated.

Equipment Needed: Rectal thermometer, cotton ball, lubricant.

Procedure	Principle
1. Assemble thermometer, lubricant, and cotton ball.	1. Prepared equipment is an aid to efficiency.
2. Close door to examining room.	2. Privacy prevents needless embarrassment.
3. Identify patient and explain procedure.	3. Proper identification and explanation can

reduce risk of error and provide assurance to anxious patients.

4. Place adult patients in a Sims (side-lying) position, if possible, and drape properly. Infants are positioned on their backs with their legs held firmly at the ankles.

4. Proper positioning and draping will provide comfort and assure safety.

5. Select a rectal thermometer and check the mercury at eye level. If necessary shake down the mercury.

5. If mercury is above 96°F, it is shaken down to ensure accurate reading. Hold firmly between thumb and forefinger and shake downward with snapping wrist movement.

6. Having the thermometer well lubricated 1 inch above the bulb, separate the buttocks so that the anal sphincter is seen clearly, and insert thermometer gently for approximately 1½ inches. Allow buttocks to fall back in place.

6. Lubrication reduces friction and thereby facilitates insertion of the thermometer and minimizes irritation of the anal canal. If the thermometer is not placed directly into the anal opening, it may cause injury to the sphincter.

7. Hold the thermometer in place for 3 to 5 minutes. Do not leave the patient for any reason without removing the thermometer.

7. Holding the thermometer in place prevents accidents. Allowing sufficient time for the thermometer to register results in more accurate measurement.

8. Remove the thermometer and wipe it once, from the fingers to the mercury bulb with a firm twisting motion.

8. Fecal matter on the thermometer makes reading difficult. Friction helps loosen foreign material from a surface. Prior cleansing of an area where there are numerous organisms minimizes the spread of organisms to cleaner areas.

9. Read thermometer and record on designated form or chart as you would for oral. When recording rectal temperature, add an R next to the numerals. Place thermometer in proper container.

9. Prompt reading prevents mistakes. Knowing it is a rectal temperature reading, the physician will make the proper interpretation.

10. Wash hands.

10. Washing prevents the transfer of microorganisms to other patients and the medical assistant.

TAKING AXILLARY TEMPERATURE

Purpose: To obtain body temperature when both oral and rectal temperature procedures cannot be accomplished, or when directed.

Equipment Needed: Oral thermometer (or thermometer designated for use as axillary), cotton ball.

Procedure	*Principle*
1. Select a thermometer. Check the level of mercury. If above 96°F, shake down.	1. Checking ensures an accurate temperature reading.
2. Identify patient and explain procedure.	2. It is important to explain what you will be doing to reduce the patient's anxiety related to the procedure.

3. Insert the thermometer in the axilla. The area must be dry. Instruct patient to hold thermometer in place by tightly pressing arm against chest.

3. The area must by dry (free of perspiration) to prevent the thermometer from slipping. The area should be tightly closed to ensure a more accurate reading.

4. Leave the thermometer in place for 10 minutes.

4. This longer time is needed to secure a temperature reading in the axilla because the area is subject to air currents.

5. Remove the thermometer. Wipe dry with a cotton ball in a twisting, downward manner from stem to bulb.

5. Wiping removes perspiration, makes calibrations visible, and prevents the transference of microorganisms to the medical assistant.

6. Read the thermometer and place in proper container after shaking down below 96°F.

6. Proper care prevents contamination of clean thermometers and utensils.

7. Record on designated form or chart. Include name, time, date, and reading. Indicate that the temperature reading is axillary by placing an A after the numerals.

7. Immediate recording is necessary to prevent error. The temperature must be indicated as axillary to facilitate the physician's interpretation.

8. Wash hands.

8. Handwashing is essential between all procedures to prevent spread of microorganisms to other patients and the medical assistant.

Summary

Vital signs are the body's own health barometers and are an important aspect of almost every visit to the doctor's office. Body temperature, the vital sign discussed here, is the balance between heat production and heat loss. The body temperature usually rises (fever) when illness occurs. However, there are normal variations in temperature produced by emotional state, time of day, environment, physical exercise, and age. Any normal condition or illness which increases metabolic rate will raise body temperature. Many terms are used to signify the various stages of fever. Oral temperatures are most commonly taken. The medical assistant is responsible for performing the task of taking the patient's body temperature.

PULSE

Skills Objectives

Upon completion of this section you will be able to:

1. Define and describe the physiology of pulse.

2. Recognize, interpret, and describe the meaning of physiologic fluctuations in pulse.

3. Explain and assess the characteristics of pulse: rate, rhythm, and volume.

4. Perform the procedure required to count and evaluate the pulse.

5. Report and record the information acquired.

Definition of Pulse

The pulse beat is another vital sign or indicator of the state health in the human body. The rate and characteristics of pulse are dynamic physiologic necessities which provide clues to the condition of the cardiovascular system. The medical assistant's ability to count and interpret pulse characteristics accurately is utilized by the physician as an integral component in patient assessment.

Pulse can be defined as the wave of alternate expansion and relaxation of the arterial walls with each beat or contraction of the *left ventricle* of the heart. Each time the heart beats, blood is forced into the arteries; the arteries expand as the wave of blood passes through and then return to their previous state. This is referred to as the pulse and can be felt or palpated by lightly placing the fingertips over the artery.

Physiology of Pulse

The heart is divided into four chambers (Fig. 16-4). The left ventricle is the chamber which when filled with fresh (oxygenated) blood contracts or pumps and forces blood into the major artery, the aorta, and flows into all the arteries of the cardiovascular system. Therefore, the pulse beat in any of the arteries will reflect and be the same as the actual heart beat. The arteries of the system are composed of a muscular wall which has the capacity to be elastic. The normal pulsating artery is soft and pliable; the abnormal artery is hard or knotty. When

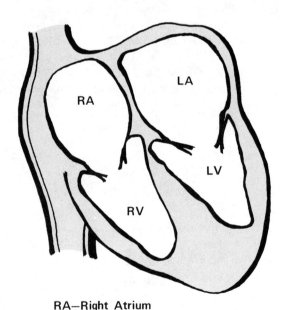

RA—Right Atrium
LA—Left Atrium
RV— Right Ventricle
LV—Left Ventricle

FIGURE 16-4. Chambers of the heart.

blood is being forced through, the vessel stretches, increasing its size. As the left ventricle is filling and is in a state of rest, the walls of the arteries also are relaxing. When the pulse is counted and evaluated, the condition of the pump—the heart itself—is represented.

Variables Affecting Pulse

As was stated earlier, any change in the body's metabolism (normal functioning) will cause a noticeable change in the vital signs. Various conditions affecting the metabolism influence the rate of pulse:

1. *Disease* will cause fluctuations in the pulse rate, and certain diseases will also affect the regularity and strength of the pulse. Certain types of heart disease, hyperthyroidism, and most infections will *increase* the pulse rate; certain other types of heart disease, hypothyroidism, mental depression, and certain brain injuries will *decrease* the pulse rate. Pain tends to increase pulse rate.

2. *Age.* The heart is a muscle and like all other muscles in the body is subject to the aging process. With age, the heart can become less efficient, thereby reducing the forceful contraction of the left ventricle and reducing cardiac output. When the amount of blood pumped by the heart per unit of time is reduced, the normal pulse will be slower than the pulse rate of a younger individual. For instance, a 75-year-old woman would have a slower normal pulse rate than a 24-year-old woman.

3. *Physical activity.* Since metabolism is related to pulse rate, it is reasonable to expect that exercise which increases metabolism will also increase heart rate and pulse. For instance, the act of climbing stairs requires the body to work harder than it would in the act of sitting. There are increased demands on the entire cardiovascular system, and therefore the pulse rate during this activity would increase.

4. *Emotions.* When strong emotions are experienced, the metabolism and heart rate may increase, causing the pulse rate to increase correspondingly. Certain substances are released in the body, and the whole human mechanism becomes accelerated with stress. Feelings of anger or excitement set this process in motion. The vital signs, which include the pulse, are measurable indicators of the state of stress, both physiologic and psychologic.

5. *Body size.* There is a correlation between the pulse rate and the size of the individual. The smaller the individual, the faster the pulse rate. This inverse relationship can be explained by the degree of efficiency of the cardiovascular system. The 2-year-old child will have a faster rate than the 22-year-old man; the adult male has a slower pulse than the adult female.

6. *Medications.* Certain medications have an effect on the metabolic rate or act on specific organs to increase or decrease activity. These influence pulse rate.

Since each of the above factors influences the rate of pulse, it is obvious that pulse rate variations and fluctuations are normal. Thus it is preferable to speak of *normal ranges* of pulse rate rather than normal pulse rates.

Characteristics of Pulse

Pulse has three major characteristics: rate, rhythm, and volume. A pulse rate (numerical value) alone is an inadequate determination of pulse as a vital sign. Judgments regarding the other characteristics are also necessary.

1. *Rate* refers to the number of beats per minute. The usual adult pulse rate ranges from 60 to 90 beats per minute. A pulse rate of 80 is considered to be the clinical average. (Clinical averages for non-adults are: infants: 110 to 130 beats per minute; children aged 1 to 7: 80 to 120 beats per minute; children over 7: 80 to 90 beats per minute.)

2. *Rhythm* is the term used to describe the pulse tempo. The pulse should have a regular pattern of beats occurring in a smooth, evenly paced sequence.

3. *Pulse volume* refers to the palpatable strength of the beat. When the pulse is being felt, the wavelike sensation of blood pulsating through the artery can be described as weak, strong, thready, full and bounding, or alternating between strong and weak pulsations. The pulse should feel full and strong and be easily perceptible by gentle pressure of the fingertips.

Arrhythmias

The term *arrhythmia* refers to an absence of rhythm or unrhythmic occurrences in the cardiac muscle. The prefix "a" signifies without, and "rhythm" signifies movement which can be measured.

Cardiac arrhythmias are not necessarily abnormalities. Certain arrhythmias are considered normal in the healthy functioning heart. Usually, however, when an arrhythmia is detected, the physician will attempt first to rule out the presence of heart disease. Arrhythmia is not a disease in itself but rather a potential sign. The medical assistant needs to become acquainted with the terminology and patterns of arrhythmias because she or he may be the first and perhaps the only individual who discovers the occurrence during the routine procedure of obtaining the vital signs.

1. *Tachycardia.* The prefix "tachy" means rapid, and the suffix "cardia" refers to the heart. Therefore, the arrhythmia tachycardia is characterized by the rapid but regular pulse due to excessive rapidity of the heart action. A pulse rate of over 90 beats per minute is usually considered tachycardia. Tachycardia is, however, normally produced during periods of exercise such as running. Tachycardia, at rest, may also be stress-related. The physician must determine the causative link.

2. *Bradycardia.* The prefix "brady" means slowness. Bradycardia is an arrhythmia characterized by a slow pulse due to slowed heart action. A pulse rate below 60

beats per minute is usually considered bradycardia. Bradycardia can be a normal by-product of athletic development. Again, the physician must first rule out an organic cause.

3. *Extrasystole.* "Systole" means contraction. In extrasystole, the arrhythmia is characterized by extra contractions or beats. What actually evolves is that immediately after the heart beats normally, a premature contraction of the heart follows and simulates in the pulse sensation that of a skipped beat.

4. *Cardiac flutter.* This arrhythmia is characterized by several premature beats (extrasystoles) occurring in a regular or irregular pattern.

5. *Auricular fibrillation.* This arrhythmia involves a serious disorder of the heart in which the pulse beat is less than the heart rate. In this condition, the left ventricle is not contracting forcefully enough to force the blood from the heart. The pulse is felt to be weak, rapid, and irregular in both volume and rhythm. The patient experiencing auricular fibrillation is seriously ill and should be admitted to the hospital.

6. *Heart block.* This is another extremely serious arrhythmia that is reflected in the pulse rate. Impulses are not transmitted from the atria of the heart (upper chambers) to the ventricles, and therefore the ventricles seek their own rhythm. The pulse rate is then excessively slow, perhaps 30 to 40 beats per minute.

The medical assistant's responsibility is to report the detection of an arrhythmia to the physician immediately. The physician will then proceed with the assessment.

Obtaining the Pulse Reading

Pulse readings may be obtained anywhere on the body where the pulse is near the surface of body and lies over a bone (Fig. 16-5). The most common pulse reading is the radial pulse, so named because the radial artery which is palpated lies over the radius bone at the wrist. Two fingers are gently applied and the pulsations can be felt. The radial pulse is favored because it is easily accessible and most comfortable for the patient.

Other pulse sites are utilized when the radial pulse is not conveniently accessible. Among these are the temporal, carotid, popliteal, femoral, and dorsalis pedis arteries.

The temporal pulse is located in the area of the temples at eye level (Fig. 16-6). At this location, the temporal artery passes over the temporal bone.

The carotid artery is the large artery that arises from the base of the neck on either side of the trachea (windpipe). By exerting gentle pressure under the chin and slightly to the side of the neck, the carotid pulse can be detected (Fig. 16-6). The popliteal pulse is located in the crevice behind the knee.

The dorsalis pedis and femoral arteries are also, but infrequently, used for pulse readings. The dorsalis pedis artery is located on the dorsal side or back of the foot, near the ankle. The femoral artery is located in the flexible (groin) area of the hip between the thigh and abdomen (Fig. 16-7).

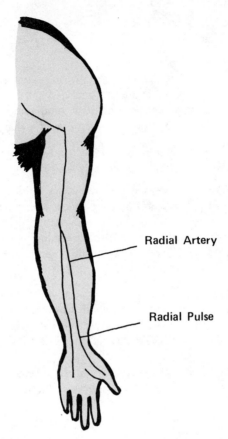

FIGURE 16-5.   Pulse sites.

TAKING A PULSE READING

Procedure	*Principle*
1. Patient must be at rest, either sitting or lying down. Pulse is usually taken over the radial artery, but the temporal, carotid, dorsalis pedis, or femoral arteries can also be utilized when necessary. The radial pulse can be taken while the oral thermometer is in the patient's mouth.	1. A resting position is necessary to ensure a more accurate reading. Exertion and excitement promote an increase in the pulse rate. Any large superficial artery that lies directly over a bone can be palpated, but the radial artery is most convenient. Determining the temperature, pulse and respiration (TPR) is usually a simultaneous procedure for the sake of time efficiency and patient comfort.
2. Apply gentle pressure over the artery with the tips of the first two fingers. When the palm is turned upward, the radial pulse can be detected by following the thumb to its base on the wrist.	2. Light pressure allows the normal pulsation to occur: expansion and contraction. Too much pressure would distort or obliterate the pulse. The fingertips are used instead of the thumb because the fingertips are most sensitive to the

Procedure	*Principle*
	sensation, and the thumb itself has a slight pulsation which can be falsely perceived to be the patient's pulse.
3. Count the beats for 30 seconds and multiply by two when the pulse is regular. If irregular, count the pulse for a full minute.	3. When rhythm and volume appear normal, 30 seconds is sufficient to determine an accurate pulse reading.
4. Record the readings immediately.	4. The physician will use the vital signs as significant factors to be considered in determining the diagnosis or health status. These must be recorded accurately when recording the TPR. The pulse reading follows the temperature reading and precedes the respiratory rate (Example: 98.6—72—16).

Summary

The rate and other characteristics of pulse are generalized reflections of the state of health of the individual, and, in particular, the cardiovascular system. The medical assistant must understand the physiology of pulse and should be competent in performing the procedure. These capabilities will ensure an accurate determination of the pulse reading to serve as essential data for compiling the patient's health profile.

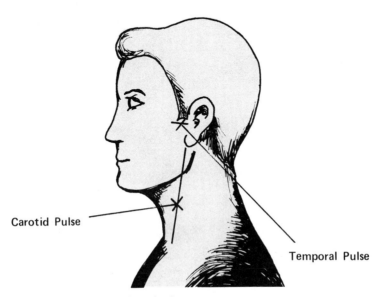

Carotid Pulse

Temporal Pulse

FIGURE 16-6. Common upper body pulse locations.

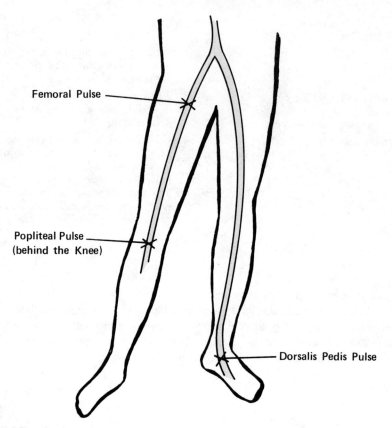

FIGURE 16-7.   Common lower body pulse locations.

RESPIRATION

Skills Objectives

Upon completion of this section you will be able to:

1. Define respiration and describe its physiology.

2. List and explain variables which affect respiration.

3. Describe the characteristics of respiration.

4. Define descriptive terms related to respiration.

5. Accurately perform and record the procedure for obtaining the respiratory reading.

Definition of Respiration

The vital sign which is representative of the general state of the respiratory system is termed respiration. Together with temperature and pulse, respiration is an essential measurement in the standard TPR procedure.

Comprehension of physiology and development of procedural skill are required in order for the medical assistant to assume full responsibility for the accurate determination of the respiratory rate and its characterization.

The act of respiration consists of two major phases: inspiration and expiration, otherwise called inhalation and exhalation. Respiration is the term used to designate the body's physiologic need for the inspiration, or breathing in, of oxygen (fresh air) and the expiration, or breathing out, of carbon dioxide (CO_2), a gaseous waste product. The complete cycle of inspiration and expiration constitutes respiration.

Physiology of Respiration

Breathing is an essential physiologic process which provides the body with the oxygen needed for most of the chemical reactions in the body.

Respiration is both internal and external. External respiration refers to the exchange of gases (oxygen and carbon dioxide) which takes place in the lungs when air is inspired and expired. Internal respiration refers to the utilization of oxygen carried by the blood stream to all the cells of the body and the subsequent production of carbon dioxide given off as waste in the chemical process of metabolism.

The major center in the brain which controls the functions of the respiratory system is located in the medulla oblongata. This center is affected by the nervous system and impulses initiated elsewhere in the body, as well as the body's temperature and the chemical composition of the blood flowing through the center. The nervous system influences the rate of respiration and responds to the body's changing needs for oxygen.

Chemical control is achieved by the chemical content of the blood which directly affects the brain center's response. Thus, even though respiration can be willfully controlled by voluntary messages sent to the brain to "hold the breath" or "breath slowly," voluntary control is limited, and chemical control maintains the involuntary function of breathing during sleep and other periods when breathing must be an automatic process. The proper balance of oxygen and carbon dioxide is maintained by the response of the brain center to increasing and decreasing levels of these gases in the blood stream and the lungs. The pons of the brain houses two other respiratory centers that participate in maintaining normal respiratory function.

Variables Affecting Respiration

Respiration is affected by most of the same variables that affect the other vital signs.

1. *Disease*. Depending on the type of illness present, the rate and characteristics of respiration may be affected. Lung and circulatory diseases *increase* respirations, while certain brain and kidney diseases *decrease* respirations.

2. *Age.* With increasing age, the efficiency of the nervous system and organs involved in the respiratory process diminishes, and slowed responses are expected.

3. *Physical activity.* As with the other vital signs, any increase in metabolic activity (digestion, muscular activity) will increase the rate and depth of respirations.

4. *Emotions.* Psychologic stresses trigger physiologic reactions. In periods of excitability or irritability the respiratory rate is increased.

5. *Medications.* Certain medications can increase or decrease the respiratory rate.

Characteristics of Respiration

The characteristics of respiration affected by the foregoing variables include rate, rhythm, depth, and special descriptive factors such as audibility.

1. *Rate.* The adult normal or average range for the number of breaths per minute is 14 to 20 complete cycles of inspiration and expiration. The ratio of one respiration to four pulse beats is usually expected when the patient is at rest. This ratio is also relevant when trying to stimulate normal functioning in cardiopulmonary resuscitation (CPR). The clinical average for infants is 30 to 38 respirations per minute; for children aged 1 to 7 it is 20 to 26 respirations per minute.

2. *Rhythm.* A regular, even breathing pattern is considered normal. Voluntary breath-holding or involuntary and automatic interruptions in the breathing pattern, such as sighing, are also considered normal.

3. *Depth.* The depth of respirations refers to the amount of air being inhaled and exhaled. When the patient is at rest and when no abnormality is present, respirations have a consistent depth, with the chest expanding and contracting at a normal rate with even depth. By contrast, when exercising, the breath may be more rapid and shallow. Rapid shallow breathing also occurs in some disease states.

4. *Special descriptive characteristics of respiration.* These include audibility of the breathing process. Normally there are no noticeable breath sounds. Breathing is quiet. In certain diseases, particularly of the respiratory system, the breath sounds become noisy. Snoring is an example of noisy respirations which are considered normal. When referring to noisy respirations the term "stertorous" is applied. An individual with blockage of the nasal passageway may have stertorous breathing. Other descriptive characteristics of breathing are represented by use of specific terminology. *Rales,* for instance, is the term used to denote abnormal bubbling or crackling sounds audible during the respiratory cycle with the aid of a stethoscope.

Descriptive Terminology

Certain terms are used to denote special types of breathing patterns. These states of respiration are not disease conditions in themselves but merely describe the type of disruption in the normal breathing pattern. In all the terms which follow, the suffix "pnea" refers to breathing.

1. *Eupnea.* "Eu" means good, thus the combined term denotes normal breathing.

2. *Dyspnea.* "Dys" means difficult. The individual experiencing dyspnea will have labored breathing. It will be difficult for this individual to breathe normally. Rate and depth are often affected and increased when the patient is dyspneic.

3. *Apnea.* "A" refers to the absence of something. This term signifies the cessation of breathing. It is usually applied to a temporary interruption rather than a permanent cessation of respiration.

4. *Orthopnea.* "Ortho" means upright or straight and refers to normal anatomic structure. Individuals with certain diseases affecting the heart and lungs can breathe comfortably only in the upright or sitting position.

5. *Polypnea.* "Poly" means many, and with its suffix is the term used to refer to the condition of rapid, panting breaths.

6. *Hyperpnea.* "Hyper" means increased, and with its suffix is the term used to refer to increased rate of respirations. The term hyperventilation is applied when the individual is experiencing rapid but less shallow breathing than that occurring with polypnea.

Other terms not ending in "pnea" are used to describe various other types of breathing. "Cheyne-Stokes" breathing, named for the physicians who first noted the syndrome, is a type of breathing which occurs in patients approaching death. This condition is characterized by respirations gradually increasing in rapidity, subsiding and then ceasing for prolonged periods (up to 50 seconds) before beginning again. Although this condition is rarely seen in the physician's office because it is critical, the medical assistant should be familiar with the terminology.

A medical term frequently used to describe an effect of respiratory difficulty is "cyanosis." When an individual cannot inspire enough oxygen to supply all the body's cells with oxygenated blood, the normal pink skin coloring, particularly around the lips and on the nail beds, is replaced by a bluish tinge. The bluish tinge represents the increased level of carbon dioxide which is present in the blood.

The respiration terms discussed above are those most frequently encountered by the medical assistant in the office setting.

Obtaining the Respiration Rate and Characteristics

Procedure	*Principle*
1. Patient should be at rest in a sitting or lying position. The respirations are counted after the pulse has been counted for 30 seconds	1. The patient needs to be at rest because the respiratory rate is increased during activity and excitement. Respirations are *counted with-*

and while the fingertips remain on the pulse as though the rate of pulsation were still being measured.

out the patient's awareness since staring at the chest would cause the patient discomfort and affect the accuracy of the measurement. When conscious of their breathing, patients may unknowingly alter their usual rate.

2. Observe the rise and fall of the chest and count each complete cycle as a single respiration. Count for 30 seconds and multiply by two.

2. The rise of the chest represents inspiration, and the fall of the chest represents expiration. When the respirations are regular and the rate normal, 30 seconds is sufficient to obtain an accurate reading.

3. Count irregular respirations for 1 full minute while keeping fingertips on radial pulse.

3. A full minute is necessary to count respirations when the breathing pattern is uneven. This allows sufficient time to confirm the irregularity or other characteristics which may be present.

4. Record the respirations accurately.

4. The respiratory rate follows the pulse rate and is designated in this manner: 98.6—72—18.

Summary

The respiratory rate, rhythm, depth, and other characteristics, as with other vital signs previously described, are generalized representations of the state of health of the individual. Medical assistants must be familiar with the physiology, as well as skilled in the proper method for obtaining the measurement, so that they can obtain and report accurate information related to respirations.

THE COMPLETE TPR PROCEDURE

The temperature, pulse, and respiration measurements are generally considered by clinicians to be a set or group of measurements which are taken together. The following outline suggests the proper approach or sequence for combining the TPR procedure.

Using the proper methods as instructed and understanding the principles stated:

1. Identify the patient.

2. Insert the oral thermometer.

3. Place the fingertips on the radial pulse, count for 30 seconds, and multiply by two (when normal).

4. While the fingertips are in place on the radial pulse, count the respirations for 30 seconds and multiply by two (when normal).

5. Remove the fingertips and record the pulse and respirations.

6. Wait until 3 minutes have expired from the time the thermometer was inserted.

7. Remove the thermometer, wipe and read, and record the temperature.

8. Shake down and cleanse the thermometer, or place in the appropriate solution.

BLOOD PRESSURE

Skills Objectives

Upon completion of this section you will be able to:

1. Define blood pressure and explain its physiology.

2. Demonstrate the proper procedure for taking blood pressure.

3. List and explain the normal blood pressure standards.

4. Demonstrate the proper care of blood pressure measuring equipment.

Introduction

The measurement of blood pressure is yet another vital sign of great significance to the diagnosis and treatment of patients. In fact, since hypertension, a disease in which the blood pressure is elevated beyond the normal range, is asymptomatic (without symptoms), it is common practice to obtain a blood pressure reading for all patients each time they visit the office, regardless of the purpose. It is the only vital sign used as a screening device. Obtaining TPR readings may be reserved for patients with suspected infection or other specific conditions, but they are not obtained routinely and are not as reliable an indication of disease as is the blood pressure reading.

The medical assistant must have a thorough knowledge of the pertinent physiology and be competent in the procedural skills in order to obtain an accurate measurement, facilitate the physician's goals for patient care, and answer the patient's questions regarding blood pressure.

Blood pressure measures the amount of force or pressure exerted on the walls of the arterial blood vessels as the blood, which is pumped by the heart, is pushed through these arteries. The cardiac cycle (or pump cycle) is the term which is used to refer to the two phases of heartbeat: contraction and relaxation. Blood pressure measures the pressure in the arteries during both phases. The phase of cardiac contraction is systole; *systolic blood pressure* is a measurement of the pressure in the arteries when the left ventricle of the heart contracts. Diastole is the phase of cardiac relaxation; *diastolic blood pressure* measures the pressure in arteries when the left ventricle is at rest.

Physiology of Blood Pressure

Perhaps the greatest aid in understanding the physiology of blood pressure is the comparison of the physiologic activity of the heart and blood vessels to that of a faucet tap and hose. The activity of the left ventricle can be simulated by alternately turning the faucet taps on and off (contraction and relaxation). The water in the adjoining hose is flowing forward and sideways when the tap is turned on. The hose offers resistance since it has a limited expandable capacity, and thus the pressure in the hose (arteries) is a result of the lateral pressure and the wall resistance. When the tap is turned off and the hose is lying on the ground, the water in the hose is not moving because there is no pressure difference in the parts of the hose lying on the ground. The heart, however, maintains continuous pumping action, and the pressure is always different in the parts of vessels.

Using the "tap and hose" analogy, when the "tap" (left ventricle of the heart) is turned on, (contracting) pressure is greatest in the "hose" connection (aortic blood vessel) closest to the tap because it is receiving the full pressure of the flow (Fig. 16-8). The flow continues from a point of high pressure to a point of lesser pressure. Because of this pressure difference or gradient, the pressure in the veins (vessels carrying blood back to the heart) is lower than the pressure in the arteries (vessels carrying blood away from the heart).

The systolic pressure is the measurement of the lateral pressure exerted in the vessel when the left ventricle contracts. The diastolic pressure is the measurement of the lateral pressure exerted on the vessel by the blood flowing through when the ventricle is at rest.

There are other physiologic factors which determine the blood pressure.

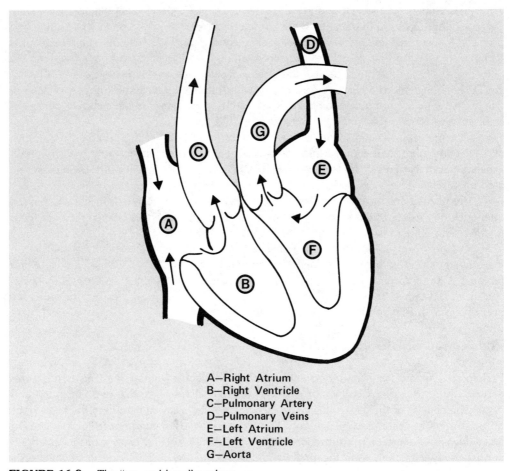

A—Right Atrium
B—Right Ventricle
C—Pulmonary Artery
D—Pulmonary Veins
E—Left Atrium
F—Left Ventricle
G—Aorta

FIGURE 16-8. The "tap and hose" analogy.

1. *Volume* is the amount of blood in the arteries. An increase in blood volume would increase blood pressure, and the correlation is also true in reverse. For example, an individual who has been injured in an accident and is hemorrhaging will have a lowered blood pressure because the volume of blood has decreased. With each contraction of the left ventricle, since it is not filling to full capacity, the volume of blood (cardiac output) will be lessened and the pressure in the vessels lowered.

2. *Peripheral vascular resistance* is the term used to refer to the resistance of the arteries to the flow of blood. The diameter of this artery is related to the degree of resistance: *the smaller the diameter, the greater the resistance.* For example, an individual with atherosclerosis (fatty deposits lining the walls of the vessels) will have an increased blood pressure because of the narrowed diameter of the vessel. The diastolic pressure is an important indicator of the state of the vessels since the left ventricle is at rest in this phase, and an increased diastolic pressure would mean that even though the heart was now relaxed, the vessel pressure was greater than normal, indicating the probability of diseased vessels.

3. *Condition of the heart muscle* is an important factor related to blood volume as a strong, forceful pump will work efficiently and will tend to normalize blood pressure.

4. *Vessel elasticity* refers to the capacity of the vessel to alternately expand and contract. The vessel condition of arteriosclerosis (hardening of the arteries) would increase resistance and thereby increase blood pressure.

Normals and Influential Factors

Although blood pressure varies with age, in the average adult at rest, the arterial blood most commonly exhibits enough pressure to raise a column of mercury to the height of 120 mm during systole and 80 mm during diastole when a sphygmomanometer (air-inflated cuff) is applied. The normal range extends from 110/70 to 140/90.

AGE

As vessels become more rigid in the natural process of aging, blood pressure increases, but not usually beyond the outer limits of the normal range.

ACTIVITY

Daily fluctuations in blood pressure are expected and considered normal. Since metabolism plays a significant role in all the vital signs, when metabolism is increased (as it is during physical activity), the blood pressure is increased. Even without pronounced activity, metabolic activity and blood pressure increase gradually during the day or after awakening and decrease during the hours of sleep. In some individuals, blood pressure can be raised or lowered by changing from a sitting to a standing position.

STRESS

Emotional changes can be reflected in blood pressures, usually causing an increase, especially in those individuals hereditarily predisposed to high blood pressure (hypertension). Certain emotions can, however, cause the blood pressure to fall. Intense pain, shock, and grief are examples. Diseases, categorized as physical or physiologic stresses, can either raise or lower blood pressure. Obesity increases blood pressure. Some endocrine disorders and certain drugs will increase physiologic stress and increase the blood pressure. Other endocrine disorders and drug therapy will decrease blood pressure. Cancer, anemia, and some infections also tend to lower blood pressure.

Descriptive Terminology

The following terms are commonly used to describe the specific measurements related to blood pressure:

1. *Hypertension.* A systolic reading over 140 mm with a diastolic reading over 90 mm is considered to be above normal and is termed high blood pressure, or hypertension. One or both (systolic and diastolic) can be elevated in hypertension. Diagnosis of hypertension is never made as a result of one reading. Rather the blood pressure pattern, ideally taken about the same time of day in a regular sequence (daily or weekly) will be examined in order to determine a conclusive diagnosis. Frequent blood pressure screening, however, is essential in uncovering abnormally high readings which then become suspect for hypertension.

2. *Hypotension.* A systolic reading under 110 mm with a diastolic reading under 70 mm (some authorities say 60 mm) is considered to be below normal and is termed low blood pressure, or hypotension. Hypotension is not regarded in most cases to be as significant a health problem as hypertension.

3. *Mean pressure.* Although the medical assistant will not usually be asked to determine the mean pressure, understanding of the term is important in a general knowledge of blood pressure. Mean pressure is the term used to express the arithmetic average of the combined systolic and diastolic pressure. It is an important figure to the physician as it represents the average rate at which blood is being circulated throughout the body.

4. *Venous pressure.* The medical assistant will *never* obtain the measurements of venous pressure; however, the probability of exposure to the term warrants discussion. Venous pressure is the pressure of blood in the veins. It is measured by inserting a needle into the vein, allowing the venous blood to flow into the manometer (measurement column); the height of the column of blood indicates venous pressure: normal values are 60 to 100 mm of water. It is a procedure not commonly performed as arterial pressure is considered to be a more conclusive determinant of the state of health of the heart and vessels.

Equipment for Measuring Blood Pressure

The stethoscope and the sphygmomanometer are the two major instruments used to obtain blood pressure.

The stethoscope is used to listen to the sounds of the blood in the artery. Although a stethoscope with a bell-shaped end can be used to detect blood pressure sounds, a stethoscope with a round end or diaphragm is more commonly used because the diaphragm covers a greater area, is easily secured, and pulse sounds can be more readily located and heard. The sound is conducted to the ears by the two pieces of tubing which end in earpieces. The flexible rubber tubing connects to the metal neck piece to which the rubber earpieces are attached. The earpieces are turned slightly forward and placed in the ear. The forward position facilitates the hearing of sounds as the ear canal runs forward toward the hose. The stethoscope is not sterilized, but the ear tips can be removed and placed in disinfectant solution when necessary.

The sphygmomanometer is the instrument used in conjunction with the stethoscope to measure blood pressure. "Sphygmo" means pulse, and a "manometer" is an instrument which measures pressure. The sphygomanometer apparatus includes a rubber bag encased in cloth with metal hooks and eyes or adhesive strips for fastening of the cuff. Also included are a pressure gauge (manometer) and a pressure bulb which has a control valve (usually a screw or dial).

The pressure gauge can be either of the aneroid or the mercury type. In an *aneroid* gauge, the movement of the dial is controlled by the amount of air pumped (Fig. 16-9). The *mercury* gauge, while controlled by the amount of air pumped, seeks a level in a scaled glass tube which corresponds to the amount of external pressure exerted (Fig. 16-10).

The mercury manometer is more accurate; the measurement is more readily identified, and for these reasons it is most frequently used. Most physicians' offices have mercury manometers installed on the wall at eye level in each examination room. The blood pressure is measured in millimeters of mercury, abbreviated as Hg mm.

The *blood pressure cuff* is the cuff containing the air-inflatable rubber bags. The cuff is snugly applied to the patient's upper arm. There are three sizes of cuffs to fit various individuals:

1. Medium: for the adult of average size.
2. Small: for children and adults with small upper arm diameters.
3. Extra large: for the obese adult. This cuff can be applied to the thigh for adults with very large upper arm diameters.

The *pressure bulb* is a hollow bulb that is used to pump air into the bag. The bulb fits into the palm of the hand, and the control valve attached to the bulb (usually a screw type) can be manipulated by the thumb and forefinger.

The patient assumes a sitting position with the arm slightly flexed and resting on a surface in order to expose the antecubital space in which the brachial artery will be located.

The cuff is wrapped snugly around the patient's upper arm, and the earpieces of the stethoscope are inserted in the medical assistant's ears. The MA then locates the brachial

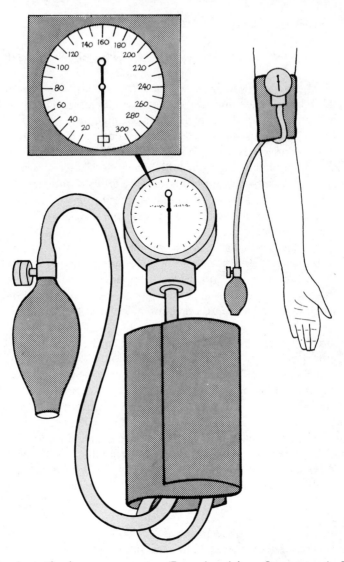

FIGURE 16-9. Aneroid sphygmomanometer. (Reproduced from Saperstein, A. B., and Frazier, M. A.: *Introduction to Nursing Practice*. F. A. Davis, Philadelphia, 1980.)

pulse, places the diaphragm of the stethoscope over the artery, tightens the control valve, and pumps air into the rubber bag.

What is occurring physiologically is that external pressure is being applied to the vessel by means of the inflated cuff. The air is pumped to approximately 180 mm Hg in order to completely compress the artery. When the cuff is properly positioned on the upper arm it is level with the heart. When the cuff is inflated, blood circulation in the artery ceases. The heart, however, continues to pump blood into the vessel. Pressure is increased, and the vessel increases in size.

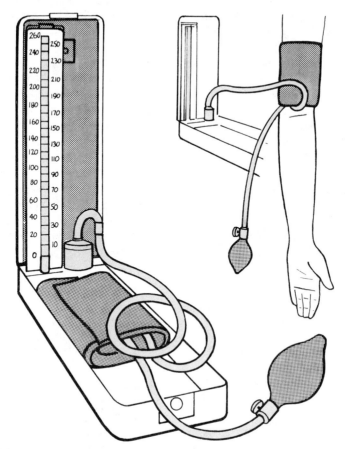

FIGURE 16-10. Mercury sphygmomanometer. (Reproduced from Saperstein, A. B., and Frazier, M. A.: *Introduction to Nursing Practice.* F. A. Davis, Philadelphia, 1980.)

At this point, no sounds will be heard through the stethoscope. There is greater pressure in the cuff than in the artery.

When the cuff is gradually deflated by manipulating the control valve, blood begins to push or spurt through the artery because the cuff pressure and the artery pressure become equalized. Sounds are now audible. When the bag is deflated further and the pressure in the cuff is less than the pressure in the artery, no further sounds are discernible.

The sounds heard when the cuff is deflated have a definite beat and rhythm (pulsation), but the discernibility and volume fluctuate. There are five phases of sounds, together called the *Korotkoff sounds*, named for the physician who identified them. These sounds are heard between the systolic and diastolic levels. *It is important to note that the systolic reading corresponds to the very first distinctly audible sound, and the diastolic reading refers to the very last distinctly audible sound.* The sounds in between are not easily categorized or differentiated but are explained here to broaden the medical assistant's understanding of blood pressure.

As pressure declines in the cuff, the sounds of phase 1 appear as faint tappings that gradually increase in intensity. During phase 2, the sounds develop a squeaking quality. Phase 3 is characterized by crisp sounds which increase in volume. In phase 4, the sounds are muffled, and they disappear altogether in phase 5.

While the Korotkoff sounds are sometimes distinctly recognizable, they are not separately measured. Again, only the first distinctly audible beat which occurs in two consecutive beats and the last distinctly audible beat comprise the systolic and diastolic readings. The Korotkoff sounds are considered in order that the changes in volume and quality can be anticipated and accepted as a normal occurrence.

Recording the Blood Pressure

Whether an aneroid or mercury sphygmomanometer is used, the instrument will have a numerical scale usually ranging from 0 to 240, incremented in tens. The first distinct sound heard will have a corresponding numerical value; likewise the last sound heard will have a corresponding numerical value. Blood pressure is abbreviated BP and is recorded with the systolic measurement placed over the diastolic measurement.

OBTAINING BLOOD PRESSURE

Procedure	*Principle*
1. Assemble necessary equipment: Sphygmomanometer and stethoscope.	1. Equipment readiness facilitates efficiency.
2. Assist the patient to assume a comfortable position with the forearm and palm supinated at heart level.	2. This position facilitates placing the stethoscope on the brachial artery in the antecubital space and promotes an accurate measurement.
3. Wrap the cuff around the upper arm about 1 inch above the elbow, placing the tubing toward the outer aspect of the arm.	3. The cuff must be properly placed and secured to obtain compression of the brachial artery. Tubing must be placed out of the way to prevent rubbing with stethoscope and occluding sounds.
4. Place stethoscope in ears.	4. The stethoscope should be in place prior to pumping the pressure bulb to free the hands in proceeding with the next steps.
5. Palpate the brachial pulse and place the diaphragm of the stethoscope over it.	5. The pulse is palpated first to assume proper location. An aid is to trace the little finger to the antecubital space. The pulse will be on the inner aspect of the arm.
6. Squeeze the (pump) inflator bulb after tightening the valve to prevent leakage until the necessary level rises to approximately 180 mm Hg. An alternative method is for the MA to place her fingertips on the radial pulse while pumping and inflating the cuff. When the radial pulse is obliterated, the cuff is pumped to a level 30 mm higher than the point at which the radial pulse was obliterated.	6. Sufficient cuff pressure must be applied to obliterate the brachial artery pulse. It is possible to obtain the systolic pressure by the palpation method *without* the use of auscultation. Placing fingertips over the radial pulse and pumping air into the cuff 30 mm above the point at which the radial pulse is obliterated identifies the systolic pressure.

7. With thumb and forefinger regulating the valve, slowly release the pressure in the cuff.

7. Blood has now collected in the artery and upon gradual release will begin to proceed forcefully.

8. Note the first distinctly audible pulse sound heard—the systolic pressure.

8. Systolic pressure is that point at which the blood in the brachial artery is first able to proceed through the artery, exerting lateral pressure while moving forward in the artery and against the external pressure exerted on the vessel by the inflated cuff.

9. Note the last distinctly audible sound heard —the diastolic pressure.

9. Diastolic pressure is that point at which the blood is flowing through the brachial artery without the imposition of external pressure. Pressure in the cuff is now less than pressure in the artery.

10. Allow the remaining air to escape by completely opening the control valve.

10. This hastens the completion of the procedure and promotes patient comfort.

11. Remove equipment, put in order, and record immediately.

11. The measurements should be recorded immediately to avoid error.

12. Earpieces and diaphragm can be cleansed with an alcohol sponge.

12. Alcohol cleanses earwax lodged in the tips and reduces bacterial invasion on the earpieces and diaphragm, readying the equipment for use with the next patient.

If a beat irregularity is detected, this should be noted. When an unsatisfactory or high reading is obtained, it is advisable to permit the patient to rest and attempt a second reading shortly thereafter. This serves as a check on the accuracy of measurement. Repeating the procedure in the same arm in a consecutive pattern will in itself elevate the pressure due to the subsequent discomfort.

Summary

The blood pressure reading is another vital sign which offers the physician a general perspective regarding the condition of the heart and vessels.

In order for the medical assistant to acquire the necessary procedural skill and discretionary judgment in applying these skills, knowledge of the physiology of blood pressure is required. Since obtaining the vital signs is a primary function of the clinical medical assistant, MAs must have confidence in their theoretical and practical expertise. Understanding the principles and the reasons underlying them is imperative to the development of confidence and professional competence.

HEIGHT AND WEIGHT

Skills Objectives

Upon completion of this section you will be able to:

1. Define height and weight and explain the relationship between these and the other vital signs.

2. Demonstrate the proper procedure for measuring the height and weight.

3. Demonstrate the proper care of the balance scales.

Introduction

Although the patient's height and weight are not routinely taken after the initial physical examination unless ordered, they are considered here as vital signs in the sense that they are indicators of the state of general health, particularly weight gain and loss.

Weight measurements may, however, be routinely obtained (1) for patients following special diets to monitor results; (2) for maternity patients to detect weight loss or gain possibly due to dietary habits, or weight gain possibly due to water retention; and (3) for children as indicators of growth patterns and general signs of their state of health. Desirable weights for men and women, determined according to height, are given in Table 16-1.

In this chapter only the procedures are described. National influences on height and weight and related disease conditions are discussed in subsequent chapters.

Equipment for Measuring Height and Weight

A balance scale is used to obtain both the height and weight measurements. There are several kinds of balance scales available, but these basically fall into two categories—mechanical and electronic. Mechanical scales essentially use the principle of the fulcrum or lever to arrive at a precalibrated set of weights which equalize the patient's total weight. Electronic scales (which are technically not balance scales) are coming into increasing popularity because they save the operation of adjusting the balance of weights. Most electronic scales provide an immediate digital readout when the patient steps on the scale.

Recording the Data

The height and weight are recorded by using the abbreviations for height (Ht) and weight (Wt) followed by the numerical measurement; for example: Ht 5'9" Wt 170 lbs. The physician determines the significance of the measurements, taking into account the time of day, dress (clothing or examination gown), weight history, dietary habits, activity, and other factors specific to the individual. The medical assistant records only the measurements; interpretations are the physician's responsibility.

MEASURING HEIGHT AND WEIGHT

Procedure	Principle
1. Check to make certain that bar weights (both 50-lb and per-pound increments) are on zero.	1. If the bar weights are not properly positioned, the accuracy of measurement will be affected.
2. Place a paper towel on the footrest of the scale.	2. The towel affords protection from possible foot disease transmitted by other users of the scale.

TABLE 16-1. Desirable Weights for Men and Women Aged 25 and Over*

Women†

Height (with shoes on) 2-inch heels Ft.	In.	Weight (in pounds fully clothed)‡ Small Frame	Medium Frame	Large Frame
4	10	92-98	96-107	104-119
4	11	94-101	98-110	106-122
5	0	96-104	101-113	109-125
5	1	99-107	104-116	112-128
5	2	102-110	107-119	115-131
5	3	105-113	110-122	118-134
5	4	108-116	113-126	121-138
5	5	111-119	116-130	125-142
5	6	114-123	120-135	129-146
5	7	118-127	124-139	133-150
5	8	122-131	128-143	137-154
5	9	126-135	132-147	141-158
5	10	130-140	136-151	145-163
5	11	134-144	140-155	149-168
6	0	138-148	144-159	153-173

Men

Height (with shoes on) 1-inch heels Ft.	In.	Weight (in pounds fully clothed) Small Frame	Medium Frame	Large Frame
5	2	112-120	118-129	126-141
5	3	115-123	121-133	129-144
5	4	118-126	124-136	132-148
5	5	121-129	127-139	135-152
5	6	124-133	130-143	138-156
5	7	128-137	134-147	142-161
5	8	132-141	138-152	147-166
5	9	136-145	142-156	151-170
5	10	140-150	146-160	155-174
5	11	144-154	150-165	159-179
6	0	148-158	154-170	164-184
6	1	152-162	158-175	168-189
6	2	156-167	162-180	173-194
6	3	160-171	167-185	178-199
6	4	164-175	172-190	182-204

*Courtesy of Metropolitan Life Insurance Company.
†For young women between ages 18 and 25, subtract 1 pound for each year under 25.
‡To convert pounds to kilograms, multiply the number of pounds by 0.45; to convert kilograms to pounds, multiply the number of kilograms by 2.2

303

3. Lift the height bar and raise it to the expected level above the patient's head.

3. This practice avoids possible injury to the patient caused by manipulating the bar after the patient is on the scale.

4. Direct the patient to remove his shoes.

4. Keeping the shoes on would yield an inaccurate height measurement.

5. Instruct the patient to step on the scale and stand erect.

5. Standing erect ensures an accurate measurement.

6. Gently lower the height bar in place, protecting the patient's head, and rest the bar on the crown of the head.

6. This technique avoids injury to the patient by dropping the height bar.

7. Note the height measurement.

7. Remember the number of inches for later conversion into feet and inches.

8. Move the large weight bar to the nearest 50-lb weight differential anticipated. (Example: move bar to 150 lbs for a man expected to be somewhere between 150 and 200 lbs.)

8. Moving the smaller bar first is inefficient and will be inaccurate. This procedure ensures efficiency of time and motion.

9. Move the smaller weight to the number which will permit the pointed end of the bar to maintain an even middle position of balance.

9. Careful bar manipulation is essential to obtain a precise measurement of weight.

10. Note the weight measurement.

10. Remember the exact weight; do not round off as this will distort the measurement.

11. Lift the height bar gently from the patient's head and hold secure.

11. This practice prevents injury.

12. Instruct the patient to step off the scale and put on shoes.

12. Patient involvement in the procedure is completed.

13. Move the weight bars to zero, return the height bar to resting position, and dispose of the paper.

13. This readies the scale for use by the next patient.

14. Immediately record the height and weight.

14. Committing results to memory for long periods of time may result in recording distorted data. Recording accurately provides the physician with significant data regarding patient's general state of health.

Summary

The height and weight of the patient are important considerations for the physician in assessing the general state of health as well as in determining medication dosage and prescribing diet therapy and exercise plans. The role of the medical assistant is to accomplish this procedure accurately and with concern for the patient's sensitivities.

APPLICATION EXERCISES

The following application exercises are grouped into five sets, one for each of the major sections of this chapter.

Body Temperature

Five different situations are listed below that relate to body temperature. Discuss which of them would increase or decrease body temperature, and how you would proceed in completing the task of obtaining the patient's temperature. Refer to the principles in the chapter.

1. You enter the room and note that the patient is walking around the room. What effect, if any, would this have on body temperature and how would you proceed?

2. The patient tells you that he has just consumed two cups of hot coffee. What effect, if any, would this have on body temperature and how would you proceed?

3. You have inserted the thermometer in the patient's mouth. The patient is talking continuously.

4. You enter the examining room and are about to insert an oral thermometer. You note that the patient is holding an iced drink.

5. You enter the examining room and note that another medical assistant is rinsing off a thermometer in hot water and is about to take the patient's temperature.

Record the following temperature readings:

1. One hundred and four and two tenths.

2. Ninety-nine and two tenths.

3. Ninety-eight and six tenths.

4. Ninety-seven.

5. Ninety-nine (rectal).

Consider the following situations and provide explanations as needed:

1. Will a person who sleeps during the day and works all night have a lower temperature reading than one who works during the day and sleeps all night? Give two reasons for your answer.

2. A patient complains of feeling cold after bathing and begins to shiver. Would the temperature reading be higher or lower than before the bath? Why?

3. A patient comes to the office extremely angry after an argument with his wife. How may this affect his temperature reading?

4. Will an 11-month-old infant usually have a temperature level higher or lower than an adult? Why?

Discuss the possible effects of the following situations:

1. A chipped thermometer.

2. Worn calibrations on a thermometer.

3. An axillary temperature reading recorded after 3 minutes.

4. A rectal thermometer used for an oral temperature.

5. A chemical solution is not rinsed off before inserting the thermometer in the patient's mouth.

Pulse

1. Locate the (a) radial, (b) temporal, (c) carotid, and (d) popliteal pulse on your own body with the aid of the instructor. You have found the artery when the pulsation is felt to be strong and bounding.

2. Form partner groupings. Locate the radial pulse on your partner. Apply heavy pressure (not gentle). Discuss results.

3. In the partner groupings, take and record your partner's radial pulse using the procedure outlined in this chapter.

Discuss the following situations and try to achieve class consensus concerning the answers and solutions:

1. A 25-year-old patient comes to the office, and, as you are taking the vital signs, states that he ran 5 miles in 3 hours before his visit. What would you expect of his pulse rate, rhythm, and volume?

2. You determine the patient's pulse rate to be 100. What would be your initial reaction? Would you ask the patient questions or retake the pulse? Discuss your response.

3. You are taking the patient's pulse for 30 seconds and you notice some skipped beats. What is your initial response?

4. While taking a patient's pulse, you determine the rate for 30 seconds is 35. The pulse is difficult to palpate and feels thin under the fingertips. Record the rate and characteristics.

5. The pulse rate of a 45-year-old woman is recorded as 52 beats per minute. The rhythm is irregular and the volume weak. Does this patient's pulse fall within the normal range? Identify the arrhythmia.

Respiration

1. Sit down and for 30 seconds each: (a) breathe rapidly and deeply (hyperpnea); (b) hold your breathe (apnea). Discuss the physiologic concepts demonstrated by this exercise.

2. Sit down and for 60 seconds breathe as rapidly and as deeply as possible. Discuss the

physiologic concepts demonstrated in this exercise. Pay particular attention to the consequences of breathing in this pattern: urges and feelings.

3. Form partnerships and take turns observing the rise and fall of each other's chest. Discuss your feelings. Count for 30 seconds and multiply by two. With the use of a stethoscope listen to your partner's chest sounds.

4. Perform the procedure as described previously in the chapter and obtain the TPR readings simultaneously.

5. Discuss your response to the following situation: You are obtaining the patient's TPR, and even though you kept your fingertips on the pulse while counting respirations, the patient asks you why you are glancing at her chest while you are counting the respirations.

Blood Pressure

In discussing the following questions, determine whether the expected blood pressure reading would be high or low. Explain your answers.

1. A patient comes to the office with a vaginal hemorrhage.

2. A 65-year-old woman and her 25-year-old daughter are having their blood pressure taken. What would you expect the comparison to illustrate?

3. A patient in the examining room has been crying. You are about to take her blood pressure.

4. A patient has been standing in the examining room while awaiting your entrance. You ask him to sit down, and you wait 5 minutes before taking his blood pressure. Why?

5. After beginning to take the patient's blood pressure, you notice the cuff is too loose. If you continued to take the blood pressure, what would your expectation be?

An Experiment Relating to Venous Pressure:

Hang one hand down at your side until the veins of the hand become distended. Now raise the hand above the heart. Discuss observations.

Procedure Preparation:

1. Identify all the parts of the stethoscope.

2. Insert earpiece and listen to your own heart beat.

3. Fold the cuff so that it fits into the palm of your left hand. Grasp tightly. Place the bulb in your right hand and with your thumb and forefinger tighten the control valve. Pump until the mercury level reaches 180. Slowly release. Tighten the valve at 152. Release. Tighten at 144. Release. Tighten at 136. Release. Be certain that you can read the scale correctly.

Procedure Practice:

Select a partner. Referring to the procedure/principle outline on blood pressure, obtain your partner's blood pressure using the stepwise approach. Record the systolic and diastolic blood pressure.

After your partner obtains your blood pressure reading, switch partners and compare readings on the same individual. Readings should be within 6 to 8 mm of one another.

Height and Weight

1. Select partners and perform the procedure for obtaining height and weight on one another.

2. Form groups and then discuss several different weight and height charts. Attempt to answer these questions:

   a. How is optimum weight determined?
   b. Do charts differ or is there a universal standard?
   c. Cite the common factors or patterns evident?
   d. What conclusions can be formed?

3. Assign roles and discuss what messages are being conveyed by the role-players and what objectives are realized.

   a. Mrs. R. is coming to the office for a complete physical examination. She is about to be weighed. She asserts that she doesn't want to be weighed. What is your response?

   b. Mr. P. has been weighed. You are recording the data. He states, "I've had a ferocious appetite but don't seem to be gaining. In fact, I think I've lost weight." What is your response?

   c. After her child is weighed and measured, a mother asks you, "Is he normal size? He's the smallest kid in his class." What is your response?

   d. A woman on a reducing diet is weighed and no weight loss is recorded for the week. She complains, "See, it's just not working. Nothing works. I give up." What is your response?

COMPLETING THE LEARNING LOOP

As you have learned in the course of this chapter, the vital signs, height, and weight are critically important indicators of the state of health. As a student you will have many opportunities to learn and share information about the vital signs. You should take a new interest in learning more about these measures. When you have an opportunity, you should ask questions and seek information which relates to these functions.

BIBLIOGRAPHY

Anthony, C. P., and Thibodeau, G. A.: *Textbook of Anatomy and Physiology*, ed. 10. C. V. Mosby, St. Louis, 1978.

Blainey, C. G.: "Site Selection in Taking Body Temperature." *American Journal of Nursing* 74:1859, 1974.

Guyton, A. C.: *Textbook of Medical Physiology*, ed. 6. W. B. Saunders, Philadelphia, 1981.

McInnes, B.: *The Vital Signs with Related Clinical Measurement*, ed. 3. C. V. Mosby, St. Louis, 1979.

17

GOWNING, POSITIONING, AND DRAPING

SPECIFIC OBJECTIVES

Upon completion of this chapter you will be able to:

1. Demonstrate the proper procedure for gowning the patient.

2. List the types of examination gowns which are available.

3. Demonstrate the basic examination positions.

4. Instruct a patient in the proper procedure for assuming each of the examination positions.

INTRODUCTION

The medical assistant prepares the patient for examination by obtaining the vital signs, history, and interview, and by gowning, positioning, and draping appropriately.

These procedures are the prelude to any examination. Since each patient who visits the office will probably require some degree of physical examination, learning and applying the proper procedures for preparing the patient must be within the scope of the MA's skill development and judgment acquisition. In this chapter the most common positioning, gowning, and draping techniques are described. Other positions used with specific procedures and examinations will be discussed in later chapters.

Among the important factors inherent in all procedures related to patient preparation is the patient's need for privacy and personal comfort. This must become the medical assistant's foremost concern.

GOWNING

Purpose

In order for the physician to perform an adequate examination, the patient must disrobe and wear a gown which will facilitate the procedure by exposing only the part to be examined. The type of examination to be performed, the patient's age and sex, and the inaccessibility of the clothing worn are the factors to be considered in gowning. The patient's privacy and comfort are also significant concerns.

Types of Gowns

Either a partial gown or a full gown may be used, depending upon the factors present. Gowns can be made either of cloth, which must be laundered, or of paper, which is disposable. The doctor's preference in these matters is, of course, the major determinant.

Partial gowns cover only the shoulders, chest, and back. Street clothing is worn from the waist down. *Full gowns* are at least knee length, with a back opening extending the full length of the gown and closed by ties or velcro strips. All clothing is removed.

Selection Criteria

The medical assistant decides what disrobing instructions to give the patient after the following criteria are reviewed:

1. *First visit.* A patient visiting the office for the first time will almost always receive a complete physical examination. Since this type of examination involves a check of all body systems, a full gown is required.

2. *Purpose of the visit.* The purpose of the visit will determine the extent of disrobing and gowning necessary. The patient's presenting symptoms or reason for the visit will give clues as to the type of examination the doctor will perform. If, for example, a patient is coming to the office because of a persistent cough, congestion, and sore throat, a partial gown is the appropriate choice because only the chest needs to be exposed for examination. The medical assistant's capacity to anticipate the type of examination to be performed will develop as she builds and integrates her knowledge of clinical medical assisting and clinical medicine. Subsequent discussions on the methods of examination and actual work experience will expand the medical assistant's judgment competencies.

3. *Sex and age.* The sex and age of the patient help determine the extent of disrobing and gowning. Using the previous example of the patient with respiratory tract complaints, an adult male or an infant male or female may not require gowning.

4. *Individual need for privacy.* Some patients are reluctant to disrobe and even after gowning directions have been given they will retain some clothing. All individuals have needs for privacy, but to varying degrees. When these individual variances are known and anticipated, special handling of the patient is facilitated. Allow the patient to retain clothing as desired if it will not interfere with the process of examination.

Patient Instruction

Gowning instructions should be thorough and clear to save time and relieve patient anxiety. Instructions should be geared to the patient's level of understanding. Obviously, the extensiveness of instruction would differ for a 4-year-old's annual checkup and a 40-year-old's monthly visit. Some patients will need assistance in disrobing. Others can be given the gown and drape sheet along with precise instructions and left alone to carry out the procedure. There are several important points to remember whenever instructions are given for disrobing and gowning:

1. Consider the age and level of understanding.

2. Assess the need for assistance.

3. Always give clear, detailed instructions.

4. Individualize instructions for patients with specific diseases, injuries or handicaps to prevent pain or further injury.

POSITIONING AND DRAPING

Purpose

The purpose of assisting the patient to assume certain positions is, like gowning, to facilitate the examination. Depending on the type of position used, certain body parts became more accessible, patient comfort becomes more obtainable, exposure is achieved, and the physician's examination is accommodated.

Positioning the patient is the medical assistant's responsibility and an essential component of patient preparation.

Types of Positioning

Many types of positions are used in medical procedures, depending on the type of examination and the sex of the patient. Those discussed here are the most basic and are illustrated in Figure 17-1. Other positions are used in conjunction with medical specialties and in specialty examinations and procedures. These, however, are usually modifications of the basic positions described in this chapter.

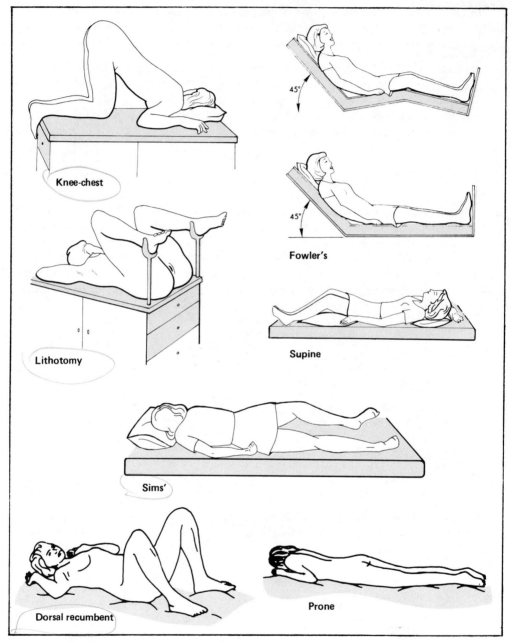

FIGURE 17-1. Common examination positions. (Adapted from Saperstein, A. B., and Frazier, M. A.: *Introduction to Nursing Practice.* F. A. Davis, Philadelphia, 1980.)

1. In the *sitting* position, the gowned patient simply sits upright on the examination table, with legs dangling over the table or feet placed on a footstool and covered by a drape sheet. The head and chest (heart, lungs, and upper extremities) can be examined in this position. It should be remembered that whenever possible the patient should begin the office visit in the sitting position, and, as the examination progresses, be assisted in assuming the proper positions. The underlying principle of this procedure is related to achieving the patient's physical and psychological comfort. When the patient first greets the physician in the sitting position, ease in relating to the physician is effected. When the visit begins in this manner, the patient usually feels that he or she can converse more freely and that time is being taken to treat the individual rather than a disorder.

2. In the *supine* position, the patient is lying flat on the back with arms at the sides and covered by a drape sheet. The chest, abdomen, and extremities can thus be examined. The head can be examined in this position as well as in the sitting position. Procedures performed on the head are usually accomplished when the patient is supine. Neurologic reflexes are also tested in this position.

3. In the *dorsal recumbent* position, the patient is supine, but the legs are sharply flexed at the knee, feet on the table, rather than lying flat and extended as in the supine position. The drape sheet is adjusted to cover and wrap each leg (with corners of the sheet) and to cover the chest and abdomen and the pubic area (with the remaining corners). The corner covering the pubic area is lifted and turned onto the abdomen when the examination is initiated to expose the genital area. The vagina and rectum can be examined in the female and the rectum in the male.

4. In the *lithotomy* position, the female patient assumes the dorsal recumbent posture but rather than having the feet on the table, they are placed in stirrups. The patient's knees are still flexed, the buttocks moved to the edge of the table, and the feet placed in stirrups. This is the position of choice for the vaginal examination and the pap smear procedure, and when a vaginal speculum (an instrument to increase the vagina's width for proper visualization) is used. Draping is the same as in the dorsal recumbent position.

5. In the *Sims'* position, the patient is instructed to lie on the left side with the left arm behind the body and the right arm forward flexed at the elbow. Both legs are flexed at the knee, but the right leg is sharply flexed and positioned next to the left leg which is slightly flexed. A drape sheet covers the patient from the waist to the toes and is adjusted when necessary to expose the anal area. In the male, the rectum can be examined in this position, and in the female, the rectum and vagina. This position is frequently used to administer an enema.

6. In the *prone* position, the patient is lying flat on the abdomen with the head turned slightly to the side. The arms can be positioned above the head and extended, or alongside the body. The back, spine, and lower extremities can be examined in

this position. A drape sheet extends from the waist to the knees and is adjusted for adequate exposure when necessary.

7. In the *knee-chest* position, the patient is assisted to assume a kneeling position with buttocks elevated and head and chest on the table with arms extended above the head and flexed at the elbow. A small pillow can be used under the chest to promote patient comfort as this position is uncomfortable, particularly for an extended period of time. The rectum is examined in this position in both males and females, and specific examination procedures using a sigmoidoscope (an instrument to visualize the color of the bowel) can be performed. Draping may require use of two sheets to cover the back and wrap the legs.

8. In the *Fowler's* position, the patient sits on the examination table, the back supported and the legs outstretched on the table, a drape sheet covers the patient's legs. This position is used in particular for patients with dyspneic conditions.

9. In the *proctologic jack-knife* position, the knee-chest posture is assumed more sharply with the use of a special table usually found in the office of a proctologist (a physician specializing in diseases of the rectum). Draping is the same as in the knee-chest position. Proctologic examination procedures are performed in this position in both male and female patients.

Selection Criteria

The position chosen is dependent on the following variables:

1. *Symptomatology.* The patient's presenting symptoms will be significant clues for the medical assistant in anticipating the type of examination to be performed. For example, a patient with respiratory complaints will most probably begin the examination in the sitting position to facilitate examination of the respiratory system.

2. *Type of examination and procedure.* The patient may be scheduled for a certain type of examination or a specific procedure. The medical assistant then proceeds to assist the patient in assuming the proper position. For example, a patient scheduled for vaginal examination would assume a lithotomy position.

3. *Age and sex.* The age and sex of the patient are important considerations in positioning. For example, a rectal examination can be performed in one of several positions; the position chosen would fit the age and sex of the individual patient.

Patient Instruction

The reason for assuming a particular position should be briefly explained to the patient and instructions given clearly and precisely to enable the patient to assume the position with minimal assistance.

The considerations for patient instruction in positioning are identical to those for gowning. It is important to emphasize, however, that handicaps or disease conditions would alter the assumed position. Patient safety and comfort are always the first priority.

Procedures for Positioning

Most of the procedures for assisting the patient to assume positions for examination do not require a detailed, stepwise description. However, procedural guides are included for the lithotomy and knee-chest positions as improper technique in these cases can greatly affect patient comfort.

ASSISTING PATIENTS IN THE LITHOTOMY POSITION

Procedure	*Principle*
1. Instruct the patient to lie flat on her back.	1. This provides a comfortable first-step transition.
2. Ready stirrups.	2. Proper positioning of the stirrups prior to inserting the patient's feet saves time and promotes comfort.
3. Instruct the patient to bend her knees and place her feet on the corners of the table.	3. Muscular strain is reduced when the position is assumed in gradual steps.
4. Instruct the patient to slide the buttocks down as close to her feet as is comfortable.	4. Again muscular strain is reduced.
5. Place the patient's feet one at a time in stirrups by placing one hand over the ball of the foot and cupping the ankle just above the heel with the other.	5. Muscular spasm is reduced and the feet are prevented from injury when handled in this manner.
6. Instruct the patient to slide the buttocks further until they are at the edge of the examining table.	6. This provides greatest accessibility to the regions to be examined.
7. Properly drape and separate the legs.	7. This affords privacy while increasing exposure.
8. Following the examination, instruct the patient to slide the buttocks up on the examination table to a comfortable position where the legs are extended.	8. Gradual resumption of normal positioning reduces muscular spasm.
9. Lift the feet out of the stirrups simultaneously and place on the examination table.	9. Removing the feet individually increases the potential for muscular cramping in the inner thigh. Cramps which do occur can be resolved by placing the leg flat on the table and pressing down on the knee with the palm of one hand while pulling up on the ball of the foot with the palm of the other hand.
10. Assist the patient to a sitting position.	10. This position is most comfortable to the patient and signals the procedure's completion.

ASSISTING PATIENTS IN THE KNEE-CHEST POSITION

Procedure	Principle
1. Instruct the patient from a sitting or supine position to assume a kneeling position.	1. Gradual steps in positioning promote the patient's understanding and cooperation.
2. Instruct the patient to lay the head and chest on the table, placing the hands above the head, flexed at the elbow. Place a small pillow under the head and chest.	2. This affords greatest comfort and prevents the arms from getting in the way of examination.
3. Instruct the patient to bring the knees up to the chest as far as is comfortably possible. Stand by the patient to offer assistance.	3. This affords greatest accessibility to the region to be examined. The same assistance may be necessary so that the patient does not fall from the table.
4. Properly drape the patient.	4. Draping affords privacy and comfort. This position should be assumed just prior to the examination procedure, with the patient completely covered until it is necessary to expose the region.
5. Assist the patient to a sitting position.	5. This signals that the procedure is over and allows for greater patient comfort.

SUMMARY

The medical assistant's role in preparing the patient for examination includes gowning, placing the patient in the appropriate position, draping, and applying the proper techniques to ensure privacy and comfort for the patient.

The assistant's responsibilities include psychological preparation as well, and this consideration should underlie all physical activities.

As the medical assistant acquires an understanding of how the physical examination proceeds and what it includes, as related to the purpose of the visit and the age and sex of the patient, anticipation of the physician's needs regarding gowning, positioning, and draping of the patient will become routinized.

APPLICATION EXERCISES

Problem-Solving Discussion Questions

Attempt to isolate the major objectives which underlie your approach to each of the following situations:

1. A patient has fractured her left arm which is in a cast. How would you approach gowning? Would you give any special instruction to the patient?

2. All patients coming to Dr. Jones' office are given a full gown and instructed to completely disrobe. Mrs. Smith does not remove her underwear. Describe your approach.

3. John A. is 2 years old. He is visiting the doctor with complaints of cough, congestion, runny nose, and fever. How would you approach gowning?

4. Mrs. Alberts is wearing a necklace and earrings. She is gowned and awaiting a complete physical examination. Would Mrs. Alberts be asked to remove her jewelry? Defend your response?

5. Mr. Pole is 76 years old and awaiting a rectal examination. Which position would Mr. Pole most likely assume? Defend your response.

Practice Exercise

Form partners and place each other in all the positions discussed following a demonstration from your teacher (refer to Figure 17-1). Using disposable drapes, properly drape according to the position assumed.

After everyone has had an opportunity to position and be positioned, discuss feelings associated with the positions. Determine the existence of common denominators in the comments expressed.

COMPLETING THE LEARNING LOOP

Part of the success of gowning, positioning, and draping lies in the medical assistant's ability to gently communicate both the techniques and the reasons for each procedure. The MA should be aware of the anxiety which a patient will normally feel during an examination and be prepared to use communications skills in directing the patient's efforts.

A properly instructed and prepared patient makes the work of the physician significantly easier. The next unit will focus on the methods of examination and the medical assistant's role.

BIBLIOGRAPHY

Broer, M.: *Efficiency of Human Movement.* W. B. Saunders, Philadelphia, 1973.
Brunner, L. S., and Suddarth, D. S.: *Textbook of Medical Surgical Nursing.* J. B. Lippincott, Philadelphia, 1975.
Matheney, R. V., et al.: *Fundamentals of Patient Centered Nursing.* C. V. Mosby, St. Louis, 1972.
Seedor, M. M.: *Body Mechanics and Patient Positioning.* Teachers College Press, New York, 1977.

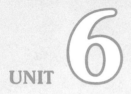

ASSISTING WITH THE PHYSICAL EXAMINATION

The clinical medical assistant is responsible for assisting the physician with the physical examination. These responsibilities include preparation of the patient, the room, and the equipment, as well as providing any assistance needed by the physician and the patient during the process of examination.

To effectively carry out these functions, the assistant must anticipate the physician's needs regarding the type of examination to be performed, the specific equipment needed, and the extent of patient assistance required. Anticipation of needs assumes adequate judgment based on a reasonable understanding of the process of the general and specific physical examinations, the methods and equipment used, and the related role of the medical assistant.

Included in this unit is a discussion of the common symptomatic reactions to disease in each system. The medical assistant who has a reasonable understanding of the body systems and the symptoms produced when they are diseased can more effectively anticipate the physician's approach to the examination and respond to the needs encountered. Upon hearing the patient's reason for the visit, the medical assistant can independently prepare the patient, ready the room and the equipment, and provide other assistance as required. To function successfully in the clinical setting, the medical assistant must perform the role of facilitator. Integration of the knowledge and skills essential to the role of facilitator is the goal of this unit.

UNIT OBJECTIVES

Upon completion of this unit you will be prepared to:

1. Assist the physician with both general and specific examinations.

2. Explain the examination and testing procedures to the patient.

3. Provide for equipment needs related to the examination.

4. Perform specific clinical procedures required as a result of the examination and requested by the physician.

5. Anticipate physician and patient needs based upon symptomatology.

CHAPTER **18**

THE GENERAL PHYSICAL EXAMINATION

SPECIFIC OBJECTIVES

Upon completion of this chapter you will be able to:

1. List the purposes of and procedures for the general physical examination.

2. Prepare the examination room for the physical.

3. List the basic steps which the physician will follow.

4. Prepare the patient for the examination.

5. List the commonly used equipment.

6. Care for the equipment.

INTRODUCTION

Every patient who comes to the medical office will receive a physical examination. The examination will be either general (complete) or specific (limited). This chapter focuses on the general physical examination, sometimes referred to as the comprehensive examination.

Most physicians prefer to perform a general examination on new patients in order to assess their state of health and establish some comparative base for future visits. Regular or routine examinations are performed as a preventive measure to ensure health maintenance. The major objective of routine examination is early detection of disease or the signs which indicate disease potential. The diagnosis of certain diseases depends on a check of all body parts and systems. In these cases, a general examination is performed.

The physical examination is the physician's primary diagnostic tool. In order to function in the role of the physician's facilitator, the medical assistant not only must master the skills required, but also must comprehend the process of the physical examination, its purpose and methods. It is this combination of understanding and skill development which will enable the MA to apply discretionary judgment to the varying situations encountered when assisting with the general physical examination.

PURPOSE OF THE PHYSICAL EXAMINATION

The purpose of the general physical examination is to determine the overall state of health. The entire body is examined including all body openings, all major organs and all body systems. Upon completing the examination, the physician interprets the findings and forms a judgment called the *diagnosis*.

Laboratory and other diagnostic tests are used concurrently to supplement physical findings. Laboratory testing is an essential component of the general physical examination and of specific examinations as well. These laboratory tests and diagnostic testing procedures will be described and discussed in Chapter 26.

THE DIAGNOSIS

The physical examination is the cornerstone of the diagnostic process upon which all other nonphysical findings rest. Pieced together, the physical examination findings, the vital signs, laboratory and other diagnostic test results, the patient's voiced symptoms, and the physician's general perceptions give shape and substance to the diagnostic puzzle. The physician studies and interprets these factors and forms a judgment, concluding a diagnosis.

There are three basic categories of diagnosis that the physician may select to represent his own conclusions:

1. *Differential diagnosis.* In this category, the physician attempts to rule out certain possibilities. From these alternative diagnoses the final diagnosis may emerge. A differential diagnosis is usually written in the following manner:

   Differential Diagnosis: 1) RO appendicitis
                            2) RO gastroenteritis
                            3) RO colitis

2. *Tentative diagnosis.* In this category, the physician has not yet reached a conclusion, and the diagnosis is therefore temporary and subject to change as the physician gains further insights from other diagnostic tools such as consultation with

other physicians or further laboratory studies. The tentative diagnosis is usually written in the following manner:

>Diagnosis: Possible bowel obstruction

3. *Final diagnosis.* The final diagnosis is the conclusion the physician comes to after the results of all diagnostic tools have been integrated and evaluated. The final diagnosis is written in the following manner:

>Diagnosis: Gastritis

EXAMINATION METHODS

In order to establish a diagnosis, the physician will utilize one or more of four methods of examination. Each requires the use of all the examiner's senses. Attention is fully concentrated upon uncovering any abnormality. The physician uses these methods collaboratively during the entire procedure.

1. *Inspection.* The physician visually inspects body parts with or without the use of illumination and magnification, depending on the part being inspected. During the process of examination, the physician will inspect the skin, ears, mouth, throat, and, with illumination and use of instruments, will examine the cervix and vaginal wall in the female patient. In certain patients a sigmoidoscopic examination may also be performed. (The sigmoid is part of the colon.)

2. *Palpation.* The physician locates and feels with fingers and hand the major organs of the body and lymph node pathways. During the process of examination, the physician will palpate lymph nodes in the neck, axilla (underarms), breast, and abdominal organs.

3. *Percussion.* During the neurologic examination, the physician will tap certain body parts for reflexes by using a percussion hammer. During the process of the general physical examination body parts are percussed by using the fingers or knuckles. The chest wall and abdomen will be examined in this manner. Through the use of percussion, certain sounds are generated and the physician evaluates their normalcy.

4. *Auscultation.* The physician listens to certain body sounds through the use of a stethoscope. During the process of examination, the physician listens to the sounds made by the heart and respiratory actions, and for bowel sounds in the intestines.

EQUIPMENT USED IN THE PHYSICAL EXAMINATION

Special instruments are required for the physical examination. These instruments are designed to enable the physician to listen, inspect, visualize, and test the body parts. The instruments are readily accessible in a special tray or are positioned permanently in each examination room.

The instruments most commonly used for a complete physical examination are described below and illustrated in Figure 18-1.

1. *Ophthalmoscope.* This instrument is used to inspect the eye. The physician checks for any abnormality of the parts of the eye, detected by focusing light through a magnifying lens of the ophthalmoscope.

2. *Otoscope or nasal speculum.* This instrument enables the physician to inspect the inner ear. Light is focused through a magnifying lens. The nasal canals also can be inspected with the same instrument by changing the speculum. Ear speculums are long and narrow, while the nasal speculum is short and wide.

3. *Pocket flashlight or headlight.* This piece of equipment is needed to supply light during various phases of the examination.

4. *Ruler or flexible tape measure.* These measuring devices are used to determine the size of an abnormality when appropriate (such as lesions). In infants the circumference of the head is measured to note progress.

5. *Tongue depressors.* A tongue depressor is used to hold down the tongue in order to visualize the throat.

6. *Stethoscope.* This instrument is a listening device and is used in the examination of various parts of the body, specifically the heart and lungs.

7. *Gloves and lubricant.* Plastic gloves (usually disposable) are used to protect the patient and physician from invading microorganisms while the physician palpates the inner structures of the vagina and rectum in the female, and the rectum in the male.

8. *Vaginal speculum.* This instrument is used by the physician to dilate and expand the vaginal opening to facilitate examination of the vaginal wall and the cervix.

9. *Reflex hammer.* This instrument is used to test neurologic reflexes, usually in the tendons of the knees.

10. *Tuning fork.* A judgment by the physician related to the degree of auditory acuity is possible through the use of this instrument. The vibration of the tuning fork produces a humming noise perceptible to the ears.

PROCEDURE FOR THE PHYSICAL EXAMINATION

The physician performs the physical examination aided by the medical assistant. The ability to effectively assist the physician is dependent on an understanding of how the physician proceeds through the examination. Equipped with this information, the MA can better anticipate the needs of the patient and the physician.

The procedure outlined here is, of course, not absolute. Patient needs or the physician's preference may alter the sequence of the examination. The following description is, however, a widely accepted comprehensive examination.

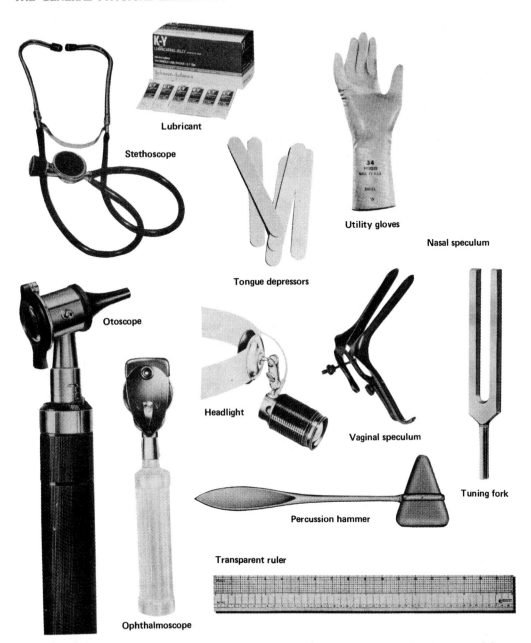

Lubricant

Stethoscope

Utility gloves

Nasal speculum

Tongue depressors

Otoscope

Headlight

Vaginal speculum

Tuning fork

Percussion hammer

Transparent ruler

Ophthalmoscope

FIGURE 18-1. Instruments commonly used in the general physical examination. (Courtesy of General Medical Corporation)

Table 18-1 compares the various areas for examination, listing the body parts, the corresponding positions of the patient, and the equipment needed for each.

Using the methods previously described, the physician assesses the general state of health of the body parts and systems. This assessment includes a general survey based on observation. Signs of distress, skin color, stature, posture, motor activity and gait, grooming, the presence of odors, facial expression, mood, body language, state of awareness and speech, all are noted by the physician as he interviews the patient.

While the patient is gowned and in a sitting position the physician will first proceed to examine the head and the neck.

Head. The hair, scalp, skull, and face are examined by inspection and palpation.

Eyes. A visual acuity test (eye chart examination) performed by the medical assistant may supplement the physician's initial examination of the eyes, which includes inspection aided by an ophthalmoscope.

Ears. The ear canals and drums are inspected by means of an otoscope. The auditory acuity is tested with a tuning fork.

Nose and sinuses. The nasal passages are examined with the use of the otoscope, and the sinuses above and below the eyes (frontal and maxillary) are palpated. The sinuses may also be illuminated by means of a light source.

Mouth and pharynx (throat). The lips, interior mucosa and roof of the mouth, the gums, teeth, tongue, and pharynx are inspected. The physician will use a light

TABLE 18-1. Areas for Physical Examination

Body Part	*Position*	*Equipment Needed*
Head and neck	Sitting	Ophthalmoscope, otoscope, nasal speculum, tuning fork, tongue blade, measuring tape
Chest (front and back), upper extremities	Sitting	Stethoscope
Abdomen	Supine and dorsal recumbent (knees flexed)	Stethoscope
Genitalia and rectum	Sims', dorsal recumbent, or lithotomy positions	Glove lubricant, vaginal speculum, slides, and curette stick (for women)
Lower extremities	Supine	None
Nervous system	Sitting	Reflex hammer

source and a tongue blade to visualize the pharynx. The mucosa of the mouth may also be palpated.

Neck. The lymph nodes that are located on both sides of the neck (cervical nodes), the trachea (windpipe), and the thyroid are inspected and palpated, and the carotid artery is auscultated bilaterally.

While the patient remains sitting, the physician examines the trunk and upper extremities.

Back. The spine and muscles of the back are palpated and inspected.

Posterior thorax (chest wall) and lungs. The chest wall and the lungs are examined by inspection, palpation, percussion, and auscultation. A stethoscope is used to auscultate the breath sounds.

Breasts. In the female patient, the breasts are inspected for symmetry and general appearance. The nodes in the axillary (underarm) region are palpated.

When the above examination steps are concluded, the patient is assisted to a supine position for the continuation of the procedure.

Breasts. The breast examination is continued in the supine position using palpation. The breasts in a male patient are examined if there is suspension or abnormality.

Anterior thorax and lungs. All four methods of examination are utilized to examine the anterior chest and lungs. Some physicians initiate this examination while the patient is in the sitting position. A stethoscope is used for auscultation.

Heart. All four methods of examination are used to examine the heart. A stethoscope is used for auscultation.

The lower body torso is examined while the patient is in the supine position.

Abdomen. All four methods are used to examine the abdomen. A stethoscope is used to auscultate bowel sounds and abdominal blood vessels.

Inguinal area. The inguinal area (the flexion point between the hips and the legs) is examined by palpation for location of inguinal nodes and subsequent assessment of the normalcy of these nodes. Blood vessels in this region are also auscultated.

Genitalia and rectal examination in men. The penis, scrotal contents, prostate, anus, and rectum are inspected and palpated. A rectal examination for both men and women may also be performed while the patient is in the Sims or side-lying position.

Genitalia and rectal examination in women. The examination of the external genitalia, vagina, cervix, and rectum can be accomplished while the patient is in the lithotomy position. A pelvic or rectovaginal examination can be achieved without the use of instruments. However, when a pap smear is performed or visualization of the vaginal wall and cervix is required, a vaginal speculum, headlight, gloves, lubricant, and wipes are needed.

Legs. The legs are inspected and palpated. Pulse sites are located. The patient then stands for further evaluation of the musculoskeletal and peripheral vascular systems.

Musculoskeletal system. The range of motion and muscle strength are noted for both upper and lower extremities and the alignment of the legs and feet, arms and hands. The patient may be asked to walk so that the physician may observe his gait.

Peripheral vascular system. The legs are inspected for varicosities (varicose veins).

Hernia. In the male patient, the inguinal area is again inspected and palpated in the standing position as the hernia may become pronounced only when upright.

Neurologic examination. Gait, the ability to do knee bends, hop, walk on toes and heels, and other procedures facilitate evaluation of the neurologic and musculo-skeletal systems. The patient assumes a sitting position when further neurologic testing is desired.

It should again be noted that the physician may delete from, or add to, the physical examination or may follow a different order based on personal preference or diagnostic perceptions.

THE ROLE OF DIAGNOSTIC TESTS IN THE PHYSICAL EXAMINATION

Diagnostic testing, including laboratory, x-ray, and other measurements, is an integral part of the general or comprehensive physical examination.

An examination of the blood and urine, a chest x-ray, and an electrocardiogram are commonly included in the diagnostic testing for evaluation of the general state of health. Here, too, the physician's own preferences and concerns would govern the choice of specific diagnostic tests as parts of the general physical examination. Detailed discussion of diagnostic tests is presented in Chapter 26.

THE ROLE OF THE MEDICAL ASSISTANT

Descriptions appear below of each of the basic responsibilities of the medical assistant during the examination process.

Room Readiness

The medical assistant is responsible for readying the examination room. Inspection of the room for cleanliness is required. The table sheet or disposable table cover should be fresh for each patient. Wastebasket contents, if odorous, sanguineous (bloody), or otherwise un-pleasant, should be removed. Contaminated instruments from previous procedures should be removed and cleaned, and counter tops should be cleaned and orderly. Equipment anticipated to be used should be assembled. Prescription pads and other material should be stored safely. The patient's file is usually placed outside the examination room door in a rack provided for the purpose. The patient's file is usually not left in the room with the patient as misinterpretation of its contents may occur. However, the patient may request to be shown the record, and the physician will respond accordingly.

Patient Preparation

Weight and height are usually recorded prior to the patient's entry into the examination room. Gowning, draping, and positioning of the patient, discussed in Chapter 17, are other responsibilities of the medical assistant in preparing the patient for the general physical examination. The patient is asked to disrobe completely and to put on a full gown after being instructed as to how it is to be worn, and is then directed to sit on the examination table. A drape sheet is provided for the legs.

If the physician approves, the MA will interview the patient for presenting symptoms, time of onset, and duration, as was discussed in Chapter 15. A history is also obtained during the first visit, as are the vital signs. The physician, as part of the general physical examination, may repeat the blood pressure procedure.

Certain diagnostic tests may be standard practice, including the CBC (complete blood count), urinalysis, and electrocardiogram. These are generally performed by the medical assistant. If certain studies are anticipated, the MA can ready the proper laboratory order sheets for the physician's use.

The medical assistant is the liaison between the physician and the patient. In preparing the patient for examination, the MA sets the tone for the visit, makes general observations concerning the patient, explains procedures, and answers questions. The medical assistant's role is clearly to create a climate of comfort and security for the patient.

The patient often shares with the medical assistant valuable information related to the purpose of the visit and the severity of symptoms, as well as personal fears and anxieties. It is not uncommon for the MA to spend more contact time with the patient than does the physician. Needless to say, the medical assistant should relate all pertinent information to the doctor in charge.

Assisting the Physician

The medical assistant's role in assisting the physician with the examination is threefold: (1) handing instruments to the physician and obtaining other instruments and materials as directed; (2) assisting the patient to assume positions and exposing body areas for examination; and (3) offering the patient reassurance and providing comfort.

While medical assistants do not perform any part of the general physical examination, their presence and assistance are extremely valuable to the physician. When the physician is aided by the MA, the examination can be performed in less time, with greater effectiveness, and with increased patient comfort.

The procedure guide which follows outlines the medical assistant's role in the general physical examination.

ASSISTING WITH THE GENERAL PHYSICAL EXAMINATION

Procedure	*Principle*
1. Prepare the room for the examination.	1. A professional environment is essential and helps to prevent the transfer of microorganisms from patient to patient. Also, an ordered work environment will facilitate the efficiency of the examination.
2. Wash hands and ready all equipment.	2. Hand-washing helps prevent the transfer of microorganisms from the assistant to the patient. Assembling the equipment will save time and will orient the physician to the purpose of the patient's visit.
3. Escort the patient to the examination room after obtaining height and weight.	3. When accompanied by the assistant, the patient avoids confusion as to which examination room to enter and feels greater comfort. Depending on the location of the scale, the weight and height may be measured prior to the patient's entry into the examination room.
4. Give the patient disrobing and gowning instructions and afford privacy.	4. If the patient does not require assistance, then personal comfort is promoted by leaving the room while the patient disrobes.
5. Re-enter the room and explain the anticipated procedure to the patient.	5. The patient's anxiety is decreased when informed of the routine and the procedures that will be performed.
6. Obtain the history and interview if directed.	6. This step saves the physician time and serves as a double-check system as the physician will further interview the patient.
7. Obtain and record the vital signs.	7. This provides the physician with data necessary to evaluate the general state of health.
8. Measure visual acuity if directed.	8. This provides the physician with data necessary to evaluate the general state of health.
9. Instruct the patient in the collection of a urine specimen if not previously obtained.	9. The patient may have brought a urine specimen to the office, or provided a specimen prior to entry into the examination room. Since urinalysis is an accepted component of the general physical examination, anticipation and execution of this procedure by the medical assistant will be valuable to the physician.
10. Ready patient for the physical examination by instructing the patient to assume a sitting position. Cover the legs with a drape sheet.	10. This is the accepted position for the initiation of the physical examination by the physician.
11. As the physician proceeds with the examination, provide the appropriate instruments; assist the patient to assume the position required; assist the physician in exposing body parts; and maintain patient comfort.	11. This manner of assistance assures the efficiency and orderliness of the examination. The more the medical assistant is able to anticipate the physician's procedures and accommodate preferences, the more valu-

12. When the examination is completed, assume followup responsibilities such as administration of medication, performing further diagnostic tests, applying dressings, or performing other clinical procedures.

13. Instruct the patient to dress, and assist if necessary. Allow opportunity for questions.

14. Escort the patient to the front desk, equipped with full instructions related to treatment and return visits. Return to the examination room, and clean and restore order.

able a time-savings resource and quality care provider the MA will become.

12. The physician usually relies on the medical assistant to carry out treatment orders. MAs can further aid the physician in providing optimum health care by assuming not only those followup procedures within their educational boundaries, but also in sharing the responsibility for patient education in the area of treatment.

13. This signals the patient that the visit is completed. Allowing and encouraging questioning ensures that the patient understands the treatment and thus increases the probability of patient compliance.

14. Patient comfort is dependent on many variables. One of prime importance is the personal treatment provided by office personnel. The examination room is cleaned to accommodate the next patient.

SUMMARY

The medical assistant's role in assisting the physician with the general physical examination is to accommodate the physician and the patient. The MA must possess a multitude of diverse skills, both clinical and interpersonal, to function in this capacity. The content of this chapter has been directed toward providing the information necessary to the development of these skills.

APPLICATION EXERCISES

Problem-Solving Exercises for Group Discussion

1. During the process of the general physical examination, the physician tests the patient's reflexes. Identify which system is being examined, what instruments the physician would need, and the patient's appropriate position.

2. The female patient being examined has very long hair. Assess what difficulty, if any, would be encountered during the examination. In what ways could the medical assistant facilitate the examination?

3. A patient is scheduled for a pelvic examination and a pap smear. She is elderly and has arthritic knees. How would you position her for examination? What other assistance would you offer?

4. The physician is examining the patient's ears in the course of a general physical examination. The doctor hands the otoscope to you and pauses a moment. What would you anticipate to be the next step in the examination? Depending on your answer to the first question, what will you do with the otoscope?

5. The physician is about to perform a pelvic examination using a speculum. What other items are needed for this examination? How would you, as the medical assistant, function in this situation in regard to room readiness, patient preparation, and assisting the physician?

Practice Exercises

After thorough study of the physical examination process, form small groups and proceed with the following role-playing exercises:

1. Each member of the group will take a turn playing the role of the medical assistant in the following exercises:

   Prepare the patient for examination: (a) greet the patient; (b) give gowning instructions; (c) orient the patient to the physical examination procedure; (d) respond to the patient's questions.

2. Each member of the group will take a turn in the following exercise:

   Assemble the equipment needed for the physical examination. Choose instruments and equipment from the collection of actual instruments or paper models supplied by the instructor.

3. With one student in the group assuming the role of the physician, another that of the patient, and another that of the medical assistant, simulate a physical examination. Use appropriate instruments if available. Other members of the group are observers who are charged with the responsibility of scrutinizing the way in which the medical assistant is functioning during the procedure. The observers should evaluate the MA's helpfulness to the physician and the patient, his or her ability to anticipate the physician's needs and respond adequately, and his or her ability to assess the patient's needs and respond adequately. All members of the group should take turns role-playing in order to add different perspectives and approaches to the medical assistant's role.

COMPLETING THE LEARNING LOOP

For many physicians the general physical examination constitutes the "core" of medical practice. In this respect the medical assistant who becomes skilled in providing support in the examination process will be an invaluable asset. Every effort should thus be made to learn to identify the equipment and anticipate the needs associated with the general examination.

The next two chapters discuss the medical assistant's role in specific examinations.

BIBLIOGRAPHY

Bates, B.: *A Guide to Physical Examination.* J. B. Lippincott, Philadelphia, 1974.

Bathory, E.: *The Physical Examination: A Feminist Perspective.* Selene Editions, Vancouver, 1980.

DeGowin, E. L., and DeGowin, R. L.: *Bedside Diagnostic Examination*, ed. 3. Macmillan, New York, 1976.

Mudgett, H. W.: *The Psychology of Physical Examination.* Arundel, London, 1978.

Saperstein, A. B., and Frazier, M. A.: *Introduction to Nursing Practice.* F. A. Davis, Philadelphia, 1980.

CHAPTER 19

SPECIFIC PHYSICAL EXAMINATIONS – I

SPECIFIC OBJECTIVES

Upon completion of this chapter you will be able to:

1. Describe the basic structure and function of the system and body part presented.

2. Identify the body's symptomatic reaction to disease relative to specific systems and body parts.

3. List and define the diagnostic studies related to the body parts and systems presented.

4. Describe the process of the specific physical examinations presented.

5. Assist the physician with specific examinations.

6. Anticipate the medical assistant's role in room and patient readiness and in examination and treatment procedures.

7. Perform the specific clinical procedures presented.

8. Provide patient instruction regarding clinical procedures.

INTRODUCTION

As was mentioned in the introduction to this unit, each patient who comes to the medical office will receive a physical examination, either general or specific. The general or comprehensive examination was explained in the previous chapter. The focus of this chapter and the one to follow will be specific examinations.

When the patient visits the office with specific symptoms, the physician will most often examine only the system or systems related to the symptomatology, provided that it is not the patient's first visit.

In order to develop the capacity to anticipate the physician's needs for assistance and to prepare the patient and the room for examination, the medical assistant must first acquire an understanding of symptomatology as the systems react to disease, and of how the examination will proceed to uncover the cause of these symptoms.

It should be noted that in this unit symptoms are discussed exclusive of signs of disease. Symptoms are the patient's subjective rendering of the physical feelings experienced as a result of the state of illness.

Signs refer to the physician's findings during examination. The doctor will listen to the patient's description of symptoms and then look for signs. The integration of the symptoms and physical findings constitutes the physician's conclusion regarding the state of health.

Common symptoms are emphasized here because medical assistants must be alert to the purpose of the visit in order to function effectively in their roles. Diagnostic testing and treatment for specific diseases are also discussed. Equipped with this theoretical base, the medical assistant will develop the skills to assist the physician with specific examinations and will also be able to reasonably predict the body parts that will be examined, the equipment that will be needed, and the treatment possibilities in which the MA may participate when informed of the patient's presenting symptoms or the purpose of the visit. To facilitate the discussion, a description of the structure and function of each system is included. While this discussion in no way serves as a comprehensive anatomy and physiology of the system, the brief description and overviews should be helpful in acquiring a more accurate visualization of the parts examined.

Certain clinical procedures performed by the medical assistant correspond to specific examinations and treatments. These are defined and described in this chapter along with the appropriate systems to which they are related.

THE RESPIRATORY SYSTEM

Structure and Function

The function of the respiratory system is to provide oxygen (air) to all the cells in the body through inhalation and to eliminate the cells' waste product—carbon dioxide—through exhalation. In the discussion on vital signs, respiration was described as the act of breathing. The exchange of gases occurs as a consequence of this act. The bloodstream carries the oxygen to all the cells of the body. The parts of the body involved in the process are the nose, pharynx (throat), trachea (windpipe), and lungs (Fig. 19-1).

The nose is lined with mucous membrane containing *cilia*, little hairs that filter

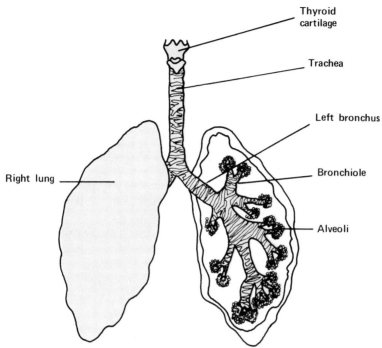

FIGURE 19-1. The respiratory system.

substances in the air. A nasal septum-cartilage divides the nose into two nostrils or external nares. As air is inhaled through the nose, it is warmed and moistened and the cilia clean the air. The air passes through the nostrils to the pharynx (throat) through two openings in the roof of the mouth called internal nares.

In the pharynx, these internal nares, the tubes which follow a pathway to the ears called eustachian tubes, the mouth cavity, the esophagus (the tube which leads from the mouth to the stomach), and the opening of the trachea called the glottis intersect.

When food enters the back of the throat, the glottis automatically closes over with the epiglottis (a small, lidlike protrusion of cartilage) and automatically opens to admit air being inhaled or exhaled.

The inspired air is channeled through the glottis through the 4- to 5-inch-long trachea. The trachea consists of a tube with cartilage rings that can be palpated. These rings prevent the trachea from collapsing, thus extinguishing the passage of air.

The inspired air then travels from the trachea into the two divisions of the trachea called *bronchi*. Cilia also line the bronchi and continuously sway, moving dust particles upward toward the throat.

Each bronchus divides into a network of bronchioles, which are smaller divisions of the bronchus. Each division of the bronchioles becomes thinner and thinner walled and the diameter becomes smaller. Each bronchiole's chamber is surrounded by *alveoli* which are minute air sacs. The exchange of carbon dioxide and oxygen takes place in the alveoli, which are connected to minute capillaries of the bloodstream. These alveoli are commonly compared to a cluster of grapes. The bronchioles and alveoli are contained in cone-shaped organs, the lungs. The lungs compress the alveoli, acting much like bellows. The right lung is divided into three lobes, the left lung into two lobes. Both lungs are covered with a membrane called the *pleura*.

All the structures of the respiratory system are vital to the objective of getting oxygen to the cells and ridding the cells of carbon dioxide. In this sense, each cell breathes.

Symptomatic Reaction to Disease

Given the structure of the respiratory system, and especially noting the throat as the center for drainage and the convergence of tubal openings, it is easier to understand how infection in one area of the respiratory system can quickly lead to infection in another area, such as the ears or larynx, the voicebox which is located in the glottis, and the sinuses located in the head.

The invasion of microorganisms not normally found in the respiratory system leads to infection when the body is vulnerable or conditions accommodating. It is important to note that there are certain microorganisms which normally inhabit the system.

Infections have both general and specific symptoms. General symptoms of infection anywhere in the body usually include fever and chills. Specific symptoms of infection in the respiratory system will include, depending on the area affected, increased pain in the part, impaired breathing, increased congestion from the swelling of mucous membranes, cough produced by excess drainage in the back of the throat, hoarseness when the larynx is affected, and chest pain when the lungs are affected. While infection is most common, these symptoms usually appear as a response to most other diseases of the respiratory tract, signaling the presence of a disturbance in the normal conditions and function.

In summary, the common symptomatic reactions to disease of the respiratory system may include:

1. fever,
2. chills,
3. pain in the affected part,
4. cough,
5. congestion,
6. discharge,
7. dyspnea (difficulty in breathing),
8. malaise (weakness or fatigue).

While one or more of these symptoms may be experienced by the patient, only the skilled physician can interpret their significance. The medical assistant can safely assume that the physician will be examining the respiratory system and therefore certain equipment must be prepared.

The Respiratory Tract Examination and the Medical Assistant's Role

An examination of the respiratory tract will usually begin with an inspection of the mucous membrane of the nose. Although the ear is not part of the respiratory system, it will also be inspected because of its proximity to the system. The sinuses, throat and lungs will also be examined (Table 19-1).

Common Diagnostic Studies of the Respiratory System

There are several traditional tests which are generally carried out in association with the respiratory system. These are listed and described in Table 19-2.

The medical assistant should become familiar with patient preparation for these studies. Except for the sputum specimen and blood work which could be collected by the

TABLE 19-1. Examination of the Respiratory System

System Part	Method and Equipment	Medical Assistant's Role
Nose and sinuses	Inspection with otoscope equipped with short, wide nasal speculum	Instruct the patient to assume a sitting position. Hand instruments to the physician and expose the parts to be examined.
Ears	Otoscope	
Pharynx and tonsils	Inspection with penlight and tongue blade	
Sinuses, neck, lymph nodes, and glands	Palpation	
Chest (lungs) and back	Auscultation (stethoscope)	

TABLE 19-2. Common Diagnostic Studies of the Respiratory Tract

Test	Description
X-ray	Visualization of lungs. Still picture of lungs which outlines lung tissue.
Fluoroscope x-ray	Visualization of lungs in motion.
Sputum specimen	Investigation of the microbial contents of sputum.
Bronchogram	Dye inserted into bronchi and x-ray examination performed.
Bronchoscopy	Examination of the bronchus by insertion of a lighted instrument containing a scope for visualization.
Respiratory function tests	Determination of respiratory capacities (how much air can be inspired and expired).
Medical technology laboratory procedures	Blood gases can be analyzed by obtaining arterial blood. Performed by medical technologist. Other blood work can also be ordered to aid in diagnosis.
Throat culture	Culture of microorganisms present in the pharnyx. Performed by medical assistant by swabing back of throat with sterile applicator.

TABLE 19-3. Common Diseases of the Respiratory Tract

Disease	Symptoms*	Treatment	Medical Assistant's Role
Acute rhinitis (common cold): inflammation of mucous membrane lining the nose may be caused by viral infection (can become chronic).	Sneezing, nasal discharge, tearing of eyes, headache.	Nonspecific treatment relieves symptoms rather than cures disease. Medication such as decongestants and analgesics (pain-relievers) may be ordered. Antibiotics cannot counteract virus.	Assist with examination; perform diagnostic studies if ordered; administer medication if ordered; patient teaching. Instruct patient to blow nose frequently but gently, keeping both nostrils open to prevent infected material from being blown into sinuses and eustachian tube, and into the middle ear. Patients with a common cold usually do not come to the office unless it has become chronic. When discharge is purulent (thick) and yellowish or greenish in color, the patient should be instructed to be seen by the physician.
Sinusitis: inflammation of mucous membrane lining the sinuses (can become chronic).	Pain and tenderness over affected area. Facial headache with infection, fever, and malaise may be present.	Medication to relieve symptoms and antibiotics if bacterial infection is present. Local application of heat. Irrigation for increased drainage. Surgery is a last resort.	General clinical assisting procedures are performed. Nasal irrigation, instillation, or spray may be employed.
Pharyngitis (sore throat): inflammation of the throat caused by irritation or infection.	Pain, difficulty swallowing, general symptoms of infection.	Medication such as antibiotics, gargle and analgesics.	General clinical assisting procedures are performed. In particular, a throat culture may be ordered.
Tonsillitis: inflammation of tonsils (adenoids may also be involved).	Symptoms same as pharyngitis.	Medication or surgery.	General clinical assisting procedures are performed. Patient teaching may be needed to prepare patient for surgery if indicated.

TABLE 19-3. *Continued*

Disease	Symptoms*	Treatment	Medical Assistant's Role
Laryngitis: inflammation of larynx (voice box) associated with infection or other disease.	Hoarseness, aphonia (loss of speech), cough, tightness in the throat, general symptoms of inflammation.	Inhalation of steam or cool mist medication. Treatment may differ depending on cause.	General clinical assisting procedures. Patient teaching may include explanation of effects of steam or cool mist vaporizer. Patient should be instructed that the nozzle should be directed over the head so that the spray falls in a mist to be inhaled.
Bronchitis: inflammation of the mucous membrane of the brochi with increased mucus production (may become chronic).	Cough, usually worse in morning; general symptoms of inflammation.	Medication.	General clinical assisting procedures. In chronic bronchitis, prescription to stop smoking may be explained and progress managed by the medical assistant when indicated.
Pneumonia: infection localized in the lungs can be bacterial or viral.	*Bacterial:* Symptoms of acute infection, fever, dyspnea (painful respirations), malaise. cough. *Viral:* Fever is usually present; dry hacking; cough initially less acute.	*Bacterial:* Antibiotics and other drugs to relieve symptoms. Hospitalization may be necessary. *Viral:* Nonspecific treatment, bedrest. Hospitalization may be necessary.	General clinical assisting procedures. Patient teaching includes instructing patient to cough into the tissue and dispose, to prevent the spread of disease.
Emphysema: air spaces or alveoli become abnormally enlarged and less elastic.	Dyspnea, persistent cough, loss of weight.	Medication, postural drainage at outpatient facility, and physiotherapy (cannot be cured, only controlled).	General clinical assisting procedures. Patient teaching includes explanation of need and procedure for mouth care as patient will usually be a mouth breather. Dietary and exercise instructions should be given and fully explained.

*Symptoms are listed which may be present, but all may or may not be present simultaneously.

medical assistant, and possible routine x-rays, additional studies must be performed by other allied health specialists or the physician.

The office manual should contain patient preparation instructions for all diagnostic tests ordered by the physician.

Common Diseases of the Respiratory Tract

Infection is the most common disease of the respiratory system. Generally, the ending "itis" denotes inflammation. Infection refers to the invasion of microorganisms and is usually accompanied by inflammation. Inflammation refers to the changes in tissue which occur as a result of disease. When attached to the medical term for a particular body part, "itis" signifies the location of the infection and/or the presence of inflamation, as, for example, sinusitis, tonsillitis, pharyngitis, laryngitis, otitis, bronchitis, bronchiolitis, tracheitis, pneumonitis, and pleuritis. Table 19-3 outlines the diseases.

Specific Clinical Procedures Involving the Respiratory System

Nasal irrigation, instillation, and the application of heat and cold to parts of the system are outlined in the following pages. The medical assistant is responsible for the performance of these procedures.

NASAL IRRIGATION

Purpose: Nasal irrigation may be ordered in conditions of rhinitis and, most specifically, sinusitis, to relieve inflammation and increase drainage. Foreign bodies inserted in the nasal canals may also be removed by irrigation.

Procedure	*Principle*
1. Wash hands.	1. Clean hands should prevent the transfer of harmful microorganisms.
2. Assemble equipment: bulb syringe, container (basin), solution ordered, gauze wipes (warmed), emesis basin, waterproof sheeting and towel.	2. Organization facilitates efficiency. The solution can be warmed by placing the closed receptacle containing the solution in a basin of warm water.
3. Prepare the patient for the procedure by (a) explaining the procedure, (b) assisting the patient to assume a Fowler's position (sitting upright with a back rest) with the head slightly forward, and (c) draping the protective sheeting and toweling "bib fashion" around the patient's shoulders.	3. The solution will drain into the basin, but may also splash onto the sheeting, which will prevent the patient from becoming wet and uncomfortable. Nasal drainage is promoted in the upright sitting position.
4. Instruct the patient to avoid speaking or swallowing during the procedure, and to breathe through the mouth.	4. Aspiration of the solution into the lungs is thereby prevented.

5. Instruct the patient to hold the emesis basin below the affected nostril.

5. The basin will collect the solution.

6. Pour the solution into the container and fill the bulb syringe by deflating the bulb prior to insertion in solution. Release pressure and the syringe will fill.

6. Pouring the solution into the basin prevents the contamination of the entire contents of the solution in its original container.

7. Instruct the patient to tilt the head slightly so that the unaffected nostril is uppermost, and insert the tip of the syringe into the unaffected nostril. Slowly and evenly squeeze the bulb. Exert only slight pressure to the bulb.

7. The solution is inserted into the unaffected nostril to prevent the transfer of infectious material from the affected nostril into the unaffected side. Solution will travel up into the nose, around the nasal system which divides the nose, and out the opposite or affected nostril. An excess of slight pressure may force the infectious material into the sinuses and eustachian tube and into the ears.

8. Repeat the insertion of solution several times or until the purpose is achieved: the foreign body is removed or the discharge is clear-colored or as the physician has instructed.

8. The objective should be made clear prior to the initiation of the procedure. If the patient should cough or choke, stop the procedure immediately and wait until coughing ceases. Begin again if irrigation is still required.

9. At the completion of the procedure, dry the patient's face with wipes and toweling. Dispose wipes and remove toweling. Assist the patient to a comfortable position.

9. These measures will increase the patient's comfort.

10. Instruct the patient not to blow his nose for 5 to 10 minutes following the procedure.

10. This prevents the remaining solution from being forced into sinuses and ears.

11. Record the time that the procedure was performed, the amount and type of solution used, and describe the characteristics of the discharge. Initial this record.

11. Proper recording is necessary for later reference and serves as protection for the medical assistant, the patient, and the physician.

12. Remove and clean the equipment.

12. The equipment is ready for reuse.

NASAL INSTILLATION

Purpose: Nasal instillation relieves congestion and softens crust formation in the nostrils. It may be ordered to relieve pain, to increase or decrease drainage, to control nasal bleeding, or to serve as an antiseptic application to irritated nostrils, such as in chronic rhinitis.

Procedure	*Principle*
1. Wash hands.	1. This prevents transfer of harmful microorganisms.
2. Assemble equipment: solution or medicine to be administered and its dropper.	2. Usually the solution or medicine ordered will include a dropper in its cap. Since the dropper will not touch the nostril, the dropper can be used.
3. Prepare the patient by explaining the procedure and assisting the patient to assume a Fowler's position, sitting upright with a back rest. Instruct the patient to blow the nostrils	3. This position facilitates the flow of solution into the nose.

together. Place a pillow under patient's shoulder and tilt the head over the pillow.

4. Fill the dropper with the prescribed amount. Hold the tip of the dropper just over the patient's affected nostril and insert the prescribed number of drops.

4. Drops will flow into the affected nose, and the dropper will not become contaminated.

5. Instruct the patient to remain in position for 5 minutes.

5. Holding the position will ensure solution reaching the nose and not reversing its flow.

6. Upon completion, assist the patient to a comfortable position and then record the procedure: medication (type and amount), time, and area of application. Initial this record.

6. Proper recording is essential for further reference.

APPLICATION OF HEAT

Purpose: Heat is applied in the form of hot compresses to the nose and sinus area to promote drainage and relieve pain.

Procedure	*Principle*
1. Wash hands.	1. The transfer of harmful microorganisms is thus prevented.
2. Assemble equipment: gauze, washcloth, basin, bath thermometer.	2. Organization facilitates efficiency.
3. Prepare the patient for the procedure: (a) explain the procedure, (b) assist to assume sitting position with back rest, (c) drape with toweling to absorb moisture.	3. These steps increase patient comfort and cooperation.
4. Tap water is usually used for external compresses. Fill the basin with the tap water and with the bath thermometer test the temperature. A temperature of approximately 105°F (41°C) is desirable.	4. Water warmed to this temperature promotes circulation and drainage as it dilates the vessels. Erythema (redness of the skin caused by dilation of the capillaries) is achieved and drainage in the nose and sinuses activated. The increased blood supply to the part acts to absorb the excess fluid in the tissues. The degree of heat and length of time applied depend on the purpose, the age of the patient, the location of the application, and the patient's general condition. These variables affect the patient's sensitivity to heat, and also to cold.
5. Completely submerge the cloth in the basin. Wring excess water from the cloth and place across the bridge of the nose and over the maxillary sinuses. If indicated, another compress can be placed over the frontal sinuses.	5. The area affected will then receive the greatest benefit. Compresses should remain in place approximately 3 minutes to achieve the desired effect. When cooled, another application is required, and the procedure is continuously repeated for a period of approximately 15 minutes.

6. Upon completion of the procedure, dry the patient's face with toweling. Remove the draping and assist the patient to a comfortable position.

7. Record the procedure in the patient's file, noting time, length of time, compresses applied, solution, the time solution was used, and site. Initial this record.

8. Remove the equipment, clean the area, and give the patient instruction, if needed, for home heat application.

6. These steps increase patient comfort. The patient may want to blow his nose and may do so gently.

7. Proper recording is essential for future reference.

8. The equipment should be ready for future use. Patient instruction is necessary if compresses are to be self-administered. The patient should be clear as to the length of time the compresses should be left in place or how long they should be continuously applied, how often, the temperature of the water, the purpose of the procedure, and its importance to treatment.

APPLICATION OF COLD

Purpose: An ice collar or ice bag may be administered in the office to relieve pain and swelling of the throat. Often the patient is instructed to perform this procedure at home.

Procedure	*Principle*
1. Wash hands.	1. This prevents transfer of harmful microorganisms.
2. Assemble equipment: ice, very cold tap water, ice bag, washcloth, and toweling.	2. Organization facilitates efficiency.
3. Prepare patient by (a) giving an explanation of the procedure and its purpose, (b) assisting the patient to a sitting position with back rest, and (c) draping the toweling over the neck and shoulders.	3. This will promote patient comfort and cooperation.
4. Fill the ice bag with ice, if available, or very cold tap water. Place the bag over toweling and directly on the throat.	4. The cold constricts or narrows the blood vessels and therefore restricts swelling by reducing fluid accumulation. It relieves pain because of the numbing effect on the nerve receptors of the skin. (It should be noted that the effects of prolonged heat or cold will cause pain and therefore prolonged application is dysfunctional.)
5. After the procedure is completed, remove and clean the equipment and assist the patient to a comfortable position.	5. These steps will ready the equipment for future use and will increase patient comfort.
6. Record the procedure and give followup instructions to the patient if required.	6. Record time, length of time applied, and initial. Followup instructions will include the length of time that the patient should use the ice collar and how often.

Respiratory Specialties

The physician who has specialized education and training in the diagnosis and treatment of respiratory disease may be referred to as a pulmonary specialist or a physician specializing in diseases of the chest and lungs if the focus of interest is in this area. Other respiratory specialists are referred to as ENT physicians, those who specialize in the ear, nose and throat.

The role of the medical assistant in the office of a specialist would differ only in the procedures done and equipment used routinely. For instance, x-ray equipment would probably be a standard feature in these offices. In the office of an ENT specialist, audiometry would be emphasized. Medical assistants working in such areas would build on their basic knowledge of clinical assisting and would apply and expand their skills in a particular specialized area.

Figure 19-2 illustrates some specific equipment that may be utilized in the office of a pulmonary specialist and an ENT specialist.

Respiratory problems may also be seen in the office of a primary care or family practice physician. Reference to Figure 19-2 will give the assistant clues as to the types of equip-

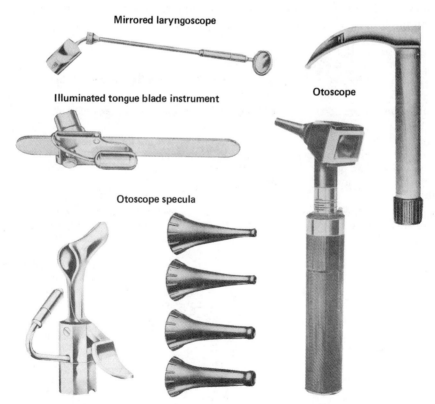

Mirrored laryngoscope

Illuminated tongue blade instrument

Otoscope

Otoscope specula

FIGURE 19-2.   Special ear, nose and throat equipment. (Courtesy of General Medical Corporation)

ment needed and the special clinical procedures and diagnostic tests which may be performed.

THE EAR

Structure and Function

The ear consists of three parts: the external ear, the middle ear, and the inner ear.

The external ear comprises the area of the ear on the outside of the head, called the auricle. The tube leading from the auricle into the inner canal is called the external canal or meatus. The tympanic membrane, or eardrum, separates the external and middle ear. Sweat glands in the canal secrete cerumen, or "earwax."

The middle ear is a small hollow in the temporal bone which is lined with mucous membrane and contains three small bones, or ossicles: malleus, incus, and stapes. These bones are more familiarly called the hammer, anvil, and stirrup because of their visual similarity to these objects.

There are five openings into the middle ear cavity. All are important in the event of infection. One opening is from the external meatus and is covered over by the tympanic membrane; two openings lead into the internal ear; one opening leads into the nostril sinuses; and the other leads into the auditory or eustachian tube. The last opening can serve as a passageway for the spread of infection from the nose or throat into the middle ear and from there into the nostril sinuses. These openings are lined with a continuous sheet of mucous membrane. In children this tube is shortened. Perhaps this accounts for the more frequent incidence of middle ear infections in children. Changes in pressure on either side of this tube will result in a disturbance of equilibrium or rupture of the drum.

Symptomatic Reaction to Disease

The ear will usually react to disease by becoming painful. Impaired hearing or discharge may also occur.

Because the eustachian tube of the ear opens into the throat, or nasopharynx, the middle ear is quite susceptible to infection. Infection of the middle ear is termed *otitis media*.

The Ear Examination and the Medical Assistant's Role

The physician will inspect the ear canal and drum with an otoscope. Although the illumination and magnification of the otoscope enable the physician to inspect the eardrum, much of the middle ear and inner ear are inaccessible to examination. The physician will test for tenderness by grasping the tip of the ear and moving it back and forth. In addition, the physician may pull on the ear lobes, again testing for tenderness.

In order for the otoscope to be inserted properly in an adult, the physician will tilt the patient's head back, grasp the auricle gently, and pull it up and back to gain visualization of the drum. In small children, the lobes will be pulled downward and backward.

The medical assistant, in preparing the equipment, should secure a clean speculum or otoscope. Specula come in a variety of sizes. Usually the physician will prefer a larger size for adults.

When the examination is completed, the assistant cleans the speculum by soaking it in disinfectant or wiping it with an alcohol swab to be ready for the next patient.

Common Diagnostic Studies of the Ear

Two common studies are associated with the ear: audiometric testing and blood counts (see Table 19-4).

The medical assistant's responsibilities lie in scheduling patients for audiometry and in performing basic laboratory procedures as ordered. Patients may be instructed to have additional blood work performed at an appropriate facility.

Common Diseases of the Ear

There are four common diseases or conditions associated with the ear: foreign body obstruction, otitis media, mastoiditis, and external otitis. These are examined in Table 19-5.

Specific Clinical Procedures Involving the Ear

Depending upon the diagnosis, the medical assistant may perform certain clinical procedures pertaining to the ear during the patient's visit. These procedures are ordered as treatment measures and include the installation of ear medications and the irrigation of the ear canal.

EAR INSTILLATION

Purpose: Medication for the ear is introduced directly into the ear canal or onto the drum. Medication may be administered to soften the earwax prior to irrigation, or may precede the application of antibiotic drops prescribed to treat infection.

TABLE 19-4. Diagnostic Tests of the Ear

Test	Description
Audiometry	An otologist or audiometrist can detect hearing loss by use of several hearing tests.
Laboratory technology	A complete blood count, or at least a white blood cell count and differential, is often ordered if infection is suspected.

TABLE 19-5.   Common Diseases of the Ear

Disease	Symptoms	Procedures	Medical Assistant's Role
Foreign body obstruction	Pain in ear, hearing loss.	Irrigation, instillation, removal.	General medical assisting procedures. Unless otherwise prescribed, children and adults should be instructed to put nothing in ears except the end of a washcloth while bathing. Instructions related to blowing the nose gently are also important in order to reduce the incidence of secondary ear infections.
Otitis media (infection of the middle ear)	Stuffy ear, pain, tinnitus (ringing in ears), general symptoms of infection.	Drug therapy, irrigation, instillation, possible myringotomy (opening into drum to relieve pressure).	
Mastoiditis (infection of the area of bone behind the ear)	Pain behind ear, headache on affected side.	Drug therapy; medical management is not successful (mastoidectomy).	
External otitis (infection of the external canal from abrasions or fungal infection)	Irritation, discomfort, possible drainage.	Antiseptic and other drug therapy; heat applied.	

Procedure	Principle
1. Wash hands.	1. This prevents the transfer of harmful microorganisms.
2. Obtain the medication using the proper procedures to ensure accuracy. Obtain several clean cotton balls.	2. The procedures for ensuring accuracy of medication administration will be discussed in Chapter 22. For the purpose of organizational efficiency, the equipment should be prepared before entry into the examination room.
3. Identify the patient and explain the procedure.	3. Patient identification is a necessary safety habit for the prevention of error. Explaining the procedure to the patient will reduce anxiety and increase cooperation.
4. The patient can be placed in a sitting or side-lying position. In the sitting position, the head is tilted toward the unaffected ear. Lying down, the patient rests on the unaffected ear.	4. The positioning facilitates the flow of medication into the drum.
5. Withdraw the medication into the dropper. Grasping the dropper with one hand, pull the auricle up and back with the other hand. Insert the medication.	5. The canal must be straightened to facilitate the flow of medication. For ear instillation in children, pull the earlobe down and back to straighten the canal. (The direction of the ear canal differs in children and adults.)
6. The patient remains in position for approximately 10 minutes.	6. Remaining in position prevents the medication from draining out of the ear.

7. A cotton wick made from a small piece of cotton, turned and elongated to fit the ear canal, is inserted only as ordered by the physician.

7. The cotton wick helps retain medication in the ear for a long period. This procedure should only be performed with the physician's supervision as improper insertion could cause ear damage.

8. Give the patient instructions for removal of the wick and continued application of medication, if ordered, and record the procedure.

8. The patient should leave the office with complete instructions for followup. This ensures properly continued patient management. Proper recording includes date, time, medication name and amount, and the assistant's initials.

EAR IRRIGATION

Purpose: Irrigation of the ear is a procedure performed to cleanse (flush out) the ear canal for the purpose of removing cerumen discharge, dislodging a foreign body, or applying a soothing antiseptic solution to the inflamed ear.

Equipment: Metal or soft rubber bulb syringe, ear basin or small emesis basin, contents for solution, cotton balls, towels, irrigation solution, sterile basin, otoscope.

Procedure	Principle
1. Wash hands.	1. The transfer of harmful microorganisms is thus prevented.
2. An otoscope may be used to visualize the ear prior to the procedure if irrigation is ordered for reasons other than reducing inflammation.	2. Visualization is important for comparison of the affected ear when the procedure is completed. If cerumen softeners have been inserted, wait 15 minutes before irrigation so that drops can achieve their effect.
3. Obtain and assemble the equipment.	3. This organizational step facilitates efficiency.
4. Identify the patient and explain the procedure.	4. Patient identification prevents error. Explanations reduce patient anxiety and promote compliance.
5. Instruct the patient to assume a sitting position.	5. The sitting position enables the irrigation solution to continuously return to the ear basin. If the patient were to assume a side-lying position for this procedure, too much pressure would be exerted on the drum from the irrigating solution.
6. Place a towel on the patient's shoulder on the side of the affected ear and fold under the ear. (Simulate a stand-up collar.)	6. This protects the patient's clothing and prevents the solution from running down the neck, chest, and back.
7. Position the ear basin under the affected ear. Instruct the patient to hold the basin in place.	7. The basin will catch the flow of solution. The patient's assistance is required here to free the hands for the procedure.
8. Cleanse the outer ear with a cotton ball dampened with the solution ordered. (A sterile normal saline solution is frequently the solution prescribed.)	8. This prevents matter on the outer ear from being introduced inside the ear.

9. Pour the solution into a *sterile* basin. Withdraw the solution into the bulb syringe, immersing the tip into the solution.

9. The solution should not be withdrawn while contained in its proper receptacle, but rather poured into the basin to prevent contamination of the entire contents of the receptacle.

10. Insert the tip of the filled syringe into the affected ear after first expelling a small amount of solution into the basin. Press the bulb to begin the irrigation.

10. A small amount of solution is expelled to prevent air from entering the ear. Air entering the ear under pressure causes discomfort. If using a metal syringe, extra caution must be undertaken to prevent insertion of the tip too far into the canal, causing injury. If using a metal syringe, less bulb pressure is exerted to avoid rupture of the tympanic membrane.

11. Repeat the irrigation, removing the syringe tip periodically to enable a free flow of returning solution.

11. Several irrigations are usually required to achieve the desired effect.

12. Dry the outer ear. Visualize the inner ear with the otoscope.

12. If a foreign body or cerumen was to be removed or discharge cleansed, the otoscope visualization will enable comparison and evaluation of results. If matter is still present, irrigation is continued. Observation of the solution in the basin will also be an evaluation tool.

13. Dry the outer ear with dry cotton balls or a towel tip when the procedure is completed, and remove the ear basin and towel.

13. This promotes patient comfort and protects clothing.

14. Instruct the patient to assume a side-lying position on the side of the affected ear. Place a towel under the ear.

14. This facilitates continued drainage of solution from the ear.

15. Record the procedure and give followup instructions to the patient.

15. Proper recording includes date, time, procedure and solution, amount of solution, and assistant's initials. Followup instructions ensure the proper continued care.

16. Clean and return the equipment.

16. Equipment is then ready for the next patient.

Ear-Related Specialties

Several related medical specialties are concerned with conditions affecting the ear. In addition to otology, which deals specifically with the ear, its anatomy, physiology, and pathology, the MA may encounter specialists in otoneurology, which concerns itself with the relationship of the ear to the nervous system; otorhinology, which deals with conditions of the nose and ear; and otorhinolaryngology, which treats diseases of the ear, nose, pharynx, and larynx.

THE CARDIOVASCULAR SYSTEM

Structure and Function

The circulatory system consists of the heart and blood vessels. The heart is a muscle that pumps blood containing oxygen (which was oxygenated in the capillaries in the alveoli) to all parts of the body through a vast network of arteries and smaller arterial vessels called arterioles. Blood which has been deoxygenated within the body's cells returns to the heart through a corresponding network of veins and smaller veins known as venules. The capillaries where the exchange of gases takes place and the lymphatics which drain lymph (a clear fluid) from the blood are also included in the circulatory system.

The Heart

The heart is the operative force of the circulatory system. It is a hollow muscle which acts as a pump. The average weight of the heart is three-quarters of a pound. As was discussed in Chapter 16, the average number of heart contractions is from 60 to 90 beats per minute with about 4,000 to 5,000 gallons of blood being pumped each day.

The heart is situated on the left side of the thoracic cavity in close proximity to the left lung. The base of the heart is lateral to (to the side of) the sternum and above the diaphragm. The apex of the heart lies about midway to the left side of the chest and just below the nipple of the left breast.

An attempt to imagine the location of the heart will be helpful to the medical assistant in performing electrocardiograms, since the positioning of leads is based on an understanding of location. The cardiopulmonary resuscitation procedure (CPR) performed in emergency situations also presumes this understanding.

The heart is divided into four chambers. These are depicted and labeled in Figure 19-3.

The auricles (atria) receive blood from the veins and the ventricles pump blood into the arteries. Both the auricles and ventricles contract. When the auricles contract, blood is forced into the ventricles. One-way valves between the upper and lower chambers prevent backflow. The tricuspid valve is between the right atrium and the right ventricle; the mitral or bicuspid valve is between the left atrium and left ventricle. When the heart is at rest, it is in the filling phase; when the heart is in the state of contraction, it is in the pumping phase. The venous blood is received into the right atrium, passes through the tricuspid valve and into the right ventricle. The blood leaves the right ventricle and flows into the pulmonary artery, which divides into two branches, one going to each lung. The artery branches in the lung into capillaries, and by means of hemoglobin in the red blood cells, the blood becomes oxygenated. Red arterial blood returns to the heart by the four pulmonary veins (two from each lung) and enters the left atrium as the cycle of circulation continues.

The heart is approximately the size of a closed fist and is composed largely of muscle tissue called the *myocardium*. The membranous lining of the heart is called the *endocardium*, and the membranous covering around the heart is the *pericardium*. The blood vessels which supply the heart muscle itself are the *coronary arteries*.

The heart beat is controlled by the sinoatrial (SA) node in the heart, otherwise known as the *pacemaker*. This node is located in the right atrium and receives stimulation from various nerve centers in the brain. Another node, the atrioventricular (AV) node, located in the interventricular septum, receives the impulse from the SA node and transmits this impulse along its fiber, known as the bundle of His, to the ventricles, causing them to contract. It is this complex mechanism which enables the medical assistant to obtain pulse measurements, for each beat of the pulse represents the contraction of the left ventricle.

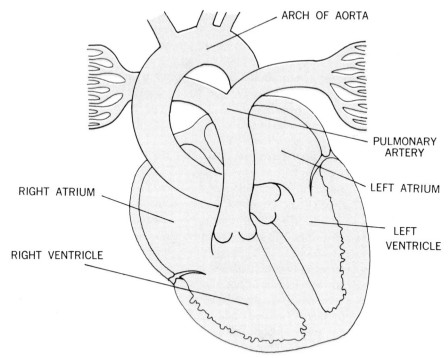

FIGURE 19-3. Interior view of the heart. (Reproduced from *Taber's Cyclopedic Medical Dictionary*, ed. 14. F.A. Davis, Philadelphia, 1981.)

This awareness of the cardiac cycle is also important to the MA as it relates to blood pressure: the systole and the diastole—contraction and relaxation.

Symptomatic Reaction to Disease

With the acquired understanding of the structure and function of the circulatory system, disturbances in its functions are regarded as indicators of disease.

Depending on the type and extent of disease, symptoms will, of course, vary. Disturbances in pulse characteristics have already been noted in the discussion on vital signs in Chapter 16. Skin color could be affected in certain diseases due to the lack of oxygenated blood which is responsible for pink coloring. Cyanosis is the term that refers to a blueness of the skin when the body is in a state of reduced intake of oxygen. This condition can occur in respiratory disease. Reduced oxygen will also cause fatigue.

A reduction of red cells will produce a decrease in oxygenated blood as well. A general term used to signify the reduced number of red blood cells or reduced hemoglobin in the red blood cell is *anemia.*

The heart itself and its surrounding structure, including the walls, can become infected. The vessels can become narrowed and clogged with substances, causing a decrease in the amount of blood circulating to the particular part, which results in pain. Clot formation in the vessel will also cause pain, and, if lodged and causing blockage of blood flow, may result in the severe pain and tissue death which occurs in myocardial infarction (heart attack).

Common symptomatic reactions to disease of the heart and vessels may include:

1. Pain as the cardinal symptom and as experienced in the chest or extremities.
2. A feeling of weakness which may impair normal functioning.
3. Headache (possible in hypertension).
4. Numbness and tingling of extremities.

The Cardiovascular Examination and the Medical Assistant's Role

The physician usually begins the examination of the circulatory system, specifically of the heart and vessels, with auscultation of the heart, noting heart sounds, rate, and rhythm. The stethoscope most commonly used has both a bell and a diaphragm (see Chapter 16). The physician will use the bell to detect lower-pitched sounds and the diaphragm for higher-pitched sounds.

Such methods of examination as percussion, inspection, and palpation will also be employed by the physician in a comprehensive examination of the heart. Palpation of the heart and chest wall is performed to detect vibrations produced by the cardiac cycle. Percussion, although more infrequently utilized, helps to detect areas of dullness outlining the heart and is helpful to the determination of cardiac enlargement. The vessels in the extremities will also be inspected, auscultated, and palpated (Table 19-6).

Common Diagnostic Studies of the Cardiovascular System

There are several diagnostic tests associated with the cardiovascular system. In addition to obtaining electrocardiographic, x-ray, and fluoroscopic findings, such procedures as angiocardiography, radiocardiography, aortography, coronary arteriography, and cardiac catheterization must be considered. These and other tests are described in Table 19-7. The medical assistant should become familiar with these procedures and should include this information in the office procedure manual for future reference.

Common Diseases of the Cardiovascular System

The medical assistant should be familiar with the most common diseases associated with the cardiovascular system. Heading the list are hypertension, coronary artery disease, myocardial infarction, and congestive heart failure. These and other cardiovascular disorders, together with their symptoms and treatment, are presented in Table 19-8.

Specific Clinical Procedures Involving the Cardiovascular System

The special clinical procedures related to cardiology for which the medical assistant assumes responsibility include obtaining the blood pressure and pulse measurements. These have been discussed as vital signs in Chapter 16.

The medical assistant is also responsible for performing the electrocardiogram (ECG). This diagnostic study will be discussed in Chapter 27.

TABLE 19-6. Examination of the Cardiovascular System*

Examination	Methods and Equipment	Medical Assistant's Role
Heart	Inspection, palpation percussion, auscultation with stethoscope.	Position, drape, expose chest, hand physician stethoscope.
Pressure	Inspection, palpation of carotid arteries, venous pressure, auscultation with stethoscope, and blood pressure readings with BP apparatus and stethoscope.	Hand physician equipment. Assist patient to change position if necessary.
Peripheral vascular system (arteries which supply arms and legs, veins in the extremities and the lymphatic system)	Palpation of pulses in arms and legs; inspection of extremities; palpation of lymph nodes.	Place patient in supine position and assist in exposing extremities.
Presence of varicosities	Inspection of backs of calves; palpation.	Assist patient to standing position. Help keep gown together to ensure privacy. Redrape and assist to sitting position when examination is completed.

* Patient is usually in the supine position or lying with upper body elevated 30 to 45 degrees.

Cardiovascular Specialties

The heart specialist is a physician trained in cardiology. Diseases of the cardiovascular system are the comprehensive focus of a cardiologist's practice, and surgery related to the treatment of heart disease is a common responsibility. The medical assistant involved in this specialty would perform electrocardiographic and, perhaps, stress tests routinely. Other assisting procedures related to office visits by cardiac patients would be practiced daily. Patient teaching would become an expanded responsibility, and emphasis on side effects and reactions to drugs used in heart disease would have to be foremost in the medical assistant's base of knowledge.

THE BREASTS AND AXILLAE

Structure and Function

The female breast tissue is composed of lobes of glands channeled into a duct which opens on the nipple, a fibrous tissue and ligament network supporting these glands, and adipose (fat) tissue which encases and surrounds the glandular and fibrous material (see Fig. 19-4).

TABLE 19-7.   Common Diagnostic Studies of the Heart and Circulatory System

Test	Description
Electrocardiogram (ECG): (called a stress test when the ECG is attached to a treadmill and measured while the patient is actively exercised)	Graphic measurement of the electrical currents produced by contraction of heart muscles. Electrodes are placed in certain areas over the heart and vessels to detect abnormalities in heart function. The medical assistant can perform the ECG in the office. In the hospital, the ECG will be performed by the ECG technician and will often be computerized to achieve an automatic readout.
X-ray and fluoroscopic examination	X-ray of the heart will present the heart's configuration. Fluoroscopic examination is x-ray of the heart as it is functioning.
Angiocardiography	An opaque dye is injected into a major blood vessel and x-ray examination performed as the dye flows through the heart, lungs, and major vessels. This procedure is performed in the hospital and special preparation of the patient is required.
Coronary arteriography	A long catheter (hollow plastic tube) is passed through an artery and into the heart. Opaque dye is injected through the catheter. Visualization through x-ray of the dye flowing through the coronary arteries is achieved. This procedure is performed in the hospital and the patient requires special preparation.
Cardiac catheterization	A catheter is inserted into a vein in the arm and passed into the heart. Blood samples can be extracted and the amount of pressure in the heart's chambers measured. This procedure is performed in the hospital and requires special preparation of the patient.
Aortography	X-ray study of the aorta. This study involves the same routine and particulars as those tests previously discussed.
Radiocardiography	Radioactive isotopes are injected into the blood stream intravenously. Their course and the timing of their arrival at the heart are measured with a special counter. Performed in the hospital with special patient preparation required.
Central venous pressure (CVP)	A catheter is inserted into the vena cava or right atrium and is attached to a measuring device that detects the amount of pressure exerted by the blood in the catheter.
Circulation time	A bitter substance is injected intravenously. The time it takes for this substance to be tested is recorded. (Also called the "arm-to-tongue" test.)
Medical technology laboratory procedures	Analysis of blood and other body substances such as sputum and feces.

TABLE 19-8. Common Diseases of the Cardiovascular System

Disease	Symptoms	Treatment	Medical Assistant's Role
Hypertension (high blood pressure)	Systolic blood pressure above 140, diastolic above 90. Headache, nervousness, vertigo (dizziness). (Usually no symptoms are present initially.)	Drug therapy, diet therapy.	General clinical medical assisting procedures. In patients with hypertension, patient teaching is extremely important. With the physician's approval, lifestyle patterns may need to be worked out with the patient. Stressing the importance of daily medication is essential as patients are reluctant to take medication when no symptoms are present. Diet instruction and planning may be the medical assistant's responsibility.
Varicose veins (dilated, knotted, and prominent veins)	Feeling of heaviness and weakness in lower legs; aching muscles of legs.	Conservative measures such as avoiding sitting or standing for long periods may be recommended. Surgery is another alternative.	General clinical medical assisting procedures. Patient teaching would include instructions such as how to wrap an ace bandage, recommendation of elastic stockings, and other precautions as the physician dictates.
Thrombophlebitis (blood clot in vein accompanied by inflammation); phlebothrombosis (clot in vein without inflammation)	Pain, warmth, redness, swelling, fever, malaise.	Drug therapy, surgery.	General clinical medical assisting procedures.
Cerebral vascular accident (CVA): arteries of brain receive reduced blood supply. (several causes)	Headaches, feeling of fullness in the head, vertigo. Could result in paralysis of part or side of body and coma.	Treatment is nonspecific. Objective is restoration and rehabilitation.	This is a medical emergency and the medical assistant needs to be alerted to the possibility when screening patients over the phone with symptoms of severe headache, etc.

TABLE 19-8. *Continued*

Disease	Symptoms	Treatment	Medical Assistant's Role
Coronary artery disease: Arteriosclerosis (narrowing of arteries by lime deposits) or atherosclerosis (narrowing of arteries by fatty deposits) can result in one of the following diseases:			
Angina pectoris: inadequate blood supply to heart muscle causes pain over pectoralis (chest muscle)	Pain under sternum (may spread down left shoulder) pain can range from discomfort to severe squeezing pain.	Drug therapy	General clinical medical assisting procedures.
Myocardial infarction (heart attack): heart tissue death from inadequate blood supply; coronary artery is occluded.	Severe vise-like pain under sternum may radiate down left arm; shortness of breath, nausea and vomiting; profuse perspiration.	Drug therapy: treatment specific to individual condition and type and amount of tissue damage.	A medical emergency that the medical assistant must be alerted to in all patients complaining of chest pain.
Infection of the heart: endocarditis, myocarditis, pericarditis	General and specific symptoms of inflammation.	Specific to location of infection.	General clinical medical assisting procedures.
Congestive heart failure: heart pump dysfunction; fluid collects in tissues.	Symptoms are dependent on which side of heart is affected.	Drug therapy, diet therapy.	General clinical medical assisting procedures.

There are variations in the proportions of these materials due to age, nutritional state, pregnancy, and other variables.

The male breast is composed of a small nipple and its surrounding areola. Breast tissue in the male is underdeveloped and usually cannot be distinguished from neighboring tissue.

In both the males and females, many of the lymph nodes drain into the axillae

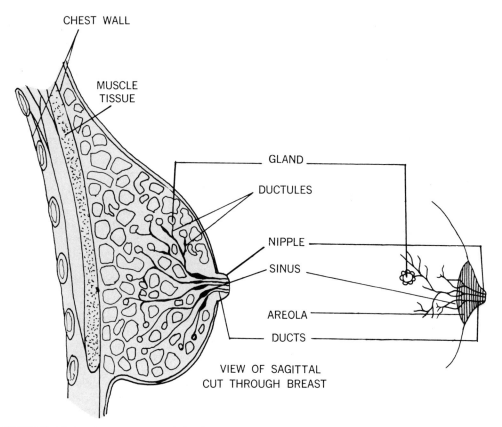

CHEST WALL

MUSCLE
TISSUE

GLAND

DUCTULES

NIPPLE

SINUS

AREOLA

DUCTS

VIEW OF SAGITTAL
CUT THROUGH BREAST

FIGURE 19-4. Interior views of the breast. (Reproduced from *Taber's Cyclopedic Medical Dictionary*, ed. 14. F.A. Davis, Philadelphia, 1981.)

(underarms). For this reason a simultaneous examination of the axillae is performed (Table 19-9). Because of the branching lymphatic pathways, disease states of the breast usually include the axillary regions of the body as well.

Symptomatic Reaction to Disease

The breasts can become infected and inflamed, and therefore the signs and symptoms of these processes can be applied to the breast: redness or swelling, pain, tenderness, discharge, and fever. Other diseases of the breast, such as carcinoma, usually do not present symptoms, but rather abnormal changes in the breast tissue. Patients themselves often detect these abnormalities and come to the office for interpretation of their findings.

Common Diagnostic Studies of the Breasts and Axillae

A frequently used diagnostic test in the evaluation of the breasts and axillae is mammography, which consists of the taking of x-ray photographs of the mammary tissues to detect the presence of abnormalities such as tumors. Though used less routinely than simple palpation, mammographic studies are an aid in the early detection of cancerous or precancerous tissues.

TABLE 19-9. Examination of the Breasts and Axillae

Body Part	Method	Medical Assistant's Role
Female breast	Inspection	Assist the patient to a sitting position and expose breasts (gown to waist). Instruct patient to keep arms at sides. The patient is then instructed by the physician to raise arms over head and then to lower arms and press hands against hips. The medical assistant may then, at the physician's request, grasp the patient's hands and extend the arms while the patient leans forward. While this procedure may cause embarrassment to the patient, it is an essential component of the examination. Changes in contour, size, symmetry, and general appearance are related by the physician. The procedure should be fully explained to the patient by the medical assistant prior to the examination to increase the patient's comfort and afford the opportunity for patient teaching.
	Palpation	Instruct and assist the patient to assume the supine position. Place a small pillow under patient's shoulder on the side to be examined. (This procedure distributes the breast more evenly on the chest wall.) The physician may instruct the patient to raise arms alternately above head. (Transfer the pillow to the side being examined.)
Male breast	Inspection and palpation	Instruct the patient to assume a sitting position and drop the drape sheet to the waist.
Axillae	Inspection and palpation	Instruct and assist the patient to assume sitting position and expose area.

Common Diseases of the Breasts and Axillae

There are a number of diseases which are associated with the breasts and axillae. Some of these may be discovered during the routine or general examination. The most frequently seen conditions are mastitis, chronic cystic mastitis, benign tumors, and breast cancer. Each of these is discussed in Table 19-10.

Specific Clinical Procedures Involving the Breasts

The clinical procedure related to the breasts for which the medical assistant is responsible is concerned with patient teaching. The MA can teach early detection of breast cancer by instructing the patient in breast self-examination (BSE). Many physicians make use of breast

TABLE 19-10.   Common Diseases of the Breasts and Axillae*

Disease	Symptoms	Treatment	Medical Assistant's Role
Mastitis: infection of the breast.	Swollen, painful breast and general symptoms of inflammation.	Drug therapy, hot or cold compress.	General clinical medical assisting procedures. May instruct patient in the use of compresses for relief of discomfort.
Chronic cystic mastitis: irregular excessive growth of normal breast tissue which results in the formation of cysts (sacs containing fluid).	Patient feels small lumps in breast and axillae, tenderness and pain.	Conservative treatment is nonspecific. Surgery, however, may be performed to remove the cyst.	General clinical medical assisting procedures. Patient usually requires extensive reassurance of benign nature of disease.
Benign tumor: abnormal growth of breast tissue (can occur in males).	Patient feels lump(s) in breast.	Biopsy performed. Surgical removal may be performed.	General clinical medical assisting procedures. Explanation of biopsy procedure and scheduling.
Breast cancer: breast tissue malignancy (can occur in males).	Patient initially notices small hard lump in breast. Signs: dimpling ("orange peel"), depressed area, or puckering. Retraction of nipple swelling.	Dependent on type and location of cancer. Alternatives: chemotherapy radiation, surgery (mastectomy).	Patient preparation, reassurance, explanation, and followup planning.

*May be discussed during routine examination.

models which contain a simulated cancerous growth. The patient is asked to locate the growth on the model. This experience helps to establish a basis of comparison.

The breast self-examination (Fig. 19-5) is reproduced here along with suggested approaches for the medical assistant to utilize in conveying the information to the patient.

1. Explain the purpose of the self-examination.
2. Assist the patient by placing her hand and arm in the proper position.
3. Demonstrate palpation of the breast.
4. Ask the patient to practice the procedure.
5. Observe the patient's self-examination.
6. Stress the importance of regular breast self-examinations and give the patient a pamphlet on the subject if one is available.

Breast-Related Specialties

The major medical specialty related to diseases of the female breast is gynecology, which encompasses all diseases of the female reproductive system. Certain cases might require the

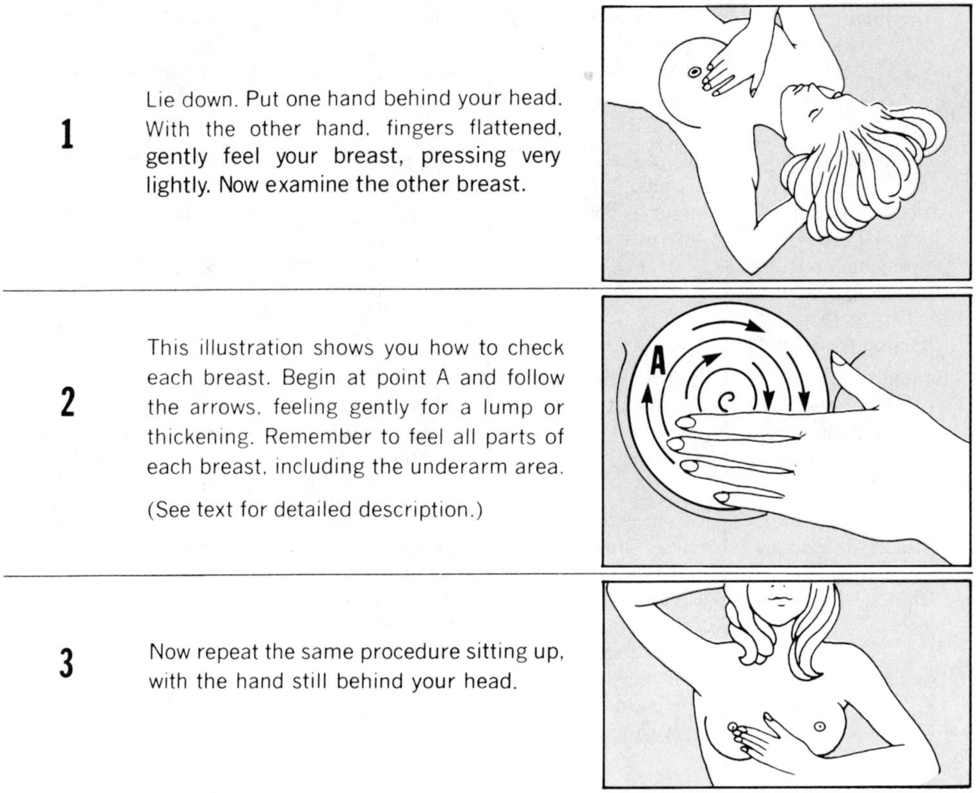

1 Lie down. Put one hand behind your head. With the other hand, fingers flattened, gently feel your breast, pressing very lightly. Now examine the other breast.

2 This illustration shows you how to check each breast. Begin at point A and follow the arrows, feeling gently for a lump or thickening. Remember to feel all parts of each breast, including the underarm area.

(See text for detailed description.)

3 Now repeat the same procedure sitting up, with the hand still behind your head.

FIGURE 19-5. Self-examination of the breast. (Reproduced from *Taber's Cyclopedic Medical Dictionary*, ed. 14. F.A. Davis, Philadelphia, 1981.)

assistance of a dermatologist, who specializes in diseases of the skin, or an oncologist, who studies the nature and development of tumors.

The medical assistant's major responsibility in the office of a gynecologist would be to assist the physician with examinations, perform patient teaching, and assist with suture removals and dressing changes.

During the discussion of diseases of the reproductive system, the special equipment utilized by the gynecologist will be illustrated.

THE ABDOMEN AND ITS CONTENTS

Structure and Function

For purposes of description of the location of symptoms, the medical assistant first must be able to identify the specific areas of the abdomen. The abdomen is generally divided into four main sections by imagining lines which cross over the umbilicus (belly button). These divisions are referred to as: right upper quadrant (RUQ), right lower quadrant (RLQ), left upper quadrant (LUQ), and left lower quadrant (LLQ). Another descriptive approach is in use which divides the abdomen into nine sections (Fig. 19-6).

Either of these methods of description may be used by the medical assistant in relating the symptomology or abnormality to the physician, as well as in charting and interpreting the physician's orders in performing procedures such as dressing changes or suture removal.

The abdomen contains in its cavity the major body organs which include the stomach, liver, pancreas, gallbladder, small and large intestines, appendix, kidneys, female and male reproductive organs, and the urinary bladder. The abdominal cavity is separated from the

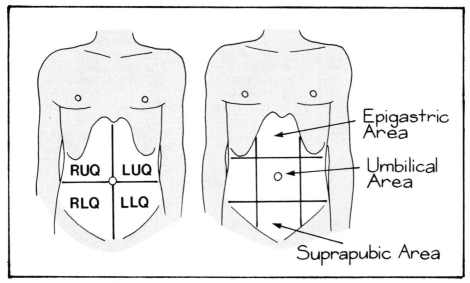

FIGURE 19-6. Divisions of the abdomen. (Reproduced from Saperstein, A.B., and Frazier, M.A.: *Introduction to Nursing Practice*. F.A. Davis, Philadelphia, 1980.)

thoracic cavity by the diaphragm. Major blood vessels also descend through the abdomen to the extremities.

The systems represented by these abdominal divisions are the gastrointestinal system, the internal organs of the reproduction system in the female, and the urinary system.

Our discussion of the examination of the abdomen will take the form of separate analyses of the gastrointestinal and urinary systems. These systems are grouped together in considering the abdomen because very frequently the patient complains of generalized distress such as pain in the abdomen. Unaccompanied by any functional disorder such as bowel changes or urinary changes, all systems and organs of the abdomen are examined initially to isolate the body part causing distress (Table 19-11). Although in the female the internal organs of reproduction are examined, this system and its examination will be covered specifically in the next section. The physical examination of the abdomen is represented here with the understanding that the physician may focus on any one system or organ contained in the abdomen (see Tables 19-12 and 19-13).

In this section, then, there will be a minor deviation from the organization of previous sections in this chapter. The method of examination and the role of the medical assistant in the examination of the abdomen will be presented *prior* to the individualized descriptions of the systems and related topics.

The Gastrointestinal System

STRUCTURE AND FUNCTION

The structure of the gastrointestinal or digestive system includes both main and accessory organs. The main organs of the system—the mouth, pharynx, esophagus, stomach, and

TABLE 19-11.   **General Examination of the Abdomen**

Body Part	Method and Equipment	Medical Assistant's Role
All regions of the abdomen	For all regions to be examined, the following methods will be utilized: inspection, palpation, percussion, auscultation with stethoscope.	Instruct patient prior to examination to empty bladder. Assist patient to assume supine position and place a small pillow under his head for comfort. Instruct patient to fold arms across chest or preferably extended at side. Pull gown up to midriff and fold under the breast line. Pull drape sheet to suprapubic edge and fold over the pubic area. Hand physician stethoscope. Warming the diaphragm in the palm of the hands increases patient comfort.

TABLE 19-12. Specific Examination of the Rectum

Body Part	Method and Equipment	Medical Assistant's Role
Rectum (In addition to the detection of abnormalities or disease of the rectum, general rectal examination can detect uterine displacement in the female, and prostatic enlargement and texture change in the male.)	Glove, lubricant, sponge forceps, sponges, rectal speculum or anoscope, applicator, culture material The physician inserts a gloved, lubricated finger in the rectum. An anoscope or speculum may be used for visualization. Sponge forceps and sponges may be used to absorb bleeding or discharge. If a culture is required, the applicator will be inserted to obtain a smear.	Instruct patient to put on a full gown. Drape and position properly. (Jack-knife position is usually preferred.) Remain with the female patient during examination. Attend to patient's comfort by recommending relaxation breathing and wiping area dry when procedure is completed.

small and large intestines—form a continuous tube with two openings: one at the mouth and one at the rectum. The terms alimentary canal and gastrointestinal tract are often used to refer to this tube. The walls of the tube consist of a mucous lining, a submucosal layer of connective tissue which encases the main blood vessels in the tract, a muscular layer, and a fibrous layer. The accessory organs of the system are the teeth, tongue, salivary glands, pancreas, liver, gallbladder, and appendix. Figure 19-7 illustrates the entire structure of the system.

The organs of the gastrointestinal system combine to perform these vital functions:

1. Preparing food for absorption of nutrients into the blood stream.

2. Altering the chemical and physical compositions of food so that it can be utilized by body cells.

3. Eliminating waste materials from the system.

The process of digestion will be described in Chapter 21, in which nutrition and diet therapy are discussed. Table 19-14 describes briefly the specific functions of each organ of the digestive system.

SYMPTOMATIC REACTION TO DISEASE

The reaction of the gastrointestinal system to disease is usually associated with a malfunction of some part of the overall system. In the upper tract, symptoms include stomach pain, nausea, vomiting, bloating (swelling), and eructation (belching). In the lower tract, pain, bloating, constipation, diarrhea, and flatulence (gas) may be present. Bleeding may be pres-

TABLE 19-13. Proctosigmoidoscopic Examination

Body Part	Equipment	Medical Assistant's Role
Rectum and lower sigmoid colon	Sigmoidoscope with obturator or proctoscope with obturator, transilluminators, rheostat, insufflator with bulb attachment, suction machine with suction tip, biopsy forceps (sterile), rubber gloves, rectal dressing forceps, gauze (4 × 4), lubricant, specimen materials	Instruct patient to take the prescribed laxative the night before the examination and to have only liquids for breakfast on the morning of the test. Administer cleansing enemas immediately prior to the examination to rid the bowel of its contents and facilitate visualization. Position and drape the patient and attend to comfort needs. Remain with the female patient during the examination. If a specimen is obtained, handle and process properly. (The physician may expect the medical assistant to attach the light source to the scope and hand the instruments. The MA will also be responsible for cleanup and instrument care.)

ent anywhere in the gastrointestinal tract and will often be observed by the patient in the form of black, tarry stools.

COMMON DIAGNOSTIC STUDIES OF THE GASTROINTESTINAL SYSTEM

The most commonly used tests associated with the gastrointestinal system include analysis of gastric contents, examination of stool specimens, x-ray examinations using barium, visualization by means of endoscopy, and examinations of the sigmoid colon, anus, and rectum. The medical assistant should be familiar with all of these procedures, which are described in Table 19-15.

COMMON DISEASES OF THE GASTROINTESTINAL SYSTEM

Among the many diseases that affect the gastrointestinal system, the most common include peptic ulcer, gastritis, appendicitis, colitis, and hernia. These and other conditions are dis-

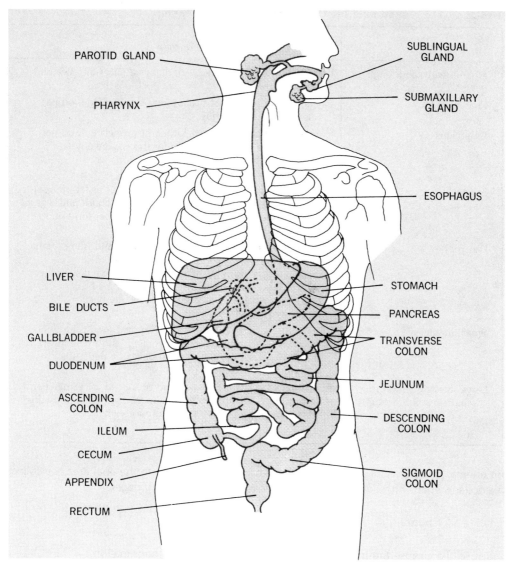

FIGURE 19-7. The gastrointestinal system. (Reproduced from *Taber's Cyclopedic Medical Dictionary*, ed. 14. F.A. Davis, Philadelphia, 1981.)

cussed in Table 19-16, together with the role of the medical assistant in the treatment of each.

SPECIAL CLINICAL PROCEDURES INVOLVING THE GASTROINTESTINAL SYSTEM

The medical assistant may perform certain clinical procedures specifically related to the gastrointestinal system. In the course of their duties, MAs may be called upon to administer

TABLE 19-14.   Function of the Organs of the Digestive System

Organ	Function
Mouth, teeth, and tongue	Food is chewed and mixed with digestive juices in saliva and then swallowed.
Pharynx	Continues the process of swallowing or propelling food particles into the esophagus.
Esophagus	Continues the process of swallowing or propelling food particles into the stomach. A term for this movement is peristalsis, a wavelike series of contractions which squeezes food down through the canal.
Stomach	An expandable sac which will hold food particles for approximately 2 hours, while gastric juices further churn and digest food particles. Peristalsis continues and moves food particles at intervals into the small intestine.
Pancreas	Secretes insulin for digestive use by the liver and is important to maintain normal blood sugar, fat and protein metabolism, and the manufacturing of important substances such as bile. The gallbladder concentrates the bile and stores what is needed by the small intestine for the process of digestion.
Small intestine	Continued churning and digestion. Digested food is brought in contact with intestinal mucosa (lining) and nutrients are absorbed. Waste materials are propelled by peristalsis into the large intestine.
Large intestine: colon, descending colon, rectum	Additional products are formed and processed for elimination in the colon. The descending colon through mass peristalsis moves the materials into the rectum for elimination.

an enema, insert a rectal suppository, apply medication topically to the anal area, or collect a stool specimen. These procedures are described in the following pages.

Giving an Enema

Purpose: To cleanse the bowel, remove impaction, and relieve constipation.

Procedure	Principle
1. Wash hands.	1. This prevents transfer of harmful microorganisms.
2. Assemble equipment: bedpan, enema container and solution, toweling and tissue, gloves. (Most frequently used in the medical office is a commercial preparation in which the enema solution is contained in a plastic squeeze bottle with an elongated tip to be inserted in the rectum.)	2. Organization facilitates efficiency.

3. Explain the procedure, and position and drap the patient. Side-lying (Sims) position is required. Place protective toweling on the examination table and under the buttocks.

3. The patient's understanding relieves anxiety and promotes cooperation. Toweling protects the examination table.

4. With one gloved hand, separate the buttocks and expose the anus. Instruct the patient to breathe slowly and evenly through the mouth and exhale through the nose.

4. Breathing in this manner relaxes the patient and relaxes the sphincter muscle of the anus, thereby providing greater ease of insertion of the nozzle.

5. Insert the complete tip of the container.

5. It is necessary to reach an appropriate length of bowel for removal of fecal contents.

6. Squeeze the container slowly until emptied and remove.

6. This induces the solution at a rate that will cause the least discomfort.

7. Instruct the patient to hold back defecation if possible for a few minutes.

7. This allows the solution a proper absorption time.

8. Escort the patient to the bathroom if possible, or place the bedpan under patient. Raise the examination table so that the patient is in Fowler's position (sitting).

8. This provides as much comfort as possible so that the patient may release fluid contents.

9. Provide tissue for the patient.

9. Tissue dries the area and promotes patient comfort.

10. Record the procedure on the patient's record, listing date, time, type of enema given, effects, and your initials.

10. The record is retained for future reference.

Note: Infrequently the enema procedure does not remove the fecal contents adequately, especially if the patient has an impaction. When this occurs, the assistant may insert a gloved hand into the rectum to locate and push out the remaining fecal matter at the end of the procedure.

Inserting a Rectal Suppository

Purpose: To administer medication when an oral or parenteral route is not desired, or for localized effect as ordered by the physician.

Procedure	*Principle*
1. Wash hands.	1. Transfer of harmful microorganisms is prevented.
2. Identify and prepare the patient. Explain the procedure and position.	2. This promotes patient comfort, and explanation reduces anxiety. A side-lying position exposes the body part.
3. Assemble equipment: rubber gloves (disposable or sterile), suppository, lubricant, gauze wipe.	3. Organization facilitates efficiency.
4. Open the suppository package (usually foil) and drop without touching with hand onto the wipe.	4. This prevents contamination of the suppository; handling would begin the melting process.

5. Pull on one glove, dip fingers lightly in lubricant. Pick up the suppository with the gloved hand.

5. Lubricant facilitates a more comfortable entry as the suppository will be pushed upward with the gloved finger.

6. With the ungloved hand, separate the buttocks, exposing the anus. Ask the patient to breath slowly through the mouth. Insert the suppository.

6. Mouth-breathing helps to relax the anus, providing a more comfortable entry for the patient.

7. Following insertion, hold the buttocks closed with the ungloved hand. Instruct the patient not to bear down.

7. This aids in absorption of the suppository.

8. With gauze wipe dry the anal area, then dispose.

8. Drying promotes patient comfort.

9. Remove the glove and dispose. Clean the work area.

9. The work area is readied for future use. Remove the glove by pulling on the cuff. The glove will be inside-out when off. This prevents contamination of the hands.

10. Record the procedure in the patient's file: medication, type and amount, time, route (rectal).

10. Recording is necessary for future reference.

TABLE 19-15.   Diagnostic Studies of the Gastrointestinal System

Test	Description
Gastric analysis	Gastric contents are analyzed after being collected through vomiting or the insertion of a nasogastric tube. The tube is passed through the mouth and into the stomach by a nurse or physician in the hospital. Vomitus can be collected and saved by the medical assistant for the physician's inspection when the patient is in the office.
Stool specimen	Bowel movement sampling is collected by the medical assistant if the patient is in the office and then sent to the hospital laboratory for examination to detect the presence of blood.
Endoscopy (esophagoscopy and gastroscopy)	Visualization of an area of the upper GI tract by passing a tube with a lighted instrument through the mouth and down into the stomach or area to be inspected. Specimens for microscopic study can also be obtained. Requires hospitalization and special patient preparation.
GI series	X-ray examination of the upper tract (barium swallow) and the lower tract (barium enema) employs a chalklike opaque substance introduced into the system for visualization of the tract outline. Performed in the hospital x-ray laboratory or special outpatient facility.
Anoscopy, proctoscopy, sigmoidoscopy	Special examination procedures performed by the physician in order to visualize the mucous membrane of the sigmoid, anus, and rectum. Special instruments are required.

TABLE 19-16. Common Diseases of the Gastrointestinal System

Disease	Symptoms	Treatment	Medical Assistant's Role
Peptic ulcer: eroded area of mucosa of upper gastrointestinal tract.	Painful, aching, burning, gnawing, or cramping sensations near the midline region under and to the left side of the sternum. Symptoms occur approximately 2 hours after ingestion of food.	Drug therapy, diet therapy, surgery	General clinical medical assisting procedures. The medical assistant should be alert to emergency conditions with any ulcer: perforation and hemorrhage. With perforation there is sudden severe pain with nausea and vomiting. Hemorrhage will produce hematemesis (bloody vomitus), bloody stools, and symptoms of shock. Patient teaching in diet instruction and avoidance of stimulants may be required.
Gastritis: inflammation of the mucous membrane lining of the stomach.	Eructation, bloating, gastric discomfort.	Drug and diet therapies	General clinical medical assisting.
Hiatal hernia: outpouching or herniation of abdomenal contents through weakness in the wall of the diaphragm.	Pain when herniation occurs. (Herniation may reverse itself automatically.)	Drug and diet therapy; surgical repair (herniorrhaphy) if required.	General clinical medical assisting procedures and dietary instruction. Patient teaching includes recommendation to patient to elevate head of bed to relieve discomfort and chance of provoking herniation.
Appendicitis: inflammation of appendage attached to the colon. The appendix has no known physiologic use.	Generalized abdominal pain or localized in the lower quadrant, with fever, nausea, and vomiting.	Surgery (appendectomy)	Emergency scheduling of patient for surgery if seen in the office.

TABLE 19-16. *Continued*

Disease	Symptoms	Treatment	Medical Assistant's Role
Colitis: inflammation of the colon; can be an ulceration (area of erosion).	Abdominal pain or cramping; frequent loose stools (diarrhea can contain pus, mucus, blood); malaise; weight loss; fever.	Diet and drug therapy; psychotherapy if indicated. Surgery if indicated (ileostomy or colostomy of part of the intestine onto abdomen).	General clinical medical assisting procedures. If patient passes stools during visit, instruct patient not to flush so that stools may be inspected.
Abdominal hernia: protrusion of the contents of the abdomen through weakness in abdominal wall.	Patient usually notices herniation, or may be detected during routine examination.	Surgical repair.	General clinical medical assisting procedures. Medical assistant should be alert for severe pain in area of hernia which signals strangulated hernia (inadequate blood supply to part).
Hemorrhoids: dilation of the veins in the anal canal or rectum; may protrude through the anus.	Anal itching; discomfort; bright red blood present upon defecation.	Drug therapy; surgery (hemorrhoidectomy).	General clinical medical assisting procedures. Explanation of preoperative and postoperative care.
Anal fissure: an ulcerated crevice in the anal wall. Fistula: an abnormal canal leading from the anus or rectum.	Pain and burning on defecation.	Nonspecific; surgery if indicated.	General clinical medical assisting procedures.

Applying Ointment to the Anal Area

Purpose: To relieve symptoms associated with hemorrhoids, anal fissures, or other irritations by administering topical medication ordered by the physician.

Procedure	Principle
1. Wash hands.	1. This prevents transfer of harmful microorganisms.
2. Prepare the patient: explain the procedure; drape and position properly.	2. Explanation reduces anxiety. A side-lying position exposes the area and is comfortable for the patient.

3. Assemble equipment: ointment or lotion and glove.

3. Organization is an aid to efficiency.

4. Put on one glove; with palm up on gloved hand, squeeze ointment onto fingertips.

4. Touching ointment with an ungloved hand or touching the opening of the tube to the gloved hand would contaminate the contents.

5. Spread ointment between gloved fingers with thumb of the same hand.

5. This distributes the ointment and prevents it from falling off the fingertips.

6. With the ungloved hand, separate the buttocks, exposing the anus. Apply gently and liberally to the affected area.

6. This distributes the medication evenly over the affected area and minimizes patient discomfort.

7. Remove the glove with appropriate technique and dispose. Record the procedure as when administering a suppository.

7. Proper technique prevents contamination. Recording is necessary for future reference.

Collecting a Stool Specimen

To obtain a stool specimen for microscopic laboratory examination, the patient is asked to defecate into a bedpan. The patient may bring the bedpan to the toilet and place it on the seat for greater comfort. A small portion of the fecal contents is then transferred, with a tongue blade, into the proper container. The lid is attached securely, and the container is labeled and placed in a paper bag. The bag, together with a request form, is then sent to the laboratory. Stool specimens are seldom collected in the medical office, most patients being given instructions for prior home collection.

GASTROINTESTINAL SPECIALTIES

A gastroenterologist is a physician specializing in diseases of the entire gastrointestinal tract, while a proctologist is a physician concerned with disorders of the lower GI tract, principally the anus, colon, and rectum. Clinical medical assistants employed in the office of physicians specializing in these areas will generally assist with examinations and other related procedures. MAs in such offices will most likely be involved with aftercare of patients during postoperative visits. Patient teaching, preparing patients for surgery, and scheduling diagnostic studies will be routine activities.

In the office of a proctologist, major differences will be encountered in the specific examination procedures and in the requisite instruments and equipment. For the proctologic examination, a table with a jack-knife capability is required in order to raise the buttocks and lower the head for adequate visualization of the lower tract. The patient lies prone on the table and then adjusts to the jack-knife contour as the table is adjusted to the needed position. The proctologic table and instruments are illustrated in Figure 19-8.

The Urinary System

STRUCTURE AND FUNCTION

The urinary system eliminates water-soluble waste products. The respiratory system, the intestinal tract, and the skin all remove waste products from the body. The urinary system

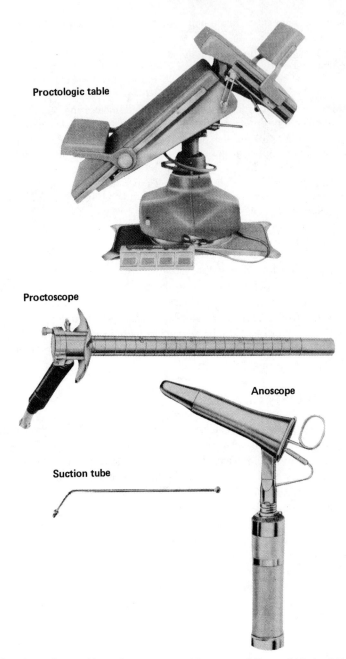

FIGURE 19-8.   Proctologic table and instruments. (Courtesy of General Medical Corporation)

removes the water-soluble waste products and maintains fluid and electrolyte balance which is essential to proper cell functioning.

The urinary system in both the male and female consists of two kidneys, two ureters, the urinary bladder, and the urethra (Fig. 19-9). In the male the urethra or urinary canal is longer than in the female since it is contained in the penis. The female urethra is approximately 1½ inches long, whereas the male urethra is approximately 8 inches in length.

The bean-shaped kidneys manufacture urine from waste materials filtered from the blood. The urine is transported from the kidneys to the bladder by the ureters. Peristalsis in the ureters assists in the downward flow of urine. The urethra leads from the bladder to the urinary meatus, the external body opening.

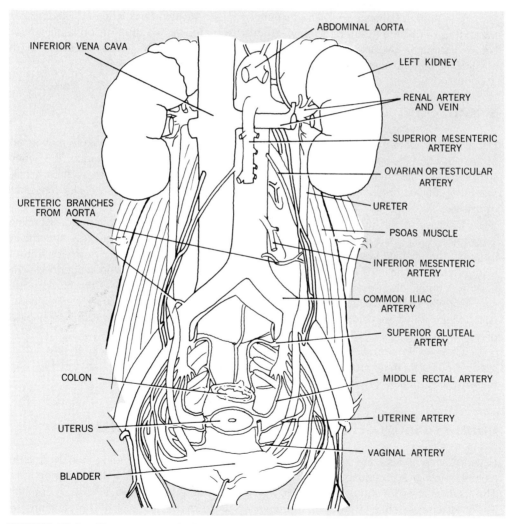

FIGURE 19-9. Urinary tract and adjacent arterial structures. (Reproduced from *Taber's Cyclopedic Medical Dictionary*, ed. 14. F.A. Davis, Philadelphia, 1981.)

The kidneys are suspended in fat and fibrous tissue. During a 1 minute period, approximately 1 quart of blood passes through the kidneys and is purified. The kidney is composed of many complicated parts, each of which plays a vital role in filtering the blood. Waste and solubles are removed from the blood, and reusable products are reabsorbed back into the blood.

The bladder is an expandable muscular sac lined with mucous membrane. Its structure is similar to that of the stomach. The bladder acts as a reservoir for urine. The bladder contracts when the nerve message or urge to void is experienced. Approximately half a pint of urine collects before the message to void is transmitted to the brain along the nerve pathways and the urge to void is experienced. Each day approximately 40 to 50 ounces (1200 to 1500 ml) are voided.

The urethra contains specialized sphincter muscles which relax when the bladder contracts, thus permitting the urine to flow. Another term for the act of urination is *micturition*. Urine has many characteristics and contains substances which can be analyzed in the medical technology laboratory.

SYMPTOMATIC REACTION TO DISEASE

Disease in the urinary tract is signaled through a number of symptoms related to malfunction of the organs of the system. Since any part of the system can become inflamed, the general symptoms of inflammation may be present. Edema, pain in the abdomen or flank (back), painful or difficult urination or bleeding, and scant or frequent urination are all symptomatic of disease.

Diseases of the urinary system and the circulatory system are often closely related since the normal physiology of urine formation is dependent on the circulatory system. For instance, the average systolic blood pressure that must be maintained in order for urine to form is approximately 70 mm of mercury. An example of the relationship is arteriosclerosis, described under diseases of the cardiovascular system. Arteriosclerosis of the blood vessels supplying the kidneys would cause malfunction of these organs. Conversely, an individual with kidney damage would have the potential for developing hypertension (high blood pressure).

Changes in normal urine constituents not only may signal disease in the urinary system, but also may provide information on the state of health in general. For these reasons, all complete physical examinations include a routine urinalysis.

COMMON DIAGNOSTIC STUDIES OF THE URINARY SYSTEM

Several different tests are associated with the urinary system, including urinalysis, urine culture, pyelogram, cystoscopy, kidney function, blood chemistry, and radiorenography. The medical assistant should be familiar with each of these tests (Table 19-17). A complete list of diagnostic studies, with comprehensive instructions for patient preparation and scheduling requirements, should be contained in the office procedure manual.

TABLE 19-17. Common Diagnostic Studies of the Urinary System

Test	Description
Urinalysis	Laboratory analysis of urine, consisting of physical, chemical and microscopic examination. Medical assistants can perform the test in the medical office if facilities and equipment are available.
Urine culture	Bacterial analysis. May also be performed in the office. Requires special training and equipment.
Pyelogram	X-ray examination using an opaque dye for visualization. Dye may be injected into the patient's vein (intravenous pyelogram), or the physician may insert a small catheter into the urethra through a cystoscope (retrograde pyelogram) and inject the dye through these catheters.
Cystoscopy	Examination of the bladder by visualization and inspection using a special instrument. The walls of the bladder and urethra can be examined. Special preparation and scheduling are necessary.
Kidney function	Various tests which determine normal kidney function: determination of waste removal capability in certain lengths of time. Special patient preparation and scheduling are necessary.
Blood chemistry studies	Medical technology study of blood substances that determines whether or not waste products are being removed from the blood stream.
Radiorenography	Dye injected as with pyelography but tagged with radioactive dye. Special patient preparation and scheduling are necessary.

COMMON DISEASES OF THE URINARY TRACT

The most commonly encountered diseases of the urinary system, including infection of the bladder, inflammation of the kidney, and kidney stones, are given in Table 19-18, together with symptoms, treatment procedures, and the medical assistant's role. As is the case with all other systems and body parts covered in this chapter, only the most frequently seen diseases are discussed. The MA's knowledge of other diseases will grow as experience is gained in the profession.

SPECIFIC CLINICAL PROCEDURES INVOLVING THE URINARY SYSTEM

The specific clinical procedures related to the urinary system that are generally performed by the medical assistant are associated with the collection of urine specimens. The procedures

TABLE 19-18.   Common Diseases of the Urinary Tract

Disease	Symptoms	Treatment	Medical Assistant's Role
Cystitis: infection of the bladder.	Urgency and frequency of burning, painful urination (dysuria); bleeding may occur (hematuria); scant voiding (oliguria).	Drug therapy; antibiotics; increased fluid intake.	General clinical medical assisting procedures. Patient teaching. With almost all infections of the urinary tract, the importance must be stressed of drinking large amounts of fluid to dilute the bacterial concentration. In women, instruction may be necessary pertaining to cleansing of the perineum after voiding or defecating to avoid urethral contamination from the rectum. *The perineum should be wiped or cleansed from front to back.*
Pyelonephritis: inflammation of the kidney which can result in serious tissue damage.	General symptoms of inflammation, pain and tenderness in the area of the kidney with frequent and painful voiding.	Drug therapy; antibiotics; increased fluid intake.	General clincial medical assisting procedures.
Nephrolithiasis: kidney stones.	Characteristic pain in the region of the kidney; hematuria may occur.	Diet therapy, drug therapy, analgesics, muscle relaxants, application of heat, increased fluid intake. Surgical removal may be necessary: nephrolithotomy (incision into kidney for removal of stone) or ureterolithotomy (incision into ureter for removal of stone).	General clinical medical assisting procedures. If a specimen is obtained from the patient, it should be screened for the presence of stones.

TABLE 19-18. *Continued*

Disease	Symptoms	Treatment	Medical Assistant's Role
Glomerulonephritis: inflammation of the kidney, especially the area composed of glomeruli. The disease may result in tissue damage.	Oliguria, hematuria: weakness, headache, anorexia (loss of appetite), edema around eyes upon awaking and edema of the feet in the evening.	Bedrest drug therapy— antibiotics, diet therapy—low sodium and moderate protein fluids restricted.	General clinical medical assisting procedures. Each time the patient comes to the office (if weight measurement is not routine) weight measurement is obtained to note fluid retention fluctuation. Patient teaching would involve stressing the importance of skin care. When skin is edematous (waterlogged), it is more susceptible to injury and infection.

which follow describe methods for obtaining a "clean-catch" specimen and a catheterized specimen. Four other types of urine specimens should be noted as well:

1. *Spot specimens*, which can be collected in a clean container at *any time of day.*

2. *First morning specimens*, collected upon arising.

3. *Postprandial specimens*, collected after meals.

4. *Timed specimens*, collected at prescribed times during the day.

Obtaining a "Clean-Catch" Urine Specimen

Purpose: To obtain a urine specimen that will not be contaminated by bacteria from the perineum.

Procedure	Principle
1. Explain purpose of the procedure to the patient.	1. Patient understanding facilitates cooperation.
2. Give the patient three gauze wipes, antibacterial soap, and a clean specimen cup.	2. These items are needed for the collection of a "clean catch" of urine.
3. Give the patient the following instructions: a. Before voiding, wet the gauze pads and suds with the special soap.	3. Give a rationale for the steps to the patient to elicit compliance. Hairs of the perineum contain bacteria. Wiping from front to back avoids cross-contamination of the urethra

b. Use one wipe and from front to back cleanse one side of the perineum. Dispose of wipe.

c. Using another wipe, cleanse the other side of the perineum from front to back. Dispose of wipe.

d. With the remaining wipe, cleanse the middle of the perineum from front to back. Dispose of wipe.

e. Instruct patient to void *briefly* into the toilet after self-cleansing has been achieved.

f. Void again and collect the urine in the specimen cup.

g. Finish voiding into the toilet.

4. Instruct the patient to bring the specimen to you. Immediately label the container, not the lid.

5. Process the specimen according to the physician's orders.

6. Record properly. (*Example*: Clean-catch specimen obtained 6/22/81 at 10:30 a.m.) Send to laboratory.

from the other perineum orifices. Each wipe is used only once to prevent contamination Voiding a small amount of urine prior to collection washes away bacteria at the urinary meatus. The urine voided in the middle will be the "clean catch." It is helpful to the patient if these instructions can be taped to the door in the bathroom for easy reference.

4. Labeling reduces the chance of error.

5. Depending on the tests to be performed, the medical assistant will perform the testing personally or will send the specimen to the laboratory.

6. Recording is necessary for future reference.

Urinary Catheterization

Purpose: To obtain a sterile urine specimen.

Procedure	Principle
1. Wash hands.	1. This prevents the transfer of harmful microorganisms.
2. Assemble equipment. Catheterization tray may be either disposable or reusable. The sterile wrapped tray contains sterile gloves, average size sterile catheter, lubricant, soap (usually foil pack), large cotton swabs, sterile collection jar and label, thumb forceps, disposable dress sheet, and waterproof sheeting. All are positioned in a deep plastic container (if disposable) which is divided into three sections, two small and one large (see Fig. 19-10).	2. Catheterization is a sterile procedure and is the method of choice for the most precise collection of urine uncontaminated by bacteria from the perineum. There may be other conditions present warranting the collection of a specimen.
3. Explain procedures to the patient and place in dorsal recumbent position.	3. Understanding facilitates cooperation.
4. Unwrap the sterile tray using the aseptic technique: opening flaps away from you,	4. This technique avoids contamination of contents.

one by one, with the thumb and forefinger grasping the tip of the flap. (Disposable set will be in plastic seal.)

5. Shift up waterproof sheeting and place under the patient's buttocks.

5. Sheeting prevents soiling of the examination table.

6. Put on glove, using sterile technique.

6. The glove avoids contamination of catheterization equipment and the introduction of harmful microorganisms into the bladder.

7. Pick up sterile soap package. Open. Pour liquid soap over the cotton swabs assembled in a section of the catheter container.

7. The soap package is sterile. A rule of thumb is sterile against sterile, nonsterile against nonsterile.

8. Place disposable window drape over the perineal area.

8. Draping creates a sterile field.

9. With thumb forceps, grasp a cotton swab and begin perineal cleansing, using the same procedure as for the "clean-catch" collection. Dispose each swab in the small empty section of the catheter container.

9. Cleansing prevents contamination.

10. Open the lubricant packet. Push up the catheter in one hand, the lubricant in the other. Twist the end to be inserted in the urethea in the foil packet to lubricate.

10. The lubricant provides greater patient comfort. Some discomfort will still be experienced by the patient. Mouth breathing during insertion helps to relax the sphincter muscle.

11. With one gloved hand, separate the labia; hold the catheter in the other hand.

11. This exposes the urinary meatus. One gloved hand is now unsterile and cannot come in contact with the catheter.

12. Insert the lubricated tip of the catheter into the urinary meatus until urine is expelled. The end of the catheter should be dangling in the specimen jar. When the desired amount is obtained in the jar, place the end into the large section of the catheterization container to finish emptying the bladder. Set aside collection jar.

12. If the bladder is not completely emptied, the patient will experience discomfort.

13. Remove the catheter and dry the perineum with the drape sheet. Remove the waterproof sheeting.

13. This completes the procedure and promotes patient comfort.

14. Assist the patient to a comfortable position and immediately label the urine specimen.

14. Labeling is necessary to avoid chance of error.

15. Record properly and care for the specimen.

15. This is necessary for future reference.

THE URINARY TRACT SPECIALTY

A physician whose practice is limited to diseases of the urinary tract and the male reproductive system is termed a urologist. Urologists perform surgery on the tract, but employ a variety of nonsurgical treatments as well.

The medical assistant's responsibilities in the office of a urologist include routine urinalysis, cultures, catheterizations, and postoperative assisting procedures such as suture removal

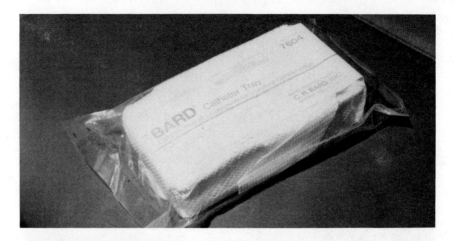

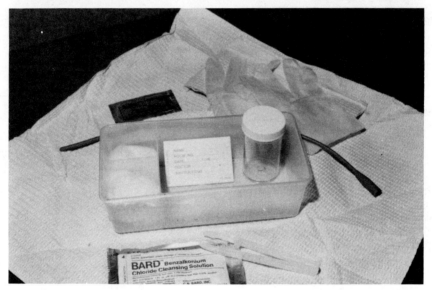

FIGURE 19-10. Catheter tray: closed package (top) and opened (bottom) to show components.

and dressing changes. The assistant must be knowledgeable in diseases of the urinary tract and diagnostic studies including related preparation and treatment procedures.

APPLICATION EXERCISES

Group Discussion and Role-Playing Exercise

The instructor will attempt to assemble the equipment that the physician will use in the examinations presented in this chapter. After groups have been formed, the instructor will assign each group one of the patients listed below. The group will then discuss (1) how the room and patient will be prepared for the examination, and (2) how to assist the physician with the examination. When called upon, three students from the group will demonstrate the group's conclusion by taking the roles of the patient, medical assistant, and narrator.

1. The narrator explains room preparation and chooses appropriate equipment.

2. The student in the role of medical assistant places the student in the role of the patient in proper position and gown (simulate) after explaining the procedure.

3. The narrator explains how the examination will proceed, and the student in the role of MA simulates the assisting procedure. (Notes from group discussion can be used.)

4. Other student groups critique.

The various patient assignments are as follows:

Patient A. Symptoms: cough, sore throat, fever.
Patient B. Symptoms: painful urination, abdominal discomfort.
Patient C. Symptoms: diarrhea for 3 days.
Patient D. Symptoms: known hypertension (routine examination).
Patient E. Symptoms: bloated stomach, belching.
Patient F. Symptoms: pain in left ear, headache.
Patient G. Symptoms: none (routine physical examination).
Patient H. Symptoms: chest pain.

Problem-Solving Activities

Discuss possible solutions to the following situations:

1. While preparing to catheterize the patient, the catheter tip touches the patient's right leg.

2. The patient is afraid of the ear irrigation procedure.

3. The physician concludes that the patient has cystitis. What do you anticipate in terms of assisting with treatment and patient teaching.

4. The patient vomits while gowning.

5. The patient asks why he is being referred to a proctologist and asks what that is.

6. The patient notices the mercury pausing at 160 mm while you are obtaining the blood pressure. The patient asks whether she has high blood pressure.

7. The patient does not want to remove her underwear. It is uncertain whether the physician will perform a pelvic examination

8. The patient is coughing and is not covering his mouth.

9. The patient asks to read her own chart.

10. While the physician is palpating the abdomen, you notice that the patient's face appears distressed.

Research Activity

The instructor will assign topics for group presentations on the description and preparation of patients for the diagnostic tests discussed in this chapter and related to particular systems.

COMPLETING THE LEARNING LOOP

While the medical assistant is not expected to have the comprehensive physiologic and medical understanding of a physician, a general awareness of diseases, symptoms, and treatments is required. The overview presented here will allow the MA to better assist both the patient and the physician.

As students, medical assistants should make a concerted effort to learn the relationships between all of the aspects of the body systems so that they will be prepared to contribute to the team efforts in the doctor's office, not only in general or family practice, but in specialties as well.

BIBLIOGRAPHY

Berne, R. M., and Levy, M. N.: *Cardiovascular Physiology*, ed. 3. C. V. Mosby, St. Louis, 1977.
Birrell, J. F.: *Logan Turner's Diseases of the Nose, Throat and Ear*, ed. 8. Year Book Medical Publishers, Chicago, 1977.
Bull, T. R.: *Color Atlas of Ear, Nose and Throat*. Year Book Medical Publishers, Chicago, 1974.
Cole, R. B.: *Essentials of Respiratory Disease*. J. B. Lippincott, Philadelphia, 1976.
Directions in Cardiovascular Medicine, Vol. 3. Hoechst Pharmaceuticals, Somerville, N.J., 1979.
Gelin, L. E., et al.: *Abdominal Pain: A Guide to Rapid Diagnosis*. J. B. Lippincott, Philadelphia, 1969.
Goss, C. M. (ed.): *Gray's Anatomy of the Human Body*, ed. 29. Lea & Febiger, Philadelphia, 1973.
Introduction to Lung Diseases. American Lung Association, New York, 1973.
Kratzer, G. L.: *The Reed and Carnick Manual on Colon and Rectal Diseases*. Reed & Carnick, Kenilworth, N.J., 1976.
Kunin, C. M.: *Detection, Prevention and Management of Urinary Tract Infections: A Manual for the Physician, Nurse and Allied Health Worker*, ed. 2. Lea & Febiger, Philadelphia, 1974.
Lipscomb, D. M.: *An Introduction to the Laboratory Study of the Ear*. Charles C Thomas, Springfield, Ill., 1974.
Rothenberg, R.: *The Complete Book of Breast Care*. Crown, New York, 1975.
Swan, K. G.: *The Cardiovascular System: Disease, Diagnosis, Treatment*. R. J. Brady, Bowie, Md., 1973.
Zarren, H. S.: *The Respiratory System: Disease, Diagnosis, Treatment*. R. J. Brady, Bowie, Md., 1973.

20

SPECIFIC PHYSICAL EXAMINATIONS – II

SPECIFIC OBJECTIVES

Upon completion of this chapter you will be prepared to list and describe the structure and function, the symptomatic reaction to disease, the examination procedures, the common diseases, and the clinical tests and procedures which are associated with:

1. The genitalia and reproductive system

2. The musculoskeletal system

3. The endocrine system

4. The neurologic system

5. The pediatric patient

6. The integumentary system

7. The eye

THE GENITALIA AND THE REPRODUCTIVE SYSTEM

Structure and Function

The *male reproductive system* consists of the scrotum and its contents, two seminal vesicles or ducts, the prostate gland, two bulbourethral glands, and the penis (Fig. 20-1).

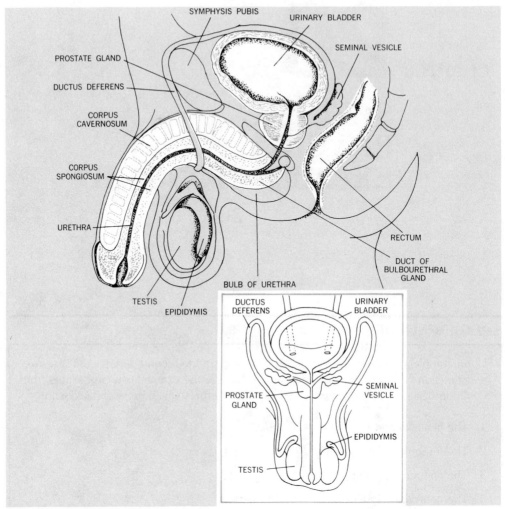

FIGURE 20-1. Male genital organs. (Reproduced from *Taber's Cyclopedic Medical Dictionary*, ed. 14. F. A. Davis, Philadelphia, 1981.)

The *scrotum* is a sac which normally contains two testes. Testes are the glands which produce the male sex hormone, testosterone, and the spermatozoa, or male germ cells (see Table 20-1).

Each *testicle* consists of two component parts: the egg-shaped testis and the winding tube surrounding the testes called the epididymis. Sperm cells are manufactured in the testes and are carried to the epididymis. By way of the seminal ducts (also called vas deferens), the cells leave the scrotum and proceed to the pelvic cavity. In the pelvic cavity each duct joins another duct from the seminal vesicle which forms the ejaculatory duct. These latter two vesicles are small sacs which store the spermatozoa and add other lubricating fluid to the sperm. The ejaculatory ducts pass through the prostate gland to the urethra.

The *prostate* is composed of muscular and glandular tissue. This gland rests between the neck of the bladder and the beginning of the urethra. It secretes a fluid added to the semen during ejaculation. The semen contains the sperm. The bulbourethral glands are located below the prostate gland and also add a substance to the semen.

The *penis* is the organ through which the ejaculatory duct passes and semen is expressed. The urethra also passes through the length of the penis (see Table 20-1).

The *female reproductive system* has both internal and external organs. The internal organs of reproduction include two ovaries, two fallopian tubes, the uterus and the vagina.

The external genitalia of reproduction are the mons pubis, labia majora, labia minora, and the clitoris. A term for these combined structures is *vulva* (Fig. 20-2).

The *ovaries* are the almond-shaped glands of reproduction which produce the hormones progesterone and estrogen. These hormones regulate menstruation and are responsible for the secondary female sex characteristics such as breast development and body contour. The ovaries contain *ova* (egg cells), one of which, when fertilized by the male egg cells

TABLE 20-1. Examination of the Reproductive System

Body Part	Method and Equipment	Medical Assistant's Role
Male: Penis	Inspection and palpation (gloves if lesion is present).	The patient is lying down with a drape sheet over the chest and abdomen. The medical assistant, if female, is usually not present during the examination of the male genitalia for purposes of avoiding embarrassment to the patient. However, since the presence of the MA is ultimately at the discretion of the physician, basic knowledge of the examination process is required.
Scrotum	Inspection and palpation. Transillumination may be required. Examining room must be darkened and a penlight used.	
Inguinal hernia (examination of ridge between abdomen and thigh)	Inspection and palpation.	Patient stands.

TABLE 20-1. *Continued*

Body Part	Method and Equipment	Medical Assistant's Role
Female: External genitalia Cervix and vaginal wall (internal examination)	Inspection. Inspection with head light or adequate overhead light, vaginal speculum, applicator or vaginal spatula, gloves, materials for bacteriologic culture, and pap smear.	The medical assistant, if female, should be in attendance and assist the physician with the examination, not only for purposes of efficiency and patient comfort, but also for legal protection. The patient should be prepared by the MA for examination by instructing the patient to empty her bladder. The patient is then placed in the lithotomy position and draped properly with only the perineum exposed. The speculum should be warmed for patient comfort. The medical assistant may place lubricant on a gauze square or squeeze it on the physician's gloves when requested. The patient's facial expressions should be observed for signs of extreme discomfort and anxiety. After the specimen is obtained, the MA may be responsible for spraying the glass slide with fixative for later laboratory examination.
Cervix, rectum (bimanual examination)	Palpation with glove, lubricant.	Instruct the patient to breathe evenly and slowly through the mouth as an aid to relaxation.

(the sperm), becomes a fetus. Each month the ovaries alternate in maturing and releasing a single ovum vulnerable to fertilization.

The ovum finds its way into the uterus by means of the *fallopian tubes.* These hollow tubes are composed of muscle tissue and are approximately 3 to 5 inches long. While one end of the tube is attached to the uterus (one on each side), the other end opens near the

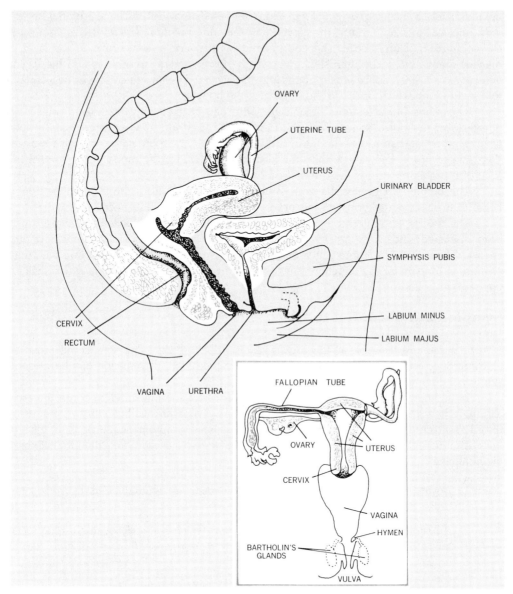

FIGURE 20-2. Female genital organs. (Reproduced from *Taber's Cyclopedic Medical Dictionary*, ed. 14. F. A. Davis, Philadelphia, 1981.)

ovary and is fimbriated (having fingerlike appendages). These ends grasp the mature ovum and propel it inside the tube to the uterus. The fallopian tubes, the uterus, and the vagina are lined with continuous mucous membrane as is the urinary tract.

The *uterus* is composed of muscle tissue which is able to expand and contract. Situated between the urinary bladder and the pear-shaped rectum is the hollow uterus. It is approximately 3 inches (7.5 cm) long and 2 inches (5 cm) wide. The uterus has several parts referred to as the fundus, the cervix, and the endometrium. The fundus is the upper, curved portion of the uterus. The endometrium is the term used to refer to the layer of mucous membrane in the uterus. The cervix (the lower portion) protrudes into the vagina and contains a small orifice which opens into the vagina. The vagina continues as a canal 3 to 4 inches long which opens to the outside of the body.

The *mons pubis* (external genitalia) is the hair-covered fatty tissue pad which lies directly over the pubic bone. From the mons pubis two outer hair-covered folds of fatty tissue separate and surround the floor of the perineum. These are called the labia majora. Two smaller inside folds are termed the labia minora. Under the mons pubis, toward the front of the labia minora, is the clitoris (see Table 20-1).

The *perineum* contains the body orifices of the female from the mons pubis (pubic bone) to the coccyx (tail bone) in this order: urinary meatus, vagina, rectal opening.

The *breasts*, also referred to as the mammary glands of reproduction, have previously been discussed since they are routinely examined during the general examination procedure. These glands become active only during pregnancy, during which time the breast changes to prepare for the secretion of colostrum (the forerunner of breast milk) and milk for the newborn following delivery.

Symptomatic Reaction to Disease

In both males and females, all the organs of reproduction are vulnerable to inflammation and infection, and thus both local and general symptoms of inflammation can be present. Abnormal discharge may also occur.

In addition, female menstrual cycle disturbances signal the onset of some diseases, although they may be caused by mechanical factors. There are various types of menstrual disorders which are not diseases in themselves but may be symptomatic reactions. In each of these disorders, the physician would determine the underlying cause and then individualize the treatment.

1. *Dysmenorrhea* is painful menstruation sometimes accompanied by headache, backache, and vomiting.

2. *Amenorrhea* is the absence of menstruation which normally occurs during lactation (breast feeding), pregnancy, and menopause. Certain disease states, however, can also produce amenorrhea.

3. *Menorrhagia* is excessive menstruation in which profuse flow or a prolonged period of menstruation may occur.

4. *Metrorrhagia* is a term for bleeding which occurs between the normal monthly menstrual periods. "Spotting" is the more common lay term used to refer to this process.

Common Diagnostic Studies of the Reproductive System

The student of medical assisting will need to be able to identify the common diagnostic tests which are associated with the genitalia and reproductive system, including biopsy, pap smear, and dilatation and curettage (D&C). These and other tests are listed and described in Table 20-2.

Common Diseases of the Reproductive System

The medical assistant should be familiar with the most common diseases of the reproductive system, including a variety of inflammations caused by bacterial infections or injuries. Table 20-3 lists these diseases together with their symptomatology and typical treatment. The role of the MA in patient management is also discussed.

Specific Clinical Procedures

The medical assistant may be responsible for irrigation of the vagina, inserting vaginal suppositories and creams, or instructing the patient on how to self-administer these medications. Creams are usually not administered in the office since an applicator can be used only by one individual. Directions for insertions are included with the medication, and the patient can usually follow these without difficulty. Irrigation solution may also be ordered and instructions again accompany the product. If homemade irrigation solutions are ordered frequently, a hand-out sheet of instructions can be designed and copies given to patients as needed.

Only the procedure for the insertion of a vaginal suppository is included in this section as it is the type of vaginal instillation most frequently encountered in the medical office.

TABLE 20-2.   Common Diagnostic Studies of the Reproductive System

Test	Description
Biopsy	Surgical removal of a piece of tissue for pathologic examination. Determines if tissue is benign or malignant (cancerous). Surgical procedure requiring special patient preparation and scheduling.
Pap smear (female)	Smear is made on culture material collected from cervical scraping to detect presence of cancer cells. Laboratory procedure.
Bacteriologic smear	Smear of vaginal discharge is made to determine the presence of bacteria. Culture can be grown in the office, and the medical assistant can monitor the growing process under the physician's supervision.
Dilatation and curettage (D&C) (female)	Surgical procedure which can also be performed as treatment measure. As a diagnostic measure, tissue of the endometrium is studied. Special patient preparation and scheduling are required.
Uterosalpingography (female)	X-ray study of the uterus and fallopian tubes accomplished by introducing a radiopaque dye into the uterus. Special patient preparation and scheduling are required.

TABLE 20-3.   Common Diseases of the Reproductive System

Diseases	Symptoms	Treatment	Medical Assistant's Role
Male: Epididymitis (inflammation of the epididymis caused by bacterial infection)	Pain, swelling, tenderness in the scrotum, fever, and malaise.	Bedrest. Patient may be instructed to apply ice bag. Drug therapy: antibiotics, analgesics (pain-relievers). Surgery (vasectomy) for recurrent disease. Increase fluid intake.	If patient is instructed to apply ice bag for relief of pain and to reduce swelling, special instruction should be given regarding keeping the bag in place for a maximum of 15 minutes every hour to prevent tissue damage.
Orchitis (inflammation of the testes caused by bacterial infection or injury)	Pain, swelling, tenderness in scrotum, fever, malaise.	Bedrest. Patient may be instructed to apply ice bag. Drug therapy: antibiotics, analgesics. Surgery (vasectomy) for recurrent disease. Increase fluid intake.	
Prostatitis (inflammation of the prostate usually caused by bacterial infection)	Dysuria (difficult and painful voiding), fever, and hematuria may occur.	Drug therapy: antibiotics, analgesics. Increase fluid intake.	
Hydrocele (collection of fluid in the scrotum which usually occurs in connection with infection of the epididymis or testes)	Scrotal enlargement without pain.	Fluid.	If procedure is performed in the office, the medical assistant will give the patient instructions to observe the dressing for signs of bleeding and to report this occurrence to the physician.

TABLE 20-3. *Continued*

Diseases	Symptoms	Treatment	Medical Assistant's Role
Female: Vaginitis (inflammation of the vagina usually caused by infection)	Itching, burning, abnormal vaginal discharge: can be white (leukorrhea), yellow, frothy, or like cottage cheese. Discharge characteristics depend on the type of microbial invasion.	Drug therapy: antibiotics (systemic and/or local). Vaginal irrigations may also be recommended.	General medical assisting clinical procedures. Patient teaching may include instructions for using a vaginal cream or inserting a suppository. Special instructions should be given the patient regarding vaginal irrigation. Be sure type of solution and amount are specified as well as the length of time to continue treatment. Instruct the patient to move irrigation tip up and down and rotate it in the vagina so as to allow the solution to infiltrate the vaginal folds.
Cervicitis (inflammation of the cervix usually caused by infection)	Abnormal discharge may or may not be present.	Drug therapy: antiseptic, antibiotic (local and systemic). Vaginal irrigation or cauterization may be required. Cauterization destroys eroded tissue by electrical current. Eroded tissue can also be destroyed by chemical application. Removal of the tissue for laboratory examination is called biopsy.	In addition to general clinical medical assisting procedures, the MA should explain cauterization to the patient if this procedure is to be performed.

TABLE 20-3. *Continued*

Diseases	Symptoms	Treatment	Medical Assistant's Role
Endometriosis (particles of the mucous membrane lining present on the ovaries and/or throughout the pelvis)	Dysmenorrhea, pelvic pain, abnormal uterine bleeding, lower abdominal and/or back pain.	Drug therapy: hormones. Surgery may be required to remove the patches or cysts which form as a consequence of the displaced tissue.	General clinical medical assisting procedures. The MA involved in the screening should be alert to certain symptoms in a patient diagnosed as having cervicitis. Symptoms that are similar to those of appendicitis would signal the occurrence of a complication such as cyst rupture.
Pelvic inflammatory disease, PID (inflammation of several of the reproductive organs)	General symptoms of infection. Large amounts of foul-smelling vaginal discharge may be present.	Drug therapy: antibiotics. Application of heat, vaginal irrigation. Surgery may be indicated.	The patient is usually hospitalized. During office visits, the medical assistant should offer patient teaching such as instructing the patient to change perineal pads frequently to avoid the spread of infection.

INSERTION OF A VAGINAL SUPPOSITORY

Purpose: To insert antiseptic or other medication for local effect to relieve symptoms of vaginitis or other diseases causing inflammation of the vaginal walls.

Procedure	Principle
1. Wash hands.	1. This prevents transfer of harmful microorganisms.
2. Explain the procedure to the patient.	2. This facilitates cooperation and reduces anxiety.
3. Assemble equipment: suppository and rubber gloves.	3. These items are necessary for carrying out the procedure. The gloves should be disposable and sterile.

4. Instruct the patient and provide assistance in assuming the dorsal recumbent position with legs wide apart. Drape properly.

4. This position exposes the vaginal orifice.

5. Open gloves using aseptic procedures. Ungloved, tear open the package containing the suppository. Without touching the suppository, drop it onto the sterile field created by the glove's wrapper or packaging. Use the sterile gloving technique described in Chapter 23.

5. Prevents contamination of the suppository and reduces the chance of introducing harmful microorganisms. If a patient is being instructed to self-administer the suppository, sterile gloving is not necessary. Washing the hands thoroughly would suffice. The medical assistant, however, is protecting both the patient and herself from contamination.

6. With one gloved hand, separate the labia minora. With the other gloved hand, pick up the suppository and insert, pushing it one finger length into the vagina.

6. The folds of labia minora must be separated to visualize the vagina.

7. Instruct the patient to remain in position for approximately 10 minutes.

7. This waiting period allows the suppository time to dissolve and prevents expulsion.

8. Remove gloves and dispose. Assist the patient to assume a comfortable position.

8. This signals the completion of the procedure and increases patient comfort.

9. Record the procedure properly in the patient's file: date, time, name of medication, route of administration. Initial the record.

9. Proper recording is necessary for future reference.

Reproductive System Specialties

The physician specializing in diseases of the female reproductive system is the gynecologist. A urologist or family practitioner usually cares for male patients as there is not a medical specialty exclusively devoted to the male reproductive tract.

The medical assistant employed in the office of a gynecologist will routinely assist with examinations and patient teaching, such as giving instruction in breast self-examination, and will most likely assist the physician with minor surgical and treatment procedures. In Chapter 23, special instruments that will most likely be found in the office of a gynecologist are pictured and their use identified.

THE MUSCULOSKELETAL SYSTEM

Structure and Function

The muscular system and the skeletal system are separate systems each with its own physiology. They are combined in this discussion because a close interrelationship exists both in providing the body with locomotion and in involvements with similar disease conditions. The physician examines the musculoskeletal system when testing range of motion and general state of locomotor function (Table 20-4).

The skeletal system is composed of bones and connective tissue. Connective tissue consists of supportive structures such as ligaments and tendons which hold the bones and muscles together. The bone network of the skeletal and muscular systems performs the functions of protection and support of vital organs as well as providing for body movement

TABLE 20-4.   Examination of the Musculoskeletal System

Body Part	Method and Equipment	Medical Assistant's Role
General systems	The physician usually instructs the patient to walk, sit, and assume various other positions and activities.	The medical assistant should be aware that a detailed musculoskeletal examination is lengthy. Usually, only the parts related to the patient's symptomatology are examined. The MA should be aware also that frequent position changes and maneuvers are undergone by the patient. For examination of the head and neck, the patient is sitting and remains so until the feet are examined. The patient then is supine.
Head and neck	Inspection and palpation. The physician may instruct the patient to rotate the neck and may give certain other directions to test the range of motion.	
Hands and wrists	Inspection and palpation. Directions to flex, extend, make a fist, and other motions.	
Elbows	Inspection and palpation. Instructions to bend, straighten, flex, and turn the elbow.	
Shoulder	Inspection and palpation.	
Feet and ankles	Inspection and palpation. Range of motion.	The medical assistant may be responsible for instructing the patient in range of motion exercises according to the physician's prescription, but is never responsible for diagnostic evaluations.

TABLE 20-4. *Continued*

Body Part	Method and Equipment	Medical Assistant's Role
Knees	Inspection and palpation. Certain other maneuvers.	The patient who has an existing joint disease or a deformity will have difficulty with some aspects of the testing and will be apprehensive. The medical assistant's role is to reassure the patient and offer the necessary assistance.
Spine	Inspection and palpation.	The patient is assisted to a standing position. The gown is opened completely at the back to allow visualization. Usually the assistant stands in front of the female patient, grasping the gown ties at each shoulder and holding the gown open for the physician. If the patient holds the gown herself, the anatomic and muscular structure may appear changed.

(Fig. 20-3). Another important function of the skeletal system is the manufacture of blood cells which takes place in the bone marrow located in the center of the bone.

Bones which fit together are called *joints.* Joints provide range of motion. *Cartilage,* a cushiony substance, helps separate the bones of the joint to absorb the force of friction in body movement. When the bones are in contact with one another the term *articulation* is applied. In addition to cartilage, the areas of articulation are also protected by a capsule-like mass called bursa which is lined with *synovial membrane.* This membrane secretes a fluid called synovia which continuously lubricates the joint. Certain joints, such as the elbow and the kneecap, are thus protected from the friction of articulation. Muscles composed of contractile tissue shorten and contract and are attached to the bones in order to effect movement. The intricate musculature of the body is depicted in Figure 20-4.

Symptomatic Reaction to Disease

The musculoskeletal system reacts to disease or injury with a variety of symptoms. Since any joint or muscle can become inflamed, general symptoms of inflammation can occur. Pain is, as usual, the most frequent response to disease or injury. In the skeletal system, injury to the bone causes pain. Muscle strains, tears, and sprains may also cause pain and

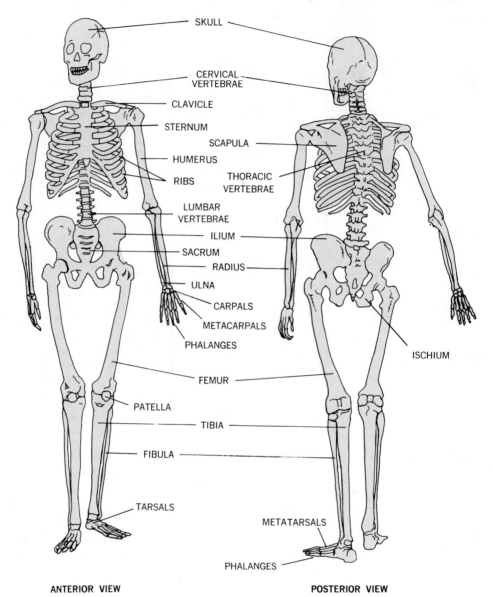

FIGURE 20-3.   The skeleton. (Reproduced from *Taber's Cyclopedic Medical Dictionary*, ed. 14. F. A. Davis, Philadelphia, 1981.)

aches and may become stiff, particularly when associated with joint disease. Deformity or impaired function is also associated with diseases of the musculoskeletal septem.

Common Diagnostic Tests of the Musculoskeletal System

The skeletal system can be visualized with the use of radiography (x-ray). Although other specific test procedures are sometimes employed, routine x-ray is the most common. Blood work may be ordered in particular instances in which blood analysis may be useful in the diagnosis of certain musculoskeletal diseases.

Common Diseases of the Musculoskeletal System

The medical assistant should be aware of the most common conditions associated with both the musculature and the skeletal system, including arthritis, bursitis, osteomyelitis, and various types of bone fractures. These are listed and described in Table 20-5 along with the typical treatment and the role of the MA.

Specific Clinical Procedures

The application of heat and cold are used frequently in treating disease and injury to the musculoskeletal system. The physician may refer the patient to the physical therapist for regular and deep heat treatment. However, the medical assistant may be responsible for applying or instructing the patient to apply various forms of heat and cold.

It should be noted that heat dilates blood vessels, increases the blood supply to the parts, and promotes healing. Heat also promotes drainage and is soothing, thereby increasing comfort.

Cold constricts blood vessels, decreases the blood supply to the part, and reduces swelling. Cold is also used to relieve pain. Prolonged application of cold, however, will have the reverse effect. Usually an application of not more than 30 minutes is recommended.

It will be remembered from the discussion on temperature in Chapter 16 that the body's reaction to heat and cold is directed at maintaining normal body temperature. When heat is applied, the vessels dilate and metabolism is increased to rid the body of excess heat. When cold is applied, the vessels constrict and metabolism is decreased to conserve heat. It is essential that the medical assistant understand these concepts before performing the related procedures. It is more likely that the MA's role will be to advise the patient in self-treatment techniques prescribed by the physician. The procedures described here are therefore presented from the patient teaching perspective.

INSTRUCTING THE PATIENT IN THE USE OF AN ICE BAG

Purpose: To enable the patient to carry out the physician's orders regarding the application of ice to relieve pain or reduce swelling.

Procedure	Principle
1. Obtain information from the physician regarding the length of time to be applied, how frequently it should be used, and the site to be treated.	1. Accurate information must be obtained to ensure proper treatment.

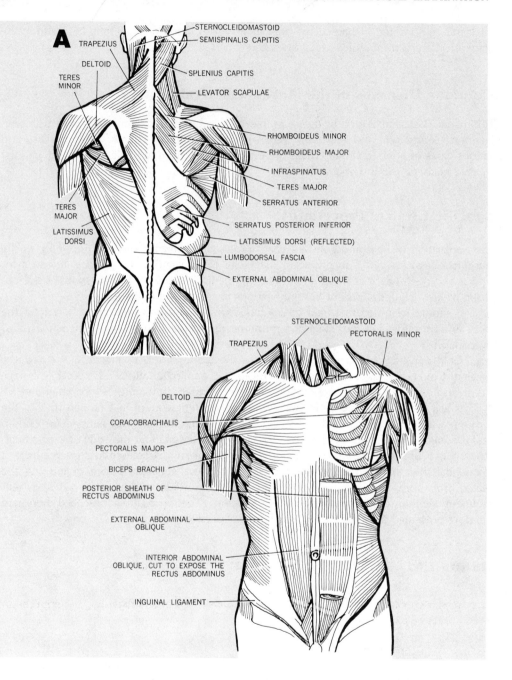

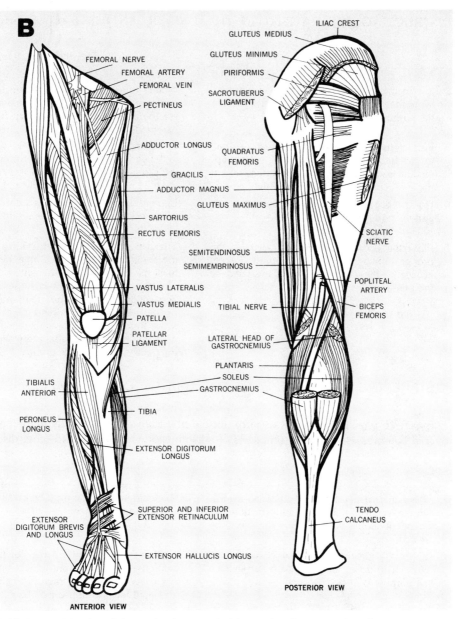

FIGURE 20-4. A. Muscles of the neck, chest, and abdominal wall. B. Muscles of the leg. (Reproduced from *Taber's Cyclopedic Medical Dictionary*, ed. 14. F. A. Davis, Philadelphia, 1981.)

INSTRUCTING THE PATIENT IN THE USE OF AN ICE BAG (Continued)

Procedure	Principle
2. Inform the patient of the physician's orders. Write them down for the patient and explain the purpose of the application.	2. Writing down the information for the patient reinforces the instruction. If these applications are routinely ordered, then instruction sheets designed for patient use may be effective.
3. Instruct the patient to fill the bag one-half to two-thirds full with ice. Expel air before capping by resting the bag on a flat surface so that the ice is level with the mouth of the bag.	3. Overfilling the bag prevents its conformity to the part. It is usually best to crush the ice for the same purpose. Air is expelled to contain the cold and also to aid flexibility of the bag.
4. Dry the bag. Place a towel between the bag and the body surface.	4. Depending on the patient's sensitivity to cold, the toweling can be used as a buffer. It also keeps the body surface dry.
5. Place the bag on the affected area for the proper duration (usually 30 minutes). Repeat procedure the number of times indicated by the physician.	5. The patient should be instructed to continue the application for the recommended time to fulfill the objectives of treatment. However, if numbness occurs or pain increases, then the applications should be temporarily suspended. Young children and the elderly tend to be more sensitive to cold; therefore these cautions should be emphasized when instructing patients in these age groups.

INSTRUCTING THE PATIENT IN THE USE OF COLD COMPRESSES

Purpose: To enable the patient to carry out the physician's orders regarding the application of cold compresses to relieve symptoms of inflammation, headache, and other disorders.

Procedure	Principle
1. Obtain information from the physician regarding the length of time to be applied, how frequently it should be used, and the site to be treated.	1. Accurate information must be obtained to ensure proper treatment.
2. Inform the patient of the physician's orders. Write them down for the patient and explain the purpose of the application.	2. Writing down the information for the patient reinforces the instruction. If these applications are routinely ordered, then instruction sheets designed for patient use may be effectual.
3. Instruct the patient to use gauze or washcloths which have been soaked in ice water and wrung out.	3. Ice water ensures that the compresses will maintain the cold for a longer period of time.
4. Apply to the affected body surface. Repeat procedures as directed and for the time specified (usually 15 to 20 minutes).	4. Compresses must be resoaked and wrung out because the body tends to warm the compress in approximately 2 minutes.
5. Instruct the patient to continue application of cold for the number of days ordered by the physician.	5. Continuing the applications is stressed to fulfill the objectives of treatment.

TABLE 20-5. Common Diseases of the Musculoskeletal System

Disease	Symptoms	Treatment	Medical Assistant's Role
Arthritis (inflammation of the joints)	Two major types: Rheumatoid (most common): general symptoms of inflammation; joint stiffness and soreness, pain and swelling; deformities may develop. Degenerative (osteoarthritis): pain, stiffness, sensitivity to weather change; bones may become larger (hypertrophy) but deformity does not usually occur.	Dependent on severity. Alternatives: Drug therapy: salicylates (aspirin), hormones, other specific groups of drugs. Application of heat. Balanced diet and exercise. Rest, sometimes immobilization of joints. Occupational therapy, Physical therapy. Surgery: synovectomy (joint removal), arthroplasty (repair of joint using synthetic materials), arthrodesis (fusion of joint surfaces).	General clinical medical assisting procedures. The patient with arthritis can be elderly or very young. In either case the patient needs information regarding care and reassurance because of the fear of deformity. Much patient teaching is directed toward helping the patient to cope with the disease since it is chronic. Patient is of extreme importance when working with arthritic patients. Personality changes are not uncommon due to the frequent periods of pain and the anxiety associated with the disease.
Bursitis (inflammation of the bursa)	Pain, often severe, especially upon movement.	Drug therapy such as cortisone. Aspiration of fluid which collects around the joint. X-ray therapy. Surgery is infrequent.	General clinical medical assisting procedures.

TABLE 20-5. *Continued*

Disease	Symptoms	Treatment	Medical Assistant's Role
Fracture (broken bone usually caused by injury) Types: Simple (broken bone with skin intact) Oblique (line of break slanted) Transverse (break line straight across bone) Compound (broken bone parts overlap) Complete (break line extends through bone) Incomplete (break line extends only part way through bone) Greenstick (resembles a "green stick" break or a splintering) Comminuted (bone broken in three or more pieces) Impacted (bones are driven together)	Pain, swelling, deformity, bleeding if compound fracture has occurred.	Alternatives: Immobilization, Surgery, Traction, Drug therapy: analgesics for pain; antibiotics if vulnerable to infection. Diet therapy (high-protein diet is usually ordered and may also be higher in calories, vitamins and minerals).	The patient with a fracture is usually not seen in the office but in the emergency facility of a hospital or medical center. However, followup visits are scheduled for the patient so that the physician may monitor progress. Patient teaching may involve explanation of the treatment alternative employed by the physician.
Osteomyelitis (localized infection of the bone)	Pain is the major symptom.	Drug therapy (antibiotics and analgesics); surgery; casting. Diet therapy (high-protein diet usually recommended.	General clinical medical assisting procedures.

INSTRUCTING THE PATIENT IN THE USE OF A HOT WATER BAG

Purpose: To enable the patient to carry out the physician's orders regarding the application of a hot water bag to relieve pain and discomfort or for the purpose specified.

Procedure	Principle
1. Obtain information from the physician regarding the length of time to be applied, how frequently it should be used, and the site to be treated.	1. Accurate information must be obtained to ensure proper treatment.
2. Inform the patient of the physician's orders. Write them down for the patient and explain the purpose of the application.	2. Writing down the information for the patient reinforces the physician's instructions. Instruction sheets designed for patient use may be effective.
3. Instruct the patient to fill the rubber bag approximately two-thirds full with heated water. Maximum water temperature should be 130°F (54.4°C). For children, 115°F is maximum. If the patient does not have a thermometer, instruct to adapt temperature to body comfort.	3. Water temperature which is too high may burn the patient. Filling the bag two-thirds full allows the bag to conform to body contour.
4. Expel the air before capping by resting the bag on a flat surface so that the water is level with the mouth of the bag.	4. This facilitates flexibility of the bag.
5. Cover the bag with flannel or cotton before applying to body surface.	5. Covering prevents burns from occurring and serves as a better conductor of heat.
6. Apply bag to body surface for the time specified and continue treatment as advised by the physician.	6. This is necessary to fulfill the objectives of treatment.

INSTRUCTING THE PATIENT IN THE USE OF A HEATING PAD

Purpose: To enable the patient to carry out the physician's orders regarding the application of a heating pad to relieve pain or discomfort, or for the purpose specified.

Procedure	Principle
1. Obtain information from the physician regarding the length of time to be applied, how frequently it should be used, and the site to be treated.	1. Accurate information must be obtained to ensure proper treatment.
2. Inform the patient of the physician's orders. Write them down for the patient and explain the purpose of the application.	2. Writing down the information for the patient reinforces the physician's instructions. If these applications are routinely ordered, then instruction sheets designed for patient use may be effective.

3. Instruct the patient to use the appliance with great caution and stress that the patient read and follow the product instructions carefully before applying.

3. Heating pads, because they are electric, are capable of incurring serious injury. The pad covering should be waterproof and well-insulated. Instructions should be read carefully to avoid body injury.

4. Apply for the length of time specified and continue use as indicated by the physician.

4. This fulfills the objective of treatment.

INSTRUCTING THE PATIENT IN THE USE OF HOT SOAKS

Purpose: To enable the patient to carry out the physician's orders regarding hot soaks to relieve discomfort and for any other purpose specified by the physician.

Procedure	*Principle*
1. Obtain information from the physician regarding the length of time to be applied, how frequently it should be used, and the site to be treated.	1. Accurate information must be obtained to ensure proper treatment.
2. Inform the patient of the physician's orders. Write them down for the patient and explain the purpose of the application.	2. Writing down the information for the patient reinforces the physician's instruction. If these applications are routinely ordered, then instruction sheets designed for patient use may be effective.
3. Instruct the patient to use the solution specified. Plain water is often recommended. Water or the solution ordered is usually heated to approximately 110°F (43.3°C).	3. High temperatures may cause burns.
4. Soak the affected body part for the time specified. Change the solution as necessary to maintain temperature. Continue treatment as directed by the physician.	4. Water will cool quickly. Even temperature is necessary to fulfill treatment objective.
5. Caution the patient to maintain good body alignment so as not to cause further injury or discomfort.	5. Use of towels or pads and comfortable positioning are necessary in order to maximize the effect of the soak. If body parts are twisted for the purpose of soaking, further discomfort will result.

INSTRUCTING THE PATIENT IN THE USE OF HOT COMPRESSES

Purpose: To enable the patient to carry out the physician's orders regarding the use of hot compresses to relieve pain, promote drainage, increase circulation, or for the purpose specified.

Procedure	*Principle*
1. Obtain information from the physician regarding the length of time to be applied, how frequently it should be used, and the site to be treated.	1. Accurate information must be obtained to ensure proper treatment.

2. Inform the patient of the physician's orders. Write them down for the patient and explain the purpose of the application.

2. Writing down the information for the patient reinforces the physician's instruction. If these applications are routinely ordered, then instruction sheets designed for patient use may be effective.

3. Instruct the patient to use gauze or washcloths which have been immersed in water or the solution prescribed and wrung out. The temperature should be as hot as the patient can tolerate unless otherwise directed: 105°F (40.6°C) is the average tolerable temperature.

3. Washcloths are the easiest, most accessible and comfortable form of compress. Caution the patient that too high temperatures will cause burning, but heat of maximum tolerance is necessary to achieve objectives.

4. Apply the moist cloth to the affected area. Change cloths frequently to maintain warmth for the time specified (usually 30 minutes).

4. Body temperature will cool compresses usually within 2 to 5 minutes.

5. Continue the procedure for the number of days directed by the physician.

5. Continuing treatment is needed to fulfill the objectives.

The Musculoskeletal Specialty

Orthopedics focuses on the diagnosis and treatment of injury and disease of the musculoskeletal system. The responsibilities of the medical assistant associated with an orthopedic practice would include the performance of general duties as well as assisting with casting procedures and perhaps obtaining x-rays. Under the physician's supervision, the MA may also be responsible for range of motion exercises and providing assistance in other specific orthopedic treatments.

The procedure for range of motion exercises is included in Chapter 25, which discusses the medical assistant's role in assisting with physical therapy procedures.

THE ENDOCRINE SYSTEM

Structure and Function

The endocrine system is composed of glands which are influential in the regulation and coordination of all body systems. The glands of this system secrete special substances called hormones. The glands manufacture these hormones by using other substances absorbed from the blood stream.

Included in the endocrine system are (1) the pituitary gland, located at the base of the skull; (2) the thyroid gland, located in the neck; (3) the parathyroid glands, positioned over the thyroid gland; (4) the adrenal glands, located above the kidneys; (5) the pineal gland, situated in the skull; (6) the sex glands (ovaries in the female, testes in the male); (7) the thymus, located in the chest under the sternum; and (8) the pancreas, located behind the stomach (Fig. 20-5).

The *pituitary* gland secretes the growth hormone which influences size. Other hormones are secreted by this gland and have specific effects on specialized body processes such as the manufacture of egg cells in both the male and female.

The *thyroid* gland can be located by placing the fingertips over the protrusion in the

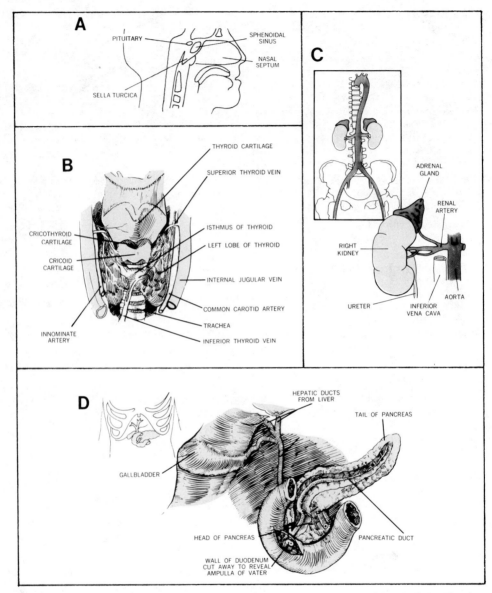

FIGURE 20-5. A. Relationship of the pituitary gland to bony structures of the skull. B. The thyroid gland and related structures. C. The adrenal glands. D. The pancreas and its relationship to the duodenum. (Reproduced from *Taber's Cyclopedic Medical Dictionary*, ed. 14. F. A. Davis, Philadelphia, 1981.)

frontal neck known as the "Adam's apple." The soft tissue behind this structure is the thyroid. It has a "bowtie" (two-lobed) appearance, and each lobe rests on the trachea. The thyroid gland depends on the pituitary for stimulation. The thyroid produces thyroxine and another less-known hormone called triiodothyronine. Thyroxine is necessary in maintaining the metabolism and oxidation rates in the cells and contains most of the body's iodine. It also influences other metabolic activity and specifically the production of enzymes.

The cortex (outer portion) of the *adrenal* glands, also stimulated by the pituitary, secretes a hormone family called corticosteroids. The most familiar are estrogen and progesterone. This family of hormones, among its many functions, maintains the body's electrolyte and water balance, is influential in the metabolism of carbohydrates, fats, and protein, and aids the body in coping with stress.

The medulla (inside portion) of the gland also produces hormones called epinephrine and norepinephrine (adrenaline and noradrenaline). Adrenaline is the body's self-manufactured defense mechanism since it is activated in times of physiologic stress to assist the body in its response.

The *pancreas* produces a hormone called insulin which is essential to the metabolism of carbohydrates (sugars and starches). Insulin converts these starches to energy and also stores carbohydrates in the form of fat on the body and glycogen in the muscles and liver for ready use when required.

Symptomatic Reaction to Disease

The endocrine system, when in a state of malfunction, produces either too much or too little of a particular hormone. Symptoms are directly related to the functions controlled by these hormones.

For instance, in a disturbance of the pituitary gland in a child, overproduction of the hormone might result in gigantism, while inadequate production might result in dwarfism. These signs are related to the growth-influencing factor of the hormone. Symptoms will be related to the specific gland that is diseased and the aspect of body functioning influenced by the hormone's increased or decreased production. The glands are interdependent. Dysfunction of one gland tends to affect the normal functioning of other glands.

The Examination of the Endocrine System

The examination of the endocrine system is specific to the gland which the physician suspects is the cause of the symptomology. The physician will use the methods of examination to determine if signs are present which correspond to malfunction of the gland. In this particular system, diagnostic studies are often the most conclusive indication of malfunction.

The medical assistant's role in an examination of the endocrine system is to expose the body part in which the gland is located using proper gowning, draping, and positioning procedures.

Common Diagnostic Studies of the Endocrine System

There are four tests which are commonly associated with the endocrine system: the basal metabolic rate, protein-bound iodine, radioactive iodine uptake, and I-urine excretion tests. Each of these is described in Table 20-6. Other less frequently used tests are available

TABLE 20-6.   Common Diagnostic Studies of the Endocrine System

Test	Description
Basal metabolism rate (BMR)	A test for thyroid function that determines the rate of metabolism of the patient at rest. Special patient preparation and scheduling are required.
Protein-bound iodine (PBI)	Blood test to determine iodine in the blood stream. A thyroid function test performed by the medical technologist.
Radioactive iodine uptake	A thyroid function test that measures the amount of radioactive iodine present in the thyroid and the urine after a small amount has been consumed. Special scheduling is necessary.
I-urine excretion test	A thyroid function test that measures the amount of the consumed substance present in the urine over a period of time, usually 48 hours.

for thyroid function determination, and highly specialized procedures have been developed to determine the functioning of other glands.

Common Diseases of the Endocrine System

The medical assistant should acquire familiarity with the most common diseases of the endocrine system, including thyroiditis, hyperthyroidism, hypothyroidism, and diabetes. Table 20-7 lists these diseases along with the symptoms and typical treatment approaches, and the medical assistant's role.

Specific Clinical Procedures

The chief area of responsibility for the medical assistant in relation to endocrine disorders is patient teaching. In addition to stressing patient compliance with the physician's instructions, this function would include explanations of specific dietary regimes, the self-administration of specific medications, and the noting of potential and observed complications in the various endocrine diseases.

The Endocrine Specialty

The physician specializing in disorders of the endocrine system is called an endocrinologist. The MA working in the office of this specialist would be expected to perform general medical assisting procedures with an emphasis on patient teaching and interaction. The endocrinologist in private practice receives patient referrals almost exclusively and is most often positioned in or closely associated with a medical center or teaching facility. Unlike specialties in which patient self-referral is the norm, the field of endocrinology tends toward consultation and research.

THE NEUROLOGIC SYSTEM

Structure and Function

The neurologic or nervous system is composed of the brain, the spinal cord, and the nerve network. Together these parts affect the regulation and integration of all of the body functions.

TABLE 20-7. Common Diseases of the Endocrine System

Disease	Symptoms	Treatment	Medical Assistant's Role
Thyroiditis (inflammation of the thyroid)	Pain in the neck which may radiate to the upper arms and chest. General symptoms of inflammation may be present.	Nonspecific. Usually subsides without drug therapy.	General clinical medical assisting procedures.
Hyperthyroidism (Graves' disease) (activity of thyroid is increased with subsequent overproduction of thyroxine)	Weakness, increased appetite with weight loss, restlessness, insomnia, tremors, and anxiety. Palpitations and dyspnea may occur.	Alternatives: Radioactive iodine, antithyroid drugs, surgery. In addition, diet therapy is employed. A high-calorie diet is usually ordered.	General clinical medical assisting procedures.
Hypothyroidism (decreased activity of the thyroid gland with subsequent decreases in the production of thyroxine)	In children cretinism (a lack of normal physical and mental development) may result. In adults myxedema may result which is a condition of dry skin and hair and sensitivity to cold. Slowed mental functions may be present. Signs: exophthalmus (protruding eyes), puffy facial appearance.	Therapy: thyroid extract	General clinical medical assisting procedures.

TABLE 20-7. *Continued*

Disease	Symptoms	Treatment	Medical Assistant's Role
Diabetes mellitus (inability of the body to metabolize carbohydrates adequately due to insufficient amount of insulin produced by the pancreas)	Major symptoms: polyuria (excessive urination), polydipsia (excessive thirst), polyphagia (excessive hunger). Major signs: increased amount of sugar in the blood, glycosuria (presence of sugar in the urine).	Combination of diet, exercise, and medication. Oral hypoglycemic agents or insulin by injection are prescribed, depending on the severity of the disease. The diet usually recommended is balanced, with restricted carbohydrates. Diet therapy may be used without drug therapy dependent on the individual disease profile.	General clinical medical assisting procedures. The MA will also be responsible for patient teaching. Diet instructions, use of an exchange list, instruction in how to self-administer insulin, and the extreme importance of patient compliance with the regime must be stressed. *

* The MA involved in patient screening for appointment scheduling must be alert to symptoms of complications in patients diagnosed as having diabetes: (1) *diabetic coma* (inability to use sugar, characterized by weakness, thirst, headache, loss of appetite, abdominal pain, nausea and vomiting), and (2) *insulin shock* or hypoglycemia (low blood sugar, characterized by hunger, weakness, nervousness, tremors, profuse perspiration, and dizziness). Diabetic coma is a medical emergency in which the physician must determine the amount of insulin necessary to metabolize the carbohydrates. Insulin coverage is inadequate, and thus the patient experiences diabetic coma. Insulin shock is a common crisis which occurs especially in newly diagnosed diabetics. Missing a meal could result in hypoglycemia. Not enough carbohydrates have been ingested to absorb the insulin coverage. In addition to wearing alerting identification, the patient should be given careful instruction about carrying sugar lumps or candy at all times to prevent insulin shock.

The nerve center (central nervous system) includes the brain and spinal cord. In this center, information regarding body function is continuously being processed. The entire body is infiltrated by a network of nerves which carry messages to and from the brain.

The brain is encased in a bone called the *cranium* (skull) to protect its delicate operational processes. The brain contains the largest mass of nervous tissue in the body.

Five parts of the brain are identified as controlling separate functions (Fig. 20-6).

The *cerebrum* is located uppermost in the cranium in the largest part of the brain. The cerebrum controls mental activities such as memory, reason, and intelligence, and sensory functions such as sight, speech, smell, and some voluntary movements.

LATERAL ASPECT

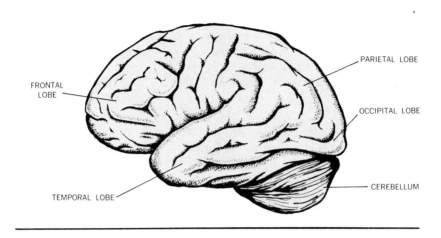

FRONTAL LOBE

PARIETAL LOBE

OCCIPITAL LOBE

CEREBELLUM

TEMPORAL LOBE

MEDIAL ASPECT

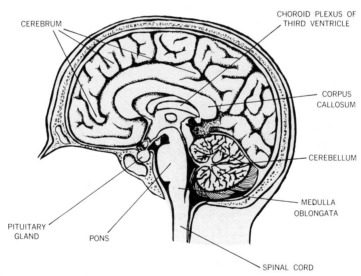

CEREBRUM

CHOROID PLEXUS OF THIRD VENTRICLE

CORPUS CALLOSUM

CEREBELLUM

MEDULLA OBLONGATA

PITUITARY GLAND

PONS

SPINAL CORD

FIGURE 20-6. The brain. (Reproduced from *Taber's Cyclopedic Medical Dictionary*, ed. 14. F. A. Davis, Philadelphia, 1981.)

The *cerebellum* is located beneath the cerebrum and assists in regulating muscle coordination and balance.

The *midbrain, pons,* and *medulla* together make up the *brain stem*. The midbrain connects the cerebrum and cerebellum to the pons; the pons connects the cerebrum to the medulla. The brain is connected to the spinal cord by the medulla. A certain group of nerves, called motor nerves since they are responsible for motion, cross in the medulla. Respiration, heart beat, and blood pressure receive automatic monitoring in the medulla.

The *spinal cord* which extends from the medulla to the region of the lower back serves as the trunk for nerve branches that act as pathways for messages (nerve impulses) between the brain and the parts of the body below the head. A liquid called cerebrospinal fluid, formed from blood capillaries in the brain, lubricates the brain and spinal cord and flows through the meninges. Both the brain and spinal cord are surrounded by protective membrane layers called the meninges. The cord is encased in a series of 33 bones called *vertebrae*. The *nerves* are bundles of nerve fiber that "plug into" the central nervous system. These nerve fibers and nerve cells are differentiated by color. White matter is made up of nerve fibers, while gray matter is made up of nerve cells. What is perhaps most significant in understanding the physiology is that nerve fibers are capable of repair. Nerve cells, however, once damaged cannot be restored.

Symptomatic Reaction to Disease

The body's response to disease in the structure of the neurologic system relates to loss of or disturbed body functioning. The characteristics and location of this disturbance depend on which part of the system is affected. The possibility of recovery from malfunction, such as paralysis of a body part, depends on whether nerve cells or nerve fibers have been damaged.

Table 20-8 describes the basic steps entailed in a standard neurologic examination, together with the medical assistant's role in the procedure.

Common Diagnostic Tests of the Neurologic System

There are four standard testing procedures which are commonly associated with the neurologic system: lumbar puncture ("spinal tap"), pneumoencephalogram, electroencephalogram, and brain scan. Each of these procedures is described in Table 20-9.

Common Diseases of the Neurologic System

The medical assistant is likely to encounter patients suffering from a wide variety of diseases associated with malfunctions of the neurologic system. These include a number of inflammatory conditions such as neuritis, encephalitis, and shingles, as well as severe pain-producing disorders such as neuralgia, sciatica, and migraine, and convulsive syndromes such as epilepsy. Each of these conditions is listed in Table 20-10 along with symptoms, treatment procedures, and the role of the medical assistant.

Specific Clinical Procedures

There are no specific clinical procedures directly related to neurology that are routinely performed by medical assistants. It is possible, however, that an MA could be instructed to

TABLE 20-8. The Neurologic Examination

Body Part and Function	Method and Equipment	Medical Assistant's Role
Mental status survey	Inspection of body posture and general appearance. Interviewing with questions directed at measuring intelligence, memory, etc.	The medical assistant is usually not present for this portion of the examination as it might interfere with the relationship between the physician and the patient. The MA, however, may provide input regarding mental status derived from time spent alone with the patient.
Face for cranial nerve status:		
Olfactory (smell)	Patient may be asked to identify common odors with eyes closed.	The MA will be present and hand the physician the items required. Patient will be sitting.
Optic (sight)	Ophthalmoscope used to examine eye. Visual acuity test may be performed to test vision capabilities.	The visual acuity test may be the responsibility of the medical assistant.
Pupil motor reaction	Flashlight inspection. Palpation of the face. Patient clinches teeth and physician palpates muscles.	
Sensory	Patient closes eyes. Physician palpates the face. Safety pin may be used.	The MA may need to assemble various items that would assist the physician to test for pain or feeling sensation. Clean safety pins and cotton balls are most frequently used. These items should be changed frequently in a tray setup.
Facial motor ability	Inspection of the face as the patient is given directions such as to frown, smile, and puff out cheeks.	The medical assistant should note the degree of patient comfort. Because the examination tends to be lengthy, rest periods are usually provided in which the physician leaves the room. The assistant can attend to the patient's comfort and remain for quiet conversation if time permits.

TABLE 20-8. *Continued*

Body Part and Function	Method and Equipment	Medical Assistant's Role
Hearing	Physician may speak in various tones to test hearing capabilities.	
Nerves of the motor system:		
Coordination and muscle strength	Patient will be asked to walk, do knee bends, walk on toes, raise hands above head, flex extremities, and push and pull against examiner's hands.	
Nerves of the sensory system:		
Arms, trunk, legs	Inspection with pin and tuning fork.	The medical assistant assists the patient to assume a supine position.
Reflexes:		
All points of reflexes such as knees, elbows, ankles	Reflex hammer.	The patient is assisted to a sitting position, then again to supine.

TABLE 20-9.   Common Diagnostic Tests of the Neurologic System

Test	Description
Lumbar puncture (spinal tap)	A procedure used to aspirate cerebral spinal fluid for examination. The physician injects a needle into a certain area of the spinal cord and withdraws fluid. The patient usually is hospitalized for this procedure. Special scheduling and patient preparation are required.
Pneumoencephalogram	In this procedure air is injected into the spinal column. The air rises to the brain and x-ray visualization is then possible. The patient usually is hospitalized for this test. Special scheduling and patient preparation are required.
Electroencephalogram (EEG)	A procedure using special equipment to trace the electrical waves of the brain. EEG can be performed in the office of a neurologist or in the hospital. Special scheduling is required.
Brain scan	A procedure involving use of radioisotopes. Highly specialized equipment is used, and the procedure is performed in a hospital or medical center.

TABLE 20-10.   Common Diseases of the Neurologic System

Disease	Symptoms	Treatment	Medical Assistant's Role
Meningitis (inflammation of the meninges caused by bacterial or viral invasion)	General symptoms of upper respiratory infection usually accompanied by headache and stiff neck.	Drug therapy: antibiotics and other drugs such as analgesics, are used to relieve symptoms.	General clinical medical assisting procedures. The patient is hospitalized and seen in the office for initial diagnosis and followup. When there is suspicion of meningitis, aseptic precautions should be carefully followed to avoid contamination.
Encephalitis (inflammation of the brain caused by infection; may be transmitted by mosquito or tick)	Headache, drowsiness, convulsion.	Drug therapy is usually not effective.	General clinical medical assisting procedures. The patient is usually hospitalized and seen in the office for initial diagnosis and followup. When there is suspicion of meningitis, aseptic precautions should be carefully followed to avoid contamination.
Neuritis (inflammation of one or more nerves; different types have different causes)	Severe discomfort or pain; weakness and/or paralysis of the part affected.	Nonspecific. Drug therapy: analgesics for pain.	General clinical medical assisting procedures. The patient is usually hospitalized and seen in the office for initial diagnosis and followup. When there is suspicion of meningitis, aseptic precautions should be carefully followed to avoid contamination.

TABLE 20-10. *Continued*

Disease	Symptoms	Treatment	Medical Assistant's Role
Herpes zoster (shingles) (inflammation of skin or mucous membrane along the course of a nerve)	Pain usually along the course of the nerve. Skin eruption may form.	Drug therapy: analgesics. Warm soaks may also be applied.	General clinical medical assisting procedures. The patient is usually hospitalized and seen in the office for initial diagnosis and followup. When there is suspicion of meningitis, aseptic precautions should be carefully followed to avoid contamination.
Epilepsy (abnormal discharge of nervous energy from the brain)	Convulsions: *Grand mal* seizures are characterized by longer-lasting loss of consciousness, while *petit mal* seizures are of short duration (5–30 seconds). Two other classifications of seizures are commonly used to describe symptoms: *Jacksonian* seizures are characterized by jerking movements in one part of the body, and *psychomotor* seizures are characterized by brief, isolated, bizarre behaviors.	If symptoms are caused by a tumor, then surgery is performed. If not, the following measures are employed: drug therapy (anticonvulsants) and family psychotherapy if indicated.	General clinical medical assisting procedures. In addition, the MA should be acutely aware of the needs of the patient and his family, and can give significant input to the physician that will assist in making judgments relating to the emotional needs of the patient.

TABLE 20-10. *Continued*

Disease	Symptoms	Treatment	Medical Assistant's Role
Migraine (pain derived from dilation of blood vessels supplying the brain)	Nausea and vomiting are the principal symptoms.	Drug therapy: vasoconstrictors	General clinical medical assisting procedures. The physician may suggest the application of an ice bag to the head on the area of the headache. The MA should be certain the patient understands how, when, why, and for how long ice should be applied.
Trigeminal neuralgia (severe pain on one side of the face which follows the pathway of a nerve branch)	Severe, incapacitating pain.	Drug therapy: analgesics, sedatives, and other specialized drugs. Surgery may be required to sever nerve impulses and relieve pain.	General clinical medical assisting procedures which include reassurance, since patient anxiety tends to be great.
Sciatica (pain which follows the pathway of the sciatic nerve)	Pain (low back and radiates down the leg). Numbness, tingling of the part, may also be present.	Dependent on cause.	General clinical medical assisting procedures. The MA should be aware that an intramuscular injection administered improperly can injure the sciatic nerve and cause sciatica (painful inflammation).

record an electroencephalogram, under a physician's supervision, as well as performing other support procedures pertinent to the treatment of patients with neurologic disorders.

Nervous System Specialties

The neurologist serves as a diagnostician for patients with suspected nervous system disease or impairment. The neurosurgeon is trained in the surgical correction of such disorders, often involving the removal of blood clots (hematomas) and tumors.

The responsibilities of the medical assistant in the office of a neurologist would include the performance of general medical assisting procedures and perhaps other tasks falling within the scope of the expanded capabilities of medical assisting for which the special supervision of the physician is required.

THE PEDIATRIC PATIENT

The pediatric patient warrants special consideration and discussion. Regardless of the type of practice, children will be frequently encountered in the office. The age range of a pediatric patient usually falls between birth and 12 years. In some pediatric practices the outside age limit may be 14 or 16.

Because of their particular stage of physiologic, psychologic, and emotional development, children require special handling to provide the best possible atmosphere in which patient comfort and quality care can be accomplished. Young children frequently form judgments regarding medical personnel and medical care that will influence their adult perceptions. Just as each adult is a unique individual, so too is each child. Obviously, however, certain general considerations are more related to one group than another.

In this section, the child is considered not in terms of physiologic structure, but rather in terms of age and behavioral expectations. The medical assistant who can relate effectively to children will be a valuable asset to the office team, facilitating the positive formation of the doctor-patient relationship.

Although information regarding ages and stages of children may differ somewhat according to the source, basic age-related behavior can be identified. The medical assistant can plan the optimum approach to the patient when a basic understanding of behavioral expectations in that patient's age range has been gained (Table 20-11).

Symptomatic Reaction to Disease in the Pediatric Patient

As with adults, symptomatic reaction to disease in children depends on the body system which is experiencing distress.

The major concern in childhood disease is that the symptoms of many diseases are quite similar. The general symptom of pain can be present in a child with pharyngitis (sore throat) and meningitis. The medical assistant responsible for patient screening in scheduling appointments must ask pertinent questions that will serve as clues to the severity and exact nature of the symptoms. The parents of small children are often alarmed when their children are ill because very young children cannot communicate the nature of their distress. Moreover, parents are often confused as to when a child should be brought to the physician.

Many pediatricians print pamphlets in which helpful information is provided. Some physicians, especially those in pediatrics, may schedule a telephone hour when parents can call for advice. Often the medical assistant assumes responsibility for initially receiving and referring the questions when necessary.

The Examination of the Pediatric Patient

The examination of the pediatric patient follows the same pattern as that for adults. Children, however, are growing and changing, and their anatomic and physiologic develop-

TABLE 20-11.   Suggested Approaches to the Pediatric Patient

Age Period	Behavior Expectations	Suggested Approach
Infancy (0-12 months)	Crying in the newborn period is expected, especially if the office visit takes place close to feeding time.	Since auscultation will be difficult when the baby is crying, encourage the mother to place the tip of her finger or pacifier in the baby's mouth when the stethoscope is being used to allow the chest sounds to be heard without distracting noises. The baby should not be fed during the examination as this would interfere with the sounds being analyzed when the stethoscope is in use. When the medical assistant is weighing the baby and performing other procedures, a gentle, quiet approach is recommended. Talking quietly and holding the baby securely are comforting.
	Infants have a short attention span and appear to be able to focus on only one stimulus at a time.	Distraction appears most successful to gain cooperation. Mobiles, body movements, a shining light, all can distract an infant. Experimentation is necessary since each child responds enthusiastically to different stimuli.
	Nudity is usually preferred.	In preparing the patient for the examination, all clothing is removed except the diaper.
	Infants need constant closeness to the mother.	The medical assistant or the mother may help position the baby during examination. When the infant is acutely ill or exhausted, and with the physician's approval, the mother can hold the baby for most of the examination.

TABLE 20-11. *Continued*

Age Period	Behavior Expectations	Suggested Approach
Early Childhood (1–5 years)	A child in this age group usually fears the office visit. The extent of the fear and behavior expressed is dependent on the patient's age and personality. However, vocal expressions of resistance such as crying, screaming, and physical struggle, and exasperated parents are common experiences.	The medical assistant is challenged to make the office visit a pleasant experience. Allowing the child to retain as much clothing as possible is comforting. Interesting toys and books in the waiting room and examining room help to reduce the child's discomfort. A gentle, quiet manner and conversation also help to gain the child's confidence. Truth is imperative. If a procedure will hurt, a brief, clear explanation of what is being done and why may be helpful, depending on age and personality. Complimentary remarks help to bridge the unfamiliarity the child feels in the presence of the office staff. If the physician prefers, the examination need not be performed on the examining table. The child may stand, or sit in the mother's, the assistant's, or the physician's lap. Demonstration of the procedure or explanation and demonstration of the examination on a doll is helpful. The medical assistant can allow the child to place the stethoscope in his ears and pretend to examine the doll or the MA. Other equipment can be handled by the patient with supervision.

TABLE 20-11. *Continued*

Age Period	Behavior Expectations	Suggested Approach
Early Childhood (continued)		First physical contacts set the stage for the child's reaction to the examination. For instance, the medical assistant may need to take a rectal temperature reading. The MA should first touch the child in a gaming situation such as counting the fingers or toes. Injections are particularly unpleasant, and the child will resist. Unpleasant procedures should be performed quickly despite patient protest. Reassurance and explanation should take place following the procedure.
Childhood (5-12 years)	Usually the school-age child is cooperative and curious, and wants to be treated as an adult.	Questions should first be directed to the child. The parent can usually add to the response.
	Privacy needs are usually well established.	Preparation for the examination includes an awareness of this need. While gowning is usually necessary, the child should be left with his mother to undress. Underpants are usually not removed until required.

ment must be closely monitored. In order to perform the comprehensive examination in children, the physician may alter the standard techniques and adapt certain other ones. The medical assistant's clinical responsibilities are also adapted. Table 20-12 outlines the general pediatric examination and the medical assistant's role.

Common Diseases of Children

Children are susceptible to most adult diseases. Respiratory tract infections are common. While there are a number of diseases prevalent in the childhood years, perhaps most useful for the medical assistant to know about are the common communicable diseases and their methods of transmission. These are described in Table 20-13.

TABLE 20-12.   **The Pediatric Examination**

Body Part or Function	Method and Equipment	Medical Assistant's Role
Vital signs	The medical assistant performs TPR, height, weight, measures head and chest circumference. Blood pressure may be omitted, depending on physician preference. If performed, a small pediatric cuff is utilized.	The medical assistant usually takes the child's temperature rectally. TPR is usually taken on every visit. The rectal temperature can be obtained by placing the young child over the lap or placing the child on the table. Spread the buttocks with one hand; with the other insert the lubricated thermometer approximately 1 inch. Upon insertion, hold the buttocks closed and the thermometer in place, as the child will have the urge to expel the thermometer. The MA's arm should lie over the child's back with the body leaning forward to secure the child. The MA's approach will greatly affect the ease in performing these procedures. Head and chest circumference is usually measured in the first two years. Blood pressure is usually obtained with a pediatric cuff at every visit when the child is over age 3. Prior to this time, if the BP is obtained, the physician usually performs the procedure.
Skin	Inspection: a magnifying glass is often used.	The medical assistant hands the physician the equipment and assists in positioning the patient.
Head and neck	Inspection. Palpation. Transillumination of the skull with a flashlight.	The medical assistant can help the mother to position the child for ease in examination. Much of the examination of the infant can occur while the mother is sitting on the examination table, holding the child.

TABLE 20-12.   *Continued*

Body Part or Function	Method and Equipment	Medical Assistant's Role
Eye	Inspection with an ophthalmoscope.	The medical assistant will most likely be responsible for visual acuity tests in young children over 3 and in early school-age children. Some resistance to covering the eye may be experienced. Again, gaming may be helpful. For example, reference to a cover as a "pirate's patch" may be helpful. (A cup cover will probably be inadequate.)
Ear	Inspection with otoscope. Otoscope with pneumatic bulb (air-inflated) may be used.	The medical assistant must provide a small speculum for the pediatric patient. In very young children, or children offering resistance, the mother may be requested to lie across or hold down the child's legs while the MA secures the patient's head. This is necessary to avoid injury to the ear.
Nose, mouth, throat	Inspection with light and tongue blade. Palpation.	Restraint of the young child may be necessary. Arms are held at sides.
Thorax and lungs	Inspection. Palpation. Percussion. Auscultation with a stethoscope.	Keeping the child quiet during this part of the examination is extremely important for the physician's accuracy in judgment.
Heart	Auscultation with a stethoscope.	Keeping the child quiet during this part of the examination is important for accuracy in judgment.
Abdomen	Inspection. Palpation. Percussion.	The medical assistant will hold the child's legs flexed in order to relax the abdomen and facilitate the physician's examination.
Genitalia and rectum	Inspection. Palpation.	The medical assistant helps the patient to maintain a supine position.

TABLE 20-12. *Continued*

Body Part or Function	Method and Equipment	Medical Assistant's Role
Musculoskeletal system	The physician puts the extremities and back through ranges of motion. The child who is able to walk is sometimes instructed to walk a short distance and is observed by the physician for abnormalities and deformities.	The medical assistant can be helpful in relaying to the physician any observation made while preparing the patient for examination.
Neurologic system: reflexes	Percussion using a hammer and specific hand movements and manipulations.	Assistance in positioning and handling instruments.

Communicable diseases are those which are easily passed from person to person, usually by direct contact. Because of the highly social nature of young children and their tendency to find themselves in close quarters with large numbers of other children in classrooms and at play, many communicable diseases have become widely known as "childhood diseases."

Pediatric Specialties

The physician specializing in the health needs of children is a pediatrician. The pediatrician will diagnose and treat diseases of childhood and, in addition, will routinely monitor the normal growth and development of children. The medical assistant positioned in a pediatric office will be responsible for record-keeping, patient teaching, and preparation of patients for examination, as well as assisting in treatment procedures and assuming other general office responsibilities.

There are other specialties with particular reference to children, such as pediatric cardiology and pediatric neurology. In these specialties, the concentration is in the related systemic diseases of pediatric rather than adult patients.

THE INTEGUMENTARY SYSTEM

Structure and Function

The integumentary system includes the layers of body covering called skin. During the general examination, the physician examines each body part and inspects its skin. There are also occasions when symptoms may suggest a specific skin examination.

The skin serves many functions. It protects the body from infection and injury, while it helps to maintain both body temperature and fluid-electrolyte balance. Touch sensations are made possible by nerve endings which are buried in the skin layers.

TABLE 20-13.   Method of Transmission of Some Common Communicable Diseases*

Disease	How Agent Leaves the Bodies of the Sick	How Organisms May Be Transmitted	Method of Entry Into the Body
Typhoid fever	Feces and urine.	Direct contact. Hands of nurse or attendant. Linen and all articles used by and about patient. Hands of carriers soiled by their own feces. Water polluted by excreta. Food grown in or washed with such water. Milk diluted with contaminated water. Flies.	Through mouth in infected food or water and thence to intestinal tract.
Diphtheria	Sputum and discharges from nose and throat. Skin lesions.	Direct contact. Droplet infection from patient coughing. Hands of nurse. Articles used by and about patient.	Through mouth to throat or nose to throat.
Streptococcal sore throat	Discharges from nose and throat. Skin lesions.	Direct contact. Hands of nurse. Articles used by and about patient.	Through mouth and nose.
Pneumonia	Sputum and discharges from nose and throat.	Direct contact. Hands of nurse. Articles used by and about patient.	Through mouth and nose to lungs.
Influenza	As in pneumonia.	As in pneumonia.	As in pneumonia.
Tetanus	Excreta from infected herbivorous animals and man.	Soil, especially that with manure or feces in it. Dust, etc. Articles used about stables.	Directly into blood stream through wounds (is anaerobe and prefers deep incised wound).

TABLE 20-13. *Continued*

Disease	How Agent Leaves the Bodies of the Sick	How Organisms May Be Transmitted	Method of Entry Into the Body
Tuberculosis, human	Sputum, lesions, feces.	Direct contact such as kissing. Droplet infection from person coughing with mouth uncovered. Sputum from mouth to fingers, thence to food and other things. Soiled dressings.	Through mouth to lungs and intestines. From intestines via lymph channels to lymph vessels and to tissues.
Tuberculosis, bovine		Milk from infected cow.	As in tuberculosis.
Cholera	Excreta from intestinal tract.	As in typhoid fever.	As in typhoid fever.
Hookworm	Feces.	Direct contact with soil polluted with feces. Eggs in feces hatch in sandy soil. Feces may also contaminate food.	Larvae enter through breaks in skin, especially skin of feet, and after devious passage through the body settle in the intestine.
Meningitis, meningococcal	Discharges from nose and throat.	Direct contact. Hands of attendant. Articles used by and about patient.	Mouth and nose. Mouth and nose.
Poliomyelitis	Discharges from nose and throat, and via feces.	Direct contact. Hands of nurse or attendant. Rarely in milk.	Through mouth and nose.
Measles (Rubella)	As in streptococcal sore throat.	As in streptococcal sore throat.	As in streptococcal sore throat.
Hepatitis, infectious viral or serum	Excreta from intestinal tract or from blood or serum.	Direct contact with feces of patient. Direct contact with equipment contaminated by blood from the patient.	Oral route or by inoculation when viral contaminated equipment such as needles and syringes are used.

TABLE 20-13. *Continued*

Disease	How Agent Leaves the Bodies of the Sick	How Organisms May Be Transmitted	Method of Entry Into the Body
Gonococcal disease	Lesions. Discharges from infected mucous membranes.	Direct contact as in sexual intercourse. Towels, bathtubs, toilets, etc. Hands of infected persons soiled with their own discharges. Hands of attendant.	Directly onto mucous membrane. Through breaks in membrane.
Ophthalmia neonatorum (gonococcal infection of eyes of newborn)	Purulent discharges from the eye.	Direct contact with infected areas as vagina of infected mother during birth. Other infected babies. Hands of doctor or nurse. Linens, etc.	Directly on the conjunctiva.
Whooping cough	Discharges from respiratory tract.	Direct contact with persons affected.	Mouth and nose.
Mumps	Discharges from infected glands and mouth.	Direct contact with persons affected.	Mouth and nose.
Smallpox	Discharges from nose and throat. Skin lesions.	Direct contact. Hands of nurse. Articles used by and about patient.	Thought to be through mucous membrane of respiratory tract.
Syphilis	Infected tissues. Lesions. Blood. Transfer through placenta to fetus.	Direct contact. Kissing or sexual intercourse. Needles and syringes.	Directly into blood and tissues through breaks in skin or membrane. Needles and syringes.
Trachoma	Discharges from infected eyes.	Direct contact. Hands, towels, handkerchiefs, possibly clothing.	Directly on conjunctiva.
Leprosy	Uncertain, may be from lesions.	Uncertain, probably via feces.	Uncertain, probably via mouth.

*Reproduced from *Taber's Cyclopedic Medical Dictionary*, ed. 14. F.A. Davis, Philadelphia, 1981.

The outer layer, or *epidermis*, is composed of dead cells which are continually being sloughed off. This layer contains no blood vessels and protects the living cells contained in the second layer, the *dermis*. The dermis lies directly below the epidermis and consists of small blood and lymph vessels, nerve endings, hair follicles, and sweat and sebaceous glands. Sweat glands secrete moisture, while sebaceous glands secrete oils which lubricate the skin. Figure 20-7 illustrates the structure of the skin.

One of the greatest fascinations related to the skin is its enormous regenerative power. In most minor skin disorders, the integumentary system repairs itself, returning to normal color and consistency.

Symptomatic Reaction to Disease

The skin responds to most disease states either by changing coloration or by erupting, or both. The skin is also susceptible to temperature changes. Extremes in heat and cold can cause injury to the skin.

Skin eruptions are classified as:

1. Macular—discolored but not elevated.
2. Papular—small, discolored and elevated (pin-point to pea size).
3. Vesicular—elevated fluid-filled blisters.
4. Pustular—elevated pus-filled eruptions.

Common Diseases of the Skin

The basic types of diseases which are commonly associated with the skin include dermatitis, burns, and various forms of sebaceous inflammation. These conditions are listed in Table

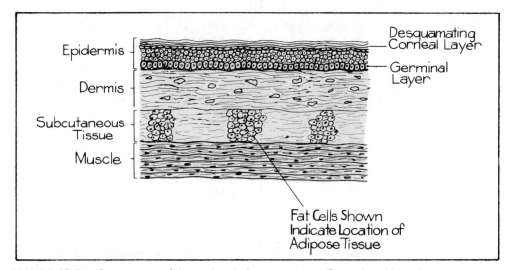

FIGURE 20-7. Cross-section of skin and underlying structures. (Reproduced from Saperstein, A. B., and Frazier, M. A.: *Introduction to Nursing Practice.* F. A. Davis, Philadelphia, 1980.)

20-14, along with symptoms, typical treatment approaches, and the role of the medical assistant.

The Skin Specialty

Dermatology is the medical specialty which studies and treats the various diseases and conditions of the skin. The medical assistant positioned in the office of a dermatologist, in addition to general medical assisting responsibilities, may administer sun lamp treatments, apply topical ointments, and assist the physician with minor dermatologic procedures.

TABLE 20-14.   Common Skin Diseases and Dermatologic Conditions

Disease	Symptoms	Treatment	Medical Assistant's Role
Dermatitis (inflammation of the skin)	Redness and any or all forms of eruption.	Dependent on type, usually ointment for specific treatment.	General clinical medical assisting procedures. MA should be aware that dermatitis is a term which encompasses a broad spectrum of dermatologic conditions. Drugs, allergies, and prolonged sun exposure are examples of causes of dermatitis. Contact dermatitis is an allergic reaction to any of the poisonous plants such as ivy or oak. In persons susceptible to allergic reactions from poisonous plants, patient teaching would include instructing the patient to thoroughly wash following exposure to such plants to prevent the reaction.

TABLE 20-14. *Continued*

Disease	Symptoms	Treatment	Medical Assistant's Role
Burns (injury to the skin and body caused by heat or other agent)	Classification: *First-degree:* redness and pain present. *Second-degree:* redness and pain and blisters occur. *Third-degree:* skin destruction is irreparable. White in appearance and no pain. *Fourth-degree:* underlying tissue destroyed. No pain.	Depends on extent of area burned and doctor's preference for treatment. First-degree burns may be covered or left open. A soothing paste of baking soda or similar substance or cool running water can be applied.	General clinical medical assisting procedures. The MA should be aware that the seriousness of burns depends on size, location, and degree. Usually minor burns are self-treated and not seen in the office. Serious burns are usually an emergency situation. Dressing changes and application of ointment may be the assistant's responsibility when the burned patient does visit the office.
		A small third-degree burn may be treated in a similar manner with a sterile dressing applied. Alternatives: Debridement (dead tissue is removed to provide an atmosphere for new growth of tissue). Isolation may be required to prevent infection and allow new growth of tissue in a sterile environment.	

TABLE 20-14. *Continued*

Disease	Symptoms	Treatment	Medical Assistant's Role
Burns (continued)		Medication may be applied such as anesthetic ointment and analgesics. Dressing impregnated with a thin layer of lubricant may be applied.	
Acne vulgaris (inflammation of the sebaceous glands causing eruptions called "pimples" and "blackheads")	Skin eruptions: papules, pustules.	Drug therapy includes topical medications specific to the type of skin and cause of acne. Sunlamp treatments may also be ordered.	General clinical medical assisting procedures. The MA should be aware that the patient is most often an adolescent and embarrassed about his or her appearance. Patient teaching should include explanation of the need for meticulous cleansing. The patient should be cautioned against squeezing the pimples since in doing this permanent injury to the pore and/or spread the inflamation may occur.

THE EYE

Structure and Function

The eye is the organ of vision. It is complex in structure and function (Figs. 20-8 and 20-9). The eye is composed of three tissue layers: (1) the *fibrous outer coat* which contains the sclera, the white of the eye, and the cornea which covers the iris and pupil; (2) the *uveal*

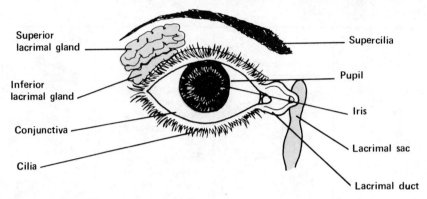

FIGURE 20-8. Front view of the eye.

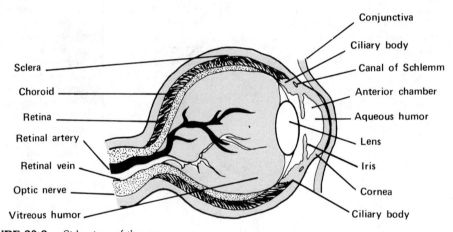

FIGURE 20-9. Side view of the eye.

tract which contains muscular tissue and blood vessels; and (3) the *retina* which contains the nerve network.

The *cornea* is the window of the eye through which light enters. The *iris* is the round, colored area of the eye which surrounds the pupil. Muscles control the narrowing and widening of the pupil. In the middle layer, a network of blood vessels lining the sclera supplies nourishment to the eye. The *retina* is a sensitive membrane containing the nerve cells which help to transfer light rays focused on the retina into an image.

In addition to these layers there are other important structures pertaining to the *eye* with which the medical assistant should become familiar:

1. *Conjunctiva:* mucous membrane which lines the eyelids and the parts of the eyeball including the cornea.

2. *Lacrimal glands:* glands located above the eyeballs which lubricate the eye surface. This lubrication is called tearing. The fluid drains into the tear ducts which open into the nasal cavity.

3. *Crystalline lens:* a transparent mass located behind the pupil which contains a jelly-like substance.

Symptomatic Reaction to Conditions and Diseases of the Eye

An individual experiencing impaired sight is said to have a visual defect. These defects are permanent conditions that can usually be resolved by use of corrective lens (glasses).

Reading difficulties are often symptomatic of these defects. Diseases of the eye are often associated with infections in which the general symptoms of inflammation are present. Other diseases may cause impairment of vision and pain.

The terminology for describing visual defects is listed and defined in Table 20-15.

Common Diseases of the Eye

The four most commonly encountered eye problems are conjunctivitis, stye, cataract, and glaucoma. Each of these is described in Table 20-16. The role of the medical assistant in the treatment of eye disorders emphasizes patient teaching and reassurance.

TABLE 20-15.   Common Visual Defects

Conditions	Definition
Myopia (nearsightedness)	Individual can see objects most accurately when close at hand. In myopia the eyeball or the crystalline lens may be contoured defectively. Corrective lenses cause light to be focused directly on the retina and thus improve sight.
Hypermetropia (farsightedness)	Individual can see objects most accurately when they are at a distance. Again, the objective of the corrective lens is to allow the light to be focused on the retina.
Presbyopia	Individual can see only distant objects clearly, but the images cloud as they are drawn closer, thus resembling farsightedness. Aging appears to be a common natural cause of presbyopia as the crystalline lens which is normally elastic becomes less accommodating. Corrective lenses can improve this condition.
Astigmatism	Individual cannot focus clearly; vision is blurred. The contour of either the cornea or the crystalline lens prevents light from being projected on the retina adequately. Corrective lenses can improve the condition.
Strabismus	Individual has difficulty directing both eyes toward the same objects. Muscle coordination in the eye is affected. Eyes may cross or turn outward. Corrective lenses and specific exercises or surgery may improve the condition.

TABLE 20-16.   Common Diseases of the Eye

Disease	Symptoms	Treatment	Medical Assistant's Role
Conjunctivitis (inflammation of the conjunctiva)	Redness and swelling, pain, increased tearing (especially is caused by allergy).	Drug therapy: ophthalmic antibiotics, anti-allergic drugs such as antihistamines. Instillation of antiseptic solutions. Eye irrigation. Warm compresses	General medical assisting clinical procedures. Patient teaching includes instruction regarding the prevention of eye strain. Emphasis on reading and writing in good light with frequent rest periods is advised.
Stye (acute inflammation on the edge of the eyelid)	Stinging pain and the presence of a hordeolum (swelling) are common.	Warm compresses. An incision may be made into the stye to allow drainage. Antibiotics may also be used.	Gazing into the distance or closing the eyes for brief periods provides rest and is recommended. Protection from the sun's rays is important to avoid destruction of the retina. Care in the purchase of sunglasses is also important. Cleanliness will help to prevent eye infection. Rubbing the eyes should be avoided.
Cataract (crystalline lens becomes clouded)	Impaired vision; spots before the eyes.	Surgical removal.	General clinical medical assisting procedures. Patient reassurance is essential before surgery.
Glaucoma (increased pressure within the eyeball with no known cause)	Pain with gradual pressure and impairment of vision.	Drug therapy. Surgery. Continuous monitoring.	Patient teaching includes emphasis on avoiding the lifting of heavy objects. Emotional stress should be avoided as this tends to increase ocular pressure.

Eye Examination and Diagnostic Testing

In addition to the ophthalmologic examination performed by the physician, the medical assistant may be responsible for testing the patient's visual acuity. Visual acuity is a term used to signify the degree of clarity or sharpness of vision. Normal visual acuity allows the individual to see without any impairment in details from short and longer distances.

There are many types of tests for visual acuity. The test most commonly used in the office and performed by the medical assistant is the Snellen eye test. The Snellen eye chart (Fig. 20-10) features letters or images in lines of decreasing size to test the patient's ability to see at measured distances, both close and far. There are charts available for non-English-speaking people, for preschoolers, and for English-speaking individuals who can read the alphabet. The chart for non-English-speaking individuals depicts the capital letter E in decreasing sizes and in various directions. The preschool chart illustrates certain common objects that children can readily identify. There is a greater margin of error, however, in the preschool test because a child may simply not recognize an object rather than have difficulty with visualization. The pattern of recognition of the objects must be carefully monitored. The child may also be tested by using cards with the letter E and instructing the child to point in the direction which corresponds to the middle line of the E. Comparing the E to a "table with three legs" is a more appealing concept to most children. The cards are then held in varying directions at the recommended distance. The charts are available either as cardboard posters or as illuminated wall-mounted or portable units.

TESTING VISUAL ACUITY

Purpose: To test the degree of visual clarity at a measured distance.

Principle	*Procedure*
1. Assemble the equipment: Snellen eye chart and eye covering (a paper cup is most commonly used). Chart should be placed at eye level.	1. A paper cup is used to cover the eyes alternately since one eye is tested at a time. Any opaque object can be used in place of the paper cup except for the patient's hand since this may not be an adequate covering, and results may be falsified. Eye level helps to ensure accurate results.
2. Prepare the room: well-lighted and with a distance marker in place. Usually the distance is 20 feet.	2. The patient must have adequate light to be able to distinguish the letters. The marker can either be fixed in place with tape or paint, or removable. Twenty feet is designated because the chart is designed to measure levels of acuity at a distance of 20 feet. The numbers on the right-hand side of the chart are depicted as fractions. The number above the line (20), which is the same all the way down the chart, represents the distance at which the test is being conducted. The number below the line represents the distance at which a person with normal vision can read the row of letters; (20/20) or line 8

is the average acuity since other patients are able to see clearly at 20 feet. (A discussion of test interpretation follows the procedure.)

3. Prepare the patient: identify and explain the procedure. If glasses or contact lenses are normally worn by the patient, testing should include their use.

3. The patient should be informed regarding the purpose and procedure of the test since this reduces anxiety. Glasses or contact lenses are used to read the chart since the test objective is to measure the patient's present visual acuity even with correction.

4. Instruct the patient to stand behind the marker and cover the right eye with the cup. Instruct the patient to keep the left eye open under the cup.

4. The patient should not be in the room with the chart prior to the testing as the tendency would be to read the chart. The letters may then be remembered rather than visualized accurately. If the eye not being examined is closed, then visual acuity of the other eye is affected. If one eye is closed, squinting occurs which temporarily increases visual clarity.

5. Stand by the chart and point to each row as the patient continues down the charts.

5. Pointing assists the patient to focus on one row at a time.

6. Instruct the patient to orally identify each letter in the row. Begin with row 3 (20/70). If the patient can read this row accurately, continue down to the last row of smallest letters that can be accurately distinguished. If the patient cannot read row 3, then proceed up the chart.

6. Other physician preferences for row order may be followed. The reading of the 20/70 line first saves time and serves as the average point of discrimination. Whatever the order, the same pattern should be followed for both eyes in order to avoid error.

7. Observe the patient's symptomatic reaction to the testing.

7. Watering eyes, tilting of the head, or squinting are examples of symptoms which may indicate difficulty with visualization.

8. When the examination of one eye is completed, proceed in the same manner to test the other eye.

8. Both eyes are tested separately for the greatest accuracy.

9. Record the results by designating the right eye as OD (oculus dexter) and the left eye as OS (oculus sinister). These Latin abbreviations are universally accepted. Note the smallest line which could be read most accurately. Refer to the number on the right-hand side of the chart. If the smallest line that could be read most accurately but with two errors was 20/25 with the right eye, then record: OD 20/25-2. Any symptoms noted by the assistant or the patient should also be recorded.

9. Accurate recording ensures proper care and treatment of the patient.

10. Return the patient to the room and a comfortable position. Answer the patient's questions regarding the testing.

10. The patient usually is interested in knowing the results. While these results are usually shared with the patient, care should be taken to properly interpret the numerical results and not to enter into diagnosis for which the assistant is unqualified. Note the discussions of interpretation of results contained in this chapter.

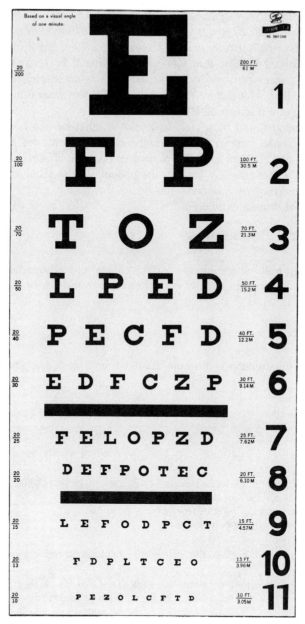

FIGURE 20-10. The Snellen eye chart.

Interpreting the Results of the Visual Acuity Test

As briefly mentioned in the foregoing section, the Snellen visual acuity test consists of rows designated by numerals on the right and fractions on the left. There are eleven rows. Each row's fraction contains the top number 20 because the test is being conducted at a distance of 20 feet. The bottom number signifies the distance at which people with normal acuity can read the row. Below the 20/20 row is the 20/15 row. If an individual standing 20 feet from the chart can read the row normally read at 15 feet, the patient has 20/15 vision in the eye examined. It is important to note that the eyes can differ from one another in degree of visual acuity. If the patient can read only the second row accurately, with the left eye the recording is OS 20/100. The patient can only see at 20 feet what individuals with normal visual acuity can see at a distance of 100 feet.

The patient being tested may wish to know whether or not he has 20/20 vision. Usually with the physician's approval, the results are shared with the patient. However, a discussion between the assistant and the patient as to what these results imply must be avoided. The physician will discuss this with the patient. The medical assistant's responsibility includes the answering of questions related to the testing procedures only, not the presence or degree of disease conditions.

Specific Clinical Procedures

The medical assistant may be responsible for the clinical procedures which involve eye irrigation, eye instillation, and applying warm compresses to the eye or instructing the patient in the technique.

EYE IRRIGATION

Purpose: To relieve inflammation, promote drainage, and wash away harmful chemicals or foreign bodies.

Procedure	Principle
1. Wash hands	1. Washing avoids transfer of harmful microorganisms.
2. Assemble the equipment: prescribed irrigation solution, bulb syringe, sterile basin in which to pour the solution, basin to receive the drainage, cotton balls, and toweling as protection for the patient's clothing.	2. Organization facilitates efficiency of procedure.
3. Identify the patient and explain the procedure.	3. Explanation reduces patient anxiety.
4. Assist the patient to the supine position.	4. This position makes the procedure more manageable. However, an eye irrigation can be performed with the patient in the sitting position.
5. Remove pillow. Drape the toweling over the patient's neck and shoulder and under the head. Place the basin next to the affected eye to catch the solution.	5. This prevents the solution from soiling or wetting the patient's clothing.
6. Assist the patient to turn his head toward the side of the affected eye.	6. This positioning is necessary to prevent the solution from running into the unaffected eye, promoting cross-contamination.

7. With a cotton ball dampened with solution, cleanse the eyelid and lashes. Cleanse from the inner (near the nose) to the outer aspect of the lid once and dispose of the cotton ball.

7. The solution should be poured over the cotton ball rather than placing the cotton ball in the solution, which would cause contamination. The lid and lashes are cleansed to avoid introducing infectious material into the eye through irrigation. The eye is cleansed in only one direction to avoid contamination. The step is repeated if necessary.

8. Pour the required amount of irrigating solution into a sterile basin. Withdraw solution into the bulb syringe by squeezing the bulb prior to insertion into the solution, then releasing the bulb when the tip is immersed in the solution.

8. The procedure facilitates sterile procedure and ease of solution withdrawal.

9. Push apart the eyelids with the index finger and thumb and hold in this position.

9. This exposes the conjunctiva and a greater area of eye surface for irrigation.

10. With the bulb syringe in the other hand, squeeze the bulb, directing the solution toward the inner contour of the eye, allowing it to flow slowly and steadily. Avoid touching the eye with the syringe. Repeat as required.

10. The flow of solution is controlled in order to avoid eye injury. It is directed toward the inner contour so that it flows over the greatest surface without injury to the cornea.

11. When the procedure is completed, dry the lid with a cotton ball from the inner to the outer canthus.

11. Drying provides patient comfort and reduces the chance of contamination.

INSTILLATION AND APPLICATION OF MEDICATION FOR THE EYE

Purpose: To apply medication such as antiseptic solution or antibiotic ointment to reduce inflammation or infection. Solution may also be instilled to dilate pupils prior to examination.

Procedure	*Principle*
1. Wash hands.	1. This prevents transfer of harmful microorganisms.
2. Assemble the equipment: medication, drape prescribed, a sterile dropper usually included in the cap of medication, gauze squares.	2. Organization facilitates efficiency.
3. Identify the patient, explain the procedure, and position. The supine or sitting positions are recommended. With the patient in the supine position, remove pillow.	3. Identification of the patient prevents medication error. Explanation of the procedure alleviates patient anxiety.
4. Instruct the patient to roll the eyes upward (look up) while pulling the lower conjunctival sac downward with fingertips placed over gauze.	4. Rolling the eyes upward prevents the chance of injuring the cornea with the dropper and distracts the patient's attention from the dropper. The sac is pulled downward to catch the drops. The gauze prevents the finger from slipping and also from contaminating the eye.

5A. For instillation of eye drops: Insert the pre-scribed number of drops into the eye directly over the center of the lower conjunctival sac. Do not touch the eye with the dropper. Allow the eye to close immediately, and instruct the patient to rotate the eyeball. Dry the excess drainage.	5A. Moving the eyeball ensures even distribution of medication.
5B. For application of eye ointment: Remove cap carefully from tube. Do not touch uncovered tip with finger. Holding the lower lid in place, squeeze a ribbon of ointment along the lower lid from the inner to the outer canthus. Do not touch tip of tube to the eye. Allow the patient to close the eye immediately and rotate eyes. Remove excess with care.	5B. These measures prevent contamination of medication.
6. Record the procedure in the patient's file, including name and amount of medication, date, and time of administration. If medication is in the form of drops, indicate which eye was treated. Initial the record.	6. Proper recording ensures quality care and is necessary for future reference.

INSTRUCTING THE PATIENT IN THE USE OF WARM COMPRESSES FOR THE EYE

Purpose: To promote drainage and soothe inflammation or irritation.

Procedure	*Principle*
1. Obtain information from the physician as to how often and how long compresses should be applied and what, if any, special solution should be used.	1. Clear understanding of directions is necessary for proper instruction and treatment times may vary with the patient.
2. Explain purpose and necessity of the procedure to the patient.	2. Proper explanation ensures greater patient compliance.
3. Inform the patient that gauze squares may be used, but unless specified by the physician, use is costly and not necessary. A washcloth may be used successfully.	3. The physician's orders and preference must be followed to ensure proper patient care. A clean washcloth, if permitted, is soft and easily cleaned for reuse.
4. Instruct the patient to soak the washcloth in warm water, or the solution prescribed, wring it out and apply to eyes for the duration recommended.	4. Keeping instructions simple helps the patient to feel confident and to remember the information.

Eye Specialties

There are several medical specialties related to the care and treatment of the eyes.

An ophthalmologist is a physician who diagnoses and treats disorders of the eye. An optometrist is a licensed practitioner (not a physician) whose expertise lies in testing visual acuity and the interpretation of results. An optician is a technician who prepares lenses according to prescription and fits them into frames of the patient's choice.

The medical assistant would most likely be employed in an ophthalmologist's office performing administrative and/or clinical functions.

APPLICATION EXERCISES

Group Discussion and Role-Playing Exercise

If available, the instructor will assemble the equipment used by the physician in the eye examination. Groups are formed, and the instructor will assign each group one of the patients listed below. The group will then discuss (1) how the room and patient will be prepared for the examination, and (2) how to assist the physician with the examination. When called upon, three students from each group will demonstrate the group's conclusion by taking the roles of the patient, the medical assistant, and the narrator.

1. The narrator explains room preparation and chooses the appropriate equipment.

2. The student in the role of medical assistant places the student in the patient's role in the proper position and simulated gowning after explaining the procedure to the patient.

3. The narrator explains how the examination will proceed, and the student in the role of MA simulates the assisting procedure. (Notes from group discussion may be used.)

4. Other student groups critique.

The various patient assignments are as follows:

Patient A. Symptoms: Painful menstruation with excessive bleeding.
Patient B. Symptoms: Swollen, painful ankle.
Patient C. Symptoms: Possible fracture of right index finger.
Patient D. Symptoms: Whitish vaginal discharge with itching.
Patient E. Symptoms: Low back pain for 5 days.
Patient F. Symptoms: Recurrent, intense headache with nausea.
Patient G. Symptoms: Raised, red rash of both forearms and trunk.
Patient H. Symptoms: Itching, discharge—left eye.

Problem-Solving Activities

Discuss possible solutions to the following situations:

1. While you are preparing the patient for a vaginal examination, she informs you that she thinks she may have VD, but asks you not to tell the doctor.

2. A male patient remarks that he hopes you will stay for the examination. He is to have an examination of the genitalia.

3. A 2-year-old child is scheduled for an ear examination. As you enter the room, she begins to cry.

4. A patient is in the office for treatment of a skin rash. You notice that she is breaking pustules open with her fingernails.

5. A patient has injured her ankle and asks you if it is broken.

6. The mother of a 14-year-old child has just been informed that her child has epilepsy. She is alone in the physician's private office. The doctor has asked you to attend to her needs.

7. A patient needs general instruction related to diabetes as she has been newly diagnosed. Discuss what you would discuss and your approach.

8. A patient is in the office with a skin rash and mentions to you that he has been having tremors and is losing weight. The physician is leaving the examination room, having completed an inspection of the skin.

Research Activity

The instructor will assign group presentations on the description and preparation of patients for the diagnostic tests discussed in this chapter and related to particular systems.

COMPLETING THE LEARNING LOOP

This chapter has served as a logical extension of the discussion presented in the previous one. Here we have considered a broader range of specific kinds of physical examinations. As a student you should strive to develop a comprehensive understanding of the kinds of examinations that are likely to be encountered. The more you learn and absorb about the presenting symptomatology of the patient and the examinations required for diagnosis, the more you will be able to anticipate the needs of the physician and patient alike. In this way you will be fulfilling and maximizing the role of a knowledgeable and efficient medical assistant.

BIBLIOGRAPHY

Alexander, M., and Brown, M.: *Pediatric Physical Diagnosis for Nurses*. McGraw-Hill, New York, 1974.
Allen, J. H.: *May's Manual of Diseases of the Eye*. R. E. Krieger, Huntington, N.Y., 1974.
Bates, B.: *A Guide to Physical Examination*. J. B. Lippincott, Philadelphia, 1974.
Catt, K. J.: *An ABC of Endocrinology*. Little, Brown, Boston, 1972.
DeAngelis, C.: *Basic Pediatrics for the Primary Health Care Provider*. Little, Brown, Boston, 1975.
Domonkos, A. N.: *Andrews' Diseases of the Skin*, ed. 6. W. B. Saunders, Philadelphia, 1971.
Gordon, D. M.: *The Fundamentals of Ophthalmoscopy*. The Upjohn Company, Kalamazoo, Mich., 1971.

Heilman, A.: *A Handbook for Differential Diagnosis of Neurologic Signs and Symptoms.* Appleton-Century-Crofts, New York, 1977.

Isselbacher, K. J., et al. (eds.): *Harrison's Principles of Internal Medicine,* ed. 9. McGraw-Hill, New York, 1979.

Kashgarian, M., and Burrow, G. N.: *The Endocrine Glands: Structure and Function in Diseases.* Williams & Wilkins, Baltimore, 1974.

King, M., and King, F.: *Primary Child Care: A Manual for Health Workers.* Oxford University Press, New York, 1978.

Leitman, J., et al.: *Manual for Eye Examination and Diagnosis.* Van Nostrand-Reinhold, New York, 1975.

Roberts, W.: *The Reproductive System: Disease, Diagnosis, Treatment.* R. J. Brady, Bowie, Md., 1974.

Rosse, C., and Clawson, D. K.: *Introduction to the Musculoskeletal System.* Harper & Row, Hagerstown, Md., 1970.

Schneider, F. R.: *Handbook for the Orthopaedic Assistant.* C. V. Mosby, St. Louis, 1972.

Spearman, R. I.: *The Integument: A Textbook of Skin Biology.* Cambridge University Press, New York, 1973.

Vaughn, V. C., et al.: *Nelson Textbook of Pediatrics,* ed. 11. W. B. Saunders, Philadelphia, 1979.

Walton, J. N.: *Essentials of Neurology,* ed. 4. J. B. Lippincott, Philadelphia, 1975.

Wilson, F. C.: *The Musculoskeletal System.* J. B. Lippincott, Philadelphia, 1975.

Wilson, J. R., and Carrington, E. R.: *Obstetrics and Gynecology,* ed. 6. C. V. Mosby, St. Louis, 1979.

UNIT 7

ASSISTING WITH TREATMENT

Once the physical examination has been completed, the next logical step in medical care is treating the patient. From the many modalities of treatment that are available, the physician must choose the one which appears most appropriate. When the selection has been made, the medical assistant will be expected to give knowledgeable support to the physician and guidance to the patient. In this unit the student will be exposed to the basic approaches to medical office treatment, including diet therapy, drug therapy, office surgery, and physical therapy. Also included is a discussion of the MA's responsibilities in common medical office emergencies.

UNIT OBJECTIVES

Upon completion of this unit you will be able to:

1. Demonstrate a working knowledge of basic nutrition.

2. Assist the physician and the patient with diet therapy.

3. Assist the physician with programs of drug therapy by administering drugs, using proper techniques.

4. Instruct patients in drug therapy.

5. Prepare for office surgery and assist the physician in office surgical procedures.

6. Utilize normal first-aid procedures in medical office emergencies.

7. Assist with physical therapy procedures.

CHAPTER 21

NUTRITION AND
DIET THERAPY

SPECIFIC OBJECTIVES

Upon completion of this chapter you will be able to:

1. List the six major nutrients, describe their function, and list the recommended allowances for each.

2. Describe the processes of metabolism and digestion.

3. List the Basic Food Groups and identify the foods contained in each group.

4. Calculate individual needs for calories and specific nutrients.

5. Apply standard diet modifications to diet plans in certain disease states.

6. Instruct the patient regarding the diet prescription.

7. Utilize and give the patient instructions in the use of the exchange list.

8. List and describe general principles of patient teaching in diet therapy.

INTRODUCTION

While prescribing the diet is the physician's responsibility, the medical assistant will be involved in aiding the patient in the process of interpreting the instructions and planning the diet. The MA will often be the resource person to whom the patient directs questions and concerns related to the diet plan. Before the medical assistant can guide the patient in diet therapy, a basic background in normal nutrition is required. Normal nutrition is the foundation of diet therapy. All therapeutic diets are modifications of the recommended daily diet which is specifically adapted to the individual physiologic needs of the patient. An understanding of the basic principles of nutrition, which this chapter provides, will enable the MA to effectively participate in the patient's dietary treatment plan.

NUTRITION

Nutrition is the term which signifies the collective processes involved in the body's intake and utilization of food. Food is a physiologic requirement for the growth, development, and maintenance of the human body.

Nutrition involves the study of the body's need for, and utilization of, special food substances called nutrients. The patient's own dietary habits, as well as injury and disease, can interfere with the intake and utilization of the essential nutrients. When essential nutrients are lacking or not supplied in sufficient quantity in the daily diet, a nutritional deficiency results.

Disease, injury, and normal physiologic states such as pregnancy cause changes in need requirements of specific nutrients. Diet therapy is the use of nutrients in specific combination, amounts, and food sources in the diet to achieve treatment objectives.

METABOLISM

Metabolism is the process of the physical and chemical changes related to the body's utilization of food. Body tissue is built up (through growth, repair, and maintenance) and broken down (through the manufacture of waste products) in the cyclic process of metabolism. The buildup process is termed anabolism, and the breakdown process is catabolism. The rate of the metabolic process differs with each individual. The individual's metabolic rate is referred to as basal metabolism—the energy required to keep the body alive when the patient is fasting and at rest. As we learned in the discussion on vital signs, certain body states change metabolic activity. Since metabolic activity produces heat and energy, normal nutrition and diet therapy are concerned with the energy produced by the nutrients combined in a particular distribution and quantity. Energy needs are referred to as caloric needs. A *calorie* is the amount of heat required to raise 1 kilogram of water 1° Celsius. Each of the nutrients supplies a certain number of calories.

Caloric needs are influenced by the state of health, age, size (weight and height), composition, sex, environment, and activity of the individual patient. In the average adult, approximately 15 calories are needed per pound of body weight to meet basal metabolic requirements.

DIGESTION

Digestion is the term applied to the physiologic process of breaking down food into substances which can be absorbed and transported throughout the circulatory system to nourish the cells. These substances are called nutrients. The process of digestion takes place in the digestive tract. The organs of digestion are illustrated in Figure 21-1. The organs are divided into two categories: major and accessory.

Food is digested through a mechanical and chemical process. The mechanical process occurs as food is chewed in the mouth and then passes down the tract, by contraction and relaxation of the muscular walls. This action (contraction and relaxation) is called peristalsis. Chemical digestion is achieved by the action of enzymes and digestive secretions which convert food in specific molecular substances.

Mechanical and chemical digestion begins in the mouth, and the total process of digestion is completed in the small intestine.

Food remains in the stomach for approximately 2 hours, and usually within 5 hours digestion has been completed.

NUTRIENTS

There are six widely used classifications of nutrients: (1) proteins, (2) carbohydrates, (3) fats, (4) vitamins, (5) minerals, and (6) water.

Proteins

STRUCTURE

Proteins are complex substances composed mainly of carbon, hydrogen, oxygen, and nitrogen. These elements are combined to form substances called amino acids. There are numerous amino acids, and several are absolutely essential for normal body functioning since human cells are composed of protein.

FUNCTION

Protein is necessary for the following functions: (1) building and repairing tissue, (2) providing disease resistance, (3) providing energy, and (4) maintaining heat. The building and repairing function is exclusive to protein and is the primary responsibility of this nutrient.

UTILIZATION

Proteins are almost completely absorbed and utilized continuously in the body; no storage occurs. However, when the amount of carbohydrates is deficient, protein is converted from building and repair activity to assume the carbohydrate and fats activity of quick energy production.

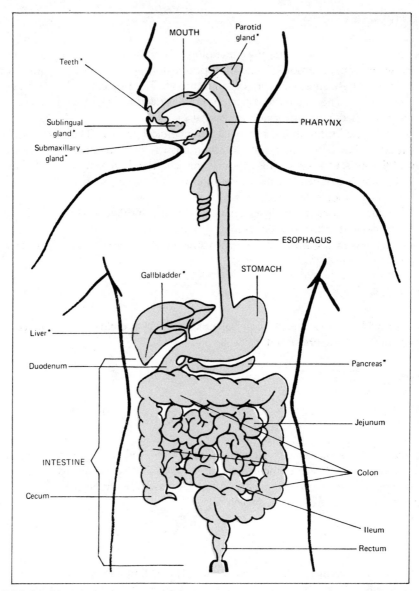

FIGURE 21-1.   Main and accessory organs of digestion. Accessory organs are starred. (Reproduced from Lewis, C.: *The Basics of Nutrition.* F.A. Davis, Philadelphia, 1976.)

SOURCES

Protein is present in a variety of food substances. Major sources of protein include eggs, milk, meat, fish, nuts, and legumes. The animal proteins are considered to be complete proteins since they contain all the amino acids. Plant protein, with the exception of soybeans, does not contain all of the essential amino acids and is considered an incomplete source.

CALORIC REQUIREMENTS

Each gram of protein produces 4 calories. The average healthy adult requires a daily intake of 1 gram of protein per kilogram of body weight. This represents approximately 10 to 15 percent of the daily caloric requirement. On the average, children require 2½ to 3 grams, and adolescents require 1½ to 2 grams. Certain conditions and disease states, such as fever and fracture, increase protein needs.

EFFECTS OF DEFICIENCY

Protein loss or deficiency can result in weight loss, dryness and scaling of the skin, lowered resistance to infection, and interference with the normal healing, growth, and development processes.

Carbohydrates

STRUCTURE

Carbohydrates, as the name implies, are composed of carbon, hydrogen, and oxygen. They are classified as monosaccharides, disaccharides, and polysaccharides.

Monosaccharides include glucose (contained in fruits and vegetables); fructose (contained in fruits, vegetables, and honey); and galactose (derived from lactose found in milk). Disaccharides include sucrose (known as table sugar and found in syrups); maltose (found in malt products); and lactose (contained in the milk of animals and humans). Polysaccharides include starches (contained in grains and vegetables); cellulose (contained in fibrous vegetables, cereals, and fruits); and glycogen (stored in the muscles and liver).

FUNCTION

Carbohydrates are the most abundant, inexpensive, and commonly used food source available. Carbohydrates (1) provide the body with a quick source of heat and energy; (2) spare protein from being converted for energy uses; and (3) enable fat to be metabolized.

UTILIZATION

The primary function of carbohydrates is to meet the body's energy expenditures. Carbohydrate which is surplus and unexpended is stored as adipose or fatty tissue. Carbohydrates provide the quickest energy source because the metabolism of many of the sugars begins in the mouth and because carbohydrates are quickly converted to glucose which requires no digestion.

SOURCES

The major sources of carbohydrates are cereals, certain vegetables such as potatoes and squash, fruits, syrups, and sugars. The sources currently recommended are fruits and whole-grain breads and cereals. Processed sugars are not considered to be of nutritional value.

CALORIC REQUIREMENTS

Each gram of carbohydrate provides 4 calories. Of the average adult calorie allowance, 40 to 50 percent should consist of carbohydrates from natural sources. These are referred to as complex carbohydrates.

EFFECTS OF DEFICIENCY

An inadequate amount of carbohydrate in the diet results principally in weight loss, protein loss, and fatigue.

Fats

STRUCTURE

Fats are also known as fatty acids. The chemical components of fatty acids are carbon, hydrogen, and oxygen. While these are the same elements contained in carbohydrates, their arrangement and proportions differ.

Fats are classified as saturated and unsaturated, and as essential and false fatty acids. Saturated fats contain the highest concentration of hydrogen and are solid at room temperature. Butter is an example of a saturated fat. Unsaturated fats are fatty acids which can absorb more hydrogen under certain conditions. Highly unsaturated fats are referred to as polyunsaturated. Unsaturated fats are soft or liquid at room temperature. Unsaturated fats can be hydrogenated, that is, additional hydrogen can be added through a special process. This hydrogenation process converts the unsaturated fat to a saturated form. Margarine is a prime example since it is hydrogenated and fortified with vitamins A and D, which give it the same food value as butter.

Essential fatty acids are the polyunsaturated fats found in butter, egg yolks, and milk. They are called essential fatty acids because they are necessary for growth and metabolism. False fats are those which have no nutritive value, such as mineral oil.

Associated with fatty acids is a nutrient called cholesterol. Cholesterol, however, is a sterol, not a true fat. It is derived from food substances as well as being manufactured in the liver. Cholesterol is closely related to fatty acids, and both cholesterol and fatty acids are considered to be *lipids*. This major grouping of fats is associated, in disproportionate amounts, with many diseases, especially hypertension.

FUNCTION

Fats provide (1) the most concentrated source of heat and energy; (2) transportation for fat in the form of soluble vitamins; (3) more satisfaction than carbohydrates and protein since they are more slowly digested; (4) a source of storage for energy; and (5) insulation and protection for body organs, in the form of adipose tissue.

UTILIZATION

Fat is stored in the body as adipose tissue. Digestion of fats is slower than that of proteins and carbohydrates. When the ingestion of carbohydrates (which are converted to fats) and fats exceeds the body's energy requirements, the amount of adipose tissue continues to expand.

SOURCES

Animal sources of fat include meat, milk, eggs, and fish. Vegetable sources include corn, olives, cottonseed, safflower, soybeans, and nuts.

CALORIC REQUIREMENTS

Each gram of fat provides 9 calories. The recommended allowance is approximately 20 percent of the daily diet.

EFFECTS OF DEFICIENCY

Dry skin, disruption of vitamin utilization, and fatigue are among the most common symptoms of fat deficiency.

Vitamins

STRUCTURE

Vitamins are organic food substances which have been identified as essential elements for growth, development, and maintenance of body systems. More commonly assigned letters of the alphabet for reference, they are also represented by chemical formulas.

Vitamins A, B, C, D, E, and K have been isolated and their functions established. Fat-soluble vitamins (those which dissolve in fat) include vitamins A, D, E, and K. Water-soluble vitamins (those which dissolve in water) consist of the B vitamins and vitamin C.

FUNCTION

Vitamins have both general and specific functions. Generally, vitamins are essential to growth, resistance to infection, and vital body functions. Specific vitamins have specific functions, characteristics, results of deficiencies, sources, and recommended allowances. These are listed in Table 21-1.

TABLE 21-1.   Summary of Vitamins Significant in the Human Diet*

Vitamin	Chief Functions	Results of Deficiency	Characteristics	Good Sources	Daily Allowances Recommended
VITAMIN A Provitamin, carotene	Essential for maintaining the integrity of epithelial membranes. Helps maintain resistance to infections. Necessary for the formation of rhodopsin and prevention of night blindness.	*Mild:* Retarded growth. Increased susceptibility to infection. Abnormal function of gastrointestinal, genitourinary and respiratory tracts due to altered epithelial membranes. Skin dries, shrivels, thickens, sometimes pustule formation. Night blindness. *Severe:* Xerophthalmia, a characteristic eye disease, and other local infections.	Fat-soluble. Not destroyed by ordinary cooking temperatures. Is destroyed by high temperatures when oxygen is present. Marked capacity for storage in the liver. *Note:* Excessive intake of carotene from which vitamin A is formed may produce yellow discoloration of the skin (carotenemia).	Animal fats butter cheese cream egg yolk whole milk. Fish liver oil. Liver Vegetable 1. green leafy, esp. escarole, kale, parsley 2. yellow, esp. carrots. *Artificial:* Concentrates in several forms. Irradiated fish oils.	*Males (Ages 11–51 yrs.):* 1000 μg retinol equivalents *Females (Ages 11–51 yrs.):* 800 μg retinol equivalents *In pregnancy:* 1000 μg retinol equivalents *In lactation:* 1200 μg retinol equivalents *Children:* 400–700 μg retinol equivalents *Infants:* 400 μg retinol equivalents
THIAMINE Vitamin B$_1$	Important role in carbohydrate metabolism. Essential for maintenance of normal digestion and appetite.	*Mild:* Loss of appetite. Impaired digestion of starches and sugars. Colitis, constipation, or diarrhea.	Water-soluble. Not readily destroyed by ordinary cooking temperature. Destroyed by exposure to heat,	Widely distributed in plant and animal tissues but seldom occurs in high concentration, exception in brewer's yeast.	*Males* (11–51$^+$ yrs.): 1.2–1.5 mg *Females* (11–51$^+$ yrs.): 1.0 to 1.1 mg

	Essential for normal functioning of nervous tissue.	Emaciation. *Severe:* Nervous disorders of various types. Loss of coordinating power of muscles. Beriberi. Paralysis in man.	alkali, or sulfites. Is not stored in body.	Other good sources are: Whole grain cereals, Peas, Beans, Peanuts, Oranges, Glandular—heart, liver, kidney, Many vegetables and fruits, Nuts. *Artificial:* Concentrates from yeast. Rice polishings. Wheat germ.	*In pregnancy:* 1.4 to 1.6 mg. *In lactation:* 1.5 to 1.7 mg. *Children:* 0.7 to 1.2 mg. *Infants:* 0.3 to 0.5 mg.
RIBOFLAVIN Vitamin B$_2$	Important in formation of certain enzymes and in cellular oxidation. Normal growth. Prevention of cheilosis and glossitis. Participates in light adaption.	Impaired growth. Lassitude and weakness. Cheilosis. Glossitis. Atrophy of skin. Anemia. Photophobia. Cataracts.	Water-soluble. Alcohol-soluble. Not destroyed by heat in cooking unless with alkali. Unstable in light, esp. in presence of alkali.	Eggs, Green vegetables, Liver, Kidney, Lean meat, Milk, Wheat germ, Yeast, dried, Enriched foods.	*Males* (11-51$^+$ yrs.): 1.4-1.7 mg. *Females* (11-51$^+$ yrs.): 1.2-1.3 mg. *In pregnancy:* 1.6 mg. *In lactation:* 1.8 mg. *Children:* 0.8 to 1.4 mg. *Infants:* 0.4 to 0.6 mg.

TABLE 21-1. *Continued*

Vitamin	Chief Functions	Results of Deficiency	Characteristics	Good Sources	Daily Allowances Recommended
NIACIN Nicotinic acid Nicotinamide Antipellagra vitamin	As the component of two important enzymes, it is important in glycolysis, tissue respiration, and fat synthesis. Nicotinic acid but not nicotinamide causes vasodilation and flushing. Prevents pellagra.	Pellagra. Gastrointestinal disturbances. Mental disturbances.	Soluble in hot water and alcohol. Not destroyed by heat, light, air or alkali. Not destroyed in ordinary cooking.	Yeast Lean meat Fish Legumes Whole grain cereals and peanuts Enriched foods.	*Males (11-51+ yrs.):* 16-19 mg *Females (11-51+ yrs.):* 13-15 mg *In pregnancy:* 17 mg *In lactation:* 20 mg *Children:* 9-16 mg *Infants:* 6-8 mg
VITAMIN B_{12} Cyanocobalamin	Produces remission in pernicious anemia. Essential for normal development of red blood cells.	Pernicious anemia	Soluble in water or alcohol. Unstable in hot alkaline or acid solutions.	Liver Kidney Dairy products. Most of vitamin required by humans is synthesized by intestinal bacteria.	*Males and Females (11-51+ yrs.):* 3.0 mcg *In pregnancy:* 4.0 mcg *In lactation:* 5.0 mcg *Children:* 2 to 5 mcg *Infants:* 1 to 2 mcg

	Function	Deficiency	Characteristics	Sources	Daily Requirements
VITAMIN C Ascorbic acid	Essential to formation of intracellular cement substances in a variety of tissues including skin, dentine, cartilage and bone matrix. Important in healing of wounds and fractures of bones. Prevents scurvy. Facilitates absorption of iron.	*Mild:* Lowered resistance to infections. Joint tenderness. Susceptibility to dental caries, pyorrhea, and bleeding gums. *Severe:* Hemorrhage. Anemia. Scurvy.	Soluble in water. Easily destroyed by oxidation; heat hastens the process. Lost in cooking, particularly if water in which food was cooked is discarded. Also loss is greater if cooked in iron or copper utensils. Quick frozen foods lose little of their vitamin C. Stored in the body to a limited extent.	Abundant in most fresh fruits and vegetables, esp. citrus fruit and juices, tomato and orange. *Artificial:* Ascorbic acid. Cevitamic acid.	*Males (11-51+ yrs.):* 50-60 mg *Females (11-51+ yrs.):* 50-60 mg *In pregnancy:* 80 mg *In lactation:* 100 mg *Children:* 45 mg *Infants:* 35 mg The infant diet is likely to be deficient in vitamin C unless orange or tomato juice or other form is added.
VITAMIN D	Regulates absorption of calcium and phosphorus from the intestinal tract. Antirachitic.	*Mild:* Interferes with utilization of calcium and phosphorus in bone and teeth formation. Irritability. Weakness. *Severe:* Rickets, may be common in young children.	Soluble in fats and organic solvents. Relatively stable under refrigeration. Stored in liver. Often associated with vitamin A.	Butter Egg yolk Fish liver oils Fish having fat distributed through the flesh, salmon, tuna fish, herring, sardines Liver Oysters Yeast and foods	*Males and Females (11-51+ yrs.):* 200-400 I.U. After age 22, none except during pregnancy or lactation. *In pregnancy:* 400-600 I.U. *In lactation:* 400-600 I.U.

TABLE 21-1. *Continued*

Vitamin	Chief Functions	Results of Deficiency	Characteristics	Good Sources	Daily Allowances Recommended
		Osteomalacia in adults.		irradiated with ultraviolet light. Formed in the skin by exposure to sunlight. Artificially prepared forms.	*Children:* 400 I.U. *Infants:* 400 I.U.
VITAMIN E Alpha tocoph-erol	Normal reproduc-tion in rats. Prevention of muscular dys-trophy in rats.	Red blood cell resist-ance to rupture is decreased.	Fat-soluble. Stable to heat in ab-sence of oxygen.	Lettuce and other green, leafy vege-tables. Wheat germ oil Margarine Rice.	*Males* (11–51+ yrs.): 8–10 mg d-α-tocopherol *Females* (11–51+ yrs.): 8 mg d-α-tocopherol *In pregnancy:* 10 mg d-α-tocopherol *In lactation:* 11 mg d-α-tocopherol *Children:* 10 to 15 I.U. *Infants:* 5 I.U.

					Requirements
VITAMIN B₆ Pyridoxine	Essential for metabolism of tryptophan. Needed for utilization of certain other amino acids.	Dermatitis around eyes and mouth. Neuritis. Anorexia, nausea, and vomiting.	Soluble in water and alcohol. Rapidly inactivated in presence of heat, sunlight, or air.	Blackstrap molasses Meat Cereal grains Wheat germ.	*Males and Females (11-51+ yrs.):* 1.8-2.2 mg *In pregnancy:* 2.6 mg *In lactation:* 2.5 mg *Children:* 0.9-1.6 mg *Infants:* 0.3-0.6 mg
FOLACIN	Essential for normal functioning of hematopoietic system.	Anemia.	Slightly soluble in water. Easily destroyed by heat in presence of acid. Decreases when food is stored at room temperature. *Note:* A large dose may prevent appearance of anemia in a case of pernicious anemia but still permit neurological symptoms to develop.	Glandular meats Yeast Green, leafy vegetables.	*Males and Females (11-51+ yrs.):* 400 µg *In pregnancy:* 800 µg *In lactation:* 500 µg *Children:* 100-300 µg *Infants:* 30-45 µg

*Reproduced from *Taber's Cyclopedic Medical Dictionary*, ed. 14. F.A. Davis, Philadelphia, 1981.

UTILIZATION

Vitamins are absorbed and utilized in the body in differing manners, depending upon the specific vitamin. Most are absorbed at some point along the gastrointestinal tract. Direct exposure to the sun is important to the production of vitamin D. Water-soluble vitamins are not stored in the body. Fat-soluble vitamins are stored; therefore excesses of these vitamins can cause dangerous side effects.

Minerals

STRUCTURE

There are numerous minerals, not all of which are essential nutrients. Minerals are chemical compounds found in the body in differing quantities. Some minerals are found in such small proportions that they are called trace minerals. Calcium, phosphorus, iron, iodine, potassium, sodium, chlorine, and magnesium represent approximately 4 percent of the body weight.

FUNCTION

The general importance of minerals to the body lies in the areas of (1) cell formation; (2) normal development of bones and teeth; (3) regulation of metabolism of enzymes; and (4) vital body functions such as iodine in the production of thyronine.

UTILIZATION

Minerals are mostly absorbed by the intestines. Most minerals are utilized by the body in the quantities needed and the excess excreted.

SOURCES

A balanced diet supplies the necessary minerals. The major sources of specific minerals are as follows:

Calcium—milk and milk products
Phosphorus—milk and milk products
Iron—liver
Iodine—seafoods
Potassium—cereals, fruits, and vegetables
Sodium—most foods contain sodium
Chlorine—seafoods, milk, meat, and eggs
Magnesium—soybeans, whole grains, and nuts

REQUIREMENTS

The average adult requires daily allowances of basic minerals:

> Calcium—800 to 1200 milligrams
> Phosphorus—800 milligrams
> Iron—10 to 18 milligrams
> Iodine—100 to 150 micrograms
> Potassium—2 to 4 grams
> Sodium—7 to 15 grams

EFFECTS OF DEFICIENCY

The results of mineral deficiency are specific to the particular mineral. Calcium is the mineral most commonly ingested in inadequate amounts since many individuals, particularly adults, do not drink milk.

Another mineral deficiency that has become less common is iodine deficiency, which results in goiter. Iodized salt has diminished this occurrence. Iron deficiency results primarily in iron-deficiency anemia.

Water

STRUCTURE

Water is composed of hydrogen and oxygen elements. Like air, water is most essential to the maintenance of normal body functioning. Water accounts for three-fourths of body weight. At least one-half of this water is found in the cells, the remainder around the cells, and approximately 5 percent in the blood.

FUNCTIONS

Water provides the body with (1) lubrication for moving parts; (2) a vehicle for elimination of wastes; (3) transportation of nutrients and body secretions; (4) a solvent for chemicals; (5) digestive aid; and (6) a regulator of body temperature.

UTILIZATION

The body absorbs and utilizes water continuously. In the average healthy adult, water intake equals water output.

SOURCES

Drinking water provides much of the body's need for water. Water is also contained in most foods.

REQUIREMENTS

The average healthy adult requires 6 to 8 cups of water daily.

EFFECTS OF DEFICIENCY

Dry lips, mucous membrane, and tongue are early signs of dehydration (water depletion). If dehydration persists for several days and a 20 percent loss is experienced, death results.

THE BASIC FOOD GROUPS

The Basic Food Groups represent the arrangement of nutrients in the daily diet. In order to provide the necessary nutrients, four food groups are recommended and their allowances specified (see Fig. 21-2). The daily dietary allowances given in Table 21-2 are the recommendations of the Food and Nutrition Board of the National Academy of Sciences.

Although fat is included in the preparation of many foods, it is not included in the Basic Food Groups. The recommended allowance for fat is a minimum of 4 teaspoons daily. Water, another nutrient not specifically identified in the Basic Food Groups, has a recommended allowance of 6 to 8 cups daily.

Processed sugars and starches are also not included and should usually be avoided. Although they provide energy, infrequent use is recommended as overconsumption tends to displace essential nutrients in the daily diet.

COMPUTATION OF CALORIC AND NUTRIENT NEEDS

The medical assistant may be responsible for planning a normal diet for the patient.

The computation formulas included in Figure 21-2 serve as the basis for determining caloric and specific nutrient needs. These computations and the recommended daily allowance (RDA) are based on weight and routine activity (see Table 21-3). Factors such as regular exercise, certain disease and normal physiologic states would alter and usually increase the caloric requirements.

Since the normal or recommended daily diet is based on the four food groups and the allowances specified, applications in diet therapy also utilize these models and the computation formulas.

Determination of Desirable Body Weight

The determination of desirable body weight begins with an established base weight for individuals of average frame and 5 feet in height. For women this base weight is 100 lbs ± 5 lbs per inch above or below 5 feet. For men the base weight is 106 lbs ± 6 lbs per inch above or below 5 feet. Ten percent of the total is added for individuals with large frames, and 10 percent is subtracted for those with small frames.

> *Example:* For a woman of average frame standing 5 feet 4 inches:
> 100 lbs (base weight) + 20 lbs (for added height) = 120 lbs.

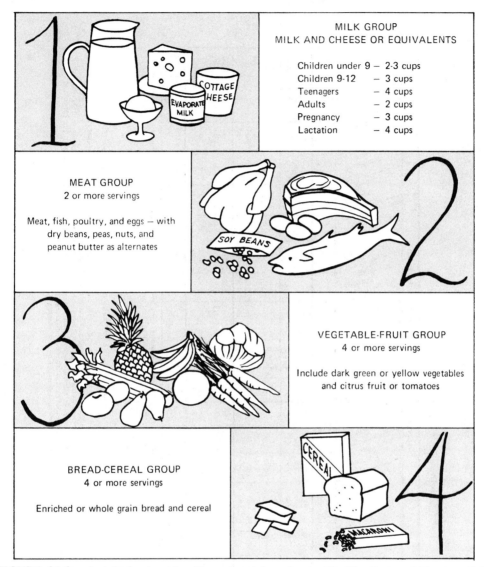

FIGURE 21-2. A daily food guide. (Reproduced from Lewis, C.: *The Basics of Nutrition.* F.A. Davis, Philadelphia, 1976.)

Determination of Frame Size: The Wrist Test

The patient places his thumb and middle finger around his wrist. If thumb and middle finger overlap, the patient's frame is considered small. If thumb and middle finger meet, his frame is medium or average, and if thumb and middle finger do not meet, the patient's frame is said to be large.

TABLE 21-2.   Recommended Daily Dietary Allowances*

	Age (years)	Weight (kg)	Weight (lbs)	Height (cm)	Height (in)	Protein (g)	Vitamin A (μg R.E.)[b]	Vitamin D (μg)[c]	Vitamin E (mg α T.E.)[d]	Vitamin C (mg)	Thiamin (mg)	Riboflavin (mg)	Niacin (mg N.E.)[e]	Vitamin B6 (mg)	Folacin (μg)[f]	Vitamin B12 (μg)	Calcium (mg)	Phosphorus (mg)	Magnesium (mg)	Iron (mg)	Zinc (mg)	Iodine (μg)
Infants	0.0-0.5	6	13	60	24	kg × 2.2	420	10	3	35	0.3	0.4	6	0.3	30	0.5[g]	360	240	50	10	3	40
	0.5-1.0	9	20	71	28	kg × 2.0	400	10	4	35	0.5	0.6	8	0.6	45	1.5	540	360	70	15	5	50
Children	1-3	13	29	90	35	23	400	10	5	45	0.7	0.8	9	0.9	100	2.0	800	800	150	15	10	70
	4-6	20	44	112	44	30	500	10	6	45	0.9	1.0	11	1.3	200	2.5	800	800	200	10	10	90
	7-10	28	62	132	52	34	700	10	7	45	1.2	1.4	16	1.6	300	3.0	800	800	250	10	10	120
Males	11-14	45	99	157	62	45	1000	10	8	50	1.4	1.6	18	1.8	400	3.0	1200	1200	350	18	15	150
	15-18	66	145	176	69	56	1000	10	10	60	1.4	1.7	18	2.0	400	3.0	1200	1200	400	18	15	150
	19-22	70	154	177	70	56	1000	7.5	10	60	1.5	1.7	19	2.2	400	3.0	800	800	350	10	15	150
	23-50	70	154	178	70	56	1000	5	10	60	1.4	1.6	18	2.2	400	3.0	800	800	350	10	15	150
	51+	70	154	178	70	56	1000	5	10	60	1.2	1.4	16	2.2	400	3.0	800	800	350	10	15	150
Females	11-14	46	101	157	62	46	800	10	8	50	1.1	1.3	15	1.8	400	3.0	1200	1200	300	18	15	150
	15-18	55	120	163	64	46	800	10	8	60	1.1	1.3	14	2.0	400	3.0	1200	1200	300	18	15	150
	19-22	55	120	163	64	44	800	7.5	8	60	1.1	1.3	14	2.0	400	3.0	800	800	300	18	15	150
	23-50	55	120	163	64	44	800	5	8	60	1.0	1.2	13	2.0	400	3.0	800	800	300	18	15	150
	51+	55	120	163	64	44	800	5	8	60	1.0	1.2	13	2.0	400	3.0	800	800	300	10	15	150
Pregnant						+30	+200	+5	+2	+20	+0.4	+0.3	+2	+0.6	+400	+1.0	+400	+400	+150	h	+5	+25
Lactating						+20	+400	+5	+3	+40	+0.5	+0.5	+5	+0.5	+100	+1.0	+400	+400	+150	h	+10	+50

a   The allowances are intended to provide for individual variations among most normal persons as they live in the United States under usual environmental stresses. Diets should be based on a variety of common foods in order to provide other nutrients for which human requirements have been less well defined.

b   Retinol equivalents. 1 retinol equivalent = 1 μg retinol or 6 μg β-carotene.

c   As cholecalciferol. 10 μg cholecalciferol = 400 I.U. vitamin D.

d   α tocopherol equivalents. 1 mg d-σ-tocopherol = 1 σ T.E.

e   1 N.E. (niacin equivalent) is equal to 1 mg of niacin or 60 mg of dietary tryptophan.

f   The folacin allowances refer to dietary sources as determined by Lactobacillus casei assay after treatment with enzymes ("conjugases") to make polyglutamyl forms of the vitamin available to the test organism.

g   The RDA for vitamin B12 in infants is based on average concentration of the vitamin in human milk. The allowances after weaning are based on energy intake (as recommended by the American Academy of Pediatrics) and consideration of other factors such as intestinal absorption.

h   The increased requirement during pregnancy cannot be met by the iron content of habitual American diets nor by the existing iron stores of many women; therefore the use of 30-60 mg of supplemental iron is recommended. Iron needs during lactation are not substantially different from those of nonpregnant women, but continued supplementation of the mother for 2-3 months after parturition is advisable in order to replenish stores depleted by pregnancy.

From: Food and Nutrition Board, National Academy of Sciences—National Research Council, Washington, D.C., 1980.

TABLE 21-3. Mean Heights and Weights and Recommended Energy Intake*

Category	Age (years)	Weight (kg)	Weight (lb)	Height (cm)	Height (in)	Energy Needs (with range) (kcal)	(MJ)
Infants	0.0-0.5	6	13	60	24	kg × 115 (95-145)	kg × .48
	0.5-1.0	9	20	71	28	kg × 105 (80-135)	kg × .44
Children	1-3	13	29	90	35	1300 (900-1800)	5.5
	4-6	20	44	112	44	1700 (1300-2300)	7.1
	7-10	28	62	132	52	2400 (1650-3300)	10.1
Males	11-14	45	99	157	62	2700 (2000-3700)	11.3
	15-18	66	145	176	69	2800 (2100-3900)	11.8
	19-22	70	154	177	70	2900 (2500-3300)	12.2
	23-50	70	154	178	70	2700 (2300-3100)	11.3
	51-75	70	154	178	70	2400 (2000-2800)	10.1
	76+	70	154	178	70	2050 (1650-2450)	8.6
Females	11-14	46	101	157	62	2200 (1500-3000)	9.2
	15-18	55	120	163	64	2100 (1200-3000)	8.8
	19-22	55	120	163	64	2100 (1700-2500)	8.8
	23-50	55	120	163	64	2000 (1600-2400)	8.4
	51-75	55	120	163	64	1800 (1400-2200)	7.6
	76+	55	120	163	64	1600 (1200-2000)	6.7
Pregnancy						+300	
Lactation						+500	

The data in this table have been assembled from the observed median heights and weights of children, together with desirable weights for adults for the mean heights of men (70 inches) and women (64 inches) between the ages of 18 and 34 years as surveyed in the U.S. population.

The energy allowances for the young adults are for men and women doing light work. The allowances for the two older age groups represent mean energy needs over these age spans, allowing for a 2% decrease in basal (resting) metabolic rate per decade and a reduction in activity of 200 kcal/day for men and women between 51 and 75 years, 500 kcal for men over 75 years and 400 kcal for women over 75. The customary range of daily energy output is shown for adults in parentheses, and is based on a variation in energy needs of ± 400 kcal at any one age, emphasizing the wide range of energy intakes appropriate for any group of people.

Energy allowances for children through age 18 are based on median energy intakes of children these ages followed in longitudinal growth studies. The values in parentheses are 10th and 90th percentiles of energy intake, to indicate the range of energy consumption among children of these ages.

* From: *Recommended Dietary Allowances, Revised 1980*, Food and Nutrition Board, National Academy of Sciences—National Research Council, Washington, D.C.

Determination of Caloric Needs

A person of normal weight requires 15 calories per pound (or 24 calories per kilogram) to maintain that normal weight. An overweight individual requires only 10 calories per pound to maintain daily caloric needs, whereas an underweight individual requires 20 calories per pound to meet his needs. The following formula may be used: weight (in pounds or kilograms) × caloric need (number specified per pound or kilogram) = daily caloric need.

> *Example:* For a woman 5 feet 4 inches tall and weighing 120 lbs:
> 15 × 120 = 1800 calories.

Determination of Protein Needs

An individual at desirable body weight requires 0.8 gram of protein per kilogram of weight. Thus weight in kilograms × 0.8 = protein need in grams.

> *Example:* For the average woman weighing 120 lbs.
> (1 kg = 2.2 lbs)
> 120 lbs ÷ 2.2 = 54.5 kilograms
> 54.5 × 0.8 = 43.6 grams.

Determination of Fats and Carbohydrate Needs

No recommended daily allowance figures have been established for fats and carbohydrates. However, calories from fats sources should constitute approximately 20 percent of total calories, while calories from carbohydrate sources should represent approximately 50 percent of the total. The remaining 30 percent is derived from protein foods.

DIET THERAPY

The arrangement of foods in the daily diet is of great significance in the prevention and treatment of disease. Much is still unknown concerning the interaction of nutrients and health status. However, the medical profession has become increasingly aware of the relationship between patterns of food consumption and disease incidence.

The modern physician is increasingly utilizing diet therapy as a treatment measure. *Diet therapy* is the term which signifies the design and prescription of diet particulars to prevent or treat disease. The normal diet is adjusted to meet the individual physiologic needs of the patient. These adjustments are based on the physician's understanding of the need and effect of certain types of foods and nutrients in the patient's condition.

In some disease states and in disease prevention plans, diet therapy may be the only treatment alternative employed. Usually, however, to control or treat disease, diet therapy is used in combination with other treatment alternatives.

The medical assistant, having acquired a basic understanding of normal nutrition, can apply and adapt these concepts in diet therapy.

Modifications of the Normal Diet

The normal diet is used as the basis for dietary adjustments. The objective in diet therapy is to meet the nutritional needs of the patient while analyzing the diet particulars required by the patient's condition.

The normal diet is modified by:

1. Adjusting the calorie allowance;
2. Changing the consistency or texture of foods;
3. Avoiding or restricting certain foods;
4. Changing the number of meals or feedings;
5. Emphasizing certain foods;
6. Increasing or decreasing certain nutrient levels.

Depending on the patient's condition, one or several modifications may be required. The physician usually prescribes a standard diet plan which includes specific modifications. For example, the physician may order a high-calorie diet for a patient with fever, or a low-fiber diet for a patient with severe diarrhea. The physician, using the standard or normal diet as the basic structure, may further individualize the diet prescription. Table 21-4 outlines the standard diet therapy models and their use in specific diseases.

Underlying concepts in diet therapy can be detected upon review of the chart. When the body's metabolism is increased, as during fever or certain growth states and diseases, energy requirements are increased. Therefore, more calories are needed. Because protein is necessary for tissue growth and repair, protein needs also increase during times when the body is experiencing growth or repair.

Certain food excesses are linked to disease. For example, overconsumption of saturated fats is associated with heart disease. Certain food consistencies and flavors are irritating to the mucous membrane lining the gastrointestinal tract when inflammation is present in diseases such as gastritis and ulcer. The integration of physiology and diet therapy will expand the medical assistant's awareness of clinical interrelationships within the human body.

General Principles of Patient Teaching in Diet Therapy

Certain general principles of effective patient teaching may be cited in connection with diet therapy. The objectives of these considerations are to gain the patient's cooperation and to assist the patient to understand the diet prescription. The medical assistant's role is to offer reassurance, give accurate information, refer certain questions to the physician, help the patient plan the diet if required, and reinforce the physician's explanations.

The medical assistant needs to understand and be capable of applying the following principles before providing instruction:

1. The MA must understand the diet prescription, the foods to be included and avoided, and the specific goals of the diet prescription.

TABLE 21-4. Standard Modifications Applied to Specific Disease

Diet Prescription	Conditions for Use	Characteristics
High-calorie	Hyperthyroidism; pneumonia; infection; fever.	A. Calorie intake increased to 3000–5000 daily. B. Increased carbohydrate and slightly increased fat food sources; maintenance of protein requirements. C. Avoidance of large servings of low-calorie foods such as lettuce.
Low-calorie	Obesity.	A. Calories are restricted but usually do not fall below 1000 calorie allowance per day. B. Carbohydrates and fats are restricted, protein maintained. C. Foods emphasized include fruits, vegetables, lean meats, and whole grains. Foods avoided include desserts, snack foods, creams, sauces, starchy foods, and refined sugars.
High-carbohydrate	Liver and gallbladder disease.	Increased carbohydrate intake by emphasis on whole-grain breads and cereals, fruits, vegetables with high-carbohydrate content, natural sugars, and starches.
Restricted or modified carbohydrate	Diabetes.	A. Carbohydrate restriction corresponds to the physician's use of drug therapy. Carbohydrate intake must be managed by the drug prescribed to control the diabetes. B. Food exchange list is most frequently utilized to assist the patient in maintaining normal nutrition.
High-protein	Fever.	A. Protein allowances are increased beyond the normal level. B. Intake of high-protein foods is increased, including milk, cheese, eggs, and meat.

TABLE 21-4. *Continued*

Diet Prescription	Conditions for Use	Characteristics
Low-protein	Kidney disease, such as nephritis; cardiac conditions.	A. Protein allowances are maintained at a low-normal level. B. Foods which are high-protein sources are restricted, and fruits, vegetables, and whole grains stressed.
Low-fat	Obesity; gallbladder disease; digestive disturbances.	A. Fats which are more easily digested are emphasized, such as lean meat, skim milk, and cottage cheese. B. Fats are restricted to include only the low-fat sources. C. Avoidance of sauces, gravies, and fatty or tough meats is encouraged.
High-fiber	Severe or continued constipation.	A. Fiber content is increased. B. Raw fruits and vegetables are stressed along with whole-grain cereals and leafy green vegetables. C. Refined foods are avoided.
Low-fiber	Severe diarrhea; ulcerative colitis; and other gastrointestinal disorders.	A. Rests the GI tract but can only be used for a brief period because of inadequacies in vitamins and minerals. B. Lean meats, fruit juice, gelatins, milk-free beverages, and fat-free soups are stressed. C. Whole grains, milk, cheese, raw fruits, vegetables, and spicy foods are avoided.
High-iron	Certain anemias.	High-iron food sources are stressed, such as liver, egg yolk, beans, and whole-grain cereals.
Bland	Peptic ulcers; gastritis; diarrhea.	A. Consistency of foods is modified. B. Small, frequent feedings are stressed. C. Pureed fruits, custards, gelatins, low spice and easily digested foods are recommended. D. Avoidance of raw fruits and vegetables is encouraged as well as strongly flavored and spicy foods.

TABLE 21-4. *Continued*

Diet Prescription	Conditions for Use	Characteristics
Soft diet	Chewing difficulties.	Strong flavors and spices are permitted, but foods must be pureed.
Clear liquid diet	Acute diarrhea.	A. Used for short periods of time because of nutritional inadequacies. B. Tea, fat-free broth, and non-citrus juices are stressed.

2. The MA must learn the patient's normal eating habits and appreciate the dietary difficulties being experienced. This is especially important if the diet is to be followed for a prolonged period of time. The diet plan cannot be successful if the patient's own eating patterns and habits are unknown or excluded. The patient's input is of extreme importance to the design of any long-term plan.

3. The patient's reaction to the diet must be considered whether the diet plan is short-term or long-term. If the assistant is aware of the patient's reactions, further explanation and reassurance can be given. The patient does not always verbalize concerns.

4. The MA should acquire an appreciation of ethnic and economic conditioning in dietary habits.

5. Care should be taken to give diet instruction within the boundaries of the MA's professional responsibility, which is to provide information and reinforcement, and not to design the prescription.

PATIENT TEACHING AND WEIGHT REDUCTION DIETS

In weight reduction diets, the physician prescribes the caloric allowance and the distribution of nutrients. The medical assistant's responsibility is to guide the patient in understanding and accepting the dietary restrictions. To achieve these objectives, the medical assistant must have an awareness of certain considerations.

Motivation

The medical assistant needs to be aware of the importance of self-motivation in the weight reduction diet. The MA's approach should help to provide an environment in which the patient can develop self-motivation. The patient may need the opportunity to discuss personal feelings. Weight reduction is an emotional issue. Much controversy surrounds the concept of weight reduction and the reasons for overeating. The medical assistant needs to be empathetic and appreciative of the real personal difficulties in overcoming the habit of overeating. Patients with disease-linked reasons for reducing their weight tend to be more successful in that their motivation is greater.

Support

The patient involved in a weight reduction diet requires much support. The MA should draw the family into the supportive network formed by the physician and the medical office staff. Family members should be included in the discussions. This is especially important if the individual will not be preparing his own meals.

Information

Before effective instruction of the patient can begin, the medical assistant must possess a reliable body of information concerning weight reduction.

FAD DIETS

A vast amount of misinformation clouds and distorts the issue of weight reduction. The medical assistant should caution the patient not to abandon the diet prescription for a "quick weight loss" diet. There are no magic formulas for losing weight. Calories and the arrangement of essential nutrients are the keys. Calories not expended become adipose tissue. When more energy is expended than the number of calories ingested, weight reduction results.

Special arrangements of restricted food allowances are important in weight loss diets to meet nutritional needs. A successful weight reduction diet will be well-balanced and provide adequate nutrition while reducing the number of calories.

OPTIMAL LOSS

Optimal weight loss is considered to be a steady, gradual process. Usually a loss of 2 pounds weekly is recommended.

COMPUTATION

The physician determines the appropriate calorie allowance by (1) multiplying the patient's desired weight by 10 (calories allowed per pound), or (2) multiplying the patient's present weight by 15 (which equals the number of calories needed to maintain present weight) and subtracting 600 calories daily per pound of loss to be achieved. Six hundred calories represents the number needed to maintain 1 pound of body weight.

STANDARD ALLOWANCE

An allowance of 1000 calories appears to be the allowance most frequently utilized by physicians, as this level can still provide adequate nutrition; allowances below 1000 calories usually cannot.

HOLISTIC PROGRAMS

The physician usually takes a comprehensive approach to the patient on a weight reduction diet by developing a program which includes exercise and some aspects of behavior modification and counseling. Maintenance of the weight loss is perhaps the single most difficult aspect of weight reduction and requires specialized patient care beyond diet instruction.

PATIENT TEACHING AND THE DIABETIC DIET

The patient with diabetes presents special challenges to the medical assistant. The MA must fully understand the crucial relationship between diet and disease in diabetes. The patient needs to acquire this same understanding. Because the diabetic diet is continued for a lifetime, the patient will need to become expert in all aspects of the diet and the disease. The general principles of diet therapy apply to the diabetic diet.

The foods in a diabetic diet are often weighed to ensure proper portions. The medical assistant may be responsible for instructing the patient in the use of the weighing scale if required, the intimate relationship between diet and drug therapy, and the exchange list.

The *exchange list* is a standard diet model for the diabetic patient. It can, however, be used by the patient on a weight reduction diet as well. The physician specifies the calories and the amounts of carbohydrate allowable. The exchange list provides a convenient and practical reference for the patient in determining an accurate intake of the specified calories, carbohydrates, proteins, and fats without the use of a scale, since household measures are used.

The patient is instructed to make allowable substitutions or "exchanges" within the allowable ranges of calories and carbohydrates from the list provided. All foods in the portions specified contain a predetermined number of calories and an amount of nutrients in grams. The exchange list provided in Table 21-5 is based upon the recommendations of the American Dietetic Association.

The diabetic patient is instructed to eat only those foods which are allowed on the exchange list, never to skip a meal, and to eat all of the portion specified. The exchange list enables the diabetic patient to experience the greatest freedom of choice possible in dietary decisions characteristic of normal living.

SUMMARY

The role of medical assistants in diet therapy is of great importance to physicians in the management of their own time. MAs who understand the concepts of basic nutrition and diet therapy, and who can make successful applications in patient teaching, free physicians

TABLE 21-5. Food Exchange Lists

Vegetable Exchange

Group A: These vegetables contain very small amounts of carbohydrate, fat, and protein. Because there are so few calories, unlimited amounts of the raw vegetable are permitted. If vegetable is cooked, limit the serving to 1 cup.

Asparagus	kale
Broccoli	mustard
Brussels sprouts	spinach
Cabbage	turnip
Cauliflower	Lettuce
Celery	Mushrooms
Chicory	Okra
Cucumber	Pepper, green
Eggplant	Radishes
Escarole	Sauerkraut
Greens	String beans
beet	Summer squash
chard	Tomato
collard	Watercress
dandelion	

Group B: Each serving of these vegetables contains 7 grams of carbohydrate and 2 grams of protein, which equals 36 calories. Each 1/2 cup serving equals one exchange.

Beets	Pumpkin
Carrots	Rutabaga
Onions	Squash, winter
Peas, green	Turnips

Fruit Exchange

Each serving contains 10 grams of carbohydrate and 40 calories.

Apple	1 (2-inch diameter)
Applesauce	1/2 cup
Apricots	2 medium
Apricots, dried	4 halves
Banana	1/2 small
Blackberries	1 cup
Blueberries	2/3 cup
Cantaloupe	1/4 (6-inch diameter)
Cherries	10 large
Dates	2
Figs	
dried	1 small
fresh	2 large
Grapefruit	1/2 small
Grapefruit juice	1/2 cup
Grapes	12
Grape juice	1/4 cup
Honeydew mellon	1/8 (7-inch diameter)
Mango	1/2 small
Nectarine	1 medium
Orange	1 small

TABLE 21-5. *Continued*

Fruit Exchange (Cont.)

Orange juice	1/2 cup
Papaya	1/3 medium
Peach	1 medium
Pear	1 small
Pineapple	1/2 cup
Pineapple juice	1/3 cup
Plums	2 medium
Prunes	2
Raisins	2 tablespoons
Raspberries	1 cup
Strawberries	1 cup
Tangerine	1 large
Watermelon	1 cup

Bread Exchange

Each serving contains 15 grams of carbohydrate, 2 grams of protein, and 68 calories.

Bread	1 slice
biscuit, roll	1 (2-inch diameter)
cornbread	1 (1/2-inch cube)
muffin	1 (2-inch diameter)
Cereal	
cooked	1/2 cup
dry (flakes, puffed, etc.)	3/4 cup
Crackers	
graham	2
oyster	20
saltine	5
soda	3
round	6 to 8
Flour	2 1/2 tablespoons
Ice cream (omit 2 fat exchanges)	1/2 cup
Rice or grits, cooked	1/2 cup
Spaghetti, noodles, etc.	1/2 cup
Sponge cake, plain	1/2-inch cube
Vegetables	
baked beans, no pork	1/4 cup
beans (dry, cooked)	1/2 cup
corn	1/3 cup
parsnips	2/3 cup
Peas (dry, cooked)	1/2 cup
Potatoes	
sweet	1/4 cup
white, baked or boiled	1 (2-inch diameter)
white, mashed	1/2 cup

Meat Exchange

Each serving contains 7 grams of protein, 5 grams of fat, and 73 calories. Remove bone and other wastes when measuring.

TABLE 21-5. *Continued*

Meat Exchange (Cont.)

Cheese	
cheddar, American	1 ounce slice
cottage	1 cup
Codfish, mackerel, haddock	
halibut, etc.	1 ounce slice
Cold cuts	1 1/2 ounces
Egg	1
Frankfurter	1
Meat and poultry	
(beef, lamb, pork, chicken)	1 ounce slice
Oysters, shrimp, clams	5 small
Peanut butter (limit to one	
exchange per day unless	
carbohydrate is allowed)	2 tablespoons
Salmon, tuna, crab, lobster	1/4 cup
Sardines	3 medium

Fat Exchange

Each serving contains 5 grams of fat and 45 calories.

Avocado	1/8 (4-inch diameter)
Bacon, crisp	1 slice
Butter or margarine	1 teaspoon
Cream	
heavy	1 tablespoon
light	2 tablespoons
Cream cheese	1 tablespoon
French dressing	1 tablespoon
Mayonnaise	1 teaspoon
Nuts	6 small
Oil or cooking fat	1 teaspoon
Olives	5 small

Milk Exchange

Each serving contains 12 grams of carbohydrate, 8 grams of protein, 10 grams of fat, and 170 calories.

Buttermilk	1 cup
Evaporated milk	1/2 cup
Powdered milk	1/4 cup
Skim milk (add 2 fat exchanges)	1 cup
Whole milk	1 cup

---

to use their office time more effectively. While the medical assistant is not a nutritionist or a professional diet therapist, the basic principles and information contained in this chapter are well within the MA's scope of practice. The medical assistant's role is clearly to reinforce the patient in carrying out the diet prescription ordered by the physician.

APPLICATION EXERCISES

Provide solutions to the following situations and discuss the approach utilized.

1. Calculate the nutritive value of your own diet on a sample day: (a) record all that was eaten for 1 day; (b) refer to the Basic Food Groups to check the number of servings of specific foods recommended; (c) calculate the total number of calories using a reference chart on the composition of foods; (d) compare nutrient levels of carbohydrate, protein, and fats in your diet with the recommended allowances; (e) record the findings; and (f) write out a diet plan to correct any deficiencies or unhealthy patterns cited.

2. Mrs. Jones is 45 years old, 5 feet 4 inches tall, and weighs 180 lbs. She has gone on diets repeatedly without success. The physician has recommended a weight reduction diet of 1200 calories. How much can she expect to lose per week? What patient teaching principles would apply?

3. Mr. Khun has been diagnosed as having diabetes. The diet prescription calls for:

   Breakfast:

   2 fruit exchanges
   2 bread exchanges
   2 meat exchanges
   1 milk exchange
   1 fat exchange
   coffee or tea

   Lunch:

   2 meat exchanges
   2 salad exchanges
   1 vegetable (group A)
   1 vegetable (group B)
   1 fruit exchange
   1 milk exchange
   1 fat exchange
   coffee or tea

   Dinner:

   2 meat exchanges
   2 bread exchanges
   1 vegetable (group A)
   1 milk exchange
   1 fat exchange
   coffee or tea

Calculate the total number of calories per day and plan menus for 2 days which differ from one another.

Role-Playing Exercise

Students form groups and the instructor assigns three roles: a patient, a medical assistant, and an evaluator for each of the situations which follow. Explain the diet and its purpose to the patient and answer questions the patient may express. (Some research may be necessary.)

1. Mr. Alberts has hypertension and has been ordered on a low-fat diet.

2. Mrs. MacIntosh has severe diarrhea, and the physician has ordered clear liquids.

3. Mr. Aaron has a high fever, and the physician has ordered a high-protein, high-calorie diet.

4. Mrs. Semple is allergic to milk products, and the physician has asked you to discuss alternative sources of protein with her.

5. Mr. Mole is 21, and a college athlete. He is curious as to how many calories he needs. He is 6'1" and weighs 165 lbs. The physician suggests that perhaps Mr. Mole is underweight and not receiving sufficient nutrients because of his energy needs.

COMPLETING THE LEARNING LOOP

Diet therapy is a treatment alternative available to the physician which requires significant use of the medical assistant's knowledge and skills. As with most skills, dietary information is best communicated to patients when the MA has first understood and internalized the principles of proper nutrition. The task of incorporating proper dietary habits in ones own daily eating pattern is a continuous process and will require an alertness to new concepts in the ever-expanding field of nutrition.

The next chapter discusses another important treatment alternative—drug therapy.

BIBLIOGRAPHY

Anderson, L., et al.: *Nutrition in Nursing.* J.B. Lippincott, Philadelphia, 1972.
Bennion, M.: *Clinical Nutrition.* Harper & Row, New York, 1978.
Caliendo, M.A.: *Nutrition and Preventative Health Care.* Macmillan, New York, 1980.
Lewis, C.M.: *Nutrition: Proteins and Carbohydrates.* F.A. Davis, Philadelphia, 1976.
Lewis, C.M.: *Nutrition: Vitamins and Minerals.* F.A. Davis, Philadelphia, 1976.
Robinson, C.H.: *Basic Nutrition and Diet Therapy,* ed. 4. Macmillan, New York, 1980.
Williams, S.R.: *Self-Study Guide for Nutrition and Diet Therapy,* ed. 2. C.V. Mosby, St. Louis, 1978.

22

PHARMACOLOGY AND DRUG THERAPY

SPECIFIC OBJECTIVES

Upon completion of this chapter you will be able to:

1. Describe the legal standards and modes of enforcement for drug administration.

2. Explain how drugs are named and list sources, define effects and actions, list variables which affect action, and describe drug routes and forms.

3. Interpret the medication order and list, and the parts of the prescription.

4. Calculate drug dosages.

5. Prepare the patient and the drug for administration of the medication.

6. List sites and types of drug administration.

7. Perform the procedure for oral administration.

8. Perform the procedure for administration of intramuscular, intradermal, and subcutaneous procedures.

9. Instruct the patient in the use of medication.

10. Be alert to undesired effects of drugs.

INTRODUCTION

Drug therapy is the most widely used treatment alternative. Almost every patient, in every type of practice situation, leaves the office with one or more prescriptions for medication. Many individuals also use nonprescription drugs which may be purchased in drug stores and supermarkets. This chemical technology is so predominant in modern society that the use of drugs is taken quite casually. This attitude, however, must be avoided by health care personnel. Although the use of drugs is so prevalent, chemical intervention in human body processes always includes some element of risk. Medical assistants must acquire an appreciation for the serious responsibility they assume in the administration of drugs. This clinical function carries with it a greater potential for error and calamity than all other clinical functions within the scope of medical assisting. MAs need to acquire an understanding of basic pharmacology concepts and applications in drug therapy in order to manage their role successfully. The assistant's responsibility in drug therapy includes not only the administration of drugs, but also the awareness of side effects, the interpretation of the prescription for the patient, and the reinforcement of the physician's instructions.

LEGAL STANDARDS AND ENFORCEMENTS

Definite legal standards govern the sale, distribution, and use of drugs. Since 1906, with passage of the Pure Food and Drug Act, the federal government has imposed regulations to monitor the manufacture of drugs. It was not until 1938, however, following the death of 100 individuals who had taken a toxic drug, that the Food, Drug and Cosmetic Act was passed. The Act mandates that all drugs must be substantially tested prior to marketing and distribution. Amendments to the Act have provided that prescription drugs be labeled as such and that drug refills can only be authorized by the physician.

A special class of drugs, labeled narcotics, is monitored under the Controlled Substances Act and the Drug Abuse Control Act. The manufacture, sale, transport, importation, distribution, administration, and prescription of narcotic drugs is federally controlled. Every narcotic substance administered must be recorded on special forms requiring the patient's name, the physician's name and narcotic licensure number, the drug, dosage, route, date, time of administration, and the medical assistant's signature.

The implementation of these acts is the responsibility of the U.S. Department of Health and Human Services. The branch of this department specifically responsible for drug management is the Food and Drug Administration (FDA). The Federal Trade Commission is the overseer of the appropriate marketing and advertising of manufactured drugs. The Drug Enforcement Administration enforces the laws related to narcotics under the U.S. Department of Justice. The medical assistant must be aware of these regulations and their implications in medical practice.

To ensure that legal standards are followed, the MA's responsibility, in addition to the accurate administration of drugs, includes (1) keeping appropriate records, (2) safeguarding prescription forms, (3) proper and safe storage of drugs, (4) removing drugs whose shelf life has expired, and (5) monitoring the currency of the physician's registration and licensure to dispense medication.

DRUGS

Definition and Listing of Drugs

According to the Food, Drug and Cosmetic Act, the term *drug* refers to any article and substance other than food that is intended to affect the structure or any function of the body and that is recognized and approved by the FDA. Drugs are listed according to their *generic* name or *trade* name. The generic name is the chemical composition of the drug, while the trade name is that assigned by the manufacturer. A physician may prescribe drugs in either their trade or generic form. (For example, Wyeth Laboratories manufactures Equanil, whose generic name is meprobamate.) Many physicians are beginning to order drugs by their generic names, since they are less expensive for the patient. If a trade name is ordered, the pharmacist cannot make a generic substitution at the patient's request except in California.

Drug Sources

It is important for the medical assistant to have some understanding of drug sources and the influence of these sources on the preparation and dosage of the drug in order to answer the patient's questions concerning these factors.

ANIMAL SOURCES

Certain substances in the tissue, organs, and body fluids of animals (including man) are extracted and usually serve as replacements or substitutions for glandular deficiencies. Insulin, thyroxine, antitoxins, serums, and gammaglobulin are examples.

PLANT SOURCES

Plant constituents comprise the most widely used substances in drug therapy. Digitalis and morphine are examples.

MINERAL SOURCES

Metals, salts, and clays can be converted to drug compositions. Iodine and magnesium sulfate (Epsom salts) are examples.

SYNTHETIC DRUGS

Synthetic drugs are man-made substances prepared in a chemical laboratory. Unlike many drugs derived from natural sources, synthetic drugs are more economical to manufacture. Sulfonamides, certain antibiotics, and vaccines derived from microorganisms are produced in the laboratory. Penicillin, an antibiotic, and the Sabin (polio) vaccine are examples of drugs derived from cultured microorganisms which are causative agents of the diseases to be treated.

Effects and Actions of Drugs

Drugs are classified by various methods in order to make generalizations related to their use and physiologic effects. The two major classifications are (1) drugs which affect specific body parts or systems, and (2) drugs which have isolated functions or effects. Examples of the first classification include diuretics (water retention reducers) which act specifically on the kidney. Examples of the second classification include vasodilators (blood vessel dilators), analgesics (pain relievers), and antibiotics (bacteria destroyers).

Drug actions are categorized as (1) affecting cellular activity, and (2) affecting absorption. Drugs depress or increase the normal processes of the cell. In addition, drugs are known to have either *local* or *systemic* actions. A drug having a local action is absorbed only at the contact site, while a drug having a systemic action is absorbed and circulated by the blood stream and distributed to all body parts.

Variables Affecting Drug Action

While the effects and actions of drugs are tested, and therefore predetermined, sometimes individual differences in reaction occur. Certain variables will affect the action of drugs:

1. *Potency.* All drugs carry an *expiration date.* If used after the date of expiration, the drug may be altered or decompose, becoming toxic or impotent. *Environmental* factors, such as lack of refrigeration when required, may also result in decomposition.

2. *Route of Administration.* Each drug activity is dependent upon the recommended route of administration. When routes other than those specified are used to administer the drug, the desired action may not occur or not occur at the rate preferred.

3. *Physiologic Variances.* Presence of food in the stomach, the rate of peristaltic activity, and unknown hypersensitivity to the drug can affect drug activity. Age, body weight, physical condition, and emotional state can influence the effects of the drug.

4. *Additive Effects.* The presence of other drugs taken simultaneously may alter individual drug action. Two drugs which work together to produce effects greater than the sum of their individual effects are called *synergistic. Potentiation* is the term used when drugs having dissimilar individual actions give a greater total effect when combined. When drugs taken together counteract the effects of one another, the result is known as antagonism. A drug which is absorbed faster than it is disposed has a *cumulative* effect. This may be due to physiologic variances, the number of dosages, or the continuous use of the drug.

Side Effects of Drugs

Although a drug is prescribed to achieve a desired therapeutic effect, all drugs have side effects. These side effects are results which are not specifically intended as the primary purpose for administration but are normal physiologic accompaniments to the desired effects of the drug. Not all side effects are undesirable. Although unintended, some side effects are harmless and even useful. An example of the production of positive side effects is aspirin. A side effect of aspirin, a pain reliever, is mild sedation. An individual with pain will also experience a state of mild relaxation if aspirin is administered. While sedation is not the purpose of the prescription, it is usually beneficial to the patient.

An *untoward* effect is a side effect which is undesirable. Unexpected or unusual reaction to a drug is termed *idiosyncrasy*. An abnormal reaction which occurs repeatedly is termed an *allergic reaction*. Other unintended effects of drug administration are related to physical and psychological responses.

Certain drugs, when used for prolonged periods, can become ineffectual in their action. While this is an undesired effect, the patient builds up a *tolerance* to the drug. Dosages must be steadily increased to achieve the desired results. *Cross-tolerance* can occur when one drug increases the body's resistance to the effects and actions of other similar drugs. Occasionally, *physical dependence* on a drug will occur, in which the cells are unable to function without high levels of the drug circulating through the blood stream. Emotional need which results in steadily increasing dosages is termed *addiction*. *Habituation* to a drug is also based on emotional need but without a tendency to increased dosage needs.

A drug may also produce certain effects that warrant special categorization. These special effects are identified as *contraindications*. This term applies to certain conditions under which the drug should not be administered.

Precautions are sometimes included in the packaging of a drug in order to list those conditions which could arise as contraindications. An example of a contraindication would be the warning "do not take with other medication" or "do not administer to a patient with hypertension." A further example of a precaution would be a directive to "take the medication with milk" or a statement that "alcohol will complicate the effects of this medication."

Drug Routes and Forms

Medication can be administered by various routes and in a variety of forms. The *drug route* refers to the site at which the drug will be administered. The *drug form* refers to the type of substance to be administered.

The choice of a drug route is based upon several considerations:

1. Desired effects and action:
   a. Local or systemic effect.
   b. Slow or rapid absorption drugs administered intravenously are most rapidly absorbed; drugs administered to dissolve in body orifices are also rapidly absorbed; drugs administered by injection are more rapidly absorbed than oral medication.
   c. Long or short duration.

2. The patient's physical and emotional state:
   a. Level of consciousness.
   b. Physical limitation.
   c. Emotional difficulties.

3. Characteristics of the drug:
   a. Safety of desired dosage and route relationship.
   b. Expense entailed.
   c. Availability of the drug in the desired form and route.

The form of a drug is determined by (1) the nature and properties of the drug, (2) the intended purpose, and (3) the availability of the drug for the desired route of administration.

ORAL ROUTE AND FORMS

The oral route is perhaps the most widely used method of administering and prescribing medication because of certain advantages:

1. The convenience of not requiring special equipment.
2. The relative inexpensiveness of the drug.
3. The diminished likelihood of trauma to body processes and structures because the rate of absorption is relatively slow.

Oral administration includes medication which can be swallowed or otherwise dissolved when placed inside the cheek or under the tongue. Drugs placed inside the cheek are termed *buccal* and are slowly absorbed through the capillaries in the mucous membrane lining the cheek. Drugs placed under the tongue are termed *sublingual* and are rapidly absorbed through the capillary network under the tongue.

Several forms of drugs are available for oral administration:

1. *Tablets:* powdered or granulated substances molded into a particular shape (round, oval, etc.). Tablets can be *uncoated*, which will allow the medication to dissolve rapidly, or *coated*, which protects the drug from destruction by acidic secretions in the stomach (enteric) and provides a longer shelf life for the drug. Enteric coated tablets can also be layered in such a way as to release a staggered dosage. Certain drugs, such as vitamins, are flavored and manufactured in chewable form.

2. *Capsules:* drug substances placed in a palatable gelatinous container. Hard capsules consist of two halves and contain powdered substances; soft capsules are sealed liquid substances. Capsules are sometimes called *spansules* because they contain tiny pellets which are released over a span of time for staggered dosage release.

3. *Troches (lozenges):* drug substances mixed with mucilage and sugar and molded into desired shapes. The drug is slowly released as it is sucked and dissolved in the mouth.

4. *Solutions:* drug substances contained in a homogenous mixture with water (solute and solvent). Several types of solutions are available: (a) *saturated* solutions, which are more concentrated; (b) *aromatic* solutions, which usually contain a volatile oil to disguise the taste of the drug substance; (c) *liquors*, which contain

nonvolatile material as the vehicle; and (d) *syrups*, which are flavored sugar solutions used to palatably carry the drug substance.

5. *Suspensions:* insoluble drug substances contained in a liquid. The suspension of two liquids which cannot be mixed together is termed an *emulsion*. A solid inorganic or mineral substance suspended in water is termed a *gel* or *magma*.

6. *Alcohol solutions:* a drug substance (solute) mixed with alcohol (solvent) to enhance the drug's properties and act as a vehicle for drug delivery. Several types of alcohol solutions are available: (a) *elixir*, a solution containing the drug substance, sugar, alcohol, water, and flavoring; (b) *spirits*, a solute consisting of volatile materials; (c) *fluidextract*, a concentrated plant preparation of 100 percent strength in solution; (d) *extract*, a very concentrated syruplike fluid; and (e) *tincture*, a drug dissolved in alcohol and available in 10 to 20 percent strength.

PARENTERAL ROUTES AND FORMS

Parenteral is the term used to refer to administration of medication by injection. There are two main advantages to the introduction of medication by the parenteral route: (1) rapid drug action is produced, and (2) the route offers a necessary alternative when drugs cannot be taken orally because of drug properties or the patient's condition.

Although injection is a required or desired route for certain medications and for administering medications in certain conditions, it carries the greatest risk. When a drug is injected, the rate of absorption cannot be altered. When oral medication is administered, the drug can be retrieved or diluted with food and water and absorption slowed if untoward effects develop. In addition, penetration of the skin carries with it the potential hazard of introducing bacteria, as well as traumatizing the tissue when the procedure is performed incorrectly.

There are several types of injections available for drug administration (Fig. 22-1):

1. *Intravenous injection.* An intravenous injection is the injection of medication directly into the vein for the most rapid absorption of the drug. It is, therefore, the most dangerous method of injection. The method is seldom employed in the physician's office and is not administered by the medical assistant.

2. *Subcutaneous injection.* Any injection into the fatty tissue beneath the skin (the subcutaneous layer) is termed a subcutaneous injection. A maximum of 2 ml of solution can be given to an adult in this manner.

3. *Intradermal injection.* An intradermal injection is the introduction of a small amount of drug substance into the dermis, the layer just beneath the skin. Absorption is very slow, and drug action is local rather than systemic. Antiallergic drugs are commonly administered intradermally.

4. *Intramuscular injection.* This route of injection is second only to intravenous injection in rate of absorption. The medication is injected into muscle tissue. Since not as many nerve endings are distributed in muscle as in fatty tissue, intramuscular injections are less painful than subcutaneous ones. A maximum of 5 ml of solution is

recommended for injection into a large muscle mass. Solution for injection which would be irritating to subcutaneous tissue is administered into muscle tissue. Antibiotics, for example, are commonly given intramuscularly.

INHALATION

Gas or vapors of a drug are inhaled and passed into circulation through the capillaries in the mucous membrane lining of the nose and lungs. Usually, the drug action is specific to the respiratory tract. Medication can be administered by inhalation in various forms:

1. *Nebulizer:* usually a hand-held atomizer which produces a fine mist.

2. *Vaporizer:* a device which produces a fine moist mist, either warm or cool.

3. *Inhaler:* a device with an open tip to insert into the nostrils for inhalation of medication.

4. *Spray bottle:* a bottle held upright and squeezed to release mist.

5. *Aerosal:* a forceful spray operated by depressing a valve on the container.

6. *Ampule:* a very small bottle which is serrated and when broken will release vapors.

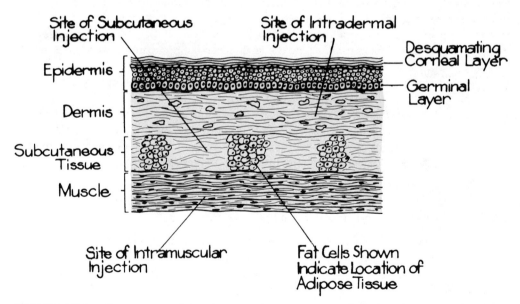

FIGURE 22-1. Cross-section of skin showing subcutaneous, intradermal, and intramuscular injection sites. (Reproduced from Saperstein, A. B., and Frazier, M. A.: *Introduction to Nursing Practice.* F. A. Davis, Philadelphia, 1980.)

TOPICAL ROUTES AND FORMS

Drugs administered topically—to the outer or external body surface—have a local action. Topical drug forms most frequently include:

1. *Creams:* drug substances contained in semisolid preparations applied to the skin in long strokes following the direction of hair growth.

2. *Lotions:* medicated liquid suspensions applied to the skin in a thin layer using long strokes.

3. *Ointments:* drug substances usually contained in an oily base which liquifies upon contact with the skin. Application of ointments is similar to that for creams and lotions.

Topical drugs are most frequently applied to dermatologic conditions.

VAGINAL ROUTES AND FORMS

Drugs administered vaginally—inserted into the vaginal canal—have primarily a local action. Vaginal drug forms most frequently include tablets (compressed powder); suppositories (compressed gel); creams (thick, semisolid liquids); and solutions (liquids instilled through a douching procedure).

Drugs can also be inserted into the urethra (the canal which leads to the bladder) but are seldom administered in office practice because of specialized application and patient discomfort.

RECTAL ROUTE AND FORMS

Drugs administered rectally may have a local or systemic action and are usually in the forms of suppositories or solutions instilled through the enema procedure. Antiemetics (drugs for control of nausea and vomiting) and local analgesics (pain relievers) are commonly administered using this route.

OPHTHALMIC ROUTE AND FORMS

Drugs applied to the eye exert a local action. Common forms of ophthalmic drugs include solutions for irrigation, suspensions, and ointments packaged in bottles, squeeze vials, or tubes. Ophthalmic medication is sterile and must be applied according to correct procedure.

OTIC ROUTE AND FORMS

Drugs applied to the ear have a local action and are usually in the form of drops or solutions for irrigation.

NOSE AND THROAT ROUTES AND FORMS

Drugs applied to the nose and throat exert a local action and are usually in the form of sprays and nose drops. Drugs specific to treatment of throat conditions may be administered in the form of sprays, applications for throat painting, and gargles.

THE LANGUAGE OF PHARMACOLOGY

A well-defined system of codes and terminology is used to exchange information in pharmacology. Some general terminology has already been presented. A specific code exists, however, for expressing the medication order to be administered by the medical assistant and another to be interpreted by the pharmacist. The specific classification of drugs listed according to drug action is another aspect of the language of pharmacology. Most traditional abbreviations and terms have Latin or Greek roots. These designations are universal and serve as a standard for communications related to pharmacology.

The Medication Order

The physician must put all orders for medication in writing. For drugs administered in the medical office, the order is placed on the patient's record. For drug orders to be filled by a pharmacist, the physician must write a prescription. Drugs administered in the medical office are usually *"stat"* orders. "Stat" means immediately. The drug is given in a single dose to the patient at the time of the visit. Although the medication order should always be in writing, there are times when the MA must administer the drug on the verbal rather than written order of the physician. As soon as possible, the physician must write down the order previously given verbally. When a medication is administered on a verbal order, the medical assistant writes the order on the patient's file as given by the physician, signs the physician's name, writes "verbal order" in the appropriate space, and countersigns the notation. When recording the procedure, MAs write "VO" before their initials.

The written requirements for the patient's record and for the prescription form include certain needed information:

1. The date that the order was written;
2. The name of the drug (usually the generic designation);
3. The dosage specified;
4. The route of administration;
5. The specific instruction regarding how frequently the drug is to be taken;
6. The physician's signature.

The Prescription

Although the prescription contains all the essential components of the medication order and the directions written specifically for the pharmacist's interpretation, the arrangement of the information and the language of the prescription require the medical assistant's consideration. The patient will ask questions regarding the prescription; therefore, the MA's familiarity with the procedure is necessary.

The prescription is actually a set of instructions for the pharmacist's use, indicating how the drug should be prepared and supplied. The information included in the prescription is as follows:

1. The patient's full name and address.

2. The date that the prescription is issued.

3. The *superscription* or symbol ℞ (Latin: to take or receive), which indicates that the information which follows is the "recipe."

4. The *inscription*—the name and quantity of the drug.

5. The *subscription*, or the directions for preparing or mixing the drug, when necessary.

6. The *transcription* (indicated by SIG, derived from the Latin *signare*: to mark), which contains the directions to the patient that will appear on the label, as well as the number of refills permitted.

7. The issuing physician's name.

An example of a prescription is illustrated in Figure 22-2. The prescription becomes the property of the pharmacist and is a legal document.

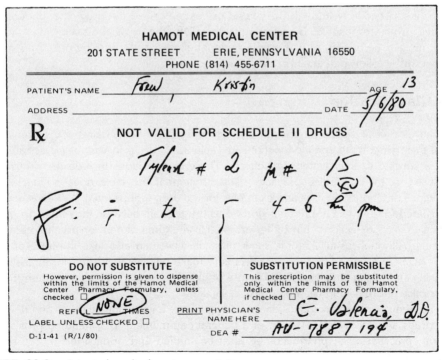

FIGURE 22-2. A typical medical center prescription.

Abbreviations Related to Pharmacology

Certain abbreviations are universally used in pharmacology to exchange information. The use of this "shorthand" saves time and space. The abbreviations listed in Table 22-1 are those most commonly used in pharmacologic practice.

Drug Information

The *Physician's Desk Reference* (PDR) is the most widely used reference source of specific information related to drugs. This text is published annually in order to include all drugs in current use.

The information in this reference guide includes (1) the names, addresses, and telephone numbers of most of the drug manufacturers in the United States; (2) an alphabetic index of the trade names of drugs; (3) the classification of drugs in broad categories; (4) the generic or chemical name of each drug; (5) color pictures of the drug products presented; (6) detailed information on each drug, citing composition, indications for use, action and effects, precautions, warnings, contraindications and side effects, recommended dosage and route, and dosage and route supplied; (7) an index of diagnostic products; and (8) a guide to the management of drug overdose. This comprehensive guide is an essential inclusion in the physician's library and is an invaluable resource for the medical assistant. The MA will need to refer to the PDR whenever an unfamiliar drug is to be administered.

No medication should be administered by the medical assistant unless sufficient information is first obtained. Although the physician has prescribed the drug, the amount, and the route, errors are possible. By referring to the PDR, the medical assistant may save the patient from a drug overdose or promote optional effects of the drug by providing specific instruction or by following certain procedures in administration.

Drug Classification

Drugs can be classified according to their effects and actions on certain body systems or in terms of their general therapeutic function. In Table 22-2, drugs in various classes are categorized according to their action and effects. These classifications include the drugs commonly used in medical office practice. Please note that the table does not include all classifications or all possible uses and examples for the drug groups listed. *Placebos* have not been included, and in fact are not categorized as drugs at all, because they have no specific physiologic effects or actions, but rather are selectively administered for psychological purposes only. Although usually simple sugar pills, placebos can also take the form of sterile water or saline injections. The desired effect is to make patients feel better in the assurance of receiving and taking "medication." The use of placebos is uncommon in modern medical office practice and has long been a controversial issue.

The study of pharmacology is an ongoing process. Each day new drugs and new uses for old drugs are discovered. As part of a general commitment to continuing professional education, practical office pharmacology must be studied and understood by the serious medical assistant.

TABLE 22-1. Common Abbreviations Used in Pharmacology*

Abbreviation	Meaning	Abbreviation	Meaning
ā	before	os	mouth
aa	equal parts	OU	both eyes
ac	before meals	oz	ounce
ad	up to; to	p̄	after
ad lib	freely as desired	pc	after meals
am	morning	per	by; through
amt	amount	po	by mouth
aq	water	PRN	as necessary
bid	twice a day	pt	pint
c̄	with	pulv	powder
cap	capsule	q	every
cc	cubic centimeter	qam	every morning
cm	centimeter	qd	every day
comp	compound	qh	every hour
d	day	q2h	every two hours
dc (D/C)	discontinue	qid	four times a day
dr	dram	qn	every night
elix	elixir	qod	every other day
ext	extract	qs	as much as is required
fl	fluid		
Gm	gram	R	rectal
gr	grain	℞	treatment or therapy
gtt	drop	s̄	without
h or hr	hour	sat	saturated
(H)	hypodermic	Sig or S	write on label
hs	hour of sleep (bedtime)	sol	solution
		sos	one dose if necessary
IM	intramuscular	sp	spirits
IV	intravenous	ss (s̄s̄)	one half
L	liter	stat	immediately
lb	pound	syr	syrup
m	minim	tab	tablet
mg	milligram	tid	three times a day
MOM	milk of magnesia	tinct or tr	tincture
NPO	nothing by mouth	TO	telephone order
N/S	normal saline	U	unit
OD	right eye	ung	ointment
OS	left eye	VO	verbal order

*Reproduced from Saperstein, A. B., and Frazier, M. A.: *Introduction to Nursing Practice.* F. A. Davis, Philadelphia, 1980.

TABLE 22-2. Classification of Drugs

Class	Effects and Actions	Common Use	Examples
Adrenergics	Affect heart muscle, increasing the rate and strength of contractions. Act as vasoconstrictors, dilate pupils, and relax the muscular walls of gastrointestinal and urinary tracts. Dilate bronchi.	Treatment of bronchitis, asthma, allergic conditions, and nasal congestion. Used in the treatment of shock to increase blood pressure	Isuprel Sudafed Neo-Synephrine Visine Epinephrine
Adrenergic blocking agents	Accomplish vasodilation, increase peripheral circulation, decrease blood pressure, and increase the tone of the muscle walls of the gastrointestinal tract.	Treatment of hypertension, migraine headache, peripheral disease.	Aldomet Ergotrate
Analgesics	Relieve pain and lower blood pressure. Vasodilation results. Decrease peristalsis, constipation, and nausea and vomiting.	Narcotic and non-narcotic analgesics are used to relieve varying intensities of pain.	Aspirin Talwin Tylenol Darvon Demerol
Anesthetics	Block nerve impulses to the brain to achieve loss of consciousness. Dilate pupils, decrease respiration, pulse, and blood pressure.	Can be used for general or local anesthesia in minor or major surgery. In local anesthesia there is loss of pain sensation without loss of consciousness. In general anesthesia, loss of consciousness also results.	Pentothal (general) Xylocaine (local)
Antacids	Neutralize the hydrochloric acid in the stomach.	Treatment of hyperacidity (indigestion) and peptic ulcers.	Aluminum hydroxide Sodium bicarbonate

TABLE 22-2. *Continued*

Class	Effects and Actions	Common Use	Examples
Anthelminthics	Rid the body of parasitic worms by paralyzing or killing action or inhibiting growth.	Treatment of roundworm, tapeworm, and other infestations.	Povan Vermox
Antiarrhythmics	Act in various ways to regulate the heart beat.	Treatment of cardiac arrhythmias.	Digoxin Dilantin
Antibiotics	Kill microorganisms, or inhibit or prevent their growth.	Treatment of diseases caused by bacteria (gram positive or negative), spirochetes, and rickettsiae. Used prophylactically in viral infections to reduce vulnerability to bacterial infection. Antibiotics, however, cannot kill viruses.	Penicillin Tetracycline Erythrocin Bacitracin (topical)
Anticholinergics	Increase heart rate, relax smooth muscle, reduce peristalsis, decrease glandular secretions, and dilate pupils.	Used to reduce muscle spasm (antispasmotic), to treat bronchial asthma, peptic ulcers, and hypermobility of the gastrointestinal tract.	Bentyl Banthine Pro-Banthine
Anticoagulants	Inhibit blood coagulation (blood clotting).	Treatment of thrombophlebitis, other specialized usages.	Dicoumaril Coumadin Heparin
Anticonvulsants	Prevent seizures or convulsions by depressing the brain's motor center or by stimulating the seizure threshold of the central nervous system.	Treatment of epilepsy and other neurologic disorders.	Dilantin Valium Phenobarbital
Antidepressants	Mood elevators.	Treatment of psychotic and neurotic types of depression and anxiety.	Elavil Ritalin Tofranil

TABLE 22-2. *Continued*

Class	Effects and Actions	Common Use	Examples
Antidiarrhetics	Inhibit diarrhea and hypermobility of the gastrointestinal tract by affecting the tract's musculature.	Treatment of diarrhea, flatulence, and GI disorders.	Kaopectate Lomotil
Antiemetics	Prevent vomiting and reduce nausea by acting on the medulla of the brain or reducing vertigo by acting on the vestibular mechanism of the ear.	Treatment or prevention of nausea, vomiting, vertigo, and motion sickness.	Compazine Dramamine Tigan
Antiflatulents	Relief of gastric or intestinal distention by changing the surface tension of gas and causing air bubbles to coalesce (usually used in combination with antacids).	Treatment of abdominal distention.	Oil of peppermint Simethicone Ilopan
Antifungals	Kill or check the growth of fungus.	Treatment of diseases caused by fungi.	Mycostatin Nystatin
Antihistamines	Counteract the production of an abnormal amount of histine produced in the body.	Treatment of symptoms of allergies and coryza (common cold).	Dimetone Phenergan Benadryl
Antihypertensives	Reduce blood pressure by lessening resistance to blood flow, through relaxation of vasoconstricted peripheral vessels.	Treatment of hypertension, migraine, headache, arteriosclerosis, and angina pectoris.	Reserpine Aldomet Apresoline Papaverine
Antiinflammatories	Act to diminish inflammation.	Treatment of arthritis, gout, and other inflammatory conditions.	Aspirin Indocin Butazolidin Cortisone

TABLE 22-2. *Continued*

Class	Effects and Actions	Common Use	Examples
Antipruritics	Relieve itching.	Treatment of skin disorders or allergies which cause itching.	Calamine lotion Temaril Hydrocortisone ointment
Antipyretics	Reduce body temperature in a febrile state. Dilate peripheral vascular system and increase heat loss, thus returning body temperature to normal.	Treatment of pyrexia (fever).	Aspirin Tylenol
Antiseptics	Prevent growth of microorganisms and are applied to living tissue. Disinfectants have some action on nonliving tissue.	For skin irritations and cleansing.	Cepacol pHisoHex Boric acid Furacin
Antitoxins (toxoids and vaccines)	Contain specific antibiotics which provide short-term passive immunity to disease. Serum is obtained from animal blood in which the diseased animal produces the antibodies to fight the disease. (Sometimes human blood is the origin of the antibodies.) Vaccines are composed of certain "antigens" which are usually live disease-causing agents. For vaccination they are weakened or partially detoxified and cause the body to manufacture its own antibodies.	Given to prevent disease or make it less severe in an individual who has been exposed to the disease.	Sabine vaccine Diptheria and tetanus toxoids DPT Measles and mumps virus vaccines

TABLE 22-2. *Continued*

Class	Effects and Actions	Common Use	Examples
Antitussives	Protect mucous membranes from irritation by coating the membrane to prevent the cough reflex by depressing the medulla.	Cough suppressant in allergies or respiratory infections.	Hycodan Tuss-Ornade Romilar Sucrets (lozenges)
Astringents	Change the surface tension of cells. Reduce oiliness of skin and excessive perspiration. Stop bleeding from minor cuts.	Treatment of conditions and forms of dermatitis. Stop bleeding of cuts from shaving, etc.	Zinc oxide Calamine Witch hazel Aluminum acetate solution Aluminum hydroxide gel Tannic acid Styptic pencil
Cardiotonics	Increase strength of myocardial contraction. Pulse strengthens and slows.	Treatment of congestive heart failure.	Digoxin (digitalis)
Cathartics	Cause the bowel to evacuate its contents. Several types of cathartics with different actions are available: fecal softener stimulants (stimulate smooth muscle of the bowel), bulk cathartics (increase fecal matter by adding nonabsorbable substance), saline cathartics. Water is retained in intestine, which promotes peristalsis.	Treatment of constipation. Used also as a preparatory drug for certain diagnostic tests.	Fleet enema Milk of magnesia Ex-Lax Metamucil
Cytotoxins	Poisonous to both normal and cancerous cells. Interfere with cell reproduction.	Used in chemotherapy in treatment of cancer.	Cytoxan 6-Mercaptopurine L-asparaginase

TABLE 22-2. *Continued*

Class	Effects and Actions	Common Use	Examples
Demulcents Emollients Protectives	*Demulcents* protect and coat the mucous membrane. *Emollients* soften, coat, and protect the skin, and can also relieve pain and itching. *Protectives* form a film on the skin to cover raw areas.	Treatment of throat irritations, cough, ulcerations, and cracked, dry skin.	Cold cream Glycerine Tincture of benzoin
Diuretics	Increase the production of urine by their action on renal tubules in the kidney.	Control of edema in cardiac disease such as hypertension. Also control premenstral retention of fluid.	Diuril Lasix Aldactone
Emetics	Cause vomiting by irritating the mucous membrane of the GI tract.	To induce vomiting when a toxic substance has been ingested.	Ipecac
Expectorants	Assist removal of mucus by liquifying tenacious mucus.	Treatment of bronchitis and other respiratory conditions.	Robitussin Terpin hydrate Eucalyptus oil
Hematinics	Stimulate production of blood cells and increase amount of hemoglobin in the blood.	Treatment of anemias.	Ferrous sulfate Imferon
Hemostatics (coagulants)	Stop and control bleeding or hemorrhage.	Treatment of hemophilia (condition of defective clotting). Also used in surgical procedures to stop or control bleeding.	Gelfoam Fibrinogen
Hormones	Used to replace specific hormonal deficiencies in the body.	Treatment of hypothyroidism and diabetes. Other selected uses. Major constituent of oral contraceptives.	Thyroxine Insulin Ovarian hormones

TABLE 22-2. *Continued*

Class	Effects and Actions	Common Use	Examples
Hypnotics Sedatives	Act on the central nervous system and interfere with nerve impulse transmission to the cerebral cortex. Heart rate and respiration are depressed. Depending on the specific drug and dosage, drowsiness, sleep, decreased awareness, loss of muscle coordination, and other changes can occur. The difference between sedative and hypnotic effects is the dosage. Sedatives produce sleep; hypnotics facilitate a feeling of restfulness.	Treatment of convulsions and insomnia. Selected use in specific conditions.	Nembutal Seconal Doriden Placidyl
Tranquilizers	Usually do not depress the central nervous system. Calm the mind and act as muscle relaxants with anticonvulsant properties. Also reduce stress.	Treatment of tension and anxiety. Treats symptoms of neuroses and psychoses. Also used in treatment of muscle spasms.	Librium Equanil Thorazine Valium
Stimulants	Stimulate the operations of the central nervous system and increase the activity of the vasomotor and respiratory centers of the medulla. Act to elevate mood and to suppress fatigue and appetite.	Treatment of obesity, exhaustion, and specific abnormal patterns of behavior.	Benzedrine Dexedrine Tenuate Caffeine

TABLE 22-2. *Continued*

Class	Effects and Actions	Common Use	Examples
Sulfonamides	Interfere with the growth of specific bacteria.	Treatment of certain infectious disorders, especially those affecting the urinary and respiratory tracts, the vagina, and the eye.	Gantrisin Sulfa Sultrin
Vasodilators	Dilate peripheral blood vessels in the heart, skeletal muscles, and various organs. Increase circulation and blood flow to the extremities.	Specific drugs have specific actions and may be used for peripheral vascular disease, dysmenorrhea, angina, and hypertension.	Nitroglycerin Vasodilan Isordil

DRUG THERAPY AND THE ROLE OF THE MEDICAL ASSISTANT

Drug therapy is the use of natural or chemical substances in the treatment of the patient to relieve symptoms and arrest or eliminate the condition or disease. Ordering and prescribing drugs is an alternative every physician utilizes on a routine basis. The physician, although well grounded in general concepts of pharmacology, derives much of his knowledge concerning new drugs from journals and pharmaceutical representatives. This statement does not imply that the physician is deficient in pharmacologic knowledge, but rather that the physician must continually learn and be aware of new developments. The medical assistant's role in drug therapy is to assist the physician to meet the objectives of the treatment. The MA should not only prepare and administer the drug accurately, but also should share with the physician the responsibility of acquiring new knowledge and preventing errors in administration. Medical assistants enhance the physician's credibility whenever they check a reference source when concerns arise related to dosage or any other aspect of drug administration. The physician determines which drug will be prescribed and how it will be administered. The MA checks the PDR or the specific literature on the drug to confirm the order.

Obviously, individual physicians acquire certain drug preferences. As medical assistants become more familiar with the drugs used, they will gain confidence in their own knowledge of drug particulars, how various drugs should be administered, and the normal dosage ranges advised.

PREPARATION FOR DRUG ADMINISTRATION

The administration of drugs is a responsibility of the medical assistant requiring the utmost care because of the gravity of the consequences of error. Certain preparations are essential to the safe and effective administration of medication.

General Rules Concerning Medications

The medical assistant must observe several guidelines to ensure accuracy in the handling and administration of medications. All drugs kept in the office should be labeled accurately. No medication should ever be poured from a container with an illegible label. All drugs should be kept in a locked cabinet which is inaccessible to patients. Outdated or deteriorated drugs should be discarded. Whether dealing with capsules, tablets, liquids, or other forms of medication, the MA must follow these guidelines habitually.

Whenever the medical assistant is involved in the preparation of medications, full attention must be focused on the accurate performance of the task. All distractions must be tuned out since the chance of error will otherwise increase.

The written order should be read and reread to ensure proper understanding of the physician's wishes. If the patient's file cannot be removed from the examining room, the MA should write the order on a note pad. Committing the order to memory is dangerous. If calculations are required and doubt arises, guesswork should be avoided and the physician consulted. The label should be read and reread (1) when removing the drug from the medicine shelf, (2) when pouring, and (3) when returning the medication to the shelf. Liquid medication should be poured at eye level for dosage accuracy.

There is a general rule of "rights" to be observed when preparing and administering medication. The MA must be certain to have the *right medication* being given to the *right patient* at the *right time*, with the *right dosage* and the *right route*.

Dosage Calculations

To calculate dosages in pharmacology, two systems of weight and measurement are used: *metric* and *apothecary*. The medical assistant needs to know how to calculate dosages because a drug often will be ordered in one system but labeled in the other. Since the weight and measurements are not compatible, conversion is necessary and calculation required. Table 22-3 lists the commonly used approximate equivalents. Since calculations may still be necessary, the approximate equivalent weights for apothecary and metric measures are given in Table 22-4. A drug may also be ordered as part of a whole which necessitates the application of mathematical principles.

In the *metric system*, liters (L) refer to volume, grams (Gm) to weight, and meters (m) to length. The metric system is a decimal system. All other units are derived from these by dividing or multiplying by powers of 10:

1. When dividing to make subunits smaller than the basic units, Latin prefixes are used to denote the subunit: deci = 0.1 (1/10); centi = 0.01 (1/100); milli = 0.001 (1/1000).

2. When multiplying to increase the number of basic units, Greek prefixes are used: deka = 10 × unit; hecto = 100 × unit; kilo = 10 × unit.

In the *apothecary system*, the basic units of weight are grain (gr), dram (ʒ), ounce (℥), and pound (lb). Fluid measurements are represented by minims (♏), fluidrams (ʒ), fluidounces (℥), pints (pt), quarts (qt), and gallons (c). Units of measure indicated in the form of symbols are combined with Roman numerals to indicate the number of units; for example, 3 drams would be represented as ʒ iii, and 2 grains would be represented as gr ii. For subunits, however, fractions are used; for example, one-fourth of a grain would be represented as gr ¼.

Although household measurements (teaspoon, tablespoon, etc.) are not conventional medical units, these measurements are most practical when instructing patients in dosage amounts for fluids. Below is a sampling of commonly used household measurements and their metric and apothecary equivalents.

Metric	Apothecary	Household
4-5 ml	1 fluidram	1 teaspoon
15 ml	1 fluidounce	1 tablespoon
240 ml	8 fluidounces	1 glassful

RULES OF CALCULATION

To accurately calculate dosage, both the prescribed amount of the drug and the dosage amount available must be expressed in the same system of measurement. Table 22-3 should be consulted for quick conversion. When the prescribed dosage and amount available are expressed in the same system of measurement, calculation of dosage is possible.

TABLE 22-3. Commonly Used Approximate Equivalents*

Weight		Volume	
Metric	Apothecary	Metric	Apothecary
1 Gm =	15 gr	1 ml =	15-16 minims
0.06 Gm =	1 gr	1 cc =	1 ml
4 Gm =	1 dram	0.06 ml =	1 minim
30 Gm =	1 oz	0.5 ml =	8 minims
1 kg =	2.2 lbs	0.3 ml =	5 minims
		4 ml =	1 fluidram
		30 ml =	1 fl oz
		500 ml =	1 pt
		1000 ml (1 L) =	1 qt

*Reproduced from Saperstein, A. B., and Frazier, M. A.: *Introduction to Nursing Practice.* F. A. Davis, Philadelphia, 1980.

TABLE 22-4.   Approximate Equivalent Weights*

Apothecary			Metric		
gr xv	=	1.0	Gm	=	1000 mg
gr x	=	0.6	Gm	=	600 mg
gr 7½	=	0.5	Gm	=	500 mg
gr v	=	0.3	Gm	=	300 mg
gr iii	=	0.2	Gm	=	200 mg
gr 1½	=	0.1	Gm	=	100 mg
gr 1	=	0.06	Gm	=	60 mg
gr ¾	=	0.05	Gm	=	50 mg
gr ½	=	0.03	Gm	=	30 mg
gr ¼	=	0.015	Gm	=	15 mg
gr ⅙	=	0.010	Gm	=	10 mg
gr ⅛	=	0.008	Gm	=	8 mg
gr 1/12	=	0.005	Gm	=	5 mg
gr 1/15	=	0.004	Gm	=	4 mg
gr 1/20	=	0.0032	Gm	=	3 mg
gr 1/30	=	0.0022	Gm	=	2 mg
gr 1/40	=	0.0015	Gm	=	1.5 mg
gr 1/50	=	0.0012	Gm	=	1.2 mg
gr 1/60	=	0.001	Gm	=	1.0 mg
gr 1/100	=	0.0006	Gm	=	0.6 mg
gr 1/120	=	0.0005	Gm	=	0.5 mg
gr 1/150	=	0.0004	Gm	=	0.4 mg
gr 1/200	=	0.0003	Gm	=	0.3 mg
gr 1/300	=	0.0002	Gm	=	0.2 mg
gr 1/600	=	0.0001	Gm	=	0.1 mg

*Reproduced from Saperstein, A. B., and Frazier, M. A.: *Introduction to Nursing Practice.* F. A. Davis, Philadelphia, 1980.

A ratio and proportion formula is used to calculate the dosage. D = desired or prescribed dosage; H = dosage amount on hand or available; X = the amount to be administered.

The following example utilizes this formula. The physician orders Diuril 30 mg po stat. The dosage on hand is in tablet form, gr ¼ in each tablet. To calculate the dosage:

1. Convert grains to milligrams.

   ¼ gr = 15 mg
   ¼ gr × 60 (60 mg in 1 gr)
   ¼ × 60 = ^{60}/4 = 15 mg (1 tablet)

2. Calculate the dosage using the ratio and proportion formula.

   15 mg per tablet. Dr. ordered 30 mg. Give 2 tablets.

   $$\frac{30 \text{ mg (D)}}{X} = \frac{15 \text{ mg (H)}}{1 \text{ tablet}}$$

$$15X = 30 \text{ mg}$$
$$X = 2 \text{ tablets}$$

Pediatric doses are based on weight or body surface area and determined by the physician.

Preparation of the Patient

Ideally the patient should be informed by the physician that medication is to be administered. Occasionally the patient is informed of the procedure as the medical assistant walks into the room with the medication. *The patient should know what he is receiving and why,* and should be given any special instruction that is required. If a prescription is given, it should be interpreted for the patient by the physician or the medical assistant. This step provides a safety measure as the patient will then check the label for error. *The patient must always be identified prior to administering the medication,* even when familiarity exists, to avoid error. *The patient must always be asked if he is allergic to anything,* and specifically to the drug in question, to avoid a drug reaction. *The medical assistant must witness the patient consume the oral medication,* if administered in the medical office, to ensure that the drug has been taken.

Patient preparation is essential to the safe and accurate administration of medication.

ORAL MEDICATION

Oral medication includes those forms which can be taken by mouth. It is the most widely used route of administration as it is most convenient for both the patient receiving the medication and the individual administering the drug. Although no special equipment is needed, certain acceptable ways of handling and delivering the medication warrant the medical assistant's consideration.

Solid medications (such as tablets) are usually brought to the patient in a small paper cup. A cup of water is carried along with the medication. The purpose of any receptacle for containing the medication is to facilitate pouring and the transfer of the drug without contact with the hands. The medication is poured directly into the bottle cap, and the correct number of tablets are then poured into the cup. Liquids are poured into a calibrated cup. The bottle is held with the pouring side away from the label to avoid soiling it. Water accompanies most medication, whether solid or liquid, unless otherwise advised. Cough preparations, however, should not be followed by water because they have a coating action on the throat.

The general principles related to the administration of all medication are followed. The specific procedure is outlined below.

ADMINISTERING ORAL MEDICATION

Purpose: To administer drugs by mouth safely and effectively for the treatment of disease or unhealthful conditions, or to aid in the diagnosis.

Procedure	*Principle*
1. Select the proper medication and check the label against the medication order. If the drug is unfamiliar, read the insert or refer to the PDR.	1. Checking and rereading prevents error. Obtaining proper information ensures safe, effective administration.
2. Correctly calculate the dosage if necessary.	2. Correct dosage ensures proper action of the drug.
3. While pouring, check the label and if the drug is in tablet form, shake the tablet(s) into the bottle cap and then into the paper cup. Do not handle with fingers. Pour liquid drugs at eye level. Hold the bottle with the label in the palm of the hand. Do not pour back the excess. Be certain of the correct dosage. Shake the liquid first if required. Use only calibrated containers. Wipe the bottle after pouring liquid.	3. This technique avoids contact with the hands which could transfer harmful microorganisms. Liquids are poured at eye level to ensure dosage accuracy. Liquids are sometimes shaken to mix the solution. Keeping the bottle clean ensures that the label will be intact and legible.
4. Read the label when returning the drug to the shelf.	4. Rechecking prevents error.
5. Bring medication and water to the patient. State the patient's name and inquire if there are any allergies.	5. Most medications with the exception of cough syrups can be swallowed with water. Proper patient identification prevents error. Acids and iron preparations are given through a straw to avoid staining and injury to the teeth.
6. Give the medicine cup to the patient. Remain until the patient has swallowed the drug.	6. Ascertain that the physician's orders were followed.
7. Give the patient any necessary instructions and information.	7. Patient education facilitates cooperation and compliance with the physician's orders.
8. Accurately record the procedure on the patient's file: name of drug, amount, route, time, date, and sign with initials.	8. Proper recording is necessary for reference and maintaining legal standards.

PARENTERAL MEDICATION

Parenteral medication includes those forms which can be injected. There are three types of injections that the medical assistant will administer: subcutaneous, intramuscular, and intradermal. The methods of injection differ only in needle gauge and length and in site of injection.

Special equipment is needed to administer parenteral medication. The MA determines the equipment to be used on the basis of the medication order, the viscosity of the solution, the patient's body size, and the site of injection.

Special precautions must be observed when administering injections:

1. Avoid injections into burned areas, scar tissue, swollen or edematous areas, and areas in close proximity to major blood vessels, bony prominences, skin eruptions, and superficial veins and nerves.

2. Use precise technique as improper technique can result in local or systemic infec-

tion. Needles must be sterile, and the injection site and the MA's hands must be clean.

Syringes

A syringe is a barrel-shaped, calibrated container with a plunger (Fig. 22-3). Medication is withdrawn into the syringe in the amount required. Syringes are available in different capacities. Those of $2\frac{1}{2}$ and 5 milliliter capacities are most commonly used and are calibrated in tenths of a milliliter. *Tuberculin syringes* are calibrated in minims, or hundredths of a milliliter, and are used for minute doses such as those injected in tuberculin skin testing. *Insulin syringes* are calibrated in a scale of 100 units which can then be easily made compatible with the prescribed insulin dosage (usually 60 to 100 units daily). A low-dosage, 50-unit syringe is also available.

NEEDLE LENGTH

Needle length refers to how long the needle must be to penetrate the layer of tissue required to absorb the medication. The patient's size (amount of fatty tissue) must also be taken into consideration. For the average adult, a needle length of $1\frac{1}{2}$ inches is usually sufficient to penetrate the muscle layer which lies beneath subcutaneous tissue. For a subcutaneous injection, a length of five-eighths to three-fourths of an inch is usually sufficient. An intradermal injection usually requires a needle one-half inch in length.

NEEDLE GAUGE

The choice of needle gauge, or width, is based on the thickness or viscosity of the medication to be administered. There is an inverse relationship between the width and the gauge numbers assigned. Needle gauges are available in different lengths and range from 27 (thinnest) to 13 (thickest). Thick medications are usually given intramuscularly because they are

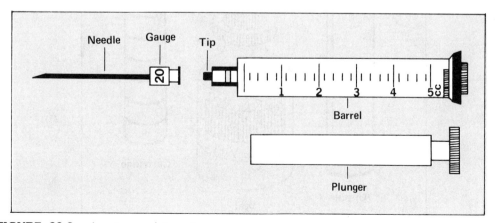

FIGURE 22-3.   A syringe and its parts.

less painfully absorbed. The average gauge for intramuscular (IM) injection is 21 or 22; for subcutaneous injections the gauges are 23 to 25. Intradermal injections require a 25 to 27 gauge needle.

Injected Medication

The medication to be administered by injection may be in the form of (1) a solution in a single or multiple vial (a small bottle with a rubber stopper), (2) a powder in a vial which must be mixed with sterile water to form solution, (3) a solution in an ampule (a small bottle scored to break so that a needle may be inserted and medication withdrawn), or (4) a solution in a cartridge (a specially designed container which fits into a special syringe). Figure 22-4 depicts these forms.

Sites of Injection

SUBCUTANEOUS

Since fatty tissue exists throughout the body, the subcutaneous injection can technically be administered anywhere on the body except the head, neck, hands, and feet. The sites most

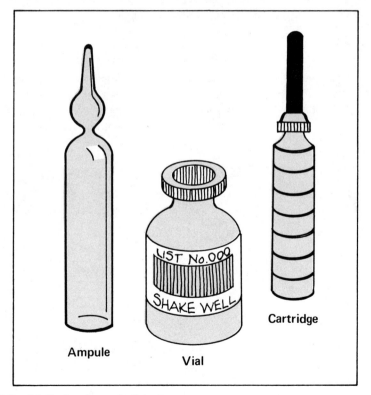

FIGURE 22-4. Medication forms for injections.

frequently used are the upper arms. When the patient must self-administer daily doses of a drug, such as insulin for diabetes, or come to the office for daily or weekly injections, the sites must be alternated and a pattern preestablished. For example, a patient may come to the office for a weekly injection, given subcutaneously. The same arm should be used only every other week to prevent tissue damage and patient discomfort. The diabetic patient usually administers daily doses of insulin in the thighs, selects a large patch on one thigh, and systematically places each daily injection in rows. Usually a month passes before the other thigh is used. The process is continuous.

INTRAMUSCULAR

Intramuscular injections can be administered in any muscle in the body. There are, however, certain preferred sites. Figures 22-5 through 22-8 depict these sites. The site most

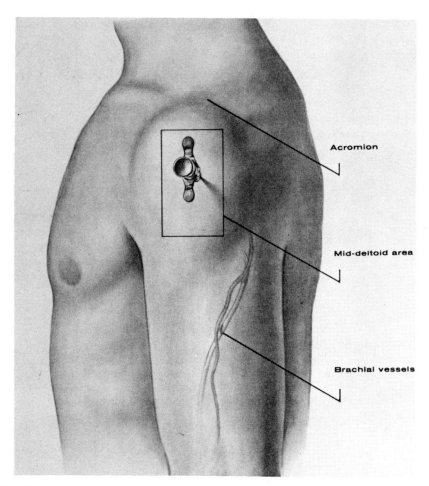

FIGURE 22-5. Mid-deltoid area intramuscular injection site. (Courtesy of Wyeth Laboratories)

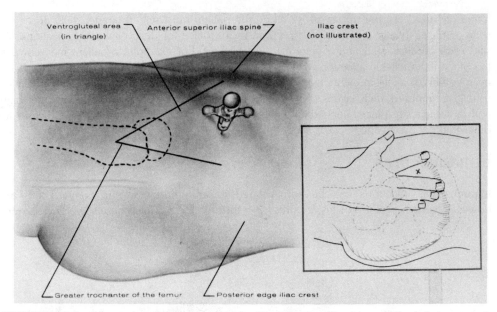

FIGURE 22-6. Ventrogluteal area intramuscular injection site. (Courtesy of Wyeth Laboratories)

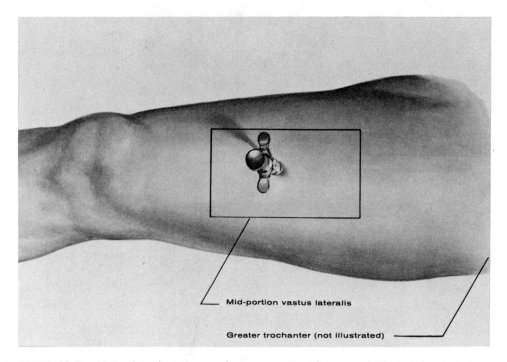

FIGURE 22-7. Vastus lateralis intramuscular injection site. (Courtesy of Wyeth Laboratories)

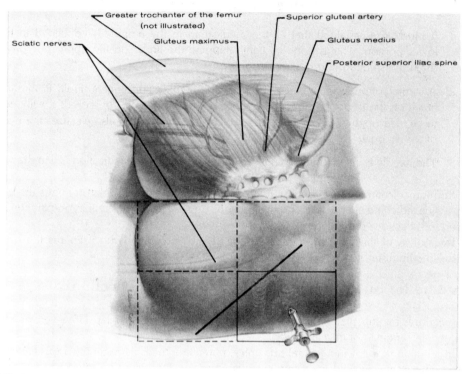

FIGURE 22-8. Gluteus medius intramuscular injection site. (Courtesy of Wyeth Laboratories)

commonly chosen for intramuscular injections is the gluteus maximus muscle in the buttocks.

INTRADERMAL

The site of choice for intradermal injections is the upper arm. The epidermis and dermis are penetrated for injection of the medication.

Preparation of Medication for Injection

Vials are the most common receptacles used to contain solution for injection. Withdrawal of medication from a vial is described in the procedure for subcutaneous injection. The medication often comes in powder form and must be mixed with sterile water to form solution. Specific directions for mixing sterile solutions from powder are enclosed with the drug package. The amount of sterile water to be injected into the powder is specified, and general instructions are given for agitating the vial to aid dissolution of the powder.

Obtaining the solution from an ampule involves the following steps:

1. It must be ascertained that all the medication in the ampule is contained in the lower portion. This is done by lightly tapping the finger on the upper portion to drain the solution into the lower portion.

2. A sterile cotton swab is placed between the ampule and fingers. Hold firmly and break off the upper portion where scored. If the ampule is not scored, it will need to be filed open. The alcohol swab protects the fingers and also cleanses the neck of the ampule.

3. The needle is inserted into the neck of the bottle and the medication is withdrawn.

Some medications for injection come packaged in a cartridge which requires the use of a special needle and syringe unit. For instructions on how to use this unit in preparation of the drug for injection, see Figure 22-9.

Regardless of the drug preparation required, the individual who prepares the drug should also administer it to avoid error.

Procedure for Subcutaneous and Intramuscular Injection

The procedures for subcutaneous and intramuscular injections are similar. However, needle gauge, length, and site of injection differ.

In addition to following general principles, parenteral medication requires specific procedures. The steps involved in giving subcutaneous and intramuscular injections are outlined in the procedure guides which follow. The major objective in the administration of any medication is to perform the procedure safely and accurately.

SUBCUTANEOUS INJECTION

Purpose: To follow the physician's orders in obtaining rapid absorption of the drug when it is inadvisable to administer it by mouth or when it would be rendered ineffective by digestive juices.

Procedure	*Principle*
1. Select the drug and equipment needed (needle, syringe, and alcohol swab). A disposable $2\frac{1}{2}$ ml syringe with a needle gauge of 25, and a needle length of $\frac{5}{8}$ inch will usually be used.	1. Organization of materials results in the economy of time and effort.
2. Check the drug against the medication order.	2. Checking prevents mistakes.
3. Properly prepare the drug. a. Cleanse the top of the vial with an alcohol swab. b. Remove the cap from the selected syringe. (Do not touch the needle with fin-	3. Proper preparation ensures correct dosage. a. Prevents contamination. b. Inserting air into the syringe and then into the vial increases the air pressure in the

gers.) While holding the syringe at eye level, withdraw the plunger to insert an amount of air in the syringe identical to the amount of required dosage to be withdrawn.

c. With the vial firmly on the work surface, insert the needle into the vial, just above the solution line, and release the air by pushing the plunger.

d. Lift up the connected vial and syringe to eye level. Hold the vial with the label and calibrated syringe facing up in the palm of one hand. With the thumb and forefinger of the other hand, grasp the plunger and withdraw the desired dosage.

e. Recap the needle.

f. Check for air bubbles. A small bubble can be expelled by tapping the syringe with the fingers and pushing the plunger slightly.

vial, facilitating the withdrawal of medication.

c. If air is inserted into the solution, bubbles will form and make removal of the medication more difficult.

d. Label faces up to check for correct medication and prevent chance of error.

e. The needle must be kept sterile. Capping reduces the chance of contamination while the syringe is being transported to the patient.

f. A large air bubble will displace medication and alter the dosage. A bubble at the top will be injected first and make the injection and absorption of medication difficult. However, some professionals advise adding 0.2 ml of air to the accurate dosage when the syringe is inverted as it would be for injection since the air bubble would now be administered after all the solution has been injected. This clears the medication from the needle and prevents leakage of fluid back through subcutaneous tissue at the site of injection.

4. Identify the patient, and question for allergies.

5. Using an alcohol swab, firmly but gently massage the site chosen for injection. Massage in a circular motion. Remove the cap from the needle.

6. Grasp the large area surrounding the site in a pinching or cushioning fashion.

7. Position one hand grasping the site with a cotton swab between the fingers for later use. Hold the syringe in a dart-like fashion in the other hand and inject the needle very quickly at a 45° angle. The entire needle should be inserted.

8. Immediately bring the fingers and thumb of the other hand to grasp the hub of the needle.

9. Withdraw the plunger slightly to check for blood.

4. Questioning prevents error and avoids complications.

5. Massage cleanses the area by friction and helps to dull the pain sensations.

6. Cushioning the subcutaneous tissue helps ensure that the needle will penetrate subcutaneous tissue.

7. The length of the needle is imbedded to ensure reaching the subcutaneous layer. Deep subcutaneous injections are administered at a 90° angle. Deep subcutaneous injections are used for solutions exceeding $2\frac{1}{2}$ ml. (See Figure 22-10.)

8. Grasping the hub prevents the needle from being withdrawn with the force of withdrawing the plunger.

9. If blood is present, then a blood vessel has been penetrated and the needle must be removed.

10. If no blood is present, push the plunger and inject the medicine.

10. Firm, steady pressure allows for continuous absorption.

11. Hold the cotton swab next to the hub. Quickly lift out and massage the area with the swab.

11. Swabbing helps distribute medication into the tissue for absorption and dulls the pain sensation.

12. Record the procedure. Name of drug, amount, route, date, and time are noted, followed by the medical assistant's initials.

12. Recording is necessary for future reference and quality health care.

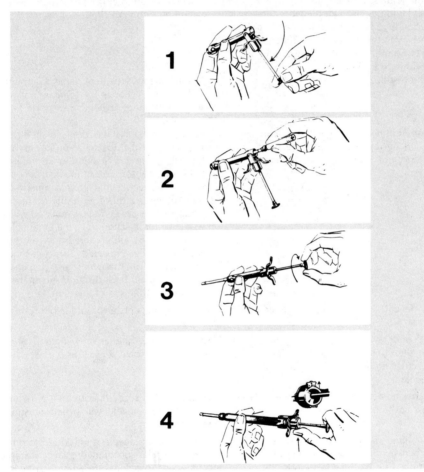

FIGURE 22-9. Loading a cartridge-needle unit syringe. 1. Grasp barrel of syringe in one hand. With other hand, pull back firmly on plunger and swing the entire handle-section downward so that it locks at right angle to the barrel. 2. Insert cartridge-needle unit, needle end first, into the barrel. Engage needle ferrule by rotating it clockwise in threads at front end of syringe. 3. Swing plunger back into place and attach end to the threaded shaft of piston. Hold metal syringe barrel—not glass cartridge—with one hand and rotate plunger until both ends of cartridge-needle unit are fully, but lightly, engaged. To maintain sterility, leave rubber sheath in place until just before use. 4. The 2-cc syringe can be used for a 1-cc syringe. Engage both ends and push the slide through so the number "1" appears. After use, the syringe automatically resets itself for 2 cc. (Courtesy of Wyeth Laboratories.)

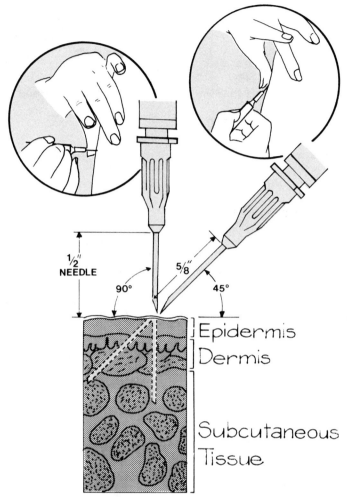

FIGURE 22-10. Subcutaneous and deep subcutaneous injections. The $^5/_8$ inch needle is injected at a 45-degree angle to the skin. The $^1/_2$ inch needle is inserted at a 90-degree angle to the skin. Because of the shortness of the needle length, it remains within the subcutaneous tissue, not the muscle. (Note inserts depicting angles of needle to subcutaneous tissue of upper arm.) (Reproduced from Saperstein, A. B., and Frazier, M. A.: *Introduction to Nursing Practice.* F. A. Davis, Philadelphia, 1980.)

INTRAMUSCULAR INJECTION

Purpose: To obtain the most rapid absorption of the drug (with the exception of IV), or when the drug cannot be tolerated in the gastrointestinal tract or injested because of patient's condition.

Procedure	*Principle*
1. Select the drug and equipment. A syringe (needle gauge 22, length 1½ inches) and an alcohol swab are usually required.	1. Organization of materials results in economy of time and effort.
2. Check the drug label against the medication order.	2. Checking prevents errors.
3. Withdraw the medication following the procedure for preparation.	3. Careful preparation ensures accurate dosage.
4. Identify the patient and question for allergies.	4. Proper questioning prevents error and complications.
5. Instruct the patient to assume the side-lying position and expose the hip. Drape properly. Draw imaginary lines as illustrated earlier.	5. The imaginary lines are drawn to avoid inserting the needle in the sciatic nerve which would cause injury and pain.
6. Massage the injection site with an alcohol swab.	6. Massaging cleanses the area and dulls the pain sensation.
7. Using the thumb and first two fingers, grasp the tissue and press down firmly.	7. Compression of tissue ensures needle entry into muscle.
8. With the cap removed from the needle, inject the syringe in a dart-like fashion at a 90° angle. (See Figure 22-11.)	8. This angle is necessary to penetrate the muscle layer.
9. With thumb and forefinger grasping the hub, aspirate the plunger to check for blood.	9. Grasping the hub ensures that the needle will not be withdrawn with the force of withdrawing the plunger. Blood in the syringe indicates that a blood vessel has been penetrated. The needle would then be withdrawn to avoid injecting the medication into the bloodstream.
10. Push the plunger down if no blood is present in the syringe. When the medication is completely injected, withdraw the syringe quickly and massage the site with an alcohol swab.	10. Quick withdrawal avoids pain and injury. Massage aids in distribution and absorption of medication and dulls the sensations.
11. Record the procedure: name of drug, amount, route, time, and date, followed by the medical assistant's initials.	11. Complete recording is necessary for continued quality care and future reference.
12. Dispose of the needle and syringe if not reusable.	12. Needles are broken to avoid being reused.

Procedure for Intradermal Injection

The administration of intradermal injections is similar to that of subcutaneous and intramuscular injections, as the following steps indicate:

1. Prepare the syringe and medication. A 27-gauge, ⅝-inch needle is used.

2. Withdraw the medication into the syringe.

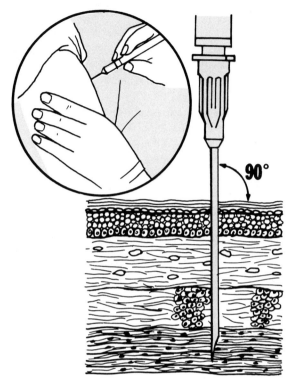

FIGURE 22-11. Intramuscular route of medication administration. (Reproduced from Saperstein, A. B., and Frazier, M. A.: *Introduction to Nursing Practice.* F. A. Davis, Philadelphia, 1980.)

3. Prepare the inner surface of the forearm with an alcohol swab.

4. Rest the patient's forearm in the palm of the hand and pull the skin tightly across the forearm with the fingers.

5. Hold the syringe parallel to the skin surface and slide the needle into the dermis.

6. Inject the medication.

7. Blot the area of injection while applying slight pressure. Massaging may alter drug response when used for allergy testing.

8. Follow the physician's instructions for determining the presence of the intended action of the drug.

9. Record the procedure.

10. Instruct the patient, if necessary, to observe the site for certain changes which will have to be reported to the physician within a specified period of time.

PATIENT TEACHING

Patient teaching related to drug administration involves informing the patient of certain aspects of drug therapy. The patient should be fully informed regarding the name and type of medication, how it is to be taken, and any precautions, contraindications, and side effects which particularly apply to the individual.

In addition, patients should be made aware of their own responsibilities pertaining to prescribed drugs. Misinformation is a frequent cause of the lack of patient compliance so prevalent in drug therapy. Emphasis should be placed on instructing the patient to take all of the drug prescribed. If the full dosage is altered for the length of time prescribed, the objectives for treatment are undermined. Accurate spacing of the drug is also imperative to successful treatment. It should be explained to the patient that taking the drug exactly as ordered will maintain adequate levels of the drug circulating in the blood stream.

Usually oral medication presents no difficulty to the patient's coping behaviors. Parenteral drugs, however, can be traumatic for the adult as well as the child. An injection given properly will not cause tremendous pain. The child will not be especially reassured when this statement is made. Pinching the top of the hand simulates an intramuscular injection and can be used for demonstration.

For adults, embarrassment is another factor to be considered when administering the injection in the buttocks. The medical assistant needs to meet the patient's needs for privacy, comfort, and reassurance when giving the injection. The procedure should be performed as quickly as possible to avoid increased apprehension.

It should be noted that many physicians keep orders for injection in the medical office to a minimum because of the irreversibility of the side effects which may occur. When administered, the medical assistant should instruct the patient to wait approximately 30 minutes after injection to be sure that the drug produces no undesired effects. Obviously, the MA needs first to be aware of the potential side effects.

The medical assistant must remember that the more the patient understands about how to take the medicine and why it is being prescribed, the greater the possibility of successful treatment.

SUMMARY

The medical assistant who will be administering drugs in the physician's office must clearly understand the basic concepts of drug administration. The responsibility of participating in this treatment alternative is perhaps the gravest of the clinical MA's functions since error could be lethal.

This chapter provides a further integration of the system of knowledge and skills for which the medical assistant is responsible. As with diet therapy, the drug classification table and other information contained in this chapter provide MAs with an expanded perception of the treatment of disease and their own involvement.

The medical assistant should not be fearful of drug administration, but rather should acquire respect for the process and respond to the challenge to continue to maintain high standards of practice.

APPLICATION EXERCISES

Solve the following dosage problems:

1. The physician orders 500 mg Diuril po stat. You have 250-mg tablets on hand.

2. The physician orders Isuprel 1 fluidounce stat. You have medicine cups calibrated in milliliters.

3. The physician orders Demerol 75 mg IM stat. The Demerol bottle on hand is labeled 50 mg per ml.

Translate the following prescription orders:

1. 250 mg Penicillin q.i.d. po.

2. 25 mg Seconal h.s. po.

3. 0.5 Gm Gantrisin b.i.d. po.

4. 10 mg Librax a.c. and h.s. po.

5. 500 mg Tetracycline IM stat.

Problem-Solving Exercises

Discuss solutions to the following situations:

1. You are about to administer an injection to Mrs. X. She refuses to cooperate.

2. After administering medication, you realize that you gave the wrong dose.

3. As you walk into the examining room, the medication spills onto the floor.

4. You are giving an injection and when you withdraw the plunger, you aspirate blood.

5. You notice that the prescription pad is missing from the examination room.

6. You are newly employed and when about to administer a drug, you notice that its expiration date has passed.

7. Mrs. J. is swallowing the medication and begins to cough. Some of the drug is spit out.

8. Mrs. L. calls the office and states that she is feeling flushed and dizzy. She was in the office three days before and was placed on medication.

Role-Playing Exercises

Students are assigned the roles of patient and medical assistant. The class discusses the responses of the student assigned to be the MA.

1. Mrs. T. calls and states that she is not feeling well and that the prescribed drug is "not working."

2. Mr. K. calls and states that his stomach is upset by the medication prescribed.

3. Mrs. C. calls and states that she needs a refill.

4. Instruct Mrs. P., a diabetic patient, how to give daily injections. Encourage the patient to ask questions.

5. Instruct Mr. Z. how to take cough syrup. Encourage the patient to ask questions.

6. Explain to Mrs. R. why it is necessary to take her medicine as directed. Encourage the patient to ask questions.

COMPLETING THE LEARNING LOOP

It is clear that the clinical medical assistant has an extremely important part in the treatment phases of office medical practice. The administration of drugs is a serious responsibility and requires an awareness of proper technique and a continuing acquisition of new knowledge.

Another treatment modality—office surgery—is discussed in the next chapter. With each presentation of new material, the medical assistant is seen to become more diversified in responsibilities and to possess ever broader competencies in the delivery of personal health care.

BIBLIOGRAPHY

Aspenheim, M. K., and Eisenhauer, L.: *The Pharmacologic Basis of Patient Care*. W. B. Saunders, Philadelphia, 1977.
Johns, M. P., et al.: *Case Studies in Drug Therapy*. Macmillan, New York, 1979.
Plein, J., and Plein, E.: *Fundamentals of Medications*. Drug Intelligence Publications, Hamilton, Ill., 1974.
Raffauf, R. F., and Warner, V. D.: *Introduction to Drug Analysis*. F. A. Davis, Philadelphia, 1978.
Rodman, M. J., and Smith, D. W.: *Pharmacology and Drug Therapy in Nursing*, ed. 2. J. B. Lippincott, Philadelphia, 1979.
Ryan, S. A., and Clayton, B. D.: *Handbook of Practical Pharmacology*. C. V. Mosby, St. Louis, 1977.
Wang, R. I.: *Practical Drug Therapy*. J. B. Lippincott, Philadelphia, 1979.
Worley, E.: *Pharmacology and Medications*. F. A. Davis, Philadelphia, 1976.

CHAPTER 23

MEDICAL OFFICE SURGERY

SPECIFIC OBJECTIVES

Upon completion of this chapter you will be able to:

1. Describe patient preparation for surgical procedures.

2. Identify surgical instruments and describe their use.

3. Define the concepts and describe the principles of asepsis.

4. Define surgical asepsis and list the techniques involved.

5. Demonstrate techniques for handwashing, gloving, and handling sterile supplies, and describe their application.

6. Describe the medical assistant's role in assisting with specific minor surgical procedures and preparing tray setups.

7. Demonstrate the application of sterile and nonsterile dressings and describe their use.

8. Define sterilization and disinfection and describe the methods of each.

INTRODUCTION

Minor surgery is sometimes performed in the medical office. Minor surgery can be defined as a surgical procedure which does not require general anesthesia. Debridement (cleansing) and suturing of lacerations, suture removal, abscess drainage, removal of infected and injured nails, and excision of small growths are examples of surgical procedures more commonly performed in the medical office.

The medical assistant must be aware of the general principles which apply to surgical procedures and must acquire certain specialized skills to effectively assist the physician.

Depending on the type of practice and the office facilities available, minor surgery may be performed only seldom or quite often. Physicians working in rural areas are more likely to perform office surgery than their urban counterparts.

PATIENT PREPARATION

Preparing the patient for office surgery includes preoperative instruction, explanation, consent forms, positioning and draping, and skin preparation.

Preoperative Instruction and Explanation

While it is the physician's responsibility to inform the patient of the need for surgery and to describe the procedure, the medical assistant must reinforce the physician by reassuring the patient, answering questions, and providing clarification. Specific instructions must be given to the patient if some of the preoperative preparation will be the patient's responsibility. For example, the patient may be requested to apply wet soaks to an abscess for a period of time prior to the scheduled surgery.

Consent Forms

Written forms giving the physician permission to perform surgery must be signed by the patient before the procedure can be initiated. While there are some exceptions to obtaining written consent, most physicians feel that written permissions provide a necessary legal protection for all concerned. *Informed consent* is the accepted standard for both major and minor surgery. As was discussed in Chapter 13, informed consent signifies that the patient has been properly and thoroughly informed as to how and why the procedure is being performed, its possible consequences, alternative methods of treatment, probabilities of success, and the expenses entailed.

Positioning and Draping

The general principles of positioning and draping apply to surgical procedures. It is extremely important, however, in anticipation of the surgical procedure to be performed, that all clothing and jewelry be removed which could possibly fall in the physician's way. In this instance, the concern for fully exposed areas is not only for the physician's convenience and visibility, but also to avoid contamination of the area. Every step should be taken to ensure the patient's comfort as the length of the procedure or required position may tend to cause the patient discomfort.

Skin Preparation

It is important to remember that the skin cannot be sterilized. Some microorganisms will remain on the skin even after thorough cleansing. The objective of presurgical skin preparation is to remove or weaken microorganisms sufficiently to reduce the likelihood of introducing infectious materials into the incised area.

If the area to be incised is covered with hair, it is removed. Because bacteria clings to hair, the area is shaved before skin cleansing begins. A wet rather than dry shave is preferred to reduce the potential for cuts and scrapes. The hair should be shaved in the direction of growth for more complete removal.

The general skin preparation procedure includes:

1. Wet prep if required.

2. Rigorous cleansing with antiseptic soap.

3. Rinsing and drying.

4. Antiseptic painting of the skin (usually an orange or red antiseptic solution such as iodine) which begins in the center and works outward without retracing the motions and is large enough in area to extend under the sterile window (fenestrated) drape which will be placed over the area.

These preparatory techniques ready the skin for surgery.

ROOM PREPARATION

If surgery is frequently performed in the office, a specially equipped room may be reserved for such use. More commonly, however, an examination room will require some preparation to facilitate the procedure.

Lighting

Adequate overhead lighting is required. After the patient's skin has been prepared, lighting should be positioned directly over the area to provide the physician with optimum visibility. During the procedure, the medical assistant may need to adjust the lighting several times as the physician would contaminate his sterile gloves were he to touch the lighting fixture. Direct light is essential to avoid error.

Work Area

A movable, height-adjustable table should be provided which will support the surgical equipment. The table should be within reasonable proximity to the physician to avoid dropping or contaminating the instruments by reaching over the patient.

SURGICAL INSTRUMENTS

Surgical instruments are precision instruments designed for use in internal operative procedures. Instruments are named according to use and manufacturer.

The medical assistant should be able to identify a large variety of surgical instruments, and must know how they are used and be able to select the correct instruments for specific procedures. The general surgical setup consists of several instruments. Figure 23-1 illustrates the tray setup for minor surgery. Some instruments are used for many purposes and procedures, while others are used only for one purpose in a specific procedure.

Scalpels

Scalpels are knives used to make incisions. They are available either as disposable or reusable instruments. There are several shapes and sizes of blades designed for creating various types of incisions in certain areas of the body. Figure 23-2 illustrates the most commonly used blades and handles.

Surgical Scissors

Surgical scissors are used primarily to cut tissue and sutures. Scissor blades touch precisely at the tips and are curved or straight to meet various needs. Blade points are either sharp or blunt and can be combined in one pair (Fig. 23-3). The probe at the end of the tip of the scissors is used to slide under bandages for cutting the dressing without injuring the skin. Stitch scissors are designed with a hook or beak to get under the suture and sever it (Fig. 23-4).

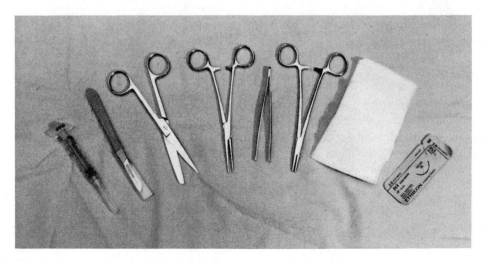

FIGURE 23-1. General surgical tray setup.

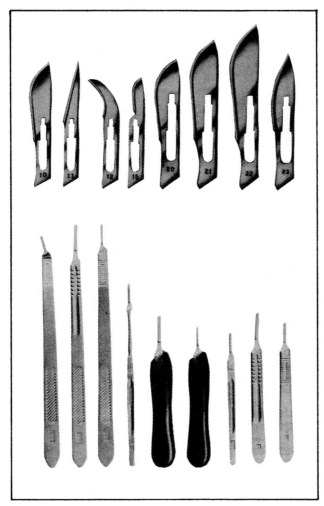

FIGURE 23-2. Scalpel blades and handles in common use. (Courtesy of General Medical Corporation)

Forceps

Forceps are instruments designed to grasp objects or tissue. There are several types (Fig. 23-5). *Hemostatic forceps,* or "hemostats," when applied to a blood vessel, grasp tightly enough to stop the flow of blood. This is an important instrument, especially in major surgery where many hemostats will be used simultaneously to hold "bleeder" vessels until they can be sutured. Their tips are straight or curved with a variety of types of serrations or teeth and different lengths and sizes to meet special needs. The handle clamps together to prevent slipping and serves to hold the hemostat in place without using hands. *Tissue*

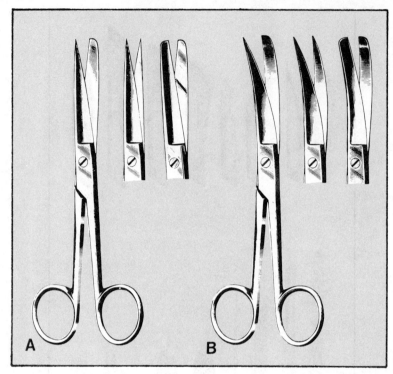

FIGURE 23-3.   Surgical scissors: (A) straight; (B) curved. (Courtesy of Herwig Surgical Instrument Company)

forceps are used specifically to grasp tissue. *Thumb forceps* are used to grasp tissue, dressings, and other sterile objects. In surgery they are primarily used to grasp and apply dressings. They are available in lengths up to 12 inches with serrations varying from coarse to fine.

  Lucae bayonet forceps are used primarily to remove foreign bodies from the ear and nose. They are curved in such a fashion as to permit the entry of scopes for visualization. Lengths up to 8½ inches are available. *Splinter forceps* are designed to grasp foreign bodies imbeded in the skin or under the nails. The tips are usually fine and pointed. *Sterilizer forceps* are used to remove sterile objects from containers and sterilizers. Objects such as syringes, metal instruments, and dressing packs can be grasped by the jaws of these forceps.

Needle Holders

One example of a needle holder, an instrument used to grasp the needle during a suturing procedure, is shown in Figure 23-6. The curved needle fits into the special slot inside the tip. The handle clamp prevents slipping. A variety of lengths and jaw sizes are available for holding various sizes of needles.

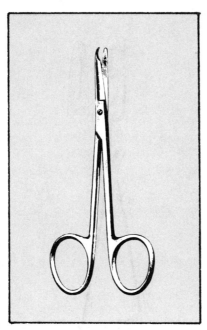

FIGURE 23-4. Spencer stitch scissors. (Courtesy of Herwig Surgical Instrument Company)

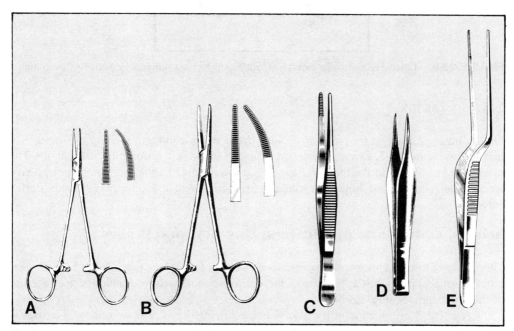

FIGURE 23-5. Hemostatic forceps: (A) Halstead-Mosquito; (B) Kelly-Murphy. C. Dressing forceps. D. Feilchenfeld splinter forceps. E. Lucae ear forceps. (Courtesy of Herwig Surgical Instrument Company)

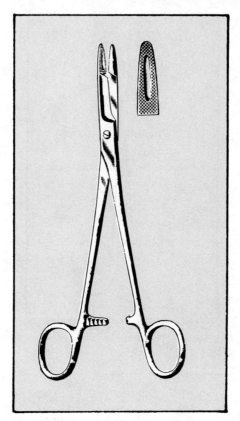

FIGURE 23-6. Olsen-Hegar needle holder. (Courtesy of Herwig Surgical Instrument Company)

Towel Clamps

One example of a clamp for grasping a sterile drape or toweling and holding it in place is illustrated in Figure 23-7. Drapes are used to create a sterile field around the surgical site. The drape can be secured to the incision flaps with a towel clamp as the sharp points can pierce tissue. The handle clasp holds the clamp in place, freeing the physician's hands during surgery.

Scopes, Obturators, Applicators, Directors and Probes

This group of instruments is used to enter body cavities for various purposes in both surgical and nonsurgical procedures. Surgery of the ear, nose, and rectum usually involves the use of these instruments (Fig. 23-8).

A *scope* is an instrument used to visualize the interior of a body orifice. It is usually equipped with a light source. A scope differs from a speculum in that a speculum has movable parts to widen the orifice and is not usually lighted. An example of the former is the sigmoidoscope; an example of the latter is the vaginal speculum.

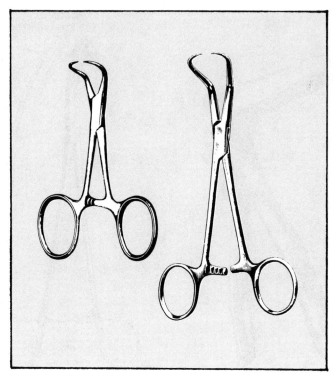

FIGURE 23-7. Backhaus towel clamps. (Courtesy of Herwig Surgical Instrument Company)

An *obturator* is an instrument which fits inside a scope and protrudes forward to guide the scope into the canal or body cavity. Some obturators also puncture tissue for insertion.

An *applicator* is a long-handled instrument used to apply medication by twisting cotton at the top. These can usually be inserted through the scope.

A *director* is an instrument, often grooved, used to guide the direction and depth of a surgical incision.

Probes are instruments used to explore cavities, wounds, or foreign bodies. The ends may be straight or curved to facilitate conformity to the shape of the canal or cavity.

Instruments with Specialized Applications

A *fingernail drill* is used to perforate the injured nail when a blood clot or infection makes drainage and pressure release necessary. *Extractors* are used to remove substances (such as comedones, or blackheads) from the superficial layer of skin (Fig. 23-9).

Ear, Nose and Throat Instruments

Various ear, nose and throat instruments are pictured in Figure 23-10. *Snares* have a sharp cutting wire which removes polyps effectively. They are available in sizes to insert in the

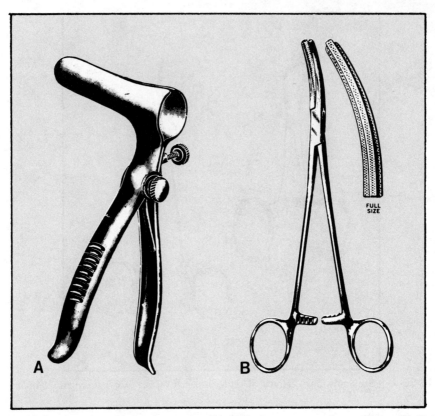

FIGURE 23-8. Rectal surgical instruments: (A) Bodenhammer rectal speculum; (B) Buie pile clamp. (Courtesy of Herwig Surgical Instrument Company)

nose or ear. *"Alligator" forceps* are so termed because of the appearance of their jaw closure. Such forceps are used to insert through a speculum in the ear or nose to remove foreign bodies. The *Wieder tongue depressor* is a metal strip which holds the tongue in place during a procedure or prolonged examination. *Ear curettes* are used to scrape accumulated or impacted cerumen from the ear canal. A *eustachian catheter* is a tube through which air can be blown into the eustachian canal, through the nasopharynx, and into the middle ear cavity. It is often used to clear an obstruction or to test the potency of the canal. *Retractors* are used to separate incisions for expanded visualization. Finally, a *trocar* is a set of instruments used to drain fluid from a cavity by piercing the site. The set consists of a cannule (outer tube) and a stylette (sharp, pointed instrument).

Biopsy Instruments

Biopsy is the removal of tissue for examination, usually for the detection of cancer cells. Biopsies are rarely performed in the medical office. If a biopsy is performed in the office,

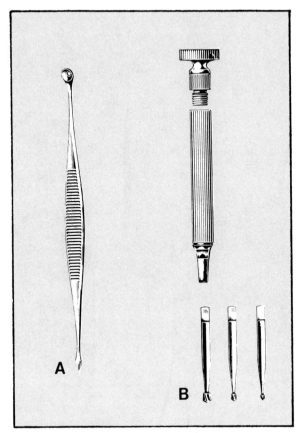

FIGURE 23-9. Instruments with special applications: (A) Saafield comedone extractor; (B) standard fingernail drill. (Courtesy of Herwig Surgical Instrument Company)

usually it will be of the rectal region and will be accomplished by inserting a *rectal biopsy punch* through a proctoscope.

Gynecologic Instruments

Various gynecologic instruments are pictured in Figure 23-11.

The *curette* is an example of an instrument used in the medical office to scrape cells from the cervix for a pap test, to remove minor polyps, and to obtain secretion samples for testing.

The *vaginal speculum* is an instrument for opening and exposing the interior of the vaginal canal for proper visualization.

Dressing forceps are used to hold a dressing in place to absorb discharge or to apply medication to the cervix and vaginal walls. Other gynecologic forceps include the vulsellum forceps and the tenaculum forceps, which are used to grasp cervical or vaginal tissue.

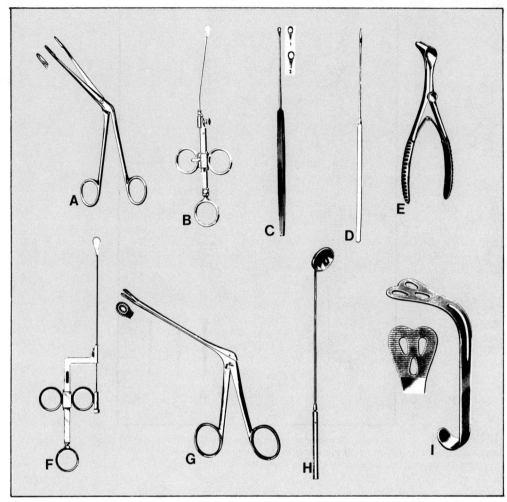

FIGURE 23-10. Ear, nose and throat instruments: (A) Hartman ear dressing forceps; (B) Krause ear snare; (C) Shapleigh ear curette; (D) myringotomy knife; (E) Vienna nasal speculum; (F) Wilde (Bruening) nasal snare; (G) Ferris-Smith alligator forceps; (H) laryngeal mirror; (I) Wieder tongue depressor. (Courtesy of Herwig Surgical Instrument Company)

The *pelvimeter* is an instrument used to measure the female pelvis to determine the adequacy of the pelvic basin for pregnancy and delivery.

ASEPSIS

A primary concern in any surgical procedure is the prevention of infection. Infectious material is airborne and can be transmitted through any activity which disturbs the air current. In major surgery, precautions are precise. In the hospital or medical center, a special surgical unit is reserved, special clothing is worn (sterile gloves, gown, face masks, caps),

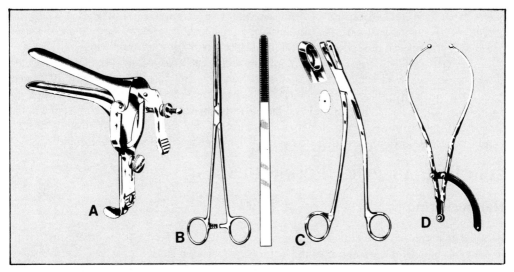

FIGURE 23-11. Gynecologic instruments: (A) Pederson vaginal speculum; (B) Bozeman uterine dressing forceps; (C) Gellhorn cervical biopsy forceps; (D) Martin pelvimeter. (Courtesy of Herwig Surgical Instrument Company)

sterile instruments are used, and the environment is specially prepared for surgical procedures.

In the medical office, minor surgery also involves the risk of infection. While minor medical office surgery does not require the elaborate preparation of major surgery, aseptic technique must be observed to control contamination by infectious substances and to prevent surgical complications.

Asepsis is a term applied to the control and elimination of all disease-producing organisms. (*A* means without, and *sepsis* means decay.) Various techniques are involved in accomplishing the objective of asepsis. Asepsis interferes with the fertility of the components necessary to promote infectious growth. These components include the *agent,* a factor which can cause the disease; the *host,* the vulnerable recipient of the agent; and the *environment,* the arrangement of conditions which support microbial life. Aseptic techniques impose changes in one or all of the components. These will be explored in this chapter, but first the medical assistant must acquire a clear understanding of the concept of asepsis.

Asepsis consists of two categories: medical asepsis and surgical asepsis.

The major objective in medical asepsis is to reduce the number of pathogens (disease-producing organisms) and inhibit their transmission. Techniques involved in medical asepsis are said to be "clean." Handwashing before performing clinical procedures is an example of medical asepsis. Removing a lid from a container which houses clean or sterile equipment and placing it upside-down on the counter top is medical asepsis, since placing it face down would increase the possibility of contamination of the inner lid. Pouring oral medication into the bottle cap rather than the hand is likewise medical asepsis.

The major objective in surgical asepsis is to free the surgical site of *all* microbial life and its spores. Techniques involved in surgical asepsis are said to be "sterile." Wearing sterile gloves to apply a sterile dressing is surgical asepsis. Using sterilized instruments in a surgical procedure also is surgical asepsis. Administering an injection requires surgical asepsis. For all surgical and special procedures, therefore, sterile techniques are observed.

Important rules to remember in applying aseptic techniques are (1) that clean must always go against clean (clean hands against a clean uniform); (2) that unclean must always go against unclean (soiled dressings in waste disposal); (3) that sterile must always go against sterile (sterile gloves for holding sterile instruments); and (4) that nonsterile must always go against nonsterile (in urinary catheterization, for example, the nonsterile gloved hand retracts the labia for insertion of the sterile catheter by the sterile gloved hand).

SURGICAL ASEPTIC TECHNIQUES

Handwashing

Because the skin, in the course of the day, continually acquires microorganisms which under the right conditions can become pathogenic (disease-causing), aseptic handwashing technique is essential. Medical aseptic handwashing becomes a surgical scrub by including the adaptations described in the procedure guide which follows.

Although sterilizing the skin is impossible, it can be rendered "clean" and prepared surgically by following the steps listed below. Upon completion of a surgical scrub, the number of microorganisms will be reduced and the transfer capability of those viable will be weakened, because the causal relationship triangle (host, agent, environment) is interrupted by the surgical scrub.

MEDICAL ASEPTIC HANDWASHING

Purpose: To reduce the number and potency of microorganisms on the hands and thereby decrease the likelihood of transfer.

Procedure	Principle
1. Remove jewelry.	1. Microorganisms can accumulate on inanimate objects.
2. Stand away from sink.	2. The sink harbors microorganisms which can be transferred to clothing or skin.
3. Open faucets and adjust to comfortable temperature.	3. Running water is one of the key elements in aseptic cleansing. Temperature of the water, however, is irrelevant since hot water does not affect the presence of microorganisms and tends to dry and chap the skin, increasing vulnerability to the lodging of microorganisms.
4. Wet the hands and wrists while keeping them directed downward.	4. This avoids contamination of the arms since water would run down from raised wet hands, thus picking up microorganisms from the arms and carrying them back down to the hands.

5. Apply a cleansing agent.

5. An agent which has bacteriostatic and oil-removal qualities is required.

6. Scrub hands and wrists vigorously, soaping and scrubbing the crevices between fingers and around fingernails for approximately 2 minutes.

6. Friction and the cleansing agent are the other key factors which disturb the activity of microorganisms. Friction is perhaps most effective because the motion dislodges many of the organisms.

7. Rinse hands thoroughly.

7. Running water rinses the organisms away.

8. Pat hands dry with paper toweling, working from the wrists to the fingertips.

8. Rubbing helps cause chapping. Hand lotion can counteract excessive dryness which occurs with frequent handwashing.

9. Turn off the faucet with a dry paper towel.

9. The faucet is unclean since the procedure began with turning it on. The toweling prevents contact.

10. Replace jewelry if cleansed.

10. Plain bands such as wedding rings and other keepsakes can be worn if they have been scrubbed and placed in disinfectant solution. It is preferable to avoid wearing hand jewelry in the medical office.

SURGICAL SCRUB

Purpose: To adapt the medical aseptic handwash in preparation for assisting with a surgical procedure.

Procedure	Principle
1. Remove jewelry.	1. Microorganisms can accumulate on inanimate objects.
2. Stand away from sink.	2. The sink harbors microorganisms which can be transferred to clothing or skin.
3. Open faucets and adjust to comfortable temperature.	3. Running water is one of the key elements in aseptic cleansing. Temperature of the water, however, is irrelevant since hot water does not affect the presence of microorganisms and tends to dry and chap the skin, increasing vulnerability to the lodging of microorganisms.
4. Wet the hands from the fingertips to the elbow.	4. The area of cleansing is extended to include the gloving area to prevent the sterile gloves from coming in contact with unprepared skin.
5. Apply a cleansing agent.	5. An agent which has bacteriostatic and oil-removal qualities is required.
6. Use a sterile scrub brush to scrub the hands and fingers, and work toward the elbow. Allow 5 minutes for each hand.	6. The brush adds further friction, and longer wash time interrupts the growth of microorganisms.

7. Raise the hands, bending the arms at the elbow, and pass under running water to rinse.

7. The hands are elevated and elbows flexed to prevent rinse water from flowing from the hands and elbows to the upper arms.

8. Pat dry with toweling. Ideally sterile toweling would be used for drying if available.

8. For major surgery, sterile toweling provides added protection against contamination. If available in the medical office, its use is recommended for minor surgery as well.

9. Turn off the faucet with a dry paper towel.

9. The faucet is unclean since the procedure began with turning it on. The toweling prevents contact.

10. Glove immediately.

10. The hands have been surgically prepared by complete surgical asepsis for wearing sterile gloves to assist with a surgical procedure or perform special clinical tasks.

Aseptic Handling of Instruments and Supplies

There are basic applications of surgical asepsis in the handling of instruments and supplies. The objective is to keep the instruments and supplies free from contamination. Again, remembering the simple precept—clean against clean, sterile against sterile—is helpful. Nothing can be almost sterile. It is either sterile or nonsterile. An awareness of these principles coupled with skillful handling of equipment will result in effective surgical asepsis.

The following techniques are required:

1. Sterile forceps are used to handle sterile instruments and supplies when sterile gloves are not worn. Often the physician is in the process of a sterile procedure and requests an instrument or other item. Putting on gloves to hand the physician the object takes too much time. Therefore, sterile forceps are usually kept standing in a container on the counter in the examination room for ready use. The handle of the forceps is nonsterile; the tips are sterile. Because forceps are usually kept in solution, the tips are wet. In order to avoid contamination by allowing the solution to run down the handle if held with the tip up, the forceps are always handled vertically, tips down. Touching the sides of the container is avoided when removing or replacing the forceps.

2. Lids removed from containers housing sterile instruments and supplies always *face up* when placed on the counter surface. The outside of the lid is nonsterile; the inside is sterile. Lids removed from containers housing sterile instruments and supplies that are not placed on the counter surface are held *face down* to avoid breathing into the inside of the lid.

3. Pouring sterile solution from a bottle requires opening the lid carefully to avoid touching the inside, pouring well above the receptacle to avoid touching the rim of the sterile receptacle with the bottle.

4. Opening commercially packaged sterile instruments and supplies requires use of the flaps provided on the package. The package is opened in one movement, pull-

ing the flaps apart and the package with the fists. The contents can be pulled out by an individual wearing sterile gloves or dropped onto a sterile field.

5. Opening sterile wrapped instruments and supplies requires placing the package on a flat surface. Grasp and open the corners with the fingertips, the farthest flaps first and then the nearest. The area inside the package becomes the sterile field. Approximately 1 inch around the edge of the wrap is considered contaminated. If equipment in the package has to be handed to a gloved individual or dropped onto a sterile field, reach under the wrap and grasp the object covered with the wrap. Lift up without dragging the corners. Gather the corners around the wrist and hold in place with the other hand.

6. The sterile gloving technique observes the principles of surgical asepsis and is described below. Sterile gloves are required for special procedures such as urinary catheterization and sterile dressing change or application, as well as for assisting with surgical procedures.

STERILE GLOVING TECHNIQUE

Purpose: To protect ones hands and the patient from the transfer of microorganisms.

Procedure	Principle
1. Wash hands using surgical aseptic technique. Remove rings.	1. Washing prevents the transfer of microorganisms.
2. Unwrap the sterile glove package (may be prepackaged and disposable) using surgical aseptic technique.	2. This creates a sterile field for completing the procedure.
3. Gloves will be cuffed with the thumbs facing toward each other. A powder packet may be provided. If a packet is provided, open it. Turn away from sterile field, powder hands, and drop the empty packet into a waste container.	3. Gloves are specially packaged to facilitate ease in pulling off. The powder packet helps ease the gloves on since it absorbs moisture which causes friction. The packet is dropped into the waste container rather than onto the sterile field (nonsterile against nonsterile).
4. For right-handed individuals, lift the cuff's folded edge with the fingertips on the glove to the left (hands cross over and turn up to match glove arrangement). While holding the glove with the fingertips, slip the right hand into the glove, palms up, holding the fingers close together and the thumb slightly extended. Lift the gloved hand off the sterile field. Do not touch body parts or any nonsterile objects. With the gloved fingers closed tightly together and the thumb extended, reach palm up under the cuff of the remaining glove. Lift up slightly and slide the hand into the glove in the same manner as the other hand.	4. This technique minimizes the chance of contamination of the glove by reducing the contact areas required in putting on the gloves.

5. Hold the hands upright, being careful not to touch any nonsterile object or surface, and then proceed.	5. The upright position avoids contact with clothing and subsequent contamination, and signifies readiness to begin the procedure.
6. When the procedure is completed, remove the gloves by grasping the cuff and pulling gloves down and off. They will be inside-out for disposal.	6. This diminishes the chance of contact with infectious materials.

UNWRAPPING STERILE PACKS

Purpose: To maintain the sterility of supplies and instruments which are wrapped and have been rendered sterile.

Procedure	*Principle*
1. Wash hands using medical aseptic technique.	1. This prevents the transfer of harmful micro-organisms.
2. Place the pack on a flat surface. ("Pack" here refers to any object which has been un-wrapped in cloth squares or disposable paper wraps.) Prepackaged (disposable) items are opened by separating the flaps and pulling open in one motion.	2. The work surface must be flat to avoid having the article slip or the corners of the wrap contaminated.
3. Check the sterilizer tape for evidence of sterility. Read the content label for identification.	3. If the tape is not properly colored, the contents have not been rendered sterile.
4. Unfold the top flaps, then the side flaps, and finally the flap which is nearest. The corners may be turned on the flaps to facilitate handling. When not turned, grasp the outside of the wrap, turn hand over, and slip hand out from under wrap.	4. This method creates a sterile field. Working away first then nearest avoids the need to reach across the wrap and possibly contaminate the field with the brushing of a cuff or fingers across the sterile field.

COMMON MINOR SURGICAL PROCEDURES

While all of the surgical procedures performed in the medical office cannot be discussed in this chapter, those described are the ones most commonly performed. Many minor procedures which could be successfully and safely handled in the office are performed instead in the hospital or medical center setting because of insurance coverage factors. The procedures discussed below are performed by the physician with the assistance of the medical assistant.

GENERAL ASSISTING PROCEDURE FOR MINOR SURGERY

Procedure	*Principle*
1. Prepare room and ready equipment.	1. Room must be clean to diminish chance of infection. Equipment readiness is essential to save time and ensure procedural safety.

2. Direct lighting, and drape and position the patient.

2. Draping, positioning, and direction of lighting will vary according to the procedure to be performed.

3. Ready the patient by explaining the procedure. (Prep is required.)

3. A basic explanation should reduce the patient's anxiety. (Prep may be necessary to provide a clean area for surgical incision.)

4. Unwrap the sterile tray setup.

4. This prepares the equipment for ready use by the physician. A sterile towel can be placed over the tray to cover the instruments until the physician arrives.

5. Unwrap and ready a pair of sterile gloves for the physician.

5. Readiness saves time. Sterile gloves are required for all surgical procedures in order to avoid infection.

6. If local anesthesia will be used, ready the vial; place a sterile needle and syringe on the tray setup.

6. Because the vial is not sterile, it cannot be placed on the sterile field.

7. When the physician is ready to begin, remove the toweling from the tray setup. If anesthesia will be used, hold the swabbed vial upside-down in the palm of your hand at the physician's eye level. Hold the vial firmly while the physician withdraws the medication.

7. Assistance is required to avoid contamination.

8. Remain with the physician to add instruments or assist as required. Anticipate the physician's needs.

8. It is usually essential that the MA remain in order to provide the physician with another set of hands for obtaining additional instruments or assisting. This cooperative effort ensures quality patient care and asepsis.

9. Reassure the patient and offer support as needed.

9. Physicians often must rely on the MA to provide patient support since their attention is necessarily focused on the surgical procedure.

10. Complete the followup procedures, which may include applying a dressing, labeling specimens, cleaning the room, equipment care, and patient instruction.

10. By assuming these followup responsibilities, the MA frees the physician to carry out the primary tasks of patient care.

Suture Removal

The surgical dressing must first be removed by the medical assistant and the incision cleansed to provide visibility of the sutures. The dressing may be matted with blood and discharge and may stick to the skin. Removal requires wetting the dressing with sterile water and then gently pulling it away from the skin. The physician may wish to remove the sutures or may delegate this responsibility to the MA.

STEPS IN SUTURE REMOVAL

Purpose: To remove sutures from the incision line.

Procedure	*Principle*
1. Remove the dressing first without touching the incision line, and then wash hands using medical aseptic technique.	1. Transfer of harmful microorganisms is prevented. The handwashing procedure is considered a surgical procedure but does not require sterile gloves.
2. Assemble equipment: thumb forceps, stitch scissors, antiseptics, and sterile sponges.	2. Organization facilitates efficiency. The suture set usually includes forceps and scissors. Sponges and antiseptics are not prepackaged.
3. Prepare the incision line by cleansing with antiseptic and pat dry. Sterile sponges are used for gentle cleansing and drying.	3. Remove matted blood and discharge for greater visibility of sutures.
4. Pick up the forceps in one hand, and scissors in the other. Do not touch the tips of instruments since they are sterile. Grasp the knot of the suture with the forceps and cut the suture as close to the skin as possible.	4. The knot of the suture provides a lever for the forceps. The suture is cut close to the skin to lessen the amount of suture that must be pulled through.
5. With the forceps gripping the knot, gently pull toward the incision line and remove.	5. The suture is pulled toward the incision line to prevent straining the incision, which would cause discomfort and possible separation.
6. Cleanse the incision line after all sutures have been removed, and follow physician's instructions for dressing.	6. Slight bleeding at suture entry points may occur. The incision is cleansed to remove particles and blood and to help prevent infection.

Toenail Resection

A toenail resection is a procedure performed in the medical office to relieve the discomfort of an ingrown toenail. Toenails which are severely ingrown require the surgical facilities of a hospital or medical center. Minor ingrown nails can be removed in the medical office with use of a local anesthetic.

The medical assistant prepares for the procedure and assists in the following manner:

1. The patient is positioned in a semi-sitting or supine position.

2. The hair on the toe is removed by shaving, and the toe and toenail are cleansed.

3. The equipment is assembled:

> local anesthetic (topical and injectable)
> sterile sponges
> scalpel
> hemostats
> needle holder
> scissors
> suture and needle
> gloves
> syringe and needle

All the supplies with the exception of the anesthetic are placed on a sterile field.

4. The medical assistant holds the local injectable anesthetic for the physician, grasping the bottle, turning it upside-down, and raising it at the physician's eye level. The physician then punctures the stopper with the needle for withdrawal of the solution into the syringe. The MA must push against the needle when it is inserted. The physician cannot touch the solution because he is wearing sterile gloves and the bottle of solution is nonsterile.

5. When the physician completes the procedures, the medical assistant gives the patient followup instructions and applies the dressing according to the physician's orders.

Abscess Drainage

An abscess is the accumulation of infectious materials contained in an area of deteriorated tissue. An abscess is commonly referred to as a "boil." Abscesses can occur anywhere on the body and are quite painful. They are usually treated by surgical incision and drainage. The medical assistant prepares for the procedure and assists by:

1. Assembling the equipment:
   antiseptic
   sterile sponges
   local anesthetic
   In the setup on the sterile field:
   gloves
   hemostats
   probes
   dressing forceps
   sterile gauze
   scalpel
   scissors
   drain

2. Cleansing the area with the antiseptic.

3. If local anesthetic is used, assisting with withdrawal by holding the bottle as described in toenail resection.

4. Disposing of contaminated sponges carefully as they will contain certain infectious materials.

5. Giving followup instructions and applying dressings according to the physician's orders.

Hemorrhoidal Excision

Excision refers to a removal, as opposed to incision which means to "cut into." Hemorrhoids are rectal varicosities which are either internal or external to the anus. They can be removed in the medical office and are routinely removed surgically in the office of a proctologist.

The medical assistant prepares for the procedure and assists by:

1. Placing the patient in a jack-knife or side-lying position.

2. Cleansing the anal area.

3. Assembling the equipment:

> coagulant
> local anesthetic (nonsterile)
> sterile gloves
> scalpel
> sponges
> dressings
> hemostat
> scissors

4. Giving the patient instructions for followup care.

Insertion of an Intrauterine Device

An intrauterine device is a contraceptive alternative. Various models and sizes are available. The patient usually is in the third day of her menstruation or is 5 to 10 days postmenstrual. The medical assistant prepares for the procedure and assists the physician by:

1. Placing the patient in the lithotomy position.

2. Cleansing the perineum.

3. Assembling the equipment:

> surgical soap
> antiseptic solution
> sterile sponges
> vaginal speculum
> sterile gloves
> single-toothed tenaculum forceps
> applicator
> suture scissors
> IUD inserter

4. Assisting the patient to a supine position following the procedure. (The patient should remain in this position for approximately 10 minutes to avoid light-headedness.)

5. Giving the patient instruction for followup care according to the physician's directives.

Cervical Biopsy

A biopsy is removal of tissue for examination, usually to determine the presence of malignancy. Biopsies are almost always performed in a hospital or medical center. Cervical and rectal biopsies, however, can be performed in the medical office. Because nerve endings that are pain receptors are absent from the cervix, there is little discomfort associated with the procedure. The medical assistant's role includes:

1. Preparing the patient by explaining the procedure.

2. Placing the patient in the lithotomy position and draping properly.

3. Assembling the equipment:

> *Nonsterile:*
> specimen bottle with preservative solution
> skin antiseptic
> *Sterile:*
> gloves
> vaginal speculum
> uterine dressing forceps
> cervical biopsy punch
> coagulant gel or foam
> sponge (dressing 4 × 4)
> uterine tenaculum
> vaginal packing

4. Providing followup instructions to the patient.

Suture Setup

Often a patient will come to the office rather than an emergency facility for surgical repair, or suturing, of a laceration. Suture setup will also be necessary to close an incision following a surgical procedure. The medical assistant's role in laceration repair includes:

1. Cleansing the wound.

2. Assembling the equipment:

> *Nonsterile:*
> local anesthetic
> dressing
> bandage and tape
> *Sterile:*
> gloves
> syringe and needle
> hemostats
> scissors
> suture and needle

forceps
needle holder

3. Dressing the wound following the procedure.

4. Instructing the patient in followup care.

As can be determined by reviewing the procedures, the medical assistant's role includes preparing the patient, the room, and the equipment for surgery; giving assistance during the procedure as needed; giving followup instructions to the patient, and applying dressings as ordered.

These role expectations are a part of every minor surgical procedure. With experience the MA will learn the equipment that is required for special procedures and the physician's preferences. Even the novice assistant, while perhaps initially unable to select the equipment precisely, will be able to apply general principles of assisting with minor surgery. If an incision is to be made, a local anesthetic, suture material, sponge, scalpel, and scissors are always required. Surgical aseptic technique and cleansing of the presurgical site will always be necessary. With experience the medical assistant will learn to anticipate the physician's "next step" and therefore the type of assistance needed.

POSTSURGICAL PATIENT CARE

Following a surgical procedure, patient care includes (1) applying dressings and bandaging to prevent infection and absorb discharge, and (2) patient instruction for avoidance of complications.

Dressing and Bandaging

The term "dressing" refers to a covering, while the term "bandaging" refers to procedures used to secure the dressing. For open wounds such as a draining abscess, the application of dressings requires sterile procedure. Closed (sutured) wounds require sterile dressing, but sterile gloves are not usually worn.

APPLICATION OF A CLEAN DRESSING

Purpose: To cover a closed wound for the prevention of infection and absorption of drainage when ordered by the physician.

Procedure	Principle
1. Wash hands using medical aseptic technique.	1. Washing prevents transfer of harmful micro-organisms.
2. Assemble supplies: bandages, scissors, adhesive tape, sterile dressings (4 × 4), antiseptic or other topical medication as ordered.	2. Organization facilitates efficiency.

Procedure	Principle
3. Plan the dressing and cut adhesive strips.	3. Planning requires that thought be given to the objective of the dressing and its anticipated appearance.
4. Apply medication to the wound if ordered.	4. Medication such as antibiotic ointment is often ordered to prevent infection.
5. Open the dressing package properly. With fingertips, grasp the corner of the dressing, lift out of the package, and apply directly on the wound site without touching any other part of the dressing.	5. The dressing remains sterile except for the edge where grasped.
6. Secure with tape from one side to another, being careful not to allow too much space between strips where the edges could curl or become loosened.	6. Adhesive or nonallergic tape is used to keep the dressing in place. The tape is applied from one side to the other rather than placed directly onto the wound. This technique avoids touching the dressing with the hand, resulting in patient discomfort.

APPLICATION OF A STERILE DRESSING

Purpose: To cover and seal the open wound to prevent infection, absorb discharge, or apply pressure.

Procedure	Principle
1. Wash hands using surgical aseptic technique.	1. Prevents transfer of harmful microorganisms.
2. Assemble equipment: sterile gloves, sterile dressing, bandage scissors, and bandage materials.	2. Organization promotes efficiency. Sterile gloves are required because the wound is open. Medication is not usually ordered for open wounds.
3. Plan the dressing and cut the adhesive tape.	3. Planning requires that some thought be given to the objective of the dressing and its anticipated appearance.
4. Using aseptic technique, open the dressing packages and create a sterile field. Using proper surgical aseptic technique, put on gloves.	4. The area must be readied for contact with gloved hands. Gloves are required for sterile procedure.
5. Apply the amount of dressing needed. (For absorption, several layers of sterile gauze dressing squares are required.) Gloved fingers touch only sterile gauze squares, not the skin or wound.	5. Touching the skin would contaminate the hands. Contaminated hands in contact with the dressing, which may saturate, will contaminate the wound.
6. Secure the dressing with a bandage that wraps and conforms to the body contour. Apply tape to the bandage to hold in place.	6. This will seal the wound and reduce the chance of contamination.

Bandages are materials used to hold the dressing in place. They are also used to support body parts by equalizing pressure. *Gauze rolls* may be used on body surfaces which are not flexible and are only slightly sloped. *Kling bandages*, which are made of a stretchy, self-adhering gauze, are used on body parts which require flexibility and expansion.

Bandages often replace extensive taping to secure a dressing, especially in the areas of the finger, hands, and feet. *Ace bandages* are elasticized and their application provides pressure to body parts such as hands, wrists, feet, ankles, and legs. Ace bandages are not stretched when applied, but rather are wrapped firmly and evenly. Stretching occurs with the patient's own movements.

Figure 23-12 provides some common examples of bandaging techniques.

Patient Instruction

Following the surgical procedure, patients must be informed of the care to be self-administered and the precautions to be observed. While specific instructions depend on the nature of the surgery, some general principles apply. The patient should be instructed to immediately report (1) excessive bleeding; (2) fever; (3) swelling, redness, or streaking around the surgical site; and (4) a dislodged drain.

The patient should be instructed to keep all dressings clean and dry. If the patient is to change the dressing at home, instructions should be given regarding how to proceed and how often dressing change is required. The physician will almost always request a followup visit with the patient to remove sutures, if necessary, and to check the healing progress.

STERILIZATION AND DISINFECTION OF EQUIPMENT

Instruments require special care and handling. After each procedure, reusable instruments which are used for specific procedures must be cleaned and sterilized.

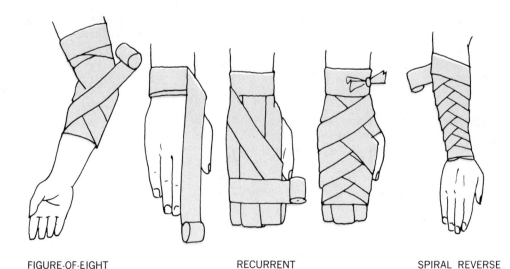

FIGURE-OF-EIGHT   RECURRENT   SPIRAL REVERSE

FIGURE 23-12. Types of bandages: left, figure-of-eight; center, recurrent; right, spiral reverse. (Reproduced from *Taber's Cyclopedic Medical Dictionary*, ed. 14. F. A. Davis, Philadelphia, 1981.)

Terminology

Before discussing the techniques of disinfection and sterilization, the terminology common to these processes must be understood.

1. *Antiseptic:* a mild disinfectant used to destroy microorganisms or render them harmless. All the spores of microorganisms, however, are not destroyed.

2. *Bacteriocidal:* a chemical which destroys bacteria.

3. *Bacteriostatic:* a chemical which prevents the growth and reproduction of bacteria.

4. *Clean:* relatively free of harmful microorganisms.

5. *Contamination:* the unclean or nonsterile rendering of previously sterile materials.

6. *Cross-contamination:* transfer of infectious material from one location to another.

7. *Disinfectant:* a chemical which destroys microorganisms, although spores may remain visible.

8. *Disinfection:* a process of destruction of microorganisms (usually excluding their spores) by chemical or physical means.

9. *Fungicide:* a chemical which destroys fungi (mold is a type of fungus).

10. *Germicide:* a chemical which destroys germs (synonymous with microorganisms).

11. *Infection:* response of the human body to the invasion of disease-causing microorganisms.

12. *Inflammation:* a living tissue's response to injury or infection.

13. *Microorganisms:* minute living organisms that can be visualized only by use of a microscope.

14. *Pathogens:* disease-producing organisms.

15. *Sanitization:* a cleansing process using water and detergents.

16. *Sterile:* completely free of all microorganisms and their spores.

17. *Sterilization:* physical and chemical methods of destroying all microorganisms and their spores.

Care of Instruments

After any special procedure requiring the use of sterile instruments, the instruments are cleansed by (1) rinsing in warm water to remove blood and other secretions, (2) washing with soap and hot water, (3) rinsing with boiling water, (4) drying, and (5) sterilizing or disinfecting, depending on the type of instrument and its anticipated use. Abrasive detergents are avoided since their use injures the finish.

If instruments cannot be cleansed immediately following a procedure, they are placed in a solution containing a blood solvent.

Physical and Chemical Disinfection

Instruments used for contact with the skin or inserted into natural body orifices and not used to penetrate tissue are usually disinfected rather than sterilized since the chance of introducing microorganisms is lessened in these instances. Examples of chemical disinfectants are 70% and 90% isopropyl alcohol and betadine. Instruments must be soaked in chemical agents for varying lengths of time to accomplish disinfection. Boiling water is a physical means of disinfection; boiling water for 15 minutes will ensure the destruction of microbial life.

It must be remembered that disinfection is never a substitute for sterilization.

Common Chemical Disinfectants

Instructions for strength of solution and time required to accomplish disinfection by chemical agents are usually listed on the container label. The chemicals described in this chapter do not represent a complete list, but rather are those in common use.

There is a seemingly endless variety of *detergents* available for use in cleansing instruments. Detergents are "wetting agents" which emulsify oily substances.

Alcohol is perhaps the chemical agent most frequently used. Alcohol also emulsifies oily substances. Other substances are often added to alcohol to increase its germicidal properties.

Ammonium compounds are also used frequently to disinfect instruments. Zephiran solution is an example of an ammonium disinfectant.

Sterilization

Sterilization is required for surgical instruments which come in contact with internal living tissue. The physical methods of sterilization most commonly used are dry heat and moist heat. Other methods of sterilization include radiation and freezing.

Chemical methods used for heat-sensitive materials include immersion in specialized solutions, such as a combination of formaldehyde and alcohol, for 3 hours or more.

DRY HEAT

Dry ovens are used to provide sufficient heat to destroy microbial life and its spores. It is most often used for those supplies for which moist heat would be impractical or damaging. Flaming a needle for splinter removal, a home sterilization technique, is a readily identifiable example of dry heat sterilization. Dry ovens require adherence to the manufacturer's instructions listed on the sterilizer.

MOIST HEAT

Moist heat sterilization in the medical office most commonly utilizes the *autoclave* (Fig. 23-13). An autoclave or sterilizer is a specially designed apparatus for providing steam under pressure, usually at 250°F, for a specified length of time. Special instructions for operating an autoclave are provided by the manufacturer and should be carefully followed.

Autoclaves provide moist heat in the form of steam which circulates in a pattern throughout the autoclave. Steam accumulates at the top of the inside chamber and moves downward from the point of entry. Cool, dry air is pushed out and down through an exhaust drain. Unwrapped instruments and supplies usually require 30 minutes at 250°F to achieve sterilization. Other materials vary in the length of time needed. The composition of the object being autoclaved and the positioning of the objects in the autoclave are factors

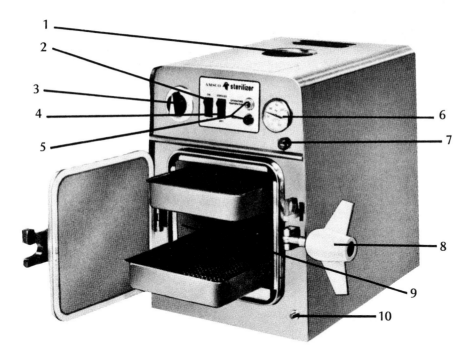

1. Reservoir fill cover
2. On-Off switch
3. Sixty-minute timer automatically turns off when cycle is completed.
4. Toggle switch changes unit from sterilizing to quick-dry cycle.
5. Pilot lights
6. Thermometer
7. Adjustable thermostat control
8. Heat-resistant handles
9. Square chamber accommodates three trays.
10. Reset button for burnout-proof cutout device.

FIGURE 23-13. Medical office sterilizer. (Courtesy of American Sterilizer Company)

which influence the time required for sterilization. The manufacturer's brochure provides the necessary information on which to base judgment.

Instruments and supplies to be autoclaved require special wrapping and positioning techniques (see Table 23-1).

Wrapping of instruments occurs following the cleansing and drying procedure. Not all instruments and supplies require wrapping or protective covering. Rubber gloves, for example, require a wrap. Certain surgical setups, such as a suture removal set, need covering to prevent contamination following the autoclave procedure during handling and storing. When items are wrapped, materials such as clean muslin, cotton, or disposable paper packaging are used.

There are several principles which apply to preparing instruments for autoclaving and for handling and storing instruments:

1. *Wrapping Techniques*
   A. Hinged instruments are opened to allow steam to penetrate all surfaces.
   B. Items to be wrapped are placed in the center of the wrap diagonal to the wrapper. The bottom corner of the wrap is placed over the object, with a small tab of the corner turned to allow grasping the corner without contaminating the object. The top corner of the wrap is placed around the object and secured with sterilizer tape. Masking tape is used to identify and date the contents of the pack. The pack should fit well but not tightly as steam needs to circulate.
   C. Instruments for immediate use or those which are kept readily available can be sterilized in trays without being wrapped separately. Usually a wrap or muslin toweling is placed under the instruments. Following the sterilization procedure, the lid is placed on the tray and instruments are ready for use. Tray "setup" for special procedures is handled in almost the same manner. No lid is used; however, instruments are neatly placed according to priority use, and the tray is wrapped.
   D. Reusable syringes are wrapped in specially designed paper containers and labeled as to type. Barrel and plunger are separated in the wrap to allow steam to circulate.
   E. Needles can be sterilized by placing each needle in a glass tube with gauze or cotton used as a stopper.
   F. Rubber gloves should be powdered before wrapping and sterilizing.

2. *Positioning in the Autoclave*
   A. Instruments and utensils should be spaced so as not to touch one another.
   B. When possible, utensils and glassware should be inverted.

3. *Removing Sterilized Objects from the Autoclave*
   A. When items are dried, they can be removed with clean, dry hands if wrapped.
   B. If unwrapped, sterile forceps or sterile gloves are required.

4. *Storing Objects Removed from the Autoclave*

A. A clean, dry storage area is required to keep sterilized items from becoming contaminated.

B. The storage area should be closed to prevent dust accumulation.

C. Storage for more than one month may necessitate resterilization as resistance to certain microorganisms diminishes.

SUMMARY

Assisting the physician with medical office surgery demands that the medical assistant acquire exacting skills. The major objective of preventing infection must be meticulously observed. In addition to the skill and knowledge of surgical asepsis and procedures, the MA

TABLE 23-1. **Wrapping and Packaging Materials for Articles to be Sterilized***

Material	Grade or Thickness	Suitable for		
		Steam	Dry Heat	Ethylene Oxide Gas
Textile				
Muslin	140 Thread count	Yes	Yes	Yes
Jean cloth	160 Thread count	Yes	No	Yes
Broad cloth	200 Thread count	Yes	No	Yes
Canvas	—	No	No	No
Paper				
Kraft-Brown	30-40 lb	Yes	No	Yes†
Kraft-White	30-40 lb	Yes	No	Yes†
Glassine‡	30 lb	Yes	No	Yes
Parchment	Patapar 27-2T	Yes	No	Yes
Crepe	Dennison Wrap	Yes	No	Yes
Cellulose Film				
Cellophane	Weck Sterilizable	Yes	No	Yes
Plastic				
Polyamide	1-2 mils	§	No	Yes
Polyethylene	1-3 mils Low-density	No	No	Yes
Polypropylene	1-3 mils	§	No	Yes
Polyvinylchloride	1-3 mils	No	No	No
Nylon	1-2 mils	§	No	No
Foil				
Aluminum	1-2 mils	No	Yes	No

* Courtesy of American Sterilizer Company.
† Papers with chlorine formulations should not be used.
‡ Glassine is a coated paper; it may adhere to hard objects when dry and may tear.
§ Difficult to eliminate air from package.

is also responsible for patient comfort. Patient education and reassurance are as essential to health maintenance as the surgical treatment exercised.

The medical assistant assuming the role of surgical assistant can be an invaluable "third arm" to the physician when the basic principles discussed in this chapter are successfully applied.

APPLICATION EXERCISES

Group Exercise

The instructor will assemble groups of instruments and other equipment for identification. Each group of students will be assigned a different group of instruments. In addition to identification, the students will discuss the use of each instrument, how it is handled, and its care and storage. One student from each group will present the group's findings to the class.

Role-Playing Exercises

The instructor will assign students in rotation the roles of patient, medical assistant, and evaluator.

1. Mrs. Jones has just been told by Dr. Askins that she is to be scheduled for office surgery for removal of a nasal polyp. Mrs. Jones expresses some fear and asks questions; the evaluator offers constructive criticism.

2. Mr. Leonard is being prepared for hemorrhoidectomy. You will be assisting Dr. Larsen with the procedure and are about to prepare Mr. Leonard. Mr. Leonard, however, appears embarrassed by your presence. What is your response?

Problem-Solving Exercises

1. While putting on sterile gloves, you accidentally touch the little finger of the left-handed glove to your uniform. Dr. Adams is involved in a procedure needing your immediate assistance. What is your response?

2. While removing sterilized instruments from the autoclave, you notice an instrument with a small particle resembling blood that has been baked on. What is your response?

3. You notice that another assistant is removing sterile gauze from a container without sterile gloves or forceps. What is your response?

4. While shaving Mr. Jones in preparation for surgery, you notice that he has been cut slightly. What is your response?

Performance Simulations

Practice gloving technique and demonstrate correct procedure as assigned by the instructor.

When assigned one of the following dressing situations, discuss the objectives and correctly apply the dressing using materials provided by the instructor. (Lacerations can be simulated with a pen.) Position and prepare the patient, room, and materials.

1. A sutured laceration of the calf of the left leg.

2. A drain in an incision of the forearm of the right hand.

3. A dime-size scrape of the top of the hand.

4. A left ankle sprain. Apply a figure-of-eight bandage.

5. A profusely bleeding wound of the right forearm.

COMPLETING THE LEARNING LOOP

Office surgery is a source of anxiety for most patients, and often evokes a high degree of tension and concern. As a medical assistant, you will be called upon to help patients prepare for minor surgical procedures by understanding and dealing with their concerns. In this regard it may be helpful to reflect on your own experiences with surgery. Regardless of where the surgery is to be performed, your empathy and communication skills will be needed to help prepare the patient. The development of proper technique is essential to ensure optimum conditions during and following surgery.

Another important aspect of clinical medical assisting has now been presented. The following chapter discusses treatment administered by the MA in emergency situations. Emergency care is not a treatment alternative; it is the care rendered when there are no alternatives.

BIBLIOGRAPHY

Galton, L.: *The Patient's Guide to Surgery*. Avon Books, New York, 1977.
Hill, G. (ed.): *Outpatient Surgery*. W. B. Saunders, Philadelphia, 1973.
Meyer, S. W.: *Functional Bandaging*. Elsevier, New York, 1967.
Molitch, M. E.: *Management of Medical Problems in Surgical Patients*. F. A. Davis, Philadelphia, 1981.
Wolcott, M. W. (ed.): *Ferguson's Surgery of the Ambulatory Patient*, ed. 5. J. B. Lippincott, Philadelphia, 1974.
Young, C. G., and Barger, J. D.: *Introduction to Medical Science*. C. V. Mosby, St. Louis, 1973.

CHAPTER **24**

MEDICAL OFFICE EMERGENCIES

SPECIFIC OBJECTIVES

Upon completion of this chapter you will be able to:

1. Define the concepts of emergency and first aid.

2. Describe the medical assistant's role in medical office emergencies.

3. List and describe the components of general patient assessment in emergency situations.

4. Identify emergency situations.

5. Administer first aid for sudden illness, wounds, shock, choking, burns, heat and cold exposure, and poisoning.

6. Assemble and maintain emergency supplies.

7. Apply accident prevention principles.

8. Describe the concept of a "safety mentality."

INTRODUCTION

Occasionally the medical assistant will be required to respond to emergency situations in the office. If the physician is not present, the MA will be responsible for the management of the emergency situation and for the administration of first aid. If the physician is present, the MA will be responsible for aiding the physician in managing the situation and caring for the patient.

Although the emergency situations discussed in this chapter are particularly relevant to medical office practice, the medical assistant will find the principles of first aid described here to be applicable in situations outside the office as well.

Because the medical assistant is a health professional, the public will depend on his or her expertise in emergency situations regardless of the setting in which they occur. The MA must therefore be prepared to handle emergencies knowledgeably and skillfully.

THE MEDICAL ASSISTANT'S ROLE IN OFFICE EMERGENCIES

An emergency situation implies that a crisis has arisen which requires immediate response. The medical assistant's role is to manage the crisis effectively by ordering priorities and demonstrating competency. The MA must make decisions that affect the physical and mental well-being of all persons involved. Each situation must be assessed apart from preconceived assumptions or past experiences. The MA must promote an atmosphere of calm control while administering first aid.

In addition to the medical assistant's knowledge and skill development in emergency medical care, sensitivity and awareness are needed to prevent crisis situations from evolving. Anticipation of potential causes of accidental injury in the medical office will reduce the incidence of emergency situations.

The medical assistant will encounter emergencies in the medical office that may include staff members, the physician, patients and their families, and other individuals visiting the office. The discussion of first aid principles in this chapter is related to these applications.

FIRST AID PRINCIPLES APPLIED TO OFFICE EMERGENCIES

Definition and Purpose

First aid is the care given immediately to a person who has suddenly become injured or ill. First aid encompasses life support measures which are temporary resolutions to a crisis.

Priority Assessment

A determination of the urgency must first be made before the type of care to be administered may be decided. Immediate attention must be given in the following cases:

1. Exposure to smoke or noxious fumes;

2. Obstructed airway;

3. Severe bleeding;

4. Poisoning and choking.

Other situations may also warrant urgent attention. The objective in priority assessment is to establish the urgency of the illness or injuries regardless of the number of individuals involved. Take, for example, the case of a patient who falls to the floor of the examination room while awaiting the doctor's return to the office and hits his head on the table. He is bleeding from a laceration of his head and is clutching his chest. Priority assessment requires first that the patient's condition be generally assessed to determine which injury is most serious or life-threatening. In the example given, the laceration may be a secondary concern if the person is having cardiac or respiratory distress. Therefore, general assessment enables the medical assistant to determine priorities.

GENERAL PATIENT ASSESSMENT

The following patient assessment guidelines should be observed in all emergency situations:

1. The individual must not be moved but allowed to remain in, or assisted to, a supine position if possible. Change of position may cause further injury. Supine position facilitates assessment.

2. Keep the individual warm. The body's metabolism will be accelerated and chilling could occur, causing further complication such as shock.

3. Obtain a description of the incident from the afflicted individual, if possible, or a bystander.

4. If the individual's medical history is unknown, check for medical identification such as a bracelet or card which identifies a chronic condition.

5. If you are unable to obtain information as to the exact nature of the illness or injury, then the individual is examined for injury by palpating the body parts and loosening or removing clothing. Never expose the individual without cause. Examine for open wounds and fractures.

6. Observe the individual's general appearance and color, especially of the inner surface of the lips, mouth, and eyelids.

7. Check the pulse for regularity and strength of beat (radial and carotid are most frequently used).

8. Determine the level of consciousness by talking to or questioning the patient.

9. In the unconscious individual, check for head injury by noting the contour of the face, body paralysis, or convulsion.

10. Observe the eyes, and especially the size and reactive qualities of the pupils. (Pupils should change in size when light is flashed on the eye.)

11. In suspected poisoning, check the mouth for stains or burns.

12. Apply first aid which corresponds to the priorities and general assessment. Use the technique that is reasonable under the circumstances.

13. Maintain calm control until the individual can be cared for by qualified persons such as the physician or the transport paramedics.

14. Never diagnose but rather administer life support measures and prevent further injury. Assessment differs from diagnosis in that assessment pinpoints the symptomatic nature of the illness or injury—wound, possible fracture, shock, respiratory or cardiac distress, poisoning, etc. Diagnosis expresses the physiologic state and cause, thus making a qualitative judgment as to the individual's condition.

The medical assistant utilizes these general principles whenever administering first aid. Perhaps the key concept underlying first aid treatment in emergency situations is to *act only with purpose and with regard to consequences.*

COMMON MEDICAL OFFICE EMERGENCIES

The medical office is not immune to accidents. Patients, other individuals, and the office staff may develop a sudden illness. Certain types of illnesses and injuries are more likely to occur in the medical office. The structure and activities of the office setting create an environment for a variety of potential accidents and injuries. For example, most of the patients visiting the office are already acutely ill and their conditions are subject to sudden changes. Everyone is susceptible to some form of sudden illness. The equipment found in the office can cause injury. Patients could fall off examination tables. Patients or staff walking on floors wet with spilled solutions or discharges could slip and fall. It is easy to imagine numerous other situations conducive to accident or illness.

All of the sudden illnesses and injuries described here can and do occur in the medical office. The medical assistant must therefore be prepared to manage and handle the emergency effectively.

Sudden Illness

FAINTING

"Fainting" is caused by a temporarily diminished supply of blood to the brain. The individual may suddenly collapse, but recovery almost always occurs within minutes if a reclining position is assumed. To prevent fainting when symptoms of weakness and dizziness occur, the head should be brought to the level of the knees with the individual in a sitting position. In the office, prepackaged smelling salts are usually kept taped to the walls or counter in each examination room. When snapped, this packet will release aromatics that will arouse consciousness.

The usual symptoms of an impending fainting attack include paleness; perspiration; clammy, cold skin; dizziness; nausea; and a numbness and tingling of the hands and feet. To prevent or arrest a fainting attack, the patient should either lower his head between his legs or be made to lie down to promote blood circulation to the head. Smelling salts may also be used at this stage.

Following a fainting attack, the individual should be kept in a reclining position to promote circulation, and his clothing should be loosened for comfort. If vomiting occurs, the individual should be rolled on his side to prevent aspiration and choking. His face should be sponged with cool water to lower body temperature. Sips of water at the individual's request should be given only if he is fully revived. If a fall was sustained, examination for injury should be made.

If the individual is a patient in the office, he should be seen by the physician as scheduled. If a patient faints in the waiting room, he should be brought to the examination room as soon as possible. Regardless of where the incident took place, the individual should be examined by a physician if underlying disease is even remotely suspected.

EPILEPTIC SEIZURES

Epilepsy is a disease characterized by convulsions of a variety of types (see Chapter 20). The individual may be known to be an epileptic or may carry identification in the form of a card or bracelet. The individual may be aware of the onset of the seizure and lie down suddenly. Those around the afflicted person may recognize certain behaviors as forerunners of the seizure. Warning signs may include sudden paleness or disorientation.

The major objective in first aid treatment of an epileptic is to keep the airway patent. During the seizure, the tongue will fall back across the trachea, obstructing the airway. An object must be placed between the teeth to hold the tongue forward and the teeth apart. In the office, a plastic airway or "resuscitube" is usually available. In addition, a tongue blade wrapped with gauze may be kept in each examination room and in a drawer of the front office.

If obstruction has occurred and difficulty in breathing is apparent, mouth-to-nose ventilation is necessary. Mouth-to-nose ventilation requires the rescuer to place her mouth over the individual's nose and breathe into the nostrils at an even rate, allowing pause for exhalation or keeping the mouth apart to facilitate exhalation.

Epileptic "attacks" can occur without seizures. Disorientation and staring may be the only symptoms. Regardless of the severity of the attack, first aid measures should be administered and subsequent examination performed by the physician. A review of the symptoms includes (1) a staring gaze; (2) slight, jerky, undefined movements; (3) collapse with violent, jerking movements; and (4) vomiting.

Basic first aid for an epileptic episode consists of the following measures:

1. Remove any objects from the surroundings which may cause injury.

2. Place and hold a soft object between the teeth, such as a rolled handkerchief or a cushioned tongue blade.

3. Loosen clothing following the convulsion to make the individual comfortable.

4. Maintain the individual in a lying position to provide rest. If the seizure occurs in the office waiting room, wait until the seizure ends and with assistance move the individual to the examination room.

5. If the individual vomits, turn the head to one side or roll on the stomach in a prone position to avoid aspiration of vomitus.

6. If breathing is obstructed, perform mouth-to-nose respiration.

7. Allow the individual to rest following a seizure.

8. If a patient, record the incident on the individual's file.

CHEST PAIN

Severe chest pain can be indicative of a heart attack and is treated as a heart-related emergency until diagnosis can be established.

Signs and symptoms include (1) ashen skin coloring; (2) profuse perspiration; (3) cyanosis of the nail beds and lips; (4) severe, crushing pain in the mid-chest region; (5) pulse usually rapid and weak; and (6) nausea.

First aid measures in a heart-related emergency are as follows:

1. Keep the patient in a position that is comfortable for him. Usually a semi-sitting position is preferred. If the attack occurs in the waiting room, move the patient to the back office. A wheelchair or a desk chair with rollers can be accommodating.

2. If the physician is present, call immediately and then prepare medication that is usually administered.

3. Administer oxygen, if previously instructed by physician.

4. If the physician is not present, call an ambulance or rescue team. Ask the patient if he has a medication which he takes for chest pain, such as nitroglycerine. Administer this medication if the reply is affirmative.

5. If the patient becomes unconscious or if breathing has ceased and pulse is absent, insert an airway, if available, and begin cardiopulmonary resuscitation. If pulse is present, omit heart-lung resuscitation and work to restore breathing action by mouth-to-mouth artificial respiration.

Figure 24-1 illustrates the mouth-to-mouth method of artificial respiration. Refer to the illustrations while learning the steps outlined in the procedure guide which follows. When cardiac arrest is apparent (as evidenced by dilated pupils and absence of pulse), *cardiopulmonary resuscitation* is required (Fig. 24-2). This procedure is outlined in the second procedure guide.

MOUTH-TO-MOUTH RESUSCITATION

Purpose: To restore breathing function.

Procedure	Principle
1. Wipe any foreign material from the victim's mouth.	1. To provide a clean, unobstructed area for mouth-to-mouth contact.

2. Bend the head back with the chin pointing up and pull the jaw outward, moving the tongue from the back of the throat.

3. Close the patient's nostrils by pinching them together with the fingers.

4. Blow three forceful breaths into the mouth, sealing the victim's mouth with your own. If the mouth is injured, hold it shut and blow into the nose. With small children, place mouth over child's nostrils and mouth and blow into both.

5. After each breath blown into the victim's mouth, turn the victim's head to one side and listen for the return rush of air.

6. Repeat the blowing procedure with approximately 12 breaths a minute for adults and 20 for children. Continue until breathing is restored or other medical personnel are available to care for the victim.

2. To establish a patent airway and to prevent the tongue from obstructing the airway.

3. To prevent air from escaping through the nose.

4. This forces air into the lungs for oxygen and carbon dioxide exchange.

5. The return flow of air signals the victim's return of breathing function.

6. The number of breaths corresponds to the average number of breaths per minute.

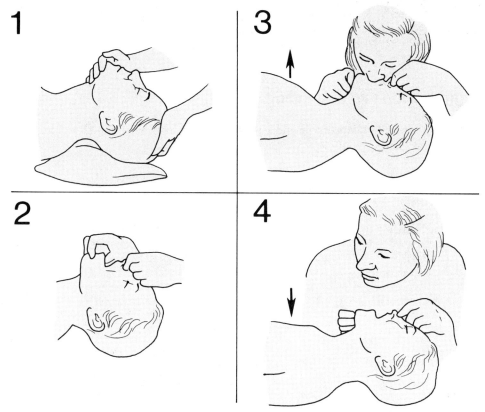

FIGURE 24-1. Mouth-to-mouth method of artificial respiration. (Reproduced from *Taber's Cyclopedic Medical Dictionary*, ed. 14. F. A. Davis, Philadelphia, 1981.)

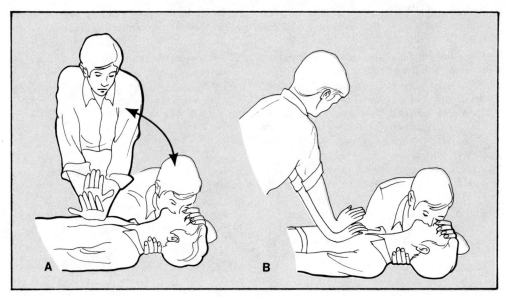

FIGURE 24-2. A. One-rescuer CPR method using fifteen chest compressions to two lung inflations. B. Two-rescuer CPR method using five chest compressions to one lung inflation. (Adapted with permission from *Standards for cardiopulmonary resuscitation (CPR) and emergency cardiac care (ECC).* J.A.M.A. (Suppl.) 227(7):846, 1974, and the American Heart Association, Inc.)

CARDIOPULMONARY RESUSCITATION

Purpose: To stimulate heart action and circulation along with breathing to restore normal heart-lung-brain functioning.

Procedure	*Principle*
1. Establish a patent airway.	1. This is necessary for ventilation of the lungs.
2. Inflate the lungs with three forceful breaths after properly situating the patient.	2. A hard and unyielding surface is necessary for CPR. Inflating the lungs provides a high concentration of oxygen.
3. Locate the heart compression points.	3. An understanding of the anatomy and physiology of the heart is necessary. The heart compression point is at the center of the lower half of the sternum, and is located by feeling the xiphoid process and the notch where the sternum attaches to the collar bone. Correct location is essential to avoid injury and provide successful CPR.
4. Place the heel of one hand over the pressure point and the heel of the other hand over the back of the first hand. The fingers of both hands are held high and outward.	4. This position of the hands prevents contact with ribs.
5. Apply pressure downward to depress the ster-	5. This procedure compresses the chest, squeezes

num 1½ to 2 inches, using all of your upper body weight. Hold for approximately one-half second.

the heart between the sternum and the spine, and forces blood into the pulmonary circulation system where it becomes oxygenated and is then carried to all parts of the body.

6. Release pressure quickly.

6. This provides suction by drawing blood into the heart from the veins and lungs.

7. Repeat the compressions at a rate of 60 to 80 per minute. Continue until normal heart-lung action is restored or qualified medical personnel arrive to manage the patient.

7. The compressions simulate a normal heart rate. Circulation is maintained as long as the procedure is continued.

8. Alternate heart compression with lung ventilation at the rate of 15 heart compresssions to 2 breaths

8. CPR necessitates the restoration of activity for both the lungs and heart. Ventilation of the lungs is accomplished by artificial respiration.

DIABETES-RELATED PROBLEMS

Diabetic coma occurs as a result of an insufficient supply of insulin circulating through the blood stream. Symptoms of diabetic coma include (1) rapid, deep, gulping respirations; (2) a flushed face; (3) dry and reddened skin; (4) apparent confusion or disorientation; and (5) "acetone breath," which has the odor of fruit or nail polish remover. Diabetic coma requires immediate hospitalization. If present in the office, the physician should be alerted as soon as an ambulance has been summoned.

Insulin shock occurs as a result of an excess of insulin and an insufficient amount of sugar circulating throughout the blood stream. The symptoms of insulin shock include (1) weak, rapid pulse; (2) profuse perspiration; (3) cold, clammy skin; (4) convulsions or tremors; and (5) restlessness and confusion.

Immediate relief can be obtained by offering the patient sugar in some available form. In the medical office, packets of sugar or soft drinks may be on hand. When in the office, the physician should be alerted immediately. When the physician is absent, transportation to the hospital should be arranged at once.

EPISTAXIS (NOSEBLEED)

Nosebleed may occur for a variety of reasons ranging from blowing the nose forcefully to hypertension. Basic first aid procedures include:

1. Elevating the patient's head and pinching the nostrils closed for approximately 10 minutes.

2. Applying a cold compress over the bridge of the nose or the back of the neck.

3. Alerting the physician when a nosebleed occurs in the medical office.

Specific Injuries

PNEUMOTHORAX

Pneumothorax, or hole in the chest wall, usually occurs as a puncture wound by an object forcefully penetrating the chest. The hole is apparent.

First aid measures are aimed at preventing air from entering the wound. Therefore the wound is sealed with a stitch or clean dressing. The dressing should be held securely until qualified medical management is possible. If the lung is also punctured, bright red, frothy blood will be expelled from the mouth. The objective of first aid is to prevent air from being sucked into the wound. An air-tight dressing is required.

EYE INJURIES

Eye injuries include foreign objects in the eye, lacerations, and burns, all of which can occur in the medical office to patients or personnel.

A *foreign object* can be removed from the eye by (1) clasping the upper lash between the thumb and forefinger; (2) folding the lash over an applicator swab at the midline of the upper lid; (3) instructing the patient to look down to expose the upper surface of the eye; and (4) using sterile water, irrigating the eye (see Chapter 20), or, if the object can be located and identified, removing it with the corner of a clean linen. A foreign object that cannot be removed by the medical assistant or the physician in the office must be removed in a medical center or hospital facility. First aid measures include covering the eye with many layers of gauze with the center cut out to contain a shield or paper cup for the purpose of avoiding contact with the object and pushing it further into the eye. Both eyes should be covered and bandaged to prevent eye movement and further injury.

Lacerations of the eyelid require a sterile pressure dressing to stop bleeding during transportation to a medical center. Laceration of the eye itself requires application of a loose dressing.

Burns of the eye require emergency treatment to prevent permanent damage. Chemicals splashed into the eye should be flushed with sterile water to dilute the strength of the chemical. In heat burns of the eye, both eyes are covered with a loose, moist dressing until the physician arrives.

HEAD INJURIES

Injuries to the skull usually include fractures and scalp lacerations. The most serious head injury results in an injury to the brain, in which case unconsciousness may occur.

Symptoms of skull fracture include (1) deformity, (2) unequal pupils, and (3) blood or clear liquid in or flowing from the eyes. Symptoms of brain injury include (1) paralysis, (2) vomiting, (3) convulsions, and (4) respiratory arrest or distress.

First aid measures in cases of head injury involve (1) maintaining an open airway, (2) covering open wounds, (3) administering oxygen with the physician's consent, (4) minimizing movement, and (5) telephoning for an ambulance.

BONE INJURIES

Fractures are the primary type of bone injury. Falls often are the cause of fractures sustained in the medical office. Fractures can be confirmed only by x-ray.

Signs and symptoms of bone injury include (1) exposed bone ends, (2) deformity,

(3) pain and tenderness, (4) swelling and discoloration, and (5) restriction or loss of movement.

First aid measures involve (1) stopping the bleeding and applying a dressing to open wounds if present; (2) immobilizing the affected body part; and (3) alerting the physician.

Wounds

Wounds appear in a great many forms, each requiring a particular kind of emergency care. Table 24-1 considers the basic types of wounds, including their history, pathology, symptoms, identifying characteristics, treatment, and complications. The types of wounds most frequently sustained in the office by patients and staff are lacerations from falls or objects, contusions, and punctures.

Shock

Any injury can stimulate the physiologic reaction of shock in which blood vessels dilate and blood volume is reduced because the heart provides inadequate circulation. The inadequate circulation is triggered by central nervous system dysfunction.

Symptoms and signs of shock include (1) cool, clammy skin; (2) ashen color; (3) dilated pupils; (4) rapid, thready, weak pulse; and (5) rapid, shallow respirations.

First aid measures are intended to restore oxygenation to the brain: (1) the feet are elevated if the procedure does not interfere with the management of the injury; (2) the patient's body is kept warm to reduce metabolic activity; (3) the physician is alerted to manage the patient; (4) the assistant may give injections as ordered by the physician.

Choking Emergencies

Choking emergencies occur as a result of the inability to completely or successfully swallow a substance. The substance becomes lodged in the trachea or pharynx and prevents the flow of air to the lungs.

The act of choking may sometimes be masked by signs of cyanosis, protruding eyes, and the waving of arms and frantic motions.

First aid measures consist of performing the *Heimlich maneuver,* illustrated in Figure 24-3. This procedure includes the following steps:

1. Wrap arms around the patient's waist from behind.

2. With one hand make a fist and place it against the victim's abdomen between the rib cage and navel.

3. With the free hand, grasp the fist and press it into the abdomen with a quick, forceful upward thrust.

4. Repeat until choking subsides.

TABLE 24-1.   Classification of Wounds*

Type	History	Pathology	Symptoms and Color	Points of Identification	Treatment	Transportation	Complications
Bite (human, animal, or insect)	Bite of a reptile or rabid human or animal. Sting or bite of poisonous insect.	Tissue degeneration at site of wound. Muscular paralysis. Venom has a drastic effect upon respiratory nerve centers.	Type of wound: Snake—two fang wound. Human—shape of denture. Dog—laceration. Patient shows rabid disposition. Insect—elevated wheal with pain and itching or burning sensation, or single or double red dot.	Shape of wound; odor of colon bacillus about the wound in human bite; presence of stinger.	Dog bite: Observe victim and dog for signs of rabies for two weeks. Pasteur treatment if necessary. Snake bite: Apply tourniquet just tight enough to prevent venous return. Use ice packs to prevent absorption of venom. Incision and suction as swelling rises. Sting: Neutralize with alkalis. Treat for shock. Respiratory stimulants for snake or insect venom	Keep patient quiet; avert apprehension; keep muscles of the area elevated and at rest.	Infection introduced by pathogenic organisms. Venom of toxic nature depresses victim. Death if delay in treatment.

Brush burns or abrasions	Friction of body against rough surface.	Surface effaced with nicks and dotted with small drops of blood.	Skin discolored. Surface peeled off with fine beadlike dots of blood. Skin may be permeated with foreign material.	Surface of the skin is brushed completely away, or remains very lightly attached to the area.	Carefully brush away loose dirt. Cleanse the wound with soap and water. Use antiseptic solutions, ointment, and apply dressings. Tetanus toxoid or antitoxin as required.	Use loose applications of sterile dressings held in place by loosefitting triangle.	Infection. May retain rough, unsightly scars.
Contusions	Blow or fall.	A bruise (hematoma) or petechial area with underlying injury.	Skin surface is rough; the area includes a large or small hematoma (depending upon the extent of injury).	Skin is not broken. Underlying tissues may be slightly or markedly crushed.	Apply cold to area for 24-48 hours.	Keep part well elevated. If there is additional abrasion, cover with loosefitting bandage.	Destruction of underlying tissue if hematoma is not aspirated early. Infection if skin is punctured or probed.
Gunshot	Accident in care of a gun. Victim of deliberate gunfire.	Wound of single outer puncture site with deep injury consisting of twisting and tearing of tissue.	Aperture is small. Powder burns occasionally are found.	Puncture site. Deep wound shows characteristic twisting of the deeper tissues.	Cleanse and irrigate. Debridement when necessary. Wet antiseptic dressings. Tetanus toxoid or antitoxin as required.	Keep patient very quiet; head slightly lower than body. Treat for shock. Watch T.P.R. and blood pressure if blood is lost or patient is in shock.	Shock; internal hemorrhage; tetanus bacillus infection.

TABLE 24-1. *Continued*°

Type	History	Pathology	Symptoms and Color	Points of Identification	Treatment	Transportation	Complications
Lacerations	Accident wherein sharp instruments have cut and torn an area of the body.	Jagged or torn and roughened edges of tissues. May include evulsion of certain parts.	Injury has produced area of two raw or bleeding edges of the skin. Blood may be oozing or spurting from the wound.	Wound edges are jagged and irregular. Wound may contain amount of debris or dirt and usually is infected.	Remove the large debris and dirt. Clean the wound by water dripping from sterile cloth, or use soap and warm water; mild antiseptics and sterile dressings.	Edges of wound may be united with flamed strip of adhesive tape. Cover the area with loose dressings held by triangle or cravat bandage. Tetanus toxoid or antitoxin as required.	Infection and septicemia. Wound usually heals with very unsightly scar if not properly sutured.
Puncture	Accidental or intentional piercing of body with a pointed object.	Tissues are pierced. Small opening through the tissues providing an excellent course or inlet for infection.	Area usually manifests no bleeding. Trauma of tissues usually evident.	Puncture site is very small. Objects usually withdrawn with fair amount of ease.	Probe the wound very carefully to enlarge bore for irrigation with antiseptic solutions. Tetanus toxoid or antitoxin as required. Treatment for prevention of gas gangrene may be required.	Cover the area with sterile dressings and triangle or cravat bandage.	Infection of the anaerobic type (Tetanus bacillus) and septicemia.

| Stab | Injury by a blunt or pointed object, incurred during a fight or acquired by a fall or push. | Size of hole in the tissues varies with the size of the instrument. Foreign material and pathogenic bacteria of anaerobic nature are usually introduced. | Evidence of the instrument that was used, such as knife, ice pick, etc. Victim shows pallor, syncope, and later collapse. | Large, very deep puncture site. Instrument may still be in wound. Victim may be pinned to an object by the force of the blow. | Cleanse and irrigate the wound when possible. Irrigation and inclusion of antiseptic drain or wet dressings. Early use of antitetanic sera. Tetanus toxoid or antitoxin as required. | Keep patient very quiet with head and chest slightly elevated. Treat for shock. If chest is involved, watch T.P.R. and blood pressure. | Internal hemorrhage from, or damage to, organs underlying site of wound, such as puncture and collapse of lung, abdominal visceral injury, or severance of a nerve. Pulmonary hemorrhage. Infection of body by anaerobic organisms. |

*Reproduced from *Taber's Cyclopedic Medical Dictionary*, ed. 14. F. A. Davis, Philadelphia, 1981.

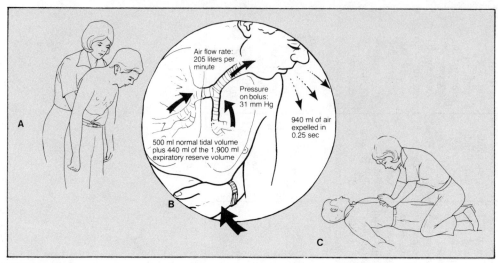

Air flow rate:
205 liters per
minute

Pressure
on bolus:
31 mm Hg

940 ml of air
expelled in
0.25 sec

500 ml normal tidal volume
plus 440 ml of the 1,900 ml
expiratory reserve volume

FIGURE 24-3. A. The Heimlich maneuver with a standing choking victim. B. Physiologic mechanism of the Heimlich maneuver. C. Application of the Heimlich maneuver to a victim in the supine position. (Adapted from Saperstein, A. B., and Frazier, M. A.: *Introduction to Nursing Practice.* F. A. Davis, Philadelphia, 1980.)

Burns

Burns occur as a result of contact with heat, chemicals, and electricity. Burns differ both in extent of injury and degree of severity.

A *first-degree burn* is a superficial injury involving the epidermis. The outer layer of skin becomes reddened. A sunburn or scalding with hot water are examples of first-degree burns.

A *second-degree burn* is an injury which involves the epidermis, the dermis, and the capillaries within the dermis. It is a deeper burn causing reddening and blister formation. Blisters form as a result of plasma seeping into the tissue, raising the top layer. Second-degree burns do not cause permanent damage to the tissue, although the patient sustaining the burn will become quite ill.

A *third-degree burn* involves the epidermis, the dermis, and subcutaneous tissue. Muscle and bone could also be involved. These burns are often called full-thickness burns because of the depth of the injury. Third-degree burns cause permanent tissue damage and require surgical treatment.

The amount of skin surface involved in a burn determines its severity. The "rule of nines" is the universally accepted formula for calculating the severity of burns. In the adult, each major body segment represents 9 percent:

    Head and neck
    Each arm
    Chest
    Upper back

Abdomen
Lower back and buttocks
Front of each leg
Back of each leg
Genital area (1%)

For children and infants, the same calculations apply with the exception of the head. For infants and small children, the head and neck comprise 18 percent of the body surface since the head is larger in proportion to body size during this time of life.

Burns are classified according to the extent of body surface involved as follows:

1. *Critical*:
   a. Second-degree burns covering more than 30 percent of the body.
   b. Third-degree burns covering more than 10 percent of the body.
   c. Burns complicated by major injury such as fracture or respiratory distress.
   d. Third-degree burns involving critical areas of the hands, face, or feet.

2. *Moderate*:
   a. Second-degree burns involving 15 to 30 percent of the body surface.
   b. Third-degree burns involving less than 10 percent of the body surface, excluding hands, feet, and face.

3. *Minor*:
   a. Second-degree burns involving less than 15 percent of the body surface.
   b. Third-degree burns involving less than 2 percent of the body surface.
   c. First-degree burns involving less than 20 percent of the body surface, excluding hands, feet, and face.

First aid measures depend on the type of agent causing the burn. *Thermal burns* are treated by (1) establishing an open airway; (2) administering pulmonary resuscitation if required; (3) covering burns with a sterile or clean dressing; and (4) treating for shock if apparent. *Chemical burns* are treated by (1) flooding the body areas affected with water; and (2) when the chemicals have been washed from the skin, covering with a sterile dressing. There are certain exceptions. *Acid burns* caused by phenol (carbolic acid) should be washed with ethyl alcohol before flooding with water, since phenol is not water-soluble. *Electrical burns* are treated by: (1) covering with a sterile dressing, and (2) administering CPR if required.

EMERGENCIES OUTSIDE THE MEDICAL OFFICE

The emergencies discussed above can and do occur in the medical office or clinical setting as well as outside the office in any aspect of daily life. The following group of emergencies, those occurring from exposure to environmental heat or cold and poisoning, do not usually take place in the office setting. Nevertheless, the medical assistant needs to be aware of first aid measures applicable in these situations.

Cold and Heat Exposure

Emergencies due to exposure to cold are usually local injuries that can cause permanent tissue damage in severe cases. The symptoms occurring from prolonged exposure to below-freezing temperatures may be delayed several hours after exposure or may appear within minutes. The conduction of heat and the presence and force of wind are major influential factors.

Emergencies from cold exposure are of two types: general cooling of the entire body surface, and local cooling of a body part.

The symptoms of general cooling include (1) shivering, (2) listlessness and apathy, (3) glassy stare, and (4) slowed pulse and respirations. First aid measures include (1) removing wet clothing; (2) applying warm clothing and blankets; and (3) the use of hot baths, hot liquids, and hot water bottles.

Local cooling emergencies are usually referred to as *frostbite*. The symptoms of frostbite include (1) reddened skin which becomes gray and blotchy, and (2) numbness. The skin becomes white when actually frozen, and no pain is felt since the nerve endings are deadened. First aid measures in cases of frostbite include the following:

1. Warming the part immediately by placing it in contact with warmed areas of the victim's body, such as under arms and between legs.

2. Immersing the part in warm water.

3. Not putting pressure on the frostbitten part.

4. Administering other comfort measures.

Coffee is beneficial in treating frostbite because it is a stimulant and will cause dilatation of blood vessels. Tobacco, however, should be avoided since it constricts blood vessels. Remember that with the application of cold, the vessels are already constricted.

It is important for the medical assistant to be able to identify and differentiate heatstroke and heat exhaustion as these two conditions are frequently encountered, especially in the summer months and in warmer climates. Table 24-2 presents a concise comparison of common heatstroke and heat exhaustion.

Poisoning

Poisoning can occur from inhalation of substances such as cleaning fluids and sprays, from ingestion of toxic substances, from absorption of substances such as insecticides, and from injection of drugs or by means of bites. (see Table 24-3).

Carbon monoxide is the most frequently inhaled poison. Symptoms of carbon monoxide poisoning include (1) headache, (2) dizziness, and (3) an unmistakable cherry-red skin color. First aid measures in cases of inhalation of poisons consist of pulmonary resuscitation and immediate transport to a medical center facility.

The first order of importance in emergencies involving ingested poisons is to ascertain what and how much was ingested (see Table 24-4). The main objective of treatment is

TABLE 24-2. Comparison of Heatstroke and Heat Exhaustion*

Heatstroke	Heat Exhaustion
Definition: A condition or derangement of the heat-control centers due to exposure to the rays of the sun or very high temperatures.	*Definition*: A state of very definite weakness produced by the loss of normal fluids and sodium chloride.
History: Exposure to sun's rays or extreme heat.	*History*: Exposure to heat, usually indoors.
Differential Symptoms:	*Differential Symptoms*:
Face: Red, dry, and hot.	*Face*: Pale, cool, and moist.
Skin: Hot, dry, with no diaphoresis.	*Skin*: Cool, clammy, with profuse diaphoresis.
Temperature: High: 106° to 110°F (41.1° to 43.3°C).	*Temperature*: Slight elevation or subnormal.
Pulse: Full, strong, bounding.	*Pulse*: Weak, thready, rapid.
Respirations: Dyspneic and sonorous.	*Respirations*: Shallow and quiet.
Muscles: Tense, possible convulsions.	*Muscles*: Tense and contracted.
Eyes: Pupils dilated but equal.	*Eyes*: Pupils normal; eyeballs may be soft.
Treatment: Absolute rest with head elevated; cold packs to promote heat loss.	*Treatment*: Keep patient quiet; head should be lowered. Keep body warm to prevent onset of shock.
Drugs: Allow no stimulants; give infusions of normal saline to force fluids.	*Drugs*: Aromatic spirits of ammonia, salt tablets, and fruit juices in abundant amounts. Intravenous isotonic saline will be required if patient is unconscious.

*Adapted from *Taber's Cyclopedic Medical Dictionary*, ed. 14. F. A. Davis, Philadelphia, 1981.

usually to rid the stomach of its contents by induced vomiting. However, certain chemicals and other substances will cause further injury if vomited. These substances include strong acids or alkalis and petroleum products. In cases where immediate elimination of the poison by vomiting can be accomplished, the following first aid measures apply:

1. Administer 1 tablespoon of ipecac syrup followed by several glasses of warm water.

2. Administer warm water in large quantities with table salt or mustard added.

3. Tickle the back of the throat to produce a reflexive action of vomiting.

Poisons absorbed through the skin must be flooded with water and the patient observed for shock and other symptoms.

Drug abuse accounts for most cases of emergencies due to injected poisons (see Table 24-5). Recognition of the symptomatology of the patient is important in determining proper first aid measures.

TABLE 24-3. Poisons and Poisoning*

Toxic Substance	Probable Lethal Dose for Adult Humans (mg./kg. body wt.)*	Symptoms of Poisoning	Emergency Measures	Supportive and Follow-up Treatment	Pathology
Acids (acetic, hydrochloric, nitric, phosphoric, sulfuric, etc.)	Variable	Immediate pain and corrosion of mucous membranes of mouth, throat, and esophagus; difficulty in swallowing; stomach pain; nausea; coffee-ground vomitus; thirst, shock syndrome with death in circulatory collapse.	Give orally, magnesium oxide, milk of magnesia, lime water, or aluminum hydroxide gel. Avoid carbonates as neutralizers. Give large amounts of water. Demulcents and morphine for pain.	Correct shock with fluids, plasma, or whole blood. Tracheotomy or gastrectomy may become necessary.	Asphyxia from glottic edema, gastric and pyloric strictures, and stenosis or perforation.
Aminophylline or Caffeine	50 to 500 mg.	Restlessness; excitement alternating with drowsiness; ringing in ears; fast pulse; nausea; vomiting; fever; diuresis; dehydration; thirst; tremor; delirium; convulsions; coma; death in cardiovascular and respiratory collapse.	Lavage, induce emesis with saline cathartic unless vomiting and purging have already begun. Treat CNS excitation with appropriate barbiturate therapy.	Oxygen and artificial respiration. Maintain fluid and electrolyte balance.	CNS stimulation and gastric ulceration.
Ammonia	Variable. Even a small amount may kill.	Irritation of eyes and respiratory tract (sometimes pulmonary edema, glottic spasm, or laryngeal edema). Other symptoms are like lye poisoning (SEE: Lye in table).	Give large amounts of diluted vinegar, lemon juice, or orange juice. Demulcents and morphine for pain. Oxygen under pressure to help prevent pulmonary edema.	Treat for shock. Tracheotomy may be needed. NOTE: Do not give drugs such as narcotics which would depress respiration.	Corrosive esophagitis and gastritis, laryngeal edema, pulmonary edema.
Antihistaminics (tripelennamine, diphenhydramine, Chlorpheniramine etc.)	5 to 50 mg.	Drowsiness; lethargy; fatigue; ataxia; dryness of mouth; fixed dilated pupils; coma. Sometimes however, only excitement is seen with tremors, anxiety, delirium, convulsions, hyperpyrexia, nausea, vomiting, diarrhea, death in cardiovascular collapse or respiratory arrest.	Lavage or induce emesis. Cautious sedation if excited. Oxygen and artificial respiration.	Ice packs and alcohol sponges for hyperpyrexia.	Mechanism of death not precisely known. Cerebral edema is described.
Barbiturates	50 to 500 mg.	Confusion; drowsiness; ataxia; vertigo; slurred speech; headache; stupor; coma; areflexia;	Establish airway, gastric lavage, artificial respiration, oxygen with	Record vital signs frequently. Correct airway obstruction. Oxygen and artificial respiration as needed. When	CNS depression with respiratory arrest. Pulmonary edema occurs in

		cyanosis; hypotension; shallow pulse; cardiovascular collapse; death in respiratory arrest.	CO_2 inhalation, maintain fluid and electrolyte balance. Use of artificial kidney to remove barbiturate has been helpful.	vital signs have stabilized and kidney function assured, induce diuresis with urea, and alkalinize urine. Antibiotic therapy if aspiration of vomitus has occurred.	prolonged coma.
Carbon monoxide	1.5% concentration in the air causes unconsciousness in a few minutes. Continued exposure will cause death. Young children are more susceptible than adults.	Mild headache; breathlessness on moderate exertion; irritability; fatigue; nausea; vomiting; confusion; ataxia; syncope with periods of convulsions; incontinence of urine and feces; death from respiratory arrest.	Artificial respiration and oxygen. Give 100% oxygen in a pressure chamber if possible. Glucose, 50% solution, I.V. for cerebral edema.	Keep patient warm. Use antibiotics at the first sign of infection. Give whole blood transfusions or washed red blood cells.	High concentrations of carboxyhemoglobin in circulating erythrocytes lead to an asphyxial death.
Chloral hydrate	50 to 500 mg.	Symptoms much like those seen in barbiturate poisoning except that large doses produce vomiting from hemorrhagic gastritis and enteritis. Combinations of chloral hydrate and alcohol (Mickey Finn) are no longer thought to exhibit more than simple additive depression.	SEE: *Barbiturates* in table.	SEE: *Barbiturates* in table.	CNS depression. May sensitize myocardium to endogenous epinephrine.
DDT	50 to 500 mg.	Vomiting (may be delayed); numbness and tickling of lips, tongue, and face; headache; sore throat; fatigue; tremors; ataxia; confusion; convulsions; coma; death from respiratory failure.	Lavage with tap water and instill saline cathartic. Phenobarbital may be given prophylactically, or parenteral short-acting barbiturates to control convulsions once they have begun. O_2 plus 5% CO_2 inhalation.	Avoid fats, oils, alcohol, epinephrine, sensory stimuli. Calcium gluconate is said to be beneficial in controlling convulsions in addition to barbiturates.	No significant pathological findings in animals except those from convulsions due to CNS excitation.
Digitalis	50 to 500 mg.	Nausea; salivation; vomiting; headache; fatigue; weakness; drowsiness; confusion; disorientation; delirium; hallucinations; visual disturbances; death from ventricular fibrillation.	Slurry of activated charcoal followed by induced emesis or gastric lavage. Disturbances in cardiac rate and rhythm can be tempo-	Nitroglycerin for anginal pain. Preserve water and electrolyte balance.	Produces cardiac arrythmia and all grades of impaired conduction. Striking lack of human pathological changes in comparison with those

TABLE 24-3. *Continued*

Toxic Substance	Probable Lethal Dose for Adult Humans (mg./kg. body wt.) *	Symptoms of Poisoning	Emergency Measures	Supportive and Follow-up Treatment	Pathology
					rarely influenced by appropriate choices from atropine, potassium or salts, quinidine, procainamide, or sodium EDTA.	seen in experimentally poisoned animals.
Ethyl alcohol	Variable: one pint to more than one quart.	Emotional instability and moods depending on personality, circumstances, and surroundings. Impaired motor coordination; slurred speech; ataxia; peripheral vasodilation with flushing, rapid pulse, and sweating; nausea and vomiting; drowsiness; stupor and coma; peripheral vascular collapse; hypotension; tachycardia; hypothermia; death from respiratory or circulatory failure.	Lavage with tap water or 3% sodium bicarbonate, mild stimulants, oxygen and artificial respiration.	Intravenous saline or lactate for circulatory collapse, dehydration, or acidosis. Mild external heat. Avoid aspiration of vomitus. Hypertonic glucose or urea for cerebral edema. Watch for hypoglycemia in young children.	Irregularly descending CNS depression leading to respiratory or circulatory failure.
Formaldehyde	500 to 5000 mg.	Pain in epigastrium; nausea; vomiting; anxiety; weak and rapid pulse; coma; collapse; death in respiratory failure.	Give 30 ml. ammonium acetate solution, 15 ml. of aromatic spirits of ammonia, or 10 to 20 drops of household ammonia diluted with water.	Treat for shock; morphine for pain; antibiotics at the first signs of infection; sodium bicarbonate or lactate for acidosis.	Inflammation and ulceration of gastrointestinal tract, acidosis, kidney damage, circulatory collapse.
Iodine	5 to 50 mg.	Burning pain in mouth, throat, and stomach; lips and mouth are stained brown; thirst; vomiting (blue vomitus if stomach contained starches); bloody diarrhea; anuria or strangury; urine containing albumin or blood. Death from circulatory collapse, asphyxia from glottic edema or aspiration pneumonia.	Immediately give orally cornstarch or flour solution, 15 gm. in 500 ml. (2 cups) water. Lavage with starch solution or 2% sodium thiosulfate. Morphine for pain and mild stimulants as indicated. Epinephrine, diphenhydramine (Benadryl) or hydrocortisone for ananaphylaxis.	Give fluids and electrolytes, supportive therapy for circulatory collapse, antibiotics for secondary infections, prepare for emergency tracheotomy.	Irritation and swelling within throat (glottic edema), esophagus, and stomach. Shock secondary to fluid and electrolyte loss. More rarely, late esophageal stenosis.

Ipecac syrup or fluid-extract	Variable. 1 to 2 ounces of fluid-extract (14 times more concentrated than the syrup).	Nausea; vomiting; diarrhea; albuminuria; abdominal cramps; bloody vomitus and feces; dehydration; myocarditis; myocardial infarction; cardiac arrest or shock secondary to cardiac depression and fluid loss.	Lavage or induce emesis if spontaneous vomiting has not occurred. Do not give additional emetic agents. Saline cathartic if purging has not occurred. Once toxin has been removed vomiting may respond to intravenous chlorpromazine.	General supportive and symptomatic measures for impending shock.	Intractable vomiting and diarrhea due to intense irritation of entire gastrointestinal tract leading to shock. Direct, specific cardiac damage.
Isopropyl alcohol	500 to 5000 mg.	Dizziness, incoordination, headache, confusion, stupor, and coma. Symptoms closely resemble ethyl alcohol intoxication. Death from circulatory collapse or respiratory failure.	Lavage with tap water; oxygen and artificial respiration; mild stimulants.	Intravenous glucose and saline. Anticipate liver or kidney injury.	Acetonuria without glycosuria is pathognomonic. Severe CNS depression. Aspiration pneumonitis.
Kerosene (Coal Oil)	500 to 5000 mg. if retained in stomach. If aspirated, a few ml. can be lethal.	Burning sensation in mouth, throat, and stomach; nausea with vomiting and diarrhea; drowsiness; restlessness; disorientation; coma. Signs of pulmonary involvement indicate grave prognosis of impending fulminating hemorrhagic bronchopneumonia.	If risks of lavage are undertaken, an endotracheal tube with inflatable cuff should be employed. Dilute sodium bicarbonate is satisfactory lavage fluid; follow with the instillation of olive oil and saline cathartic.	Antibiotics for secondary infection and positive pressure oxygen. Corticosteroids for pulmonary edema.	Severe chemical pneumonitis.
Lead or its salts	30 gm. (Chronic poisoning is much more common than acute.)	Dryness in mouth; burning pain in stomach and abdomen; constipation followed by diarrhea; muscular weakness; paralysis of extremities; skin cold and cyanotic; delayed severe anemia; death in peripheral vascular collapse or encephalopathy.	Gastric lavage with magnesium or sodium sulfate. Morphine and atropine for pain. Milk or egg white as demulcent. Intravenous calcium salts may relieve colic. Intravenous calcium disodium edetate in accordance with supplier's directions.	Keep patient quiet. Maintain fluid and electrolyte balance. Urea, 4% I.V. for encephalopathy with increased intracranial pressure.	Gastrointestinal inflammation, liver and kidney injury when sufficient lead has been absorbed. Encephalopathy is frequent in children. Precise mechanism of death is not known.
Lye, Sodium and Potassium hydroxides and Carbonates	Total dose of 10 gm. may be fatal.	Severe pain in mouth and difficulty in swallowing; gastrointestinal pain and purging; weak and rapid pulse; death in shock or asphyxia from glottic edema.	Large amounts of water by mouth; diluted vinegar or lemon juice; avoid emetics and lavage. Olive oil by mouth or milk and egg whites. Mild stimulants to prevent shock. Tracheotomy may be required.	Morphine for pain; fluids and electrolytes; cortisone. Use of bougies to prevent esophageal stricture. Broad-spectrum antibiotics.	Laryngeal or glottic edema; corrosion and possible perforation of upper gastrointestinal tract; late esophageal stenosis.

TABLE 24-3. *Continued*

Toxic Substance	Probable Lethal Dose for Adult Humans (mg./kg. body wt.)*	Symptoms of Poisoning	Emergency Measures	Supportive and Follow-up Treatment	Pathology
Meprobamate, Equanil, or Miltown	500 to 5000 mg.	Drowsiness; relaxation; stupor; sleep; coma; areflexia; muscular flaccidity; severe and persistent hypotension.	Lavage or induce emesis; plasma or pressor agents for hypotension; mild stimulants. Artificial respiration and oxygen.	Symptomatic and supportive care with frequent recording of vital signs.	No significant pathological changes in tissues.
Methyl alcohol	500 to 5000 mg.	Exhilaration accompanied by headache, muscular weakness, nausea, vomiting, and abdominal pain; delirium with visual disturbances which may progress to blindness; weak and rapid pulse; rapid and shallow respirations; cyanosis; coma; death from respiratory failure.	Gastric lavage with 5% sodium bicarbonate, leaving some solution in the stomach. Inject 3% sodium bicarbonate I.V. at the rate of 1000 ml./hour but do not continue after acidosis is corrected. To prevent formation of formic acid, give 10 ml. of ethyl alcohol orally. If poisoning is severe, give ethyl alcohol I.V. in 5% solution in bicarbonate or saline.	Bedrest, treat for shock; mild external heat, stimulants as indicated, protect patient's eyes from light. Oxygen.	Intense metabolic acidosis. Partial to complete blindness due to atrophy of the ganglion cells of the retina if patient survives.
Morphine	5 to 50 mg.	Gross overdosages produce prompt depression, but smaller doses may cause transient period of excitement before drowsiness. Weariness; loss of pain sensation; nausea; vomiting; pinpoint pupils; coma with muscular relaxation and slowing of respiratory rate; cyanosis; slow pulse; fall in blood pressure; death in respiratory arrest.	Gastric lavage, even if several hours after ingestion, with 1:10,000 potassium permanganate; saline cathartic left in stomach. Nalorphine is specific antagonist given I.V. in doses of 5–10 mg. Artificial respiration. Inhalation of oxygen with 5% CO₂	Keep patient awake with mild stimulation. Correct airway obstruction. Maintain fluid and electrolyte balance. Keep patient warm.	Pulmonary congestion. Death is from respiratory failure due to central depression, but circulatory insufficiency may be contributory.
Naphthalene (moth balls)	5 to 15 gm.	Abdominal pain; nausea; vomiting; diarrhea; headache; diaphoresis; coma with or without convulsions. Certain individuals exhibit intense intravascular hemolysis accompanied by	Induce emesis or lavage with tap water; saline cathartic, demulcents, and mild stimulants. Sodium bicarbonate every 4 hours to main-	Anemia from hemolysis may require whole blood transfusions. Supportive measures for acute renal failure. Avoid use of milk, oils, or fatty foods.	Various states of central excitement or depression. Rarely, liver necrosis. Acute hemolytic anemia.

Poison	Lethal dose	Symptoms	Treatment	Treatment (cont.)	Physiologic action
		anemia, hematuria, and renal insufficiency.	tain alkaline urine in order to prevent renal blockage with acid hematin crystals.		
Nicotine	Less than 5 mg.	Burning sensation in mouth and throat; salivation; vomiting; diarrhea; headache; sweating; dizziness; weakness; pupils contracted at first then dilated; pulse slow at first then rapid; respirations deep and rapid at first then dyspneic; death from paralysis of respiratory musculature.	Slurry of activated charcoal as lavage fluid with additional portion left in stomach. Artificial respiration and oxygen.	Control convulsions with small doses of intravenous barbiturates. Relief for visceral symptoms is obtained with atropine or phenoxybenzamine (Dibenzyline).	Transient stimulation then depression of CNS, all autonomic ganglia and nerve endings in skeletal muscle.
Salicylate (sodium, methyl, acetylsalicylic acid)	50 to 500 mg.	Mild gastrointestinal pain; nausea; vomiting; deep and rapid breathing; headache; dizziness; ringing in ears; dimness of vision; irritability; nervousness; confusion; delirium; mania; convulsions; coma and death from respiratory failure with or without cardiovascular collapse.	Induce vomiting or lavage with 5% bicarbonate solution; saline cathartic.	Determine acid-base status and if acidosis is profound, institute sodium lactate therapy. Correct dehydration and hypoglycemia if present. Barbiturates, vitamin K, dialysis procedures or exchange transfusion as indicated.	Disturbed acid-base balance. Children often exhibit metabolic acidosis while adults more commonly show respiratory alkalosis. Intense CNS stimulation followed by depression.
Turpentine	500 mg. to 5 gm.	Sensation of warmth or pain in mouth, throat, and stomach followed by abdominal pain, vomiting and diarrhea. Aspiration into lungs may cause pneumonitis. Excitement, ataxia, delirium, and stupor, followed by convulsions, coma, and death from respiratory failure.	Gastric lavage with weak bicarbonate solution, followed by demulcents and saline cathartic.	Morphine sulfate for intense pain and a short-acting barbiturate for excitement. Mild stimulation if indicated, e.g., caffeine sodium benzoate. Force fluids.	Irritation of kidneys; hematuria, albuminuria, and sometimes complete urinary suppression. Kidney symptoms appear to be related to composition of the turpentine, and often never appear.

* Adapted from *Taber's Cyclopedic Medical Dictionary*, ed. 14. F. A. Davis, Philadelphia, 1981. Most probable lethal dose values from data in Gleason, M. N., Gosselin, R. E., Hodge, H. C., and Smith, R. P.: *Clinical Toxicology of Commercial Products*, ed. 3. Williams & Wilkins, Baltimore, 1969.

TABLE 24-4.   Dose Equivalent Expressed in Household Measures*

Less than 5 mg/kg	A taste; less than 7 drops
5 to 50 mg/kg	Between 7 drops and 1 teaspoon
50 to 500 mg/kg	Between 1 teaspoon and 1 ounce
500 to 5,000 mg/kg (0.5 to 5 gm)	Between 1 ounce and 1 pint
5,000 to 15,000 mg/kg (5 to 15 gm)	Between 1 pint and 1 quart
Greater than 15,000 mg/kg (15 gm)	Greater than 1 quart

*Adapted from data in Gleason, M. N., Gosselin, R. E., Hodge, H. C., and Smith, R. P.: *Clinical Toxicology of Commercial Products,* ed. 3. Williams & Wilkins, Baltimore, 1969.

PREVENTION OF EMERGENCIES

In the medical office, safety precautions must be carefully followed. Hurried procedures increase the potential for accidents. Instruments and equipment should be well-maintained and handled with great care and proper technique. The floor should be kept free of obstructions. Patients with questionable orientation states or conditions should not be left unattended. Drugs should be kept in a locked cabinet.

Because of the nature of medical practice, many potentialities exist that can easily develop into emergency situations. The medical assistant must be aware of possible hazards in the office and work toward their prevention. Every individual in the office should consciously develop a "safety mentality."

EMERGENCY READINESS

In the medical office, supplies are readily available for most emergencies. Nevertheless there should be an area especially designated for emergency medications and special equipment. The medications should be routinely checked for expiration dates, and the equipment for proper functioning.

The following is a list of emergency medical supplies that should be preassembled:

1. Airway equipment

2. Emergency medications in individual dosages, usually including:
    Aminophylline
    Ampicillin
    Amytal
    Aramine
    Atropine sulfate
    Benadryl
    Caffeine sodium benzoate
    Calcium gluconate
    Codeine sulfate
    Compazine
    Deslanoside

      Dextrose in water
      Heparin
      Hydrocortisone succinate
      Ipecac
      Isuprel
      Methergine
      Morphine
      Nitroglycerin
      Pronestyl
      Seconal
      Sodium bicarbonate
      Sterile water

3. Laryngoscopes (infant, medium, and large sizes)

4. Thoracentesis needle (4-inch, 18-gauge bevel with stylet)

5. Laryngeal intubation tubes

6. Oxygen tank and mask

Dressings and other related supplies are usually available in the examination room.

SUMMARY

Medical office emergencies present medical assistants with yet another challenge. They must possess the knowledge and skills to meet their responsibilities. Becoming certified in first aid and CPR is essential to the development of these skills. The information presented in this chapter should serve as a basic foundation and reference in identifying and responding to medical office emergencies. Obviously the role of the medical assistant in patient management in emergency situations is determined by the presence or absence of more qualified medical personnel. It remains the MA's responsibility, however, to check and replace office emergency supplies and equipment routinely, and to initiate and monitor safety measures for accident prevention.

APPLICATION EXERCISES

Role-Playing

The instructor will assign students to the roles of patient and medical assistant. The class will evaluate response.

1. Mrs. Jones, the nurse in the office, has just cut herself with the top of a broken glass ampule. Her thumb is bleeding profusely. What is your response?

TABLE 24-5. Toxic Emergencies Produced by Abused Substances*

	CNS Excitation-Confusion	CNS Depression	Vital Signs†	Withdrawal Reaction
CNS Stimulants				
Amphetamines	Irritability, confusion, agitation, delirium, paranoia; sympathomimetic effects prominent.	Exhaustion or collapse only from prolonged excitation.	↑	"Crashes" after long excitation, otherwise mild depression.
Methylphenidate and phenmetrazine	Stimulation, possibly convulsions.		↑	No specific syndrome.
Strychnine	Spinal convulsions, rigidity, trismus, hyperacusis.	Postictal or exhaustion.	↑(↓)	None
Cocaine	Excitement, emotional instability to convulsions, sympathomimetic effects.	Muscle paralysis, coma, CV or respiratory failure.	↑(↓)	None
Hallucinogens				
Substituted indoles LSD Harmines Ibogaine DMT (bufotenine), DET, DPT‡	Anxiety, panic, hallucinations; rare convulsions or catatonia.	Coma with high overdose.	↑ or ↓	None
Morning glory derivatives	Mild LSD-like.			
Psilocybin Psilocyn	LSD-like plus fever and convulsions; rarely in children with high doses.			
Mescaline (peyote)	LSD-like, plus nausea, vomiting, sweating.		↑	None
Ditran and analogs	Resembles anticholinergics.			None
Psychotomimetic amphetamines§ DOM (STP), DOET, DOP MDA, myristicin (nutmeg), PMA	Similar to LSD and amphetamines (hallucinogenic with strong sympathomimetic effects); panic reactions greater than with LSD.	Coma with high overdose.	↑	None
Phencyclidine (PCP), derivatives, ketamine	Convulsions in most severe (early) excitation, hallucinations, rigidity, paranoia at lower than depressant doses, hyperacusis.	Coma followed by excitation and confusion, rarely respiratory depression.	↑(↓)	None
Cannabis (marijuana, THC, hashish)	Perceptual and body image distortions, rarely hallucinations.	Mild hypotension occasionally.		None
Anticholinergics datura belladonnas antihistamines (nonbarbiturate sedatives)	Disorientation, hallucinations, excitement, sympathomimetic effects; fixed, dilated pupils pathognomonic.	Coma with extreme doses, collapse after prolonged excitation.	↑(↓)	None
Methysergide amantadine	Probably LSD-like.			None
Inhalants				
Solvents	Delirium, psychosis, hallucinations, rarely sudden death.	Coma, cardiorespiratory arrest with extreme exposure, suffocation not uncommon.	↑ or ↓	None
Vasodilator-hypoxic agents, amyl and butyl nitrite	Drunken sensorium, disorientation, headache.	Coma, hypotension, methemoglobinemia, coronary insufficiency on exertion.	↓ (resp. ↑)	None

TABLE 24-5. *Continued*

	CNS Excitation-Confusion	CNS Depression	Vital Signs†	Withdrawal Reaction
Opiates and Opioids				
Morphine, codeine, heroin, and derivatives, meperidine, methadone, propoxyphene	Convulsions rarely, especially with codeine, propoxyphene, meperidine; otherwise confusional state most likely a sign of withdrawal; pinpoint pupils (except terminally) with all except meperidine.	Coma, respiratory depression, hypothermia, CV collapse.	↓	Restlessness, nausea, vomiting, diarrhea, muscle aches and spasms, weakness, chills, gooseflesh, yawning, accentuated vital signs.
Pentazocine	Like other opiates, plus delirium.			May precipitate withdrawal from another opioid.
Sedative-Hypnotics				
Barbiturates Meprobamate Glutethimide Methyprylon	Some confusional manifestations from depressant effect; no excitatory state.	CNS depression to coma, hypotension, respiratory depression, hyporeflexia, CV collapse or respiratory failure.	↓	Tremulousness, insomnia, fever, agitation, delirium, psychosis; seizures not uncommon; death is possible.
Benzodiazepines	Same as barbiturates.	Rarely, severe depression with cardiorespiratory insufficiency.	(↓)	Anxiety, restlessness, rarely convulsions.
Chloral hydrate	Resembles barbiturate poisoning.	Resembles barbiturate poisoning.	↓	Resembles mild DTs.
Alcohol	Inebriation, inhibition loss, disorientation.	Coma, hypotension, hypothermia, respiratory or circulatory failure.	↓	Delirium tremens, hallucinations, possible convulsions.
Methaqualone	From muscle spasticity and hyperactivity to convulsions; hyperacusis, vomiting, bronchial hypersecretions.	Coma, respiratory failure, rarely delayed CV collapse.		Headache, cramps, anorexia, nausea, rarely convulsions; not fatal.

*Reproduced, with permission, from *Emergency Medicine*, March 15, 1980. (Prepared by Alan K. Done, M.D.)

†Vital signs: ↑ = accentuated; ↓ decreased; sign in parentheses is less common, usually seen only in especially severe cases or as a postexcitatory depressive effect.

‡DMT = dimethyltryptamine; DET = diethyltryptamine; DPT = dipropyltryptamine.

§DOM = dimethoxymethylamphetamine (or STP: serenity, tranquility, peace); DOET = dimethoxyethylamphetamine; DOP = dimethoxypropylamphetamine; MDA = methylenedioxyamphetamine; PMA = paramethoxyamphetamine.

2. Mr. Alberts, a hypertensive patient, comes to the office for a routine BP check. While you are taking his blood pressure, he clutches his chest and falls to the floor. The doctor is not expected for an hour. What is your response?

3. Ms. Ames, another medical assistant, trips over a patient's package on the floor in the examination room. She falls and her ankle is causing her severe pain. The doctor is not present in the office. What is your response?

4. Mrs. Caine, the office receptionist, is enjoying a morning coffee break with you. She chokes on a pastry. You are not in the office but nearby. What is your response?

Demonstration and Practice

With equipment available, perform the cardiopulmonary resuscitation technique. Alternate from a solo performance of CPR to a partnership.

Research and Problem-Solving

1. For the emergency medications listed in this chapter, obtain the use, usual dosage, and route administered.

2. Write a paragraph citing two potential office hazards and how they can be corrected.

COMPLETING THE LEARNING LOOP

As a student you are likely to have found much of the information in this chapter to be of immediate practical use. To a greater degree than most other groups, students quite often find themselves in situations where emergencies arise. This is especially true for those who live in dormitories. Emergency care concepts should be continuously reviewed to ensure the dependability of one's competence and skill in the event of need.

The next chapter discusses physical therapy, a treatment alternative applicable in a variety of special circumstances. It can be seen that the clinical skills component of medical assisting is gradually expanding. Upon completion of this unit you will be able to provide entry level assistance to the physician in the treatment phase of medical practice.

BIBLIOGRAPHY

Aaron, J. E., and Bridges, A. F.: *First Aid and Emergency Care: Prevention and Protection of Injuries.* Macmillan, New York, 1972.

American National Red Cross: *Advanced First Aid and Emergency Care.* Doubleday, Garden City, N.Y., 1974.

Arnold, P.: *Check List for Emergencies.* Doubleday, Garden City, N.Y., 1974.

Birch, C. A.: *Emergencies in Medical Practice,* ed. 10. Churchill Livingstone, New York, 1976.

Giving Emergency Care Competently. Intermed Communications, Horsham, Pa., 1978.

Greenberg, M. I., and Roberts, J. R.: *Emergency Care: A Clinical Approach to Challenging Problems.* F. A. Davis, Philadelphia, 1981.

Henderson, J.: *Emergency Medical Guide.* McGraw-Hill, New York, 1973.

Miller, R. H., and Cantrell, J. R.: *Textbook of Basic Emergency Medicine.* C. V. Mosby, St. Louis, 1975.

Moore, M. E.: *Medical Emergency Manual,* ed. 2. Williams & Wilkins, Baltimore, 1977.

Shaftan, G. W., and Gardner, B.: *Quick Reference to Surgical Emergencies.* J. B. Lippincott, Philadelphia, 1974.

Snyder, D. R., et al.: *Handbook for Emergency Medical Personnel.* McGraw-Hill, New York, 1978.

Warner, C. G., et al. (eds.): *Emergency Care: Assessment and Intervention,* ed. 2. C. V. Mosby, St. Louis, 1978.

25

PHYSICAL THERAPY AND ALLIED FIELDS

SPECIFIC OBJECTIVES

Upon completion of this chapter you will be able to:

1. List the common functions of the physical therapist.

2. Assist patients with learning to use crutches.

3. Assist with hot and cold applications.

4. Define and describe physical therapy alternatives and discuss the MA's role.

5. List the functions of the occupational therapist.

6. Describe the basic aspects of psychotherapy.

INTRODUCTION

The medical assistant may sometimes be involved in performing basic physical therapy functions or assisting the physician with physical therapy procedures. In most cases, the physician will refer the patient to a physical therapist for treatment. Likewise, other therapies are utilized for the patient's treatment plan or serve as treatment alternatives. Psychotherapy and occupational therapy are also discussed in this chapter since patient referrals to these professionals are not uncommon. The topics and procedures discussed here are included for the purpose of expanding the medical assistant's awareness of these professions and their significance in comprehensive patient care.

The frequency with which the medical assistant participates in these functions, especially physical therapy, is directly related to the physician's type of practice. An orthopedic physician, for instance, may require the MA to teach patients how to use crutches or prescribe range of motion exercises that the MA must teach the patient.

Regardless of their involvement, medical assistants need to acquire a fundamental understanding of therapeutic functions and must know how to assist the physician by advising and aiding patients. MAs should also be able to reassure patients who have been referred to therapists by responding to basic questions.

There are three therapeutic areas in which physicians commonly make recommendations or specific referrals:

> *Physical Therapy*: The process of using exercise or manipulation of body parts to facilitate or assist the return of an injured body part to normal functioning.
>
> *Psychotherapy*: The process of helping individuals to better function or to develop themselves through the analysis of personality and how it affects either life processes or interpersonal interactions.
>
> *Occupational Therapy*: The process of assisting the client in training and preparation for new types of employment.

THE ROLE OF THE MEDICAL ASSISTANT

Since exercising, developing a well-balanced personality, and preparing for a meaningful new career are explicitly tied to the general quality of life, and thus become closely linked with the perceptions and aspirations of patients, many physicians will find themselves dealing with these issues. Statements such as "you should do some stretching exercises for your stiff back," or "you've been working too hard," or "you should try to spend more time talking with your wife" are common recommendations which physicians direct to patients. In most cases physicians are not acting as special therapists when they offer such advice. Instead, they are seeing the problems of the patient in an expanded light, one which views the entire process of life as relating to specific symptoms. This is why it is common practice for the doctor to make inquiries regarding problems with jobs or family relationships when a patient complains of persistent headaches. This approach is termed *holistic* medicine because the total, integrated person is recognized, accepted, and treated.

In these generalized cases it is crucial that the MA support the suggestions of the physician and help the patient to understand and deal with the advice that has been given. Quite often a gentle suggestion to do some stretching exercises can be met with patient resistance.

The MA's role is to reinforce the physician by emphasizing and restating his advice in attempting to convince the patient that the physician's suggestion, if followed, will be effective and is as important to recovery as the prescription. MAs should also apprise the physician of their observations when a patient is resisting advice or not assigning it the importance it is due.

Occasionally, patients may presume that since there is no explicit organic problem suggesting a medication or surgery they will get better automatically. To counter this common reaction the MA should emphasize the need for the patient to take an active role in his or her treatment. The patient must grasp the fact that some medical problems do not lend themselves to specific drug or surgical procedures, but that these problems must still be treated by following the practical suggestions made by the physician.

It is important that medical assistants understand their role as a liaison between patient and physician. The assistant should make it a point to help patients to understand exactly what is being suggested to them. The MA should be sure that the patient doesn't confuse a serious recommendation or general advice, such as "you ought to slow down and take time off work," with a more casual comment, such as "take it easy."

Did the patient understand the "mechanics" of the general suggestion? Has the patient taken this advice seriously? These are basic questions that medical assistants should be asking themselves each time the physician offers general advice or recommendations. Perhaps the key role of the medical assistant in all therapy situations is to provide patients with the clearest possible explanation of the procedures that they are to undergo.

Assisting with Specific Therapeutic Procedures

Often the physician will encounter a patient who requires a clearly prescribed therapeutic program. How to use crutches, exercises to recover from a back injury, and strategies to improve marital relationships are a few common examples.

The patient will often be referred to a specialty therapist such as a marriage counselor or psychologist. Depending upon the specialty area of the physician, however, the MA may be required to serve as a teacher or patient communicator relative to a specific program of therapy. While it would be impossible to detail all of the therapeutic procedures which the MA could encounter, the remaining sections of this chapter will discuss the procedures more frequently performed in the medical office.

As stated earlier, the medical assistant who is positioned in the office of a specialist, an orthopedic surgeon for example, may become responsible for many more detailed procedures than those listed.

Assisting the Therapist

It is quite conceivable that the medical assistant could actually work as an assistant to a physical therapist or psychologist. In this case the procedures which would constitute a rather complete education for most MAs will serve only as an introduction to the functions of the specialty therapist.

PHYSICAL THERAPY

The physical therapist is one who has completed at least a four-year baccalaureate program and has received state licensure. A physician who has specialized in this field is termed a physiatrist. The role of the physical therapist in the medical team is to restore or maximize function in body parts which have been damaged or injured due to disease, accident, or amputation. The physical therapist may also use physical and mechanical agents to diagnose and prevent disease. As a part of a generalized package of techniques, the physical therapist may utilize massage, exercise, application of heat and cold, electricity, and diathermy. In some cases the physician will work out a detailed program of physical therapy for a particular patient and then expect the physical therapist to follow the mechanics of the program. In other cases the physician may refer the patient and rely on the physical therapist's judgment relative to a particular program. The approach taken depends upon the physician, the physician's specialty, the patient, the nature of the physical problem, and the relationship between the physician and the therapist. The objective of physical therapy is usually to relieve pain, increase or improve circulation, increase or restore muscular function, or improve strength, range of motion, or joint mobility.

In situations where the physician prescribes an elementary, physical routine, and the expertise of the therapist is not required, the MA will be asked to instruct the patient.

Physical medicine is an enormously broad field, and any attempt to summarize the contents would surely omit large and important areas, but the following 13 subtopics have been chosen for discussion as they represent the majority of practical office applications.

Heat and Cold

Physicians commonly prescribe heating (thermotherapy), cooling (cryotherapy), or both for treatment of problems such as sprains or muscle spasms. There are several ways of applying heat, including heating pads, hot water bottles, hot packs, infrared light, and immersion. The general precautions outlined below contain guidelines for heat therapy. It should generally be noted that the application of heat causes edema, an excessive accumulation of fluid in the tissues. Thus patients who may be dysfunctioned by an increase of edema may not be able to tolerate the application of heat.

The application of cold is generally accomplished by immersion in cold water or the use of ice packs. The time limits of the prescription apply to treatments with cold since prolonged application may result in tissue damage.

The procedures related to the application of heat and cold were discussed in Chapter 20. Infrared radiation as a dry heat form, however, warrants some discussion. Infrared therapy is usually administered by heat lamp. Surface heat is transmitted which penetrates the skin to a depth of 5 to 10 mm. Lamps fitted with incandescent light bulbs also produce infrared rays. A distance of 2 to 4 feet from the area is recommended to avoid burning the skin. Exposure time is usually 15 to 20 minutes.

GENERAL PRECAUTIONS IN APPLICATION OF HEAT

Precautions	Principle
1. Great care should be taken with very young children.	1. Because infants cannot tolerate heat, young children not sufficiently matured to have acquired a normal heat tolerance may develop adverse heat reactions.

2. Elderly patients should be observed carefully.

2. Older people may find that local heating challenges cardiovascular reserves, thus reducing heat tolerance.

3. Patients should be warned of the dangers of heating pads.

3. In addition to the danger of electric shock, heating pads remain on and hot even if patients fall asleep.

4. Dosages of infrared rays should be carefully observed.

4. Too little heat does not achieve the required effect; too much can lead to skin damage.

5. Soaking or immersion should be done in water temperatures between 40° and 45°C.

5. Temperatures of 47°C or above (116°F) can cause burning.

Diathermy

Diathermy is a form of heat therapy in which the objective is deep (internal) rather than surface heating. Diathermy works by creating an electrical field in the tissues which is capable of conduction, thus heating the tissue and increasing circulation. Diathermy is commonly used in the treatment of muscular injuries and inflammatory joint disease. There are three basic approaches to diathermy:

1. *Microwave:* electromagnetic radiation is directed to the tissues.

2. *Shortwave:* high-frequency electric current is directed to the tissues.

3. *Ultrasound:* high-frequency sound waves are directed to the tissues.

Each of these forms of therapy requires the use of specific equipment. Microwave diathermy is generally the least complicated. It requires the aiming of a beam toward the affected area. Shortwave diathermy usually requires the manipulation of a semi-complex control panel, and sometimes the use of rather cumbersome and specialized appliances for application. Ultrasound utilizes a movable electrode in addition to a control panel.

Since equipment changes quite rapidly, and varies from manufacturer to manufacturer, the MA must be specifically trained to operate such equipment by the physician or the sales representative.

Because of the enormous heat which is generated in the diathermy process it is vitally important to adhere to recommended dosage allowances. A patient should never be allowed to continue a treatment beyond the prescribed time. Treatments are usually ordered for 15- to 20-minute periods.

Hydrotherapy

Hydrotherapy is the use of external water applications for therapeutic purposes. Hot and cold water immersion has previously been discussed, but physicians are also likely to prescribe whirlpool baths, contrast baths, or underwater exercise in particular applications. The patient is usually referred to the physiotherapy department of a medical center for hydrotherapy treatments.

1. *Whirlpools* provide the heat which is also available in immersion along with a gentle massage action. There are a number of different kinds of whirlpools available,

including wheelchair stalls, total body immersion baths, and smaller tubs for specific body parts.

2. *Contrast baths* employ two different containers of water, one hot and the other cold. The patient is required to move the affected body part quickly from the hot to the cold and then back to the hot baths.

3. *Underwater exercise* is often prescribed in cases of joint injuries, burns, or arthritis. In some minor cases this therapy can be carried out by the patient in a swimming pool of his choice.

These three modalities provide varying degrees of relaxation, increased or improved circulation, and mobility. For patients with burns, hydrotherapy may be prescribed for debridement purposes.

Ultraviolet Therapy

Many skin problems are treated with ultraviolet therapy, the use of heat lamps on the skin. Generally speaking, the heat instrument is one of three types: a hot quartz lamp, a cold quartz lamp, or a sun lamp. Each of these types is a complex electrical unit which has distinct characteristics. The MA need not be concerned with the types of appliance, but simply with the proper implementation of the physician's prescription. The appliance may be fixed or portable, but in either case the distance between patient and lamp is just as critical as the exposure time. Both exposure time and distance depend on the reason for use. Common medical office uses include treatment for acne, psoriasis, and superficial infections. Prior to lamp application at full dosage, the patient's sensitivity to ultraviolet light must be tested. Different areas of the body are exposed to different dosages of ultraviolet light and then compared for changes in coloration. Redness is expected, but burning would indicate increased sensitivity. The treatment usually begins with the time and distance that achieved the desired coloration. The exposure time is sometimes increased after repeated applications without ill effects. During the procedure, dark glasses are worn by the medical assistant and the patient to protect the eyes from harmful rays.

Joint Mobility

The measurement of joint motion, referred to as *goniometry,* is critical to the work of physical therapy since it allows the physician and therapist to establish base levels of disease or injury, thus helping to track the success of treatment or the progress of disease.

The traditional instrument of measurement is the goniometer (Fig. 25-1), which is a simple 360-degree protractor with a movable pointer arm. The goniometer is used to measure the joint in question, and the physical therapist has a list of standards for that particular joint. For example, the average person who lies flat on his back can move his elbow from 30 to 180 degrees, as recorded on the goniometer (Fig. 25-2).

Because many physicians carry out joint motion measurements, the MA may be required to assist with, or be instructed to assume the responsibility for, joint mobility testing. In assisting the physician with goniometry, it is important to understand the terminology used (Table 25-1).

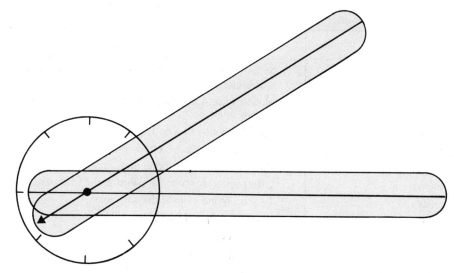

FIGURE 25-1. A universal goniometer.

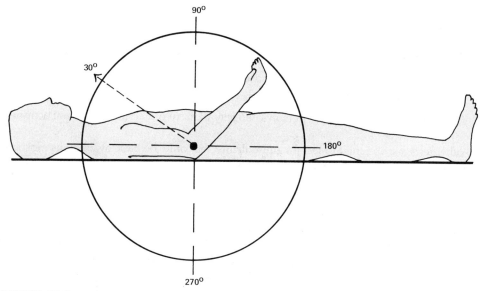

FIGURE 25-2. A standard goniometric test.

Muscle Testing

Many physicians employ manual muscle testing for the same reasons that joint mobility is measured. The general purpose is to evaluate the strength of muscle groups so that patients

TABLE 25-1. Goniometric Terminology

Term	Description
Flexion	Motion toward closing the joint or bringing two body parts together.
Extension	Motion toward opening the joint or spreading two body parts apart.
Abduction	Upward motion of a body part.
Adduction	Downward motion of a body part.
Circumduction	Circular rotation of a body part.
Pronation	Lifting up or down of the palms at the wrist joint.
Supination	Twisting of the palm at the wrist joint.
Inversion	Inward bending of foot at the ankle.
Dorsiflexion	Upward twist of foot.
Plantar flexion	Downward flex of foot.

can be assisted in the process of regaining function following injury or disease. Muscle testing usually includes:

1. *Range of motion tests*: testing which is focused upon muscle flexibility and resilience.

2. *Strength tests*: testing whose purpose is to establish the force with which a muscle or muscle group can act.

3. *Task skill tests*: testing the person's capacity to carry out certain important activities.

Many other tests are designed to test the musculature, but only the basic evaluations most frequently utilized in the medical office are listed here.

Exertherapy

Exertherapy is the use of body motion to achieve an improvement in one or more of the specific parts of the body. For the trained athlete, exercise may be used to move toward high levels of performance such as in running or jumping. In physical therapy, however, exercise is substantially more than a tool for the athlete. Exertherapy, or "PT exercise," is a therapeutic technique for helping patients to regain body function, to improve the ability to perform important motor functions, or to return to their usual occupations.

In physical therapy, the postoperative patient, the elderly individual, and the amputee are benefited by exercise, just as is the athlete. Thus the physician and the medical assistant may find themselves dealing with a 70-year-old patient who is doing exercises to regain the capacity of walking a few steps.

Exercise is a very powerful medical tool. It may have as great an effect as drug or other therapy. Thus it is important that the practitioner be knowledgeable. Exercises should never be prescribed without a thorough evaluation of the physical problem, and never by an untrained individual. Because the process of exertherapy is dynamic, the dosage (repetition frequency) must constantly be adjusted as the patient gets stronger.

The role of medical assistants in exertherapy is clearly that of a resource person. MAs should be sure that they understand the objective of any exercise which is prescribed. They should encourage and support the patient as he moves toward completion of his program.

Exercise programs may employ one or more of the following forms:

1. *Active-voluntary mobility.* The patient performs his own exercises.

2. *Passive-involuntary mobility.* The patient's body parts are moved by external force.

3. *Aided mobility.* Voluntary mobility with conducive aids, such as a therapy pool.

4. *Active resistance.* Voluntary mobility with counterpressure.

5. *Range of motion.* Active or passive joint mobility.

Massage

Massage, the manipulation of external body tissues, is one of the oldest known methods to promote healing. Various massage techniques appear to be almost instinctive in both humans and lower animals. In cases of strains, bruises, muscle soreness, lower back pain, dislocations, and other problems in which muscle relaxation and/or increased circulation is desired, the physical therapist may prescribe therapeutic massage.

There are basically three approaches to massage, and the therapist may choose one or all of them for a particular patient.

1. *Stroking*: the systematic movement of the hand across the skin. (This is the most common massage modality used in the medical office.)

2. *Compression*: the squeezing, pressing, or kneading of soft tissues.

3. *Percussion*: the alternating thumping of the skin with various parts of the hand.

Most persons regard massage as an art which should be based upon scientific understanding of the body and its injury. Often the physical therapist or physician will demonstrate a massage technique and ask that the patient or a family member carry out massage on a systematic basis.

The MA should understand the basic principles of massage therapy. These are listed and explained below.

GUIDELINES FOR MASSAGE

Principle	*Purpose*
1. The patient must be relaxed.	1. For massage to be effective, all muscles should be completely relaxed. Thus the first step is to calm the patient. Have him wear comfortable clothing, lie down, and expose only the area to be worked on.

2. A lubricating cream or oil should be utilized.

3. Pressure is transmitted through relaxed muscles, but not through tensed muscles.

2. The reduction of skin surface friction is important in helping the patient to relax.

3. A relaxed muscle has the characteristics of a liquid so that pressure is transmitted. A tense muscle will not work in this way. The patient must be relaxed.

Electrodiagnosis and Therapy

One of the more powerful and complex forms of therapy available to the physical therapist is the use of electrical stimulation of muscles or other body tissues. The use of electricity as a therapeutic tool flows logically from the electrodiagnostic approaches which are employed in physical medicine. Most therapists now regard the electromyogram as the most reliable test for muscle condition. Nerve conduction studies and muscle action potentials as well as other types of measurements are possible with electrodiagnosis.

Medical assistants will not usually be involved in electrical diagnosis or therapy since these procedures lie outside their usual expertise.

Paraffin Wax Hand Bath

This procedure consists of melting and heating wax and dipping the patient's hand into the substance. Paraffin wax baths are usually prescribed for patients with arthritis to relieve pain, increase circulation, and relax stiffness. The wax is usually melted and heated to 126°F (52°C) and is mixed with mineral oil in a proportionate amount (usually 7 to 1). A dry hand is immersed in the wax and quickly lifted out. The paraffin coating is often prescribed for home treatment. The medical assistant may be responsible for explaining the procedure and instructing the patient in the technique.

Traction

Traction, the act of pulling or stretching applied to the musculoskeletal system, is sometimes prescribed by the physician to ensure proper alignment of bones following injury or disease, to correct or prevent deformities, and to achieve other specific treatment objectives. The physical therapist applies traction according to a variety of different methods. Traction can be accomplished manually (using the hands to exert a pull), or by means of appliances, weights, or weighted pads applied to the sides of limbs. Skeletal traction may be effected by surgical insertion of pins, wires, or tongs.

Patient Assisting Devices

Quite often patients find that they require the use of a patient assisting device. The MA should be knowledgeable in the use of these supports in order to respond to the patient's questions and concerns.

WHEELCHAIRS

There are several criteria which should be considered by a patient who requires use of a wheelchair.

1. *Term of use.* Perhaps the most important issue is whether the patient will require the chair for an indefinite period or for a limited time. For short periods the patient may be best served by a rental unit, and may be able to live with standard models which have not been adjusted to his needs.

2. *Size.* Wheelchairs are available in a wide range of sizes. It is essential that the chair fit properly to offer proper support.

3. *Patient disorder.* A great many options are available, depending upon the special needs of the patient. Neck braces, specialized foot braces, and different transfer systems can be combined to facilitate the needs of individual patients.

4. *Life style.* Wheelchairs can also be purchased in "folding" models, outdoor styles, and any of a number of other forms which serve the special needs of particular patients.

The patient who faces long-term use of a wheelchair is usually referred to a medical supply house which can provide a precise chair prescription. In the long run a used or borrowed "bargain" chair does not facilitate the patient's physical or psychological needs, since the fit may be improper or the mobility hampered by the type of model. An illustration of a universal wheelchair is shown in Figure 25-3.

CRUTCHES

A patient for whom crutches have been prescribed should be assisted in understanding how to use them effectively. For the young or healthy patient with one "good" leg, the task of crutch training is uncomplicated. Most persons who spend a few moments with a pair of crutches will quickly learn how to manipulate them. Special instructions may be required in the following cases:

1. *Stairs.* Place both crutches under one arm and balance the body between the pair of crutches and the handrail (Fig. 25-4). Care should be taken so that the patient does not "jack-knife" and fall.

2. *Obstructions.* Obstructions such as curbs or steps without handrails can be approached by placing the lead crutch either up (ascending) or down (descending) and then twisting and elevating (or lowering) the body simultaneously (Fig. 25-5).

3. *Single crutch.* Patients for whom one crutch is prescribed should be advised to carry the crutch on the side of the "good" leg, not the "bad" leg. Most patients intuitively take the reverse approach.

4. *Crutch gaits.* The approach to a particular walking technique will depend upon the patient and his injury. The physician may prescribe a two-, three-, or four-point gait.

Four-point gait: a. right crutch
       b. left foot
       c. left crutch
       d. right foot
       e. repeat

Three-point gait: a. two crutches and weak leg
       b. strong leg
       c. repeat

Two-point gait: a. right crutch and left foot
       b. left crutch and right foot
       c. repeat

There are two main types of crutches: the *axillary crutch,* which is most commonly seen, and the *Lofstrand crutch,* which offers wrist support (Fig. 25-6).

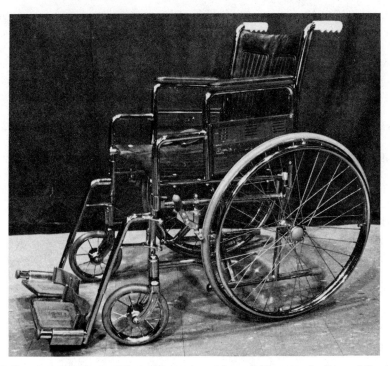

FIGURE 25-3. A universal wheelchair. (Reproduced from Saperstein, A. B., and Frazier, M. A.: *Introduction to Nursing Practice.* F. A. Davis, Philadelphia, 1980.)

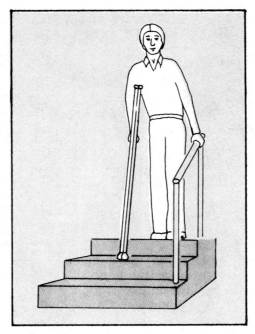

FIGURE 25-4. Descending stairs with use of crutches and a handrail. (Reproduced from Palmer, M. L., and Toms, J. E.: *Manual for Functional Training.* F. A. Davis, Philadelphia, 1980.)

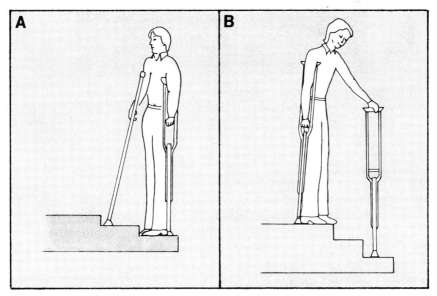

FIGURE 25-5. Left: Ascending stairs without a handrail. Right: Descending stairs with use of shoulder rests. (Reproduced from Palmer, M. L., and Toms, J. E.: *Manual for Functional Training.* F. A. Davis, Philadelphia, 1980.)

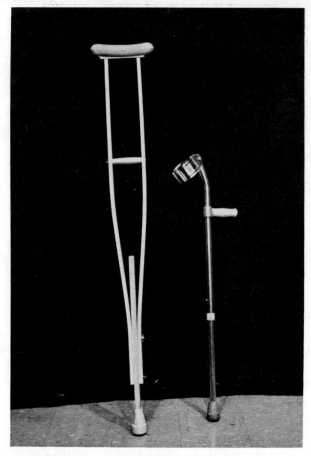

FIGURE 25-6.   Two types of crutches: axillary (left), and Canadian or Lofstrand (right). (Reproduced from Saperstein, A. B., and Frazier, M. A.: *Introduction to Nursing Practice*. F. A. Davis, Philadelphia, 1980.)

CANES AND WALKERS

The needs of some patients are best served by one of a variety of available types of canes or walkers. A few of these are illustrated in Figures 25-7 and 25-8.

BRACES

There are so many different types of braces available that it is not possible to offer a detailed discussion in this chapter. When a patient is in need of a brace, the medical assistant should make a special effort to prepare for patient teaching by learning as much as possible about the brace from the salesman or manufacturer. It is not uncommon for special representatives of brace companies to give detailed instructions to the patient.

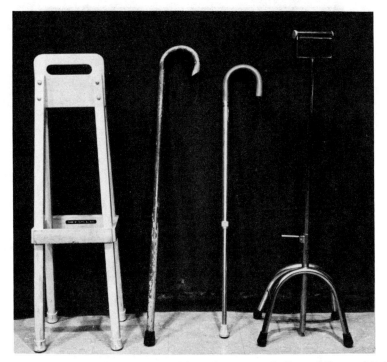

FIGURE 25-7.   Types of canes. (Reproduced from Saperstein, A. B., and Frazier, M. A.: *Introduction to Nursing Practice.* F. A. Davis, Philadelphia, 1980.)

Range of Motion Exercises

In some cases, the MA may be asked to assist with exercises which are designed to maintain patient joint mobility. These are *passive* exercises in the sense that they are performed by another person for the patient. Although these exercises do not promote muscle tone, they do help to maintain joint mobility.

Common Uses of Physical Therapy

ATHLETIC INJURY

In recent years a rather sudden and unexpected increase has occurred in the physical activities pursued by American men and women of all ages. Jogging, tennis, and weekend athletics are becoming increasingly popular. The result of this trend for physicians is an ever-growing interest in the treatment and prevention of athletic injury.

   The proper treatment of the athlete must be approached from a special perspective. The sedentary person with a sprained ankle is interested only in having his pain reduced. The tennis player with a sprained ankle wants to know when he can play tennis again and how he can "speed up" the process.

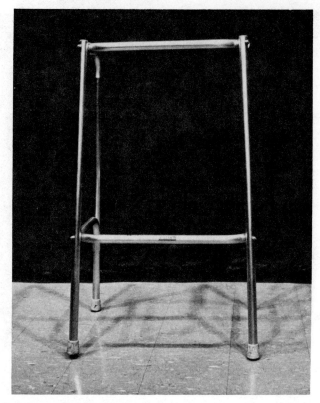

FIGURE 25-8. Standard walker. (Reproduced from Saperstein, A. B., and Frazier, M. A.: *Introduction to Nursing Practice*. F. A. Davis, Philadelphia, 1980.)

Athletes are typically willing to invest a great deal of energy in pursuing therapeutic programs which will speed their recovery. Often this zeal motivates the athlete to try to return to activity too soon, thus risking aggravation of the injury. Substitute activities are usually suggested to reduce the athlete's temptation to resume full activity prematurely. The jogger with tendinitis of the knee, for example, might be encouraged to change temporarily to a swimming program until his knee is healed.

In working with injured athletes, the role of the medical assistant is to reinforce and clarify the physician's orders.

THE AMPUTEE

A major role of physical therapy is the care of the amputee. Unless working for a physical therapist or an orthopedic specialist, the medical assistant will probably not often be involved in the care of an amputee. However, contact with patients who utilize some kind of prosthesis is inevitable. Therefore, a basic understanding of the dynamics of such devices is essential.

Many persons are erroneously convinced that amputations are followed by the fitting of an artificial limb and that after a brief training program, all problems are resolved and the patient adapts. For most amputees, the truth is far from this common assumption. The prosthesis requires constant attention; it may wear out, cause pain, become obsolete, or in other ways cause difficulties. Meanwhile, the patient almost always faces major psychological and emotional adjustment problems.

The MA must have empathy for these problems, offer the patient reassurance, and reinforce the orders of the physician or therapist.

DISEASE-RELATED USES

The physician will often consult the physical therapist and request recommendations for treatment. The physical therapist also serves as a diagnostician in some instances, collaborating with the physician in patient assessment of diseases related to the musculoskeletal system. Physical therapy procedures are often recommended for the following conditions commonly encountered in the medical office:

1. *Arthritis* — to increase circulation and maintain mobility.

2. *Cardiovascular disease* — to restore strength and increase circulation.

3. *Cerebral palsy* — to maintain mobility.

4. *Cerebral vascular accidents (CVAs)* — to restore function and strength.

5. *Low back pain* — to relieve discomfort and maintain mobility.

6. *Muscle spasm* — to relax the musculature and relieve pain.

7. *Muscle diseases and injuries* — to maintain mobility and prevent deformity.

8. *Pressure sores and infections* — to promote healing and kill microorganisms.

9. *Skin disorders* — to promote healing, reduce inflammation, and kill microorganisms.

OCCUPATIONAL THERAPY

Occupational therapists (OTRs) have earned at least a Bachelor's degree in occupational therapy. As professionals, they are concerned with the re-entry, or in some cases the initial entry, of persons into the work world. The basic premise of occupational therapy is that all persons need to be involved in meaningful, productive activities.

While there is a broad range of clients for whom the OTR offers important services, the most frequently encountered would include:

1. Skilled workers who have lost their jobs because of an illness or accident.

2. Amputees who find that they are unable to continue with their previous occupations.

3. Stroke victims who must readapt basic skills to their jobs.

4. Learning-disabled teenagers who need to move from the special education environment to the work world.

5. Young persons with birth defects who must begin to prepare for jobs.

6. Emotionally disturbed persons who are trying to seek employment.

7. Persons who are stricken with arthritis or other crippling diseases.

Occupational therapists view their functions microscopically. The task is not only one of helping persons to acquire skills and training, but also one of adaptation. Occupational therapy has been defined as:

> The art and science of directing man's participation in selected tasks to promote and maintain health, to restore, reinforce, and to enhance everyday performance, and to diminish or correct pathology caused by illness.*

As in the area of physical therapy there are two levels of problems which arise in the typical medical practice—the minor (advising) problems and the major dilemmas which require the counsel of an OTR—as well as the large gray area in between.

Many physicians make an effort to understand the delicate relationship between work and health. Thus they involve themselves in the interaction between the patient's medical problems and his occupation. The role of the medical assistant is to support the advice of the physician and to serve as counselor/facilitator for the patient. It is imperative that the patient be convinced that there is a clear link between occupational therapy and personal health.

Among the disease-related uses of occupational therapy for which the physician may refer the patient to an occupational therapist are the following:

1. *Cerebral vascular accidents (CVAs) and spinal cord injuries*—to assist the patient in maximizing function. Self-dressing and self-feeding techniques may be stressed for patients with paralysis. Application of splints to extend usefulness of body parts may also be necessary. Adaptation of automobiles and of the work and home environment may be necessary to restore the individual to independent functioning.

2. *Arthritis*—to assist the patient experiencing debilitation to maintain or restore self-care.

3. *Cerebral palsy*—to provide self-care instructions to encourage independence and maximization of functional ability.

4. *Psychiatric disorders*—to supplement psychotherapy objectives.

PSYCHOTHERAPY

There are a great many therapeutic activities which fall within the general framework of psychological treatment. As in the case of physical and occupational therapy, there are

---

*M. Abbott and M. L. Franciscus, *Opportunities in Occupational Therapy*, VMG Career Horizons Books, 1979, p. 1.

many degrees of psychological disturbance, ranging from minor adjustment or adaptation problems, which the general or family physician might encounter and treat, to extreme problems which may require specific medications, referrals for extensive therapy, or institutionalization.

Among the many participating professionals in the general area of the psychological helping professions are the following major groups:

1. *Psychiatrists*: Medical doctors who have specialized in the treatment of psychological disorders, and who utilize drug prescriptions as a part of their approach.

2. *Psychologists*: Academically trained persons (usually having doctoral degrees) who take a counseling rather than a drug prescription approach to therapy.

3. *Counselors*: Academically trained persons (usually having Master's degrees) who generally specialize in a particular problem area such as marriage counseling, drug rehabilitation, or mental health counseling.

As in the other areas, physicians will typically be drawn into psychological counseling in administrating to the needs of the patient until the nature of the problem transcends the physician's expertise. The patient is then referred to a specialist or therapist.

Again the role of the medical assistant is supportive in nature. In a case in which a patient is referred to a therapeutic specialist, the MA must encourage the patient to follow through and help him to feel comfortable and confident with such therapy.

APPLICATION EXERCISES

Group Presentations

Form groups and respond to one of the following assignments, as directed by the instructor. Upon completion, share results with the class by role-playing simulations or other creative presentations.

1. Develop a plan for teaching a patient with a right leg cast how to use axillary crutches.

2. Demonstrate range of motion of the hands (wrists and fingers). The patient is a 66-year-old woman and is arthritic. She is to continue these exercises at home. Plan the instruction.

3. Patient is a 300-lb male with a knee injury and must be confined to a wheelchair to travel long distances. The physician has instructed the MA to orient the patient to the use of the wheelchair. Develop a teaching plan.

4. The patient is 15 years old and is a football player. He has suffered a sprain of the right knee. The physician has ordered hot soaks. Discuss a teaching plan for this patient, what would be stressed, and what special problems you anticipate.

Problem-Solving Exercises

Discuss possible solutions to the following problems. Role-play where appropriate.

1. Mrs. Jones has just been informed by the physician that she needs the consultation of a psychotherapist. She is alone in the examining room and appears angry.

2. Mrs. Adams, 26, has been informed that she needs to use a cane because of a chronic debilitating condition. When the physician leaves the room, she confides that she will never use a cane. Can you anticipate what her concerns might be? What would be your response?

3. Mr. Green, a machinist, has had a cerebrovascular accident and has lost the use of one side of his body. The physician has scheduled occupational therapy for Mr. Green, who appears quite apprehensive. How would you prepare Mr. Green for his visit? What are your objectives?

4. Mrs. Roberts has been scheduled to visit a physical therapist twice a week for 3 months. This poses an inconvenience to her since she has small children at home. She is hesitant to begin treatments. How would you prepare Mrs. Roberts for therapy? What can you anticipate to be her objections in addition to the concern for her children?

COMPLETING THE LEARNING LOOP

As a student you may begin to gather information about physical and occupational therapy and psychotherapy from libraries, course descriptions, and conversations with allied health professionals. In these fields as well as in other areas of medical practice, concepts are always in the process of change or modification. It is therefore the responsibility of the professional medical assistant to keep abreast of new information that would be applicable to medical office practice.

You are now ready to begin the next unit, which exposes the aspiring medical assistant to yet another important area of responsibility—diagnostic testing.

BIBLIOGRAPHY

Banet, A. G., Jr. (ed.): *Creative Psychotherapy: A Source Book.* University Associates, San Francisco, 1976.
Binder, V., et al.: *Modern Therapies.* Prentice-Hall, Englewood Cliffs, N.J., 1976.
Competencies in Physical Therapy: An Analysis of Practice. American Physical Therapy Association, Washington, D.C., 1977.
Corsini, R. J., and Cardone, S.: *Roleplaying in Psychotherapy: A Manual.* Aldine, Chicago, 1966.
Cynkin, S.: *Occupational Therapy.* Little, Brown, Boston, 1979.
Downer, A. H.: *Physical Therapy Procedures: Selected Techniques,* ed. 3. Charles C Thomas, Springfield, Ill., 1978.
Krusin, F., Kottke, F. J., and Ellwood, P. M.: *Handbook of Physical Medicine and Rehabilitation.* W. B. Saunders, Philadelphia, 1971.
MacDonald, E. M. (ed.): *Occupational Therapy in Rehabilitation,* ed. 4. Macmillan, New York, 1976.
Palmer, M. L., and Toms, J. E.: *Manual for Functional Training.* F. A. Davis, Philadelphia, 1980.
Shestack, R.: *Handbook of Physical Therapy,* ed. 3. Springer, New York, 1977.

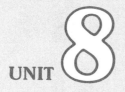

UNIT 8

ASSISTING WITH DIAGNOSTIC TESTING

The final area of mastery for the student of medical assisting is that of diagnostic testing. As the practice of medicine has evolved, the use of patient testing has greatly increased and its applications have likewise expanded. The medical assistant must be familiar with the classic testing approaches to effectively assist the physician and to properly instruct the patient. This unit focuses on the major areas of medical technology, electrocardiography, and radiography.

UNIT OBJECTIVES

Upon completion of this unit you will be prepared to:

1. List and describe the basic components and applications of medical technology.

2. Instruct the patient in the uses of clinical laboratory test procedures.

3. Assist the physician in the use of electrocardiographic equipment.

4. Instruct the patient in the process and uses of electrocardiographic testing.

5. Assist the physician in the use of radiographic equipment.

6. Instruct the patient in the nature and uses of radiographic testing.

26

MEDICAL TECHNOLOGY LABORATORY PROCEDURES

SPECIFIC OBJECTIVES

Upon completion of this chapter you will be able to:

1. Perform a skilled venipuncture.

2. Perform a skilled capillary puncture.

3. Comprehend laboratory medical terminology and recognize normal values.

4. Prepare laboratory specimens for presentation to reference laboratories.

5. Maintain proper quality control and daily worksheets.

6. Chart laboratory results and maintain a complete patient file.

7. Perform basic laboratory tests.

INTRODUCTION

The laboratory test is a valuable diagnostic tool. Specific laboratory tests can often be used to diagnose a particular disease; an abnormal glucose level, for example, may indicate diabetes. Laboratory tests are also used to monitor therapeutic drug levels for an individual patient who is being treated. Many physicians require a blood profile and a urinalysis for a yearly physical examination. Laboratory tests then act as a tool in preventive medicine.

Due to the broad scope of laboratory medicine, the field has become highly sophisticated, requiring skilled technologists and highly specialized equipment. The requirements for strict quality control, documentation, and periodic maintenance checks on equipment are too time-consuming to enable the average physician to offer a wide range of tests within the office setting. Consequently, test specimens are often sent to a regional reference laboratory for the actual testing.

The purpose of this chapter is to introduce the medical assistant to the basic concepts and techniques of laboratory medicine.

THE ROLE OF THE MEDICAL ASSISTANT IN DIAGNOSTIC LABORATORY TESTING

The role of the medical assistant as a laboratory technician is to be generally knowledgeable of laboratory medical terminology and normal test values, to be able to perform a skilled phlebotomy, to do basic laboratory testing, and to properly prepare specimens for reference laboratory testing. By comprehending the concepts and techniques of laboratory medicine, the medical assistant is able to operate more efficiently and effectively within the entire office system.

THE MEDICAL ASSISTANT AS A PHLEBOTOMIST

Phlebotomy is the making of an incision into a vein. Another term often used for this procedure is *venipuncture*, the primary purpose of which is to obtain a small sample of blood for diagnostic testing. The medical assistant must establish an environment which allows the patient to relax. Many patients view a venipuncture as a traumatic event and are very apprehensive. It is the phlebotomist's job to make the procedure as comfortable and painless as possible. The MA must maintain a professional attitude at all times, while being sympathetic to the concerns of the patient.

There are three basic groups of patients who will be encountered during a phlebotomy: the positive patient, the negative patient, and the first-time patient. Each must be approached differently.

Approaching the Positive Patient

The patient who has a positive attitude toward a phlebotomy will need little explanation as to the phlebotomy procedure and may in fact wish to tell the medical assistant how to perform it. The MA should graciously accept his suggestion as to the best vein, while exercising professional judgment in choosing an appropriate location for a venipuncture. The patient's positive attitude is usually related to the experience of skilled venipunctures in the past. This patient will appear relaxed, talkative, and confident. The medical assistant's goal as a phlebotomist must be to help every patient to develop a positive attitude.

Approaching the Negative Patient

The patient who has a negative attitude toward a phlebotomy represents a difficult problem for the phlebotomist. The medical assistant must deal not only with the present situation, but also with past events which have implanted this negative attitude. This type of patient has often experienced unpleasant, possibly traumatic events associated with phlebotomy procedures.

The individual's veins may be difficult to locate, or an unskilled phlebotomy may have been performed at an earlier time. The patient will appear nervous, apprehensive, and quite ill at ease. If the medical assistant has had an opportunity to interview the patient on his medical history, an insight into the patient's personality may already have been gained. Reviewing the patient's chart will alert the MA to any mental problems that could lead to the anxiety that the patient is experiencing. In the case of such patients, the medical assistant must make a special effort to perform the phlebotomy rapidly, efficiently, and effectively.

Medical assistant	"Mr. Jones, your doctor would like to have some laboratory work done."
Mr. Jones	"Oh, no! No blood tests for me!"
Medical assistant	"Your doctor needs these tests to aid in your diagnosis. Is there some reason you don't want the test done?"
Mr. Jones	"The last time they couldn't find a vein and after three times, you know, well, I just fainted. I said never again."
Medical assistant	"I never do more than one phlebotomy, Mr. Jones. Since you fainted before, please lie down and then you will be more comfortable."
Mr. Jones	"Well, uh, one try, understand, but that's all I'll stand for."

The medical assistant should exercise particular caution with any patient who has previously fainted. The patient must be lying down, an ammonia ampule should be readily available, and the physician should be in the office. By identifying the patient's past problem, as in the dialogue above, the MA was able to reassure the patient of her professional skill when she insisted that she would only do one venipuncture. This type of confident, firm, reassuring professional care may eventually transform negative resistance into a positive attitude toward a phlebotomy.

Approaching the First-Time Patient

The patient who has never had a phlebotomy is often apprehensive and nervous, but negative attitudes have not been formed. When dealing with this type of patient it is important to explain the procedure, answer any questions, and perform a skilled venipuncture rapidly before anxiety is allowed to build.

Medical assistant	"Mr. Green, your doctor would like you to have some laboratory tests done. Have you ever had a blood test?"
Mr. Green	"No. Why do I need blood tests? Does he think I have a serious disease?"
Medical assistant	"The blood test will just aid in your diagnosis. By obtaining a small sample of blood from your arm, an overall picture of the functioning of your body can be viewed."
Mr. Green	"What tests are ordered?"
Medical assistant	"You are to have some chemistry and hematology tests done."
Mr. Green	"How long will this take?"
Medical assistant	"I will draw the blood sample now and the doctor will have the results tomorrow. You can call the office by 3 p.m., if you would like to. Now, just have a seat and I will explain everything. I'll tie this tourniquet around your arm and locate your vein. There will be a small pinch, and I'll fill these two tubes. I will apply a bandaid, and you may leave after five minutes."

The medical assistant assures the patient by answering all of his questions. When questions concern the patient's diagnosis, very broad, nonspecific answers should be given. For instance, the MA would say, "The doctor has ordered a chemistry test," rather than "The doctor has ordered a blood sugar test because he thinks you have diabetes mellitus." It is your responsibility as a phlebotomist to make sure that each first-time phlebotomy patient leaves the office with a positive attitude toward the phlebotomy experience.

Factors Affecting a Good Venipuncture

As the foregoing discussion has shown, the phlebotomist must work rapidly and must perform a skilled venipuncture to gain the patient's confidence. There are three major factors affecting a good venipuncture: (1) the patient's attitude and the nature of his veins, (2) the equipment, and (3) the phlebotomist.

The patient is likely to arrive with firm ideas formulated about phlebotomies. Although the goal is to create a positive attitude in every patient, the phlebotomist has little initial control over the patient's feelings. The nature of the patient's veins can be assessed, but cannot be changed. A patient with difficult veins may, however, be able to alert the phlebotomist to the best location for a venipuncture.

The second factor, the equipment utilized, can be controlled to a greater degree. Most facilities use either syringes or a vacutainer system. The vacutainer is a blood collection system composed of a plastic barrel, a double-pointed needle, and interchangeable vacutainer tubes (Figs. 26-1 and 26-2). The three major advantages to the vacutainer system are

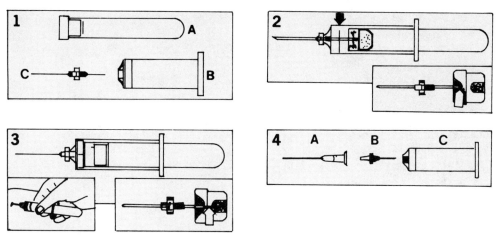

FIGURE 26-1. How to assemble a Becton-Dickinson Vacutainer. 1. Description of parts: (A) evacuated glass tube with rubber stopper; (B) plastic holder with guide line; (C) double-pointed needle. 2. Thread needle into holder and tighten firmly. Place tube in holder with needle touching stopper. 3. Push tube forward until top of stopper meets guide line and then let go. Tube stopper will retract below guide line and should be left in that position. At this stage the full point of the needle is embedded in the stopper, thus avoiding blood leakage upon venipuncture and preventing premature loss of vacuum. 4. Alternate method using (A) Luer hub needle; (B) Vacutainer adapter; and (C) plastic holder. Thread adapter into holder and tighten firmly. Attach Luer needle to adapter as a needle is attached to a syringe. Place tube in holder with needle touching stopper, then proceed to step 3 above.

that it is disposable, that it allows for multiple tubes to be drawn from a single venipuncture, and that there is less chance of labeling error and hemolysis since the blood is not transferred.

The phlebotomist is the factor allowing for the greatest measure of control. Venipuncture is a skill, and skills are developed and perfected through practice and study. It is the medical assistant's responsibility to master this skill.

The steps entailed in performing a venipuncture and a finger puncture are given below. Because of the risk of contamination by tissue fluid and the inability to repeat the test due to the small volume of blood obtainable from finger puncture, venipunctures are preferred over capillary methods. Nevertheless, the capillary method is used in cases in which the patient has extremely poor veins, or with children and newborns from whom large amounts of blood are difficult to obtain. A note should always be made on the laboratory slip when the testing specimen is from a capillary source.

PERFORMING A VENIPUNCTURE USING THE VACUTAINER SYSTEM

Purpose: To perform a skilled venipuncture so that the blood sample can be used for diagnostic testing.

Equipment: tourniquet
        sterile alcohol swab
        sterile gauze pad (2-inch square)

vacutainer holder
vacutainer tube
double-pointed vacutainer needle (19- to 21-gauge)
bandage
ammonia ampule

Procedure	*Principle*
1. Wash hands.	1. Washing prevents the spread of microorganisms.

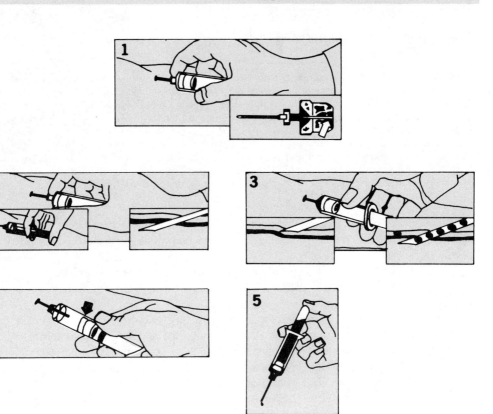

FIGURE 26-2. How to use a Becton-Dickinson Vacutainer. 1. With rear point embedded in stopper, enter tissue and immediately complete puncture of diaphragm. 2. If the needle enters a vein, blood will flow immediately. In general proceed as with a hypodermic syringe. The holder provides a finger grip and the tube acts as a plunger. 3. If tissue is entered, blood will not be drawn. Proceed until venipuncture is signaled by intake of blood into the Vacutainer tube, as shown. 4. To conserve the vacuum when the vein cannot be located, remove tube from rear cannula (see arrow) before withdrawing needle from tissue. 5. To obtain specimens for blood smears or cell counts, grasp holder as shown and press firmly on bottom of tube. After each drop is collected, remove pressure and repeat for successive drops.

2. Identify the patient and check his laboratory request form for any clerical errors.

2. Proper patient identification must be done to ensure that the right patient is being drawn.

3. Select proper test tubes for the tests requested. Ask the patient if he is fasting for those tests requiring a fasting specimen.

3. Depending on the test requested, the tubes may need to have an anticoagulant. For fasting specimens, the patient must not have eaten since midnight of the previous day.

4. Observe the patient for abnormal anxiety and explain the procedure.

4. Many patients are very nervous and anxious about a phlebotomy, and they should be reassured to reduce this anxiety level.

5. Assemble equipment. Thread the needle into the vacutainer holder and place the appropriate tube in the holder until the rubber stopper reaches the guideline.

5. The needle will puncture the rubber when inserted to the guideline, but will not break the vacuum seal in the tube. This prevents blood leakage around the rubber stopper.

6. Apply the tourniquet to the upper arm above the elbow (Fig. 26-3). Cross the ends of the tourniquet and pull upward to create tension. Tuck the upper end of the tourniquet into the tightened band.

6. The tourniquet causes physical pressure to the area which allows the veins to become more pronounced. The tourniquet must not be too tight or blood flow will be obstructed. The tourniquet should be released after 1 minute due to patient discomfort.

7. Ask the patient to open and close his fist twice. The fist should remain closed.

7. Physical pressure is increased by this movement.

8. Palpate the veins and select the venipuncture site.

8. The antecubital veins are usually used and should be easily located due to the pressure from the tourniquet and closed fist. The median basilic vein is easier to stabilize due to its centralized position.

9. Cleanse the venipuncture site with a sterile alcohol swab, using a circular motion working from the inside outward. Allow to dry.

9. The antiseptic will remove dirt and bacteria. The circular cleansing motion carries particles away from the area.

10. Hold the vacutainer system with the needle level upward. Stabilize the vein by pulling the skin tight.

10. Stabilizing the skin prevents the vein from rolling.

11. Insert the needle into the skin and vein at a 20-degree angle. Engage the vacuum tube fully.

11. Blood will flow into the vacuum tube because of the vacuum pressure once the vein is punctured. The 20-degree angle will prevent the needle from going too deep into the tissue. Pushing the vacuum tube past the guideline will ensure that the tube is properly engaged.

12. Allow the tube to fill completely.

12. Any tube with anticoagulant is based on a ratio of blood volume to anticoagulant. If a short sample is drawn, this ratio will be affected and yield inaccurate results.

13. Have the patient relax his fist. Remove the tourniquet.

13. The open fist decreases physical pressure. Release the tourniquet by pulling one end.

14. Apply a sterile gauze pad over the puncture site and withdraw the needle.	14. The tourniquet must be released prior to withdrawing the needle to avoid bleeding around the area, resulting in a hematoma.
15. Raise the patient's arm and have him hold the gauze in place until the blood has clotted.	15. This pressure will prevent a hematoma.
16. Label each tube drawn immediately with the patient's full name, the date, and the test requested. Properly mix the tubes if anticoagulants are used.	16. Properly labeled specimens are required by all laboratories.
17. Properly dispose of equipment and destroy the needle.	17. Proper disposal prevents the spread of microorganisms. (Commercial devices are available for destroying needles.)
18. Check the patient's arm and apply a bandage.	18. Observe the area for abnormal coloration or excessive bleeding.
19. Have the patient wait 5 minutes before leaving the office.	19. This time period assures that the patient is stable and no adverse reactions, such as fainting, will result.
20. Wash hands.	20. This prevents the spread of microorganisms.
21. Properly process the test tubes for testing or mailing to the reference laboratories.	21. Maintaining specimens under improper storage conditions will result in inaccurate laboratory test values.

OBTAINING CAPILLARY BLOOD FROM A FINGER PUNCTURE

Purpose: To obtain a small volume of capillary blood for diagnostic testing.

Equipment: sterile gauze pad (2-inch square)
sterile lancet
sterile alcohol swab
circular spot bandage

Procedure	*Principle*
1. Wash hands.	1. Washing prevents the transfer of microorganisms.
2. Assemble equipment quickly.	2. Many patients become apprehensive even about a finger puncture.
3. Observe the patient's finger for coldness, calluses, wounds, or rashes.	3. The patient who has poor circulation will have cold hands. Place the finger in warm water for 2 to 3 minutes. Any calluses, wounds, or rash areas must be avoided to prevent the spread of infections.
4. Choose the puncture site.	4. The lateral side of the finger is less sensitive. The most common fingers chosen are the middle finger and the fourth finger.

5. Cleanse the area with alcohol and allow to dry.

5. Alcohol will clean the area, removing bacteria. The alcohol must dry to prevent stinging once the finger is punctured.

6. Open the sterile lancet. Do not touch the tip.

6. The lancet must be sterile to prevent infection.

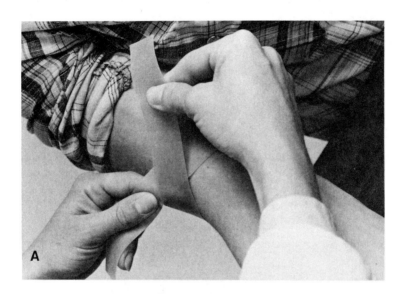

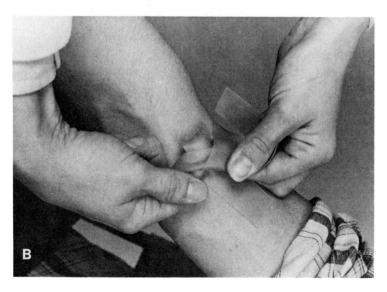

FIGURE 26-3. Applying a tourniquet. A, Cross the ends of the tourniquet and pull upward to create tension. B, Tuck the upper end of the tourniquet into the tightened band.

7. Grasp the patient's finger. Do not touch the sterilized area. Penetrate the skin approximately 2 to 3 mm with a swift wrist motion.

7. The patient's finger must be held firmly to assure that if the patient moves, his finger will remain stationary. The area must be sterile. If the area is touched, it must be recleaned. The lancet has a calibrated tip and the design is such that a deeper puncture cannot be made (Fig. 26-4).

8. Wipe away the first drop of blood with sterile gauze.

8. The first drop of blood will contain diluted alcohol and tissue fluid. Therefore, it is not an adequate blood specimen.

9. Press the finger but do not squeeze. Fill the laboratory test equipment and make dilutions. Apply gauze firmly to the puncture site to make sure bleeding has stopped.

9. Squeezing the finger will increase tissue fluid, yielding false laboratory test results.

10. Observe the site to make sure that bleeding has stopped. Apply a bandage.

10. The pressure on the gauze will cause the blood to clot. The site should be inspected to be sure that there is no bleeding. The bandage is for protection.

11. Wash hands.

11. This prevents the spread of disease.

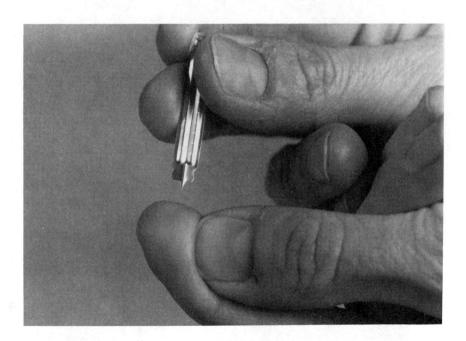

FIGURE 26-4. Procedure for obtaining blood by finger puncture. The lateral side of the finger is less sensitive, and the most common fingers chosen are the middle finger and the fourth finger. While the patient's finger is held firmly, the skin is penetrated with a sterile lancet.

UNDERSTANDING LABORATORY MEDICAL TERMINOLOGY AND NORMAL VALUES

The medical assistant must have a broad knowledge of the medical laboratory field in order to interpret the variety of laboratory data received in the medical office. Normal values will vary depending on the individual laboratory and the methods utilized. Many reference laboratories provide lists of normal values with each patient's report sent to the physician's office. When charting laboratory reports in the patient's file, abnormal values should be highlighted in red to alert the physician. A list of common laboratory abbreviations and a sample of generally accepted normal values are provided below for reference.

Common Laboratory Abbreviations

HEMATOLOGY AND COAGULATION

Baso	= polymorphonuclear (segmented) basophil leukocyte
Bl	= blood; bleeding
Bl & Coag	= bleeding and coagulation
CBC	= complete blood count (includes Hgb, Hct, WBC, RBC, MCV, MCH, and MCHC)
Diff	= differential leukocyte count of peripheral blood
EDTA	= ethylenediaminetetraacetic acid (a common blood anticoagulant)
Eos	= polymorphonuclear (segmented) eosinophilic leukocyte
ESR	= erythrocyte sedimentation rate
F Hgb	= fetal hemoglobin
Hgb, Hb	= hemoglobin
HB	= Heinz body
Hct	= hematocrit or packed cell volume (PCV)
LE	= lupus erythematosus
MCH	= mean corpuscular hemoglobin
MCHC	= mean corpuscular hemoglobin concentration
MCV	= mean corpuscular volume
PA	= pernicious anemia
PMN	= polymorphonuclear neutrophil leukocyte
PT	= prothrombin time
PTT	= partial thromboplastin time
RBC	= red blood cell count
Retic	= reticulocyte
S Hgb	= sickle cell hemoglobin
WBC	= white blood cell count

CHEMISTRY

Ab	= antibody
ACTH	= Adrenocorticotropic hormone

A/G   = albumin-globulin ratio
Ag   = antigen
Alb   = albumin
Alc   = alcohol
Alk   = alkaline
BJP   = Bence-Jones protein
BUN   = blood-urea-nitrogen
CEA   = carcinoembryonic antigen
CPK   = creatine phosphokinase
FBS   = fasting blood sugar
GA   = gastric analysis
G 6PD = glucose-6-phosphate
GTT   = glucose tolerance test
5HIAA = 5-hydroxyindole acetic acid
ICD   = isocitric dehydrogenase
IgE   = immunoglobulin E
17KS   = 17-ketosteroids
LAP   = leucine aminopeptidase
LDH   = lactic dehydrogenase
PBG   = porphobilinogen
PBI   = protein-bound iodine
PKU   = phenylketonuria
SGOT   = serum glutamic-oxaloacetic transaminase
SGPT   = serum glutamic-pyruvic transaminase
Sp Gr = specific gravity
T_3 = triiodothyronine
T_4 = tetraiodothyronine (thyroxine)
TBG   = thyroxine-binding globulin
TIBC   = total iron-binding capacity
TSH   = thyroid-stimulating hormone

SEROLOGY AND IMMUNOLOGY

ASOT   = antistreptolysin-O titer
CF   = complement fixation
CRP   = C-reactive protein
CSF   = cerebrospinal fluid
FA   = fluorescent antibody; febrile antigens
FTA   = fluorescent treponemal antibody
LE test   = a rapid slide test method for systemic lupus erythematosus (Hyland)
Mono-Spot = a test for mononucleosis
RA test   = a rapid slide test for rheumatoid arthritis
RF   = rheumatoid factor
RIA   = radioimmunoassay
rpm   = revolutions per minute

SLE   = systemic lupus erythematosus
STS   = serologic test for syphilis
TB   = tuberculin
VD   = Venereal disease
VDRT   = Venereal Disease Reference Test

Common Normal Values *

NORMAL BLOOD CHEMISTRY VALUES FOR ADULTS

Substance	Normal Values
Acetone	0.3-2.0 mg/dl
Albumin	3.5-5.0 gm/dl
Ammonia	102 ± 23 µg/dl 45-50 µg/dl
Amylase	80-150 U/dl
Ascorbic acid	0.6-2.0 mg/dl
Bilirubin (total/direct)	0.8/0.2 mg/dl
Calcium	4.25-5.25 mEq/L 8.5-10.5 mg/dl
Chloride	98-106 mEq/L
Copper	Men: 70-140 µg/dl Women: 80-155 µg/dl
Creatine phosphokinase	5-55 mU/ml
Creatinine	Men: 0.6-1.2 mg/dl Women: 0.5-1.0 mg/dl
Fibrinogen	200-400 mg/dl
Globulins	2.3-3.5 gm/dl
Glucose	90-120 mg/dl (Folin-Wu method) 65-95 mg/dl (Nelson-Somogyi method) 60-105 mg/dl (glucose oxidase method) 46-94 mg/dl (ultra-micro method)
Iron	56-183 µg/dl
Lactic dehydrogenase	200-450 U/ml (Wroblewski-LaDue method) 60-120 U/ml (Wacker method)
Lipase	0.1-1.0 U/ml
Lipids (total)	450-1000 mg/dl

---

* Modified from Widmann, F. K.: *Clinical Interpretation of Laboratory Tests*, ed. 8. F. A. Davis, Philadelphia, 1979.

Magnesium	1.4-2.2 mEq/L
	1.7-2.7 mg/dl
Nitrogen (NPN)	25-40 mg/dl
(BUN)	5-25 mg/dl
pH	Arterial: 7.37-7.42
	Venous: 7.34-7.39
Phosphatase, acid	0.5-4.0 U/dl (Babson-Read method)
	0-0.1 U/dl (Shinowara method)
Phosphatase, alkaline	1.5-4.0 U/dl (Bodansky method)
	3.7-13.1 U/dl (King-Armstrong method)
	2.2-8.6 U/dl (Shinowara method)
Phospholipids	To age 65: 175-275 mg/dl
	After age 65: 196-366 mg/dl
	Pregnancy: 205-291 mg/dl
Phosphorus, inorganic	2.6-4.8 mg/dl
Potassium	3.5-5.3 mEq/L
Sodium	135-148 mEq/L
Transaminase	
Glutamic-oxaloacetic	12-36 U/ml
Glutamic-pyruvic	6-53 U/ml
Uric acid	Men: 3.0-7.0 mg/dl
	Women: 2.0-6.0 mg/dl

NORMAL VALUES FOR URINE

Test	Normal Values
Albumin	
Qualitative	Negative
Quantitative	10-100 mg/24 hr
Aldosterone	2-23 µg/24 hr
Amino acid nitrogen	100-290 mg/24 hr
Ammonia	700 mg/24 hr
Bence-Jones protein	Negative
Bilirubin	Negative
Blood, occult	Negative
Calcium	
Qualitative	Positive 1+ (Sulkowitch method)
Quantitative	30-150 mg/24 hr
Chloride	110-250 mEq/24 hr
Creatine	Less then 100 mg in 24 hr, or less than 6% of creatinine. Pregnancy: up to 12% of creatinine. Children under 1 yr: may equal creatinine. Children over 1 yr: up to 30% creatinine.

Creatinine	Females: 0.8-1.7 gm/24 hr Males: 1-1.9 gm/24 hr
Estrogens	Females: 4-60 μg/24 hr Males: 4-25 μg/24 hr
Glucose	
Qualitative	Negative
Quantitative	50-500 mg/24 hr
Lead	0.021-0.038 mg/L
pH	4.8-7.8
Phenylpyruvic acid	Negative
Phosphorus	0.9-1.3 gm/24 hr
Porphobilinogen	Negative
Potassium	25-100 mEq/24 hr
Sodium	About 110 mEq/24 hr
Specific gravity	1.002-1.030 (single specimen) 1.015-1.025 (24-hr specimen)
Uric acid	0.5-1.0 gm/24 hr
Urobilinogen	
Semiquantitative	Up to 1 Ehrlich unit/2 hr
Quantitative	1.0-4.0 mg/24 hr
Volume	Adults: 1000-1500 ml/24 hr (about 15-21 ml/kg body weight) Children: 3 to 4 times as much as adults per kg body wt

HEMATOLOGY VALUES IN ADULTS

"Complete blood count" (CBC)	
Hematocrit (%)	Men: 40-54 Women: 37-47
Hemoglobin (gm/dl)	Men: 13.3-17.7 Women: 11.7-15.7
Red blood cells per mm^3	Men: 4.5-6.0 $\times$ 10^6 Women: 4.3-5.5 $\times$ 10^6
White blood cells per mm^3	5,000-10,0000

Mean corpuscular
    volume (MCV) as
    μ^3/cell
	80-94

Mean corpuscular
    hemoglobin (MCH) as
    pg/cell
	27-34

Mean corpuscular
    hemoglobin concen-
    tration (MCHC) as
    percent of cell volume
	31-36

Erythrocyte sedimentation rate (ESR)	Men below age 50: 1-15

Modified Westergren method, in mm/hr	Men above age 50: 1-20 Women below age 50: 1-20 Women above age 50: 1-30
Leukocyte alkaline phosphatase as arbitrary score	13-130
Reticulocytes as percent of red cells	0.5-2.5

COAGULATION VALUES IN ADULTS

Bleeding time	
Ivy	1-6
Template	3-6
Fibrinogen	150-450 mg/dl
Partial thromboplastin time (PTT)	60-85 sec
Partial thromboplastin time, activated (aPTT)	35-40 sec or within 5 sec of control
Plasminogen	10-20 mg/dl
Platelets	150,000-450,000/mm^3
Prothrombin time (PT)	11-13 sec or within 2 sec of control
Thrombin clotting time (TCT)	10-15 sec or within 1.3 times as long as control

Common Laboratory Tests and Indicated Disease States

Laboratory tests are indications of body metabolism at the time a specimen was obtained. Not all laboratory results can be correlated to a single disease state. For this reason the patient's total condition must be assessed by the physician with the aid of laboratory data.

Test	*Disease*
Acid phosphatase	Prostatic cancer
Amylase and lipase	Acute pancreatitis
Antistreptolysin-O titer (ASOT) and erythrocyte sedimentation rate (ESR)	Rheumatic fever and other streptococcal infections
Bence-Jones protein (BJP)	Multiple myeloma
Cholesterol	Atherosclerosis
Cold agglutination test	Primary atypical pneumonia
Febrile agglutins	Typhoid O and H Paratyphoid A and B Brucellosis

	Tularemia
	Dysentery
	Typhoid fever
Heterophil antibody or "mono" test	Infectious mononucleosis
PKU test (phenylpyruvic acid in urine; phenylalanine in serum)	Phenylketonuria
Prothrombin test	Anticoagulation therapy or coagulation disorders
Red blood cells, hematocrit, hemoglobin, iron, total iron-binding capacity	Anemia
Sickle cell test	Sickle cell trait or sickle cell disease
Sugar (glucose); FBS (fasting blood sugar) 2 hr P.C.	Diabetes mellitus
Glucose tolerance test (GTT)	Hypoglycemia

Many physicians will order a profile or a group of laboratory tests designed to screen a particular metabolic function. The medical assistant should have a general acquaintance with the individual laboratory tests being ordered. Reference laboratories usually provide a list that includes profile tests and specifically used normal values.

Bleeding Studies

Bleeding time
Clot retraction
Partial thromboplastin time (PTT)
Platelet count
Prothrombin time

Electrolyte Tests

Chloride (Cl)
Potassium (K)
Sodium (Na)

Kidney Function Tests

Addis count
Albumin/globulin ratio
Blood-urea-nitrogen (BUN)
Clearance tests
Creatinine
Total protein

Liver Function Tests

Albumin/globulin ratio
Alkaline phosphatase
Bilirubin
Hepatitis-associated antigen (HAA)
Lactate dehydrogenase (LDH)

Plasma proteins
Prothrombin time
Protein electrophoresis
Serum proteins
        Serum glutamic-pyruvic transaminase (SGPT)
        Serum glutamic-oxaloacetic transaminase (SGOT)
Urobilinogen

Thyroid Function Tests

Protein-bound iodine (PBI)
Triiodothyronine (T_3)
Thyroxine (T_4)
Thyroid-stimulating hormone (TSH)

Laboratory Culturing

The following is a list of common culture specimens, the method used for culturing, and the common organisms isolated from each source.

Source	Method	Organism
Blood	Blood culture tube containing transport medium and an anti-coagulant. Collected by venipuncture.	Bacteriodes, Brucella, Clostridium, Histoplasma, Listeria, Vibrio, Salmonella, Staphlococcus, Streptococcus, Pseudomonas, Pasteurella, Mycoplasma, Neisseria, Pneumococci.
Urine	First morning voided midstream. Clean-catch specimen in sterile container. Refrigerate if transportation is delayed.	Escherichia coli, Klebsiella, Enterobacter, Serratia, Proteus, Pseudomonas, Streptococcus, Staphylococcus, Candida, Neisseria.
Wounds	Culturette method	Staphylococcus, enterococci, Streptococcus, Clostridium, Bacteroides, Pseudomonas, Proteus, Escherichia coli.
Sputum	Sterile sputum collection container. The patient must obtain a sputum specimen by coughing deeply when getting up in the morning.	Diplococcus pneumoniae, Streptococcus, Staphylococcus, Mycobacterium, Haemophilus, Klebsiella, Neisseria.
Throat and naso-pharynx	Culturette swab	Streptococcus (Group A), Staphylococcus, Pneumococcus, Candida, Bordetella, Haemophilus.
Ear	Culturette swab	Staphylococcus, Streptococcus, Pneumococcus, Pseudomonas,

		Proteus, Candida, Haemophilus.
Eye	Culturette swab	Streptococcus, Staphylococcus, Pneumococcus, Neisseria, Pseudomonas, Haemophilus, Corynebacterium.
Cerebrospinal fluid (CSF)	CSF is collected by lumbar puncture. Specimens should be processed immediately. (This procedure is not done at the physician's office.)	Neisseria, Haemophilus, Proteus, Pseudomonas, Pneumococcus, Myco-bacterium, Staphyloccus, Streptococcus, Cryptococcus.
Feces	Stool specimen collected in early morning or with a rectal swab.	Salmonella, Shigella, Proteus, Pseudomonas.

QUALITY CONTROL IN LABORATORY MEDICINE

In any discussion concerning laboratory medicine, it is necessary to stress quality control. The medical assistant performing various diagnostic laboratory tests has a responsibility to record accurate, precise, and reproducible results. Quality control can be achieved by maintaining excellent technique and selecting reliable procedures, standards, and control serums. Glassware must be clean and pipettes free from chips. Instruments must be calibrated and routine maintenance checks performed. Reagents must be used within their expiration dates. Documentation of instrument calibration, routine maintenance, reagent lot numbers, and laboratory test results of standards, controls, and patients must be recorded daily.

Standards and controls are used with laboratory procedures to ensure that the reagents, temperatures, instruments, and techniques at the time the test is performed are within an acceptable range of accuracy. If only the patient's test is performed without the aid of standards and controls, there is no way to determine whether the results are valid. When standards and controls are utilized and for some reason are out of range, a source of error is recognized and identification of that source must be investigated. The first items to be checked should be the expiration dates of all reagents and, when repeating the procedure, the different lot numbers utilized, if these are available. Instrument malfunction as well as proper procedural technique should also be investigated. Laboratory test results are only as valid as the quality control used for the individual tests.

Specimen Collection

Quality control begins with a properly collected specimen. If the specimen was mislabeled or collected with the wrong anticoagulant, invalid laboratory results will be obtained. There are four basic criteria for a properly collected specimen:

1. Identification of the patient
2. Proper screening of the patient
3. Good venipuncture technique
4. Proper selection of anticoagulants

The specimen must be labeled at the time it is taken with the patient's full name, date, and the test requested. The laboratory request form must match the data on the specimen. The patient must be screened to make sure that he has followed preliminary instructions, such as fasting for certain laboratory tests. Good venipuncture technique will provide an unhemolyzed specimen. Hemolyzed specimens are to be avoided because they produce invalid results.

Many tests require whole blood or plasma. Blood will normally clot, yielding serum if anticoagulants are not added at the time of collection. The anticoagulants used will vary with the laboratory test requested. It is important to mix the blood specimen and the anticoagulant by gentle inversion. Shaking will cause the blood specimen to hemolyze.

Several basic types of anticoagulant are available, each with different effects and applications:

1. *Sodium, potassium or ammonium oxalate* prevents coagulation by removing calcium. It is unsuitable for potassium, sodium, nitrogen, and BUN determinations, and is known to alter cells in morphologic studies.

2. *Citrate* prevents coagulation by removing calcium. It is used for coagulation and sedimentation studies.

3. *EDTA (ethylenediamine tetraacetic acid)* prevents coagulation by chelating or binding calcium. It is used for routine chemistry work and hematology studies.

4. *Heparin* prevents coagulation by inhibiting thrombin formation.

5. *Sodium fluoride* acts as a preservative and inhibits enzymatic activity; therefore, it should not be used for glucose determinations or studies utilizing enzymes.

Specimen Handling

When a venipuncture is performed and the blood sample enters a test tube, various chemical changes occur due to enzymatic reactions. Because laboratory test results are expected to represent the patient's metabolic state at the time of collection, it is necessary to control or retard these changes. There are basically two means of preserving specimens: physical and chemical. Physical means, such as refrigeration and freezing, slow down these chemical changes. Freezing can only be done with plasma or serum since red blood cells will lyse, resulting in a grossly hemolyzed specimen. Chemical means, such as sodium fluoride, actually inhibit enzyme activity.

For clotted specimens it is best to allow the specimen to clot normally at room temperature for 30 minutes, centrifuge, remove the serum into a properly labeled test tube, and freeze. Most reference laboratories provide detailed instructions for specimen handling keyed to the procedures and methods employed by the individual facility.

BASIC MICROBIOLOGY

Microbiology is the study of microorganisms. Medical microbiology deals primarily with pathogenic, or disease-causing, organisms. Microbiologic laboratory tests are usually performed outside the medical office in medical laboratories. These laboratories maintain various culture media, substances used to enhance the growth of microorganisms, and specialized microbiologists to study the cultures. The medical assistant must have a general knowledge of the basic steps for studying bacterial cultures, even though these tasks may not be performed in the physician's office. The MA may be involved in the collection of various cultures from wounds and from throat, ear, eye, nasal, blood, urine, and vaginal sources. Because results in microbiologic studies are only as good as the original culture submitted for study, great care must be taken to prevent contamination when specimens are collected.

The main focus of this section will be on the use of the microscope and on specimen collection, handling and transportation of specimens, smear preparation, and Gramstaining technique. While it is beyond the scope of this discussion to consider each and every pathogen, the medical assistant will find a reference text, such as *Bergey's Manual of Determinative Bacteriology*, to be a valuable tool for interpretation of individual pathogens reported from patient cultures.

The Microscope

The microscope is an optical instrument used to magnify small structures for morphologic study. It is a vital laboratory tool and one which the medical assistant must be able to use properly. The MA should be familiar with the parts of the microscope and their function, as well as proper maintenance to keep it in good working condition.

The major parts of the microscope and their purpose are listed below and can be compared with Figure 26-5, which illustrates a binocular compound microscope.

Parts	*Purpose*
Eyepiece (ocular lens)	The eyepiece is the lens system that is closest to the eye, on which the magnification is printed.
Interpupillary distance adjuster	The binocular compound microscope has two eyepieces that can be adjusted to the width between the individual's eyes by means of the knob found between the oculars.
Body tube	The body tube directs the light path from the light source to the eyepiece.
Arm	The arm is used to carry the microscope with one hand on the arm handle and the other firmly holding the base of the microscope.
Base	The base of the microscope is its foundation or platform.
Revolving nosepiece	The revolving nosepiece holds the objectives and permits their movement for selection.
Objectives	The objectives constitute the lens system found on the nosepiece. There are usually three objectives (low-power dry, high-power dry, and oil immersion), each having the magnification engraved on the barrel.
Stage clip	The stage clip is a movable spring device used to secure a slide to the top of the stage.
Stage	The stage is a movable platform allowing the entire slide to be scanned.
Stage mechanism	The stage mechanism consists of two knobs which control the vertical and horizontal movement of the slide.

Fine adjustment	Fine adjustment provides better resolution by exact focusing with slow movement within a limited range.
Coarse adjustment	Coarse adjustment provides better resolution by approximate focusing within a wide range of movement.
Substage condenser	The substage condenser is a lens system used to increase the light and converge the rays for a sharper focus.
Diaphragm	The diaphragm is an adjustable aperture that controls the intensity of light.
Light source	An in-base illuminator usually serves as the microscope's light source.
Rheostat	Some microscopes have the light source connected to a rheostat which regulates the intensity of the light.

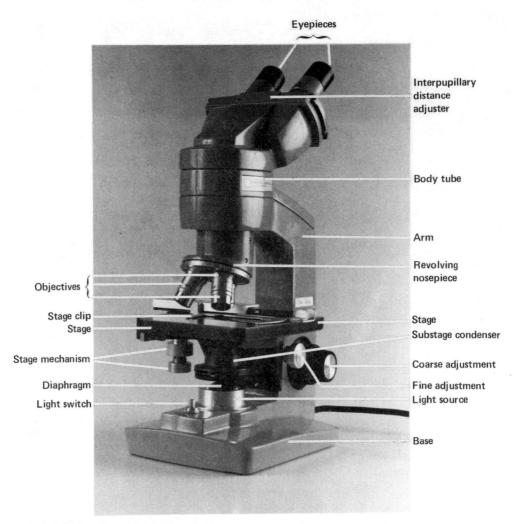

FIGURE 26-5. Parts of a microscope.

The total magnification of an object is calculated by multiplying the objective magnification engraved on the barrel with the eyepiece magnification. For example, a low-power dry objective ($10\times$) used with a $10\times$ eyepiece results in a magnification of $100\times$.

The ability of the microscope to produce a sharp image depends not only on its magnification qualities, but also on the resolving power of the lens. Resolution is the ability of the objective to present details of separate images, making them sharp and clear. The numerical aperture (NA) is an index used to indicate the resolving power of the objective. The higher the NA, the greater the resolution.

FOCUSING THE MICROSCOPE

Purpose: To learn the proper procedure for focusing the microscope and how to care for the microscope in order to keep it in good working condition.

Equipment: binocular compound microscope
slide
cover glass
lens paper
cleansing tissue
xylene
immersion oil

Procedure	*Principle*
1. Place the slide on the stage and secure it with the stage clip.	1. The stage is movable and allows the entire slide to be scanned. The spring clip causes the slide to adhere to the stage.
2. Turn the light switch on.	2. The light switch causes the light source to be illuminated.
3. Adjust the eyepieces.	3. The interpupillary distance knob is used to adjust the distance of the eyepieces to the proper width of the individual's eyes.
4. Rotate the nosepiece until the low-power dry objective ($10\times$) is directly over the slide.	4. The nosepiece allows for the objectives to be changed depending on the magnification needed. The low-power dry objective has the smallest magnification and is used to perform the initial focusing on a wide range.
5. Close the diaphragm.	5. The diaphragm controls the light intensity.
6. Use the coarse adjustment and move the stage and objective close together.	6. The stage and objective should be as close as possible to allow the slide to be readily focused.
7. Look through the eyepieces and using the fine adjustment, focus the slide on a microscopic field.	7. Rotate the fine adjustment slowly so that the distance between the stage and objective is increased. The microscopic field will come into focus.
8. Rotate the nosepiece to the high-power dry objective ($43\times$).	8. This increases the magnification of the microscopic field.

9. Focus with the fine adjustment.

9. This adjustment refines the details of the image.

10. Raise or lower the condenser to alter the light refraction and open the diaphragm.

10. The condenser is the lens system that collects the light rays and converges them. The diaphragm controls the light intensity.

11. Rotate the nosepiece until the slide is free of all objectives. Place one drop of oil on the slide. Move the oil immersion objective (97×) directly into the drop of oil.

11. The oil immersion objective is the highest magnification. The oil is used to correct light refraction (see Fig. 26-6).

12. Use the fine adjustment to focus.

12. Use only a slight adjustment because the slide should be almost in focus from the high-power dry objective adjustments made earlier.

13. Observe the slide.

13. Choose the proper objective for the type of microscopic work to be done. For example:

urinary casts—low-power objective
urine RBCs—high-power objective
differentials—oil immersion objective

Urine, blood or other body fluids observed under the high-power dry objective must be covered with a cover glass. This objective is calibrated to be used with a cover glass.

14. Rotate the nosepiece until the slide is free from all objectives. Remove the slide by releasing the spring clip.

14. This prevents the slide from scratching the objective.

15. Turn the light switch off.

15. This stops the illumination.

16. Clean the eyepieces and objectives with lens paper.

16. Lens paper is a special cleaning tissue for optical surfaces.

17. Clean the metal parts of the microscope.

17. Use a cleaning tissue, and for heavy oil film use xylene to dissolve the oil.

18. Rotate the nosepiece until the low-power dry objective is in place and the objective is as close to the stage as possible. Unplug the electric cord and wrap carefully around the base of the microscope.

18. This is the correct position for storing the microscope.

19. Cover the microscope with the protective covering.

19. A cover prevents dust from collecting on the microscope.

20. Carry the microscope to the storage area.

20. The microscope is to be carried by the arm with the base of the microscope in an upright position.

Specimen Collection

A culture specimen should be collected prior to any type of antibiotic therapy. The microbiologic laboratory test results will be an aid to medical diagnosis only if the pathogen is isolated in a culture and transported properly. External contamination should be avoided during the culture collection and aseptic technique should be used. Specimens should be collected and aseptic technique should be used. Specimens should be collected in sterile

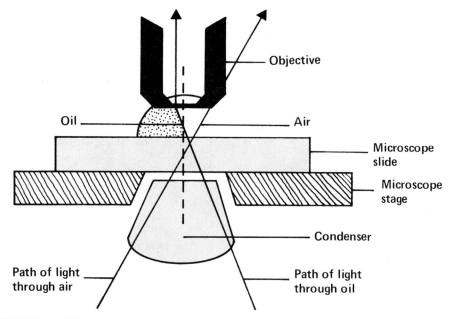

Oil

Objective

Air

Microscope slide

Microscope stage

Condenser

Path of light through air

Path of light through oil

FIGURE 26-6. When viewing a slide mounted on the microscope stage, a problem arises due to the refraction of light. When traveling through a dense material (the slide) to a less dense material (the air), the path of the light will bend toward the denser material. To solve this problem, a dense material such as oil is used between the slide and the oil immersion objective.

containers and transported promptly. Delay will result in the death of certain organisms and the overgrowth of others. Most reference medical laboratories have detailed instructions for specimen handling and transportation, and these instructions should be followed.

The "Culturette System," manufactured by Scientific Products, is a culturing packet commonly used for the collection of specimens from the throat, nose, eye, ear, and rectum, as well as from wounds and urogenital sites. The Culturette has a sterile, disposable plastic tube containing a cotton applicator swab and a sealed glass ampule of Stuart's holding medium. The holding medium is the transport medium which prevents drying and deterioration of the specimen. The plastic tube is removed from the sterile envelope, and the applicator swab is then used to collect the specimen. The swab is placed back into the plastic tube, and the ampule of Stuart's holding medium is crushed. The plastic tube is placed back into the envelope, and the envelope is properly dated and identified as to the specimen source and patient donor. This system allows for 72 hours of room temperature storage.

OBTAINING A SPECIMEN USING THE CULTURETTE SYSTEM

Purpose: To obtain a specimen for isolation and identification to aid in medical diagnosis.

Equipment: Culturette System.

Procedure	*Principle*
1. Wash hands.	1. Washing prevents the spread of microorganisms.
2. Assemble the Culturette System and label the envelope with the patient's name, date, and specimen source.	2. Proper identification of the specimen is mandatory. The Culturette envelope must be sealed to ensure that it is sterile.
3. Identify the patient and describe the procedure.	3. The patient may be apprehensive and will benefit from an explanation of the procedure.
4. Locate the infected area and position the patient.	4. The patient should be comfortable.
5. Remove the plastic tube from the envelope. Remove the plastic top from the tube and take out the cotton swab.	5. Do not contaminate the sterile swab.
6. Using aseptic technique, apply the swab to the infected area.	6. Care must be taken to avoid external contamination from other areas.
7. Insert the swab into the plastic tube and replace the top. Place the plastic tube in the envelope.	7. Immediately placing the swab in the plastic tube prevents contamination.
8. Crush the glass ampule of holding medium.	8. Stuart's holding medium prevents drying and deterioration of the specimen.
9. Staple the ends of the envelope.	9. The ends of the envelope should be stapled to prevent the plastic tube from falling out of the envelope.
10. Complete the laboratory request form.	10. The laboratory request form must be filled out completely with the patient's name, date, specimen, source, probable diagnosis, laboratory test requested, and a list of any medications that the patient is receiving.
11. Transport immediately.	11. Delay will cause the specimen to become unsatisfactory for isolation and identification of pathogens.
12. Wash hands.	12. This prevents the spread of microorganisms.

MAILING A SPECIMEN TO A REFERENCE LABORATORY

Purpose: To assure that the specimen will arrive at the destination intact.

Equipment: properly labeled specimen
mailing container
labels
laboratory request

Procedure	*Principle*
1. Obtain a properly collected specimen with a Culturette.	1. A specimen must be collected using sterile technique to ensure proper identification.
2. Label the specimen.	2. Proper patient identification is a prerequisite of all laboratory testing. The specimen will not be processed if it does not match the laboratory request.
3. Complete the laboratory request form.	3. The laboratory request identifies the culture source, date, patient, and the tests requested.
4. Pack the Culturettte with gauze and place in a metal container.	4. The gauze will protect the specimen during transportation.
5. Place the metal container in the mailing container.	5. The metal container is watertight and will prevent leakage.
6. Address properly and label "Attention: Pathology Specimen."	6. Proper address labels aid in prompt delivery.
7. Log all mailed specimens into notebook, including date, time, patient's name, and specific request.	7. If the specimen is lost in the mail, this will make it possible to trace.

Classification and Identification of Bacteria

Bergey's Manual of Determinative Bacteriology introduced a scheme of classification for microorganisms that is now used universally. It is based on the morphology and the metabolic and chemical characteristics of individual microorganisms. Bacteria generally have two names. The first name designates the genus and is capitalized. It usually indicates general structure and shape or is derived from its discoverer's name. The second name is not capitalized and designates the species. It generally refers to the color, the chemical characteristics, the specific disease produced, or its discoverer's name. In the case of *Diplococcus pneumoniae,* for example, the first name refers to spherical bacteria occurring in pairs, and the second name refers to the disease produced.

Considering the morphologic basis for classification of bacteria, five categories can be recognized: cocci, bacilli, vibrios, spirillae, and spirochetes (Fig. 26-7).

Cocci are spherical bacteria which vary according to their patterns of arrangement. Diplococci are bacteria that appear in pairs. Pneumonia, gonorrhea, and meningitis are diseases caused by pathogenic diplococci. Staphylococci appear in irregular, grapelike clusters. The pathogen *Staphylococcus aureus* is the causative agent for food poisoning, boils, abscesses, acne, osteomyelitis, and pneumonia. Streptococci appear in chains. *Streptococcus pyogenes* is a pathogen that may cause scarlet fever, rheumatic fever, sore throat, endocarditis, and glomerulonephritis.

Bacilli are straight, cylindrical rods. Examples of diseases caused by bacilli include tuberculosis, dysentery, whooping cough, food poisoning, gas gangrene, botulism, and gastroenteritis.

Vibrios are curved or sickle-shaped cells. The pathogen *Vibrio cholerae* is the causative organism for cholera.

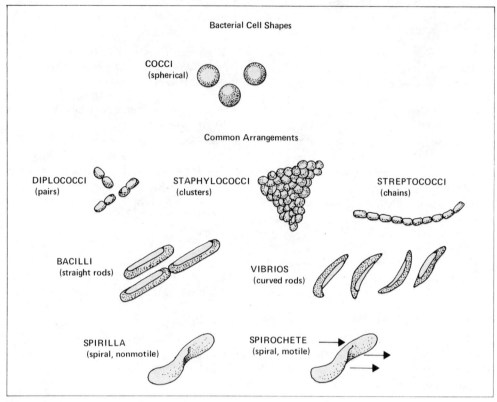

FIGURE 26-7.   Bacterial cell shapes.

Spirillae are spiral, nonmotile rods. *Spirillum minus* is a species causing rat-bite fever in humans.

Spirochetes are spiral, motile bacteria. Syphilis is caused by the spirochete *Treponema pallidum*.

Microorganism Identification by Culture and Isolation Techniques

Microorganism identification and isolation are usually the responsibility of the medical laboratory where the specimen was mailed. The medical assistant should be aware of the general procedure for the isolation and identification of pathogens. Once the specimen is received by the medical laboratory it is checked for proper patient identification and for proper collection and handling. Special media specific for the specimen source are used for the primary culture which will isolate pathogenic organisms from normal flora. Normal flora are harmless, nonpathogenic microorganisms which are found in the specimen. A small inoculum, or sample, of the specimen is streaked onto Petri dishes containing a specific medium. The choice of media is made according to the metabolic characteristics of the organisms. The primary culture is allowed to grow under controlled incubation at 37°C. A secondary culture is made by selecting isolated colonies and placing the specific colonies on selected media. This provides a pure culture containing only one type of organism. The secondary culture is again incubated at 37°C to allow the organisms to grow. Identification of the organism is made by using the pure culture to prepare special stains, and by performing biochemical tests. By observing the morphologic and chemical characteristics that are present, the organism can be correctly classified.

Sensitivity Testing

Once the organism has been isolated and identified, it is necessary to determine which antibiotic will provide the best therapeutic value. Sensitivity testing determines the susceptibility of an organism to particular antibiotics. The disc method is used routinely by most medical laboratories. A pure culture is used for sensitivity testing to be sure that only one type of organism will react with the antibiotic discs. A pure culture is placed on a Petri dish containing Mueller-Hinton agar. Antibiotic discs are placed on the agar and the Petri dish is incubated overnight at 37°C. The size of the zone of inhibition is measured to determine the sensitivity of the organism to each particular antibiotic disc. The zone of inhibition, a clear area around the disc, denotes susceptibility. The absence of a zone of inhibition denotes resistance.

PREPARATION OF A SMEAR

Purpose: To prepare a culture smear from a specimen to observe microscopically for pathogens.

Equipment: culture specimen
microscopic slides
Bunsen burner
forceps
inoculating needle

Procedure	Principle
1. Wash hands.	1. Washing prevents the spread of microorganisms.
2. Assemble equipment.	2. Having the equipment close at hand allows the procedure to be performed quickly.
3. Label a clean microscope slide with the patient's name.	3. Dirt and scratches interfere with microscopic examination.
4. Hold the slide between the thumb and index finger.	4. A half-inch allowance will prevent the fingers from becoming contaminated. Rolling the swab along the slide provides an even distribution of organisms.
5. Allow the slide to air-dry for 20 to 30 minutes.	5. Forced heating will cause the organisms to be distorted and will cause possible contamination if the specimen spatters.

6. Hold the slide with forceps or between the thumb and third finger and "heat-fix" by passing the slide over a Bunsen burner flame (see Fig. 26-8).	6. Heat-fixing the slide kills the organisms and allows them to adhere to the slide for staining techniques.
7. Allow the slide to cool before staining.	7. A hot slide would prevent proper staining.

The Gram Stain

The medical assistant must have a general knowledge of the principles involved in the Gram-staining technique. The Gram stain is a differential stain which separates bacteria into two groups: gram-positive and gram-negative. The purpose of any staining technique is to properly color the organism so that the morphology of the organism can be studied. The Gram stain was discovered in 1883 by a Danish physician, Hans Christian Gram. Although the actual staining principles are not fully understood, it is believed that an acid substance (magnesium ribonucleic acid) is present in all gram-positive organisms. This allows for the formation of an insoluble complex with crystal violet and iodine, which is not removed by decolorization with an alcohol-acetone solution. Gram-negative organisms appear to lack magnesium ribonucleic acid, and the complex is readily removed by decolorization. A counterstain, safranin, is used to stain the gram-negative organisms.

Four basic steps are involved in Gram staining: (1) smear preparation, (2) staining with crystal violet and iodine, (3) decolorization with alcohol-acetone solution, and (4) counterstaining with safranin. Gram-positive organisms are deep purple; gram-negative organisms are red.

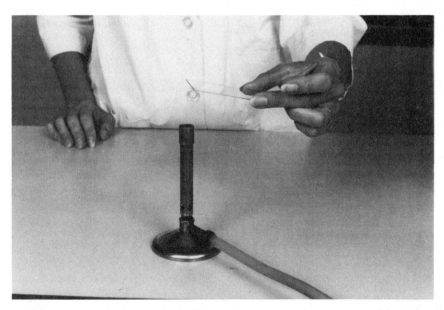

FIGURE 26-8. A slide is "heat-fixed" by being passed over a Bunsen burner flame. The heat kills the organisms and causes them to adhere to the slide for ease of staining.

Some of the more common gram-positive and gram-negative organisms are listed below:

Gram-positive organisms	*Gram-negative organisms*
Cocci:	Cocci:
Diplococcus	Neisseria
Staphylococcus	Bacilli:
Streptococcus	Arizona
Bacilli:	Bacteroides
Bacillus	Bordetella
Clostridium	Brucella
Corynebacterium	Citrobacter
Listeria	Enterobacter
Mycobacterium	Haemophilus
Fungi:	Klebsiella
Candida	Proteus
	Pseudomonas
	Salmonella
	Shigella
	Serratia
	Vibrio

GRAM-STAINING PROCEDURE

Purpose: To gram-stain a smear for differentiation of gram-negative and gram-positive organisms to aid in medical diagnosis.

Equipment: Gram-stain kit: crystal violet, Gram's iodine, alcohol-acetone solution, and safranin
      culture specimen
      microscopic slides
      Bunsen burner
      forceps
      staining rack
      wash bottle (distilled water)
      bibulous paper
      microscope
      immersion oil
      stopwatch

Procedure	*Principle*
1. Wash hands.	1. Washing prevents the spread of microorganisms.
2. Assemble equipment.	2. Gram-staining is a timed procedure which must be done rapidly.
3. Make a smear, air-dry, and heat-fix, follow-	3. A heat-fixed smear will prevent the orga-

ing the procedure for the preparation of a smear.

4. Place the slide on the staining rack, smear side up, and flood the side with crystal violet solution for 1 minute (Fig. 26-9A).

5. Tilt the slide with forceps and allow the stain to drain off the slide. Rinse with distilled water (Fig. 26-9B).

6. Flood the slide with Gram's iodine for 1 to 2 minutes.

7. Decolorize with alcohol-acetone by gentle flooding of the side for 30 seconds (Fig. 26-9C).

8. Rinse the side with distilled water.

9. Flood the slide with safranin stain for 30 seconds.

10. Rinse with distilled water and blot dry on bibulous paper (Fig. 26-9D).

11. Examine under the microscope, using the oil immersion objective.

12. Notify the physician when the gram-staining technique is completed.

nisms from washing off the slide during the staining process.

4. All cells will stain with crystal violet.

5. This will remove the crystal violet stain from the slide surface.

6. Gram's iodine acts as a mordant which combines with the crystal violet to form a soluble stain-mordant complex.

7. The alcohol-acetone solution acts as a decolorizer. Gram-negative organisms allow the stain-complex to be washed away, leaving them colorless. Gram-positive organisms, due to the chemical nature of the cell wall, retain the stain complex and will remain purple.

8. Rinsing will stop the decolorization process.

9. The safranin counterstain will stain the decolorized or gram-negative cells a pink color.

10. Rinsing removes any of the remaining counterstain. Do not wipe or the smear will rub off.

11. Gram-positive organisms will appear purple. Gram-negative organisms will appear pink or red.

12. Most physicians interpret the smears in the medical office.

PRECAUTIONS IN GRAM-STAINING TECHNIQUE

1. Gram-positive bacteria may change to gram-negative bacteria due to temperature, incubation, age of the culture, and autolysis.

2. The timing element of the Gram stain is critical and may change due to the age of the reagents and individual techniques.

3. Because many Gram stains may be misinterpreted, preliminary Gram stain results must be followed with culture and isolation techniques for organism identification and final medical diagnosis.

BASIC URINALYSIS

Urinalysis is an analysis of the urine and provides information concerning body metabolism. Abnormalities identified during a routine urinalysis may aid the physician in diagnosis. Because a routine urinalysis involves simple chemical tests requiring very little specialized equipment, it is a frequently used diagnostic tool in the physician's office.

Urine is composed of about 95 percent water and 5 percent waste products, including

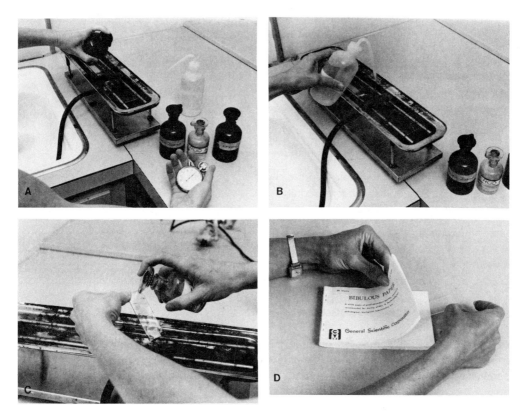

FIGURE 26-9. Gram-staining procedure. A, Flood the slide with crystal violet solution for 1 minute. B, Rinse with distilled water, then flood with Gram's iodine stain for 1 to 2 minutes. C, Decolorize with acetone-alcohol by gently flooding the slide for 30 seconds. Rinse with distilled water, then counterstain by flooding the slide with safranin stain for 30 seconds. D, Carefully blot the slide between bibulous paper, then examine under the microscope using the oil immersion objective. Notify the physician for interpretation.

urea, ammonia, creatinine, uric acid, and electrolytes. The primary function of the kidneys is to eliminate water and waste products; consequently, a urinalysis will provide an indicator for kidney function. Diseases such as cystitis (inflammation of the bladder), nephritis, (inflammation of the kidney), diabetes, endocrine disorders, and PKU (phenylketonuria) are often identified by urinalysis procedures. Other conditions such as pregnancy and drug overdoses are also studied by means of analysis of urine specimens.

Specimen Collection

Four basic types of urine specimens are used in diagnostic tests:

1. A *random specimen* is a freshly voided specimen collected in a sterile (or nonsterile) container which is properly labeled.

2. A *first morning specimen* is the first voided specimen of the day. This is the preferred specimen because it will be more concentrated.

3. A *clean-catch specimen* is collected in midstream and is used most often for microbiology studies, particularly urine cultures (see Chapter 19).

4. A *24-hour specimen* is used primarily for quantitative chemical assays.

The collection of a 24-hour urine specimen entails the following steps:

1. Have the patient empty his bladder and discard the urine.

2. Collect all urine samples during the next 24 hours in an appropriate container. (Most 24-hour specimens require a preservative which will be designated by the reference laboratory used.)

   Example:

   Patient voids at 6:00 a.m.
   Discard urine.
   Collect urine next 24 hours through 6:00 a.m. of the following day.

Routine Urinalysis Procedure

A routine urinalysis is composed of three major parts: (1) physical examination by macroscopic inspection, (2) chemical examinations using reagent dipsticks, and (3) microscopic examination of urinary sediment.

PHYSICAL EXAMINATION

The physical examination of a urine specimen rests upon a careful consideration of its appearance, its color, and its specific gravity.

Appearance

The urine may be clear, hazy, turbid, or cloudy, owing to the presence of bacteria, mucus, blood, or amorphous salts. Normal urine is translucent.

Color

The color of the urine may vary from pale yellow to brown, although normal urine is a pale, straw color. The color of normal urine is due to a urinary pigment, urochrome. Abnormal colors may result from particular diets or medications. A red color may be due to blood, while a greenish shade is associated with the presence of bile.

Specific Gravity

Specific gravity is a measurement which indicates the total solute (dissolved solids) concentration of the urine. The kidney regulates the volume of voided urine and the concentration of the solute to maintain body balance, or homeostasis of fluids and electrolytes. Urea, sodium, and chloride are the most important of the dissolved solids. The normal range of specific gravity for urine is between 1.003 and 1.030.

There are two methods of measuring specific gravity; one uses a urinometer and the other employs a refractometer. A *urinometer* is a hydrometer which is calibrated at 20°C to measure specific gravity. The device is floated in urine and the specific gravity is read on the scale from the bottom of the meniscus. The urinometer must be refilled daily with distilled water to a level reading of 1.000 (see Fig. 26-10). Certain precautions must be taken in recording specific gravity. Surface bubbles should be avoided, and the urinometer should not be allowed to touch the sides or bottom of the cylinder. This will result in inaccurate readings. Specific gravity is influenced by temperature. If the urine is not at room temperature at the time of testing, a correction of 0.001 must be made for each 3°C above or below 20°C. Corrections must also be made for protein and sugar present in the urine. For every 7 gm/100 ml of glucose or protein, 0.003 should be subtracted from the specific gravity reading.

An alternative method for measuring specific gravity employs the *refractometer*, an optical instrument that uses a single drop of urine. Light is reflected in proportion to the dissolved solids present. The reading is determined by interpreting the line representing a

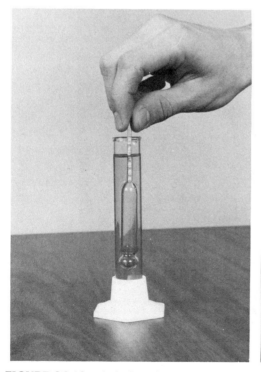 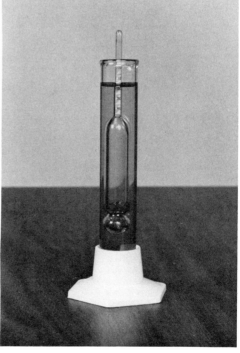

FIGURE 26-10. *Left:* Spin the urinometer to ensure that it is free-floating. *Right:* Read the bottom of the meniscus using the calibrated column of the urinometer. This reading is 1.014.

light and dark contrast area and reading the scale accordingly (Fig. 26-11). The refractometer has two advantages over the urinometer: it requires only one or two drops of urine for specific gravity readings, and, in most cases, it compensates for temperature variations and should read 1.000 with distilled water.

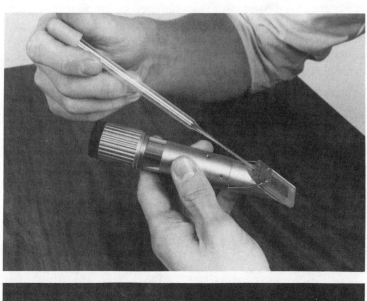

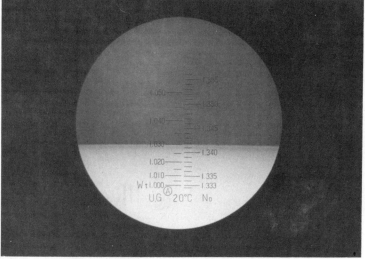

FIGURE 26-11. *Top:* Place one drop of urine in the refractometer. Hold the refractometer toward a light source and view the scale through the eyepiece. *Bottom:* The reading is determined by interpreting the line represented by a light and dark contrast area and reading the scale on the left side. This reading is 1.030.

CHEMICAL EXAMINATION USING REAGENT DIPSTICKS

Urine dipsticks are used for semiquantitation of chemical components in the urine specimen (Fig. 26-12). A urine control should be used as a quality control measure. Dipsticks must be properly stored and used to provide accurate results. Manufacturer's instructions should be followed exactly because the procedure and reagents specified will vary.

The chemical reactions between the urine specimen and the reagents on the dipstick result in color changes which are interpreted according to the manufacturer's instructions.

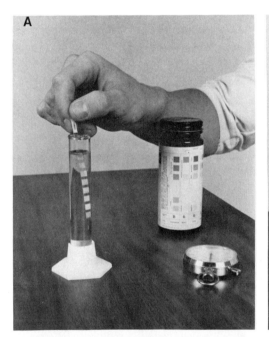

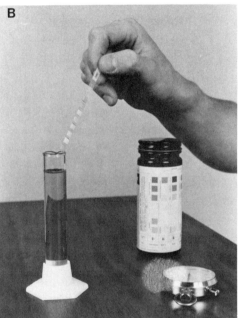

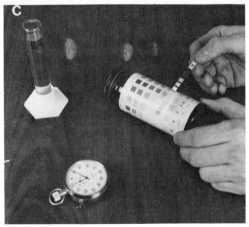

FIGURE 26-12. Urinalysis procedure. A, Place the dipstick strip into a fresh, well-mixed urine specimen. B, Drain the excess urine by gently tapping the side of the dipstick. C, Start the stopwatch and compare the chemical reactions between the urine specimen and the reagents impregnated on the dipstick. The color changes are interpreted by comparison with the color-coded chart on the reagent bottle.

Inaccurate test results will occur if the reagents are outdated or improperly stored. The lot number and expiration date of the reagents as well as the results from quality control must be recorded daily to insure accuracy.

Most dipsticks provide for the following measurements:

1. *pH*. pH is a measurement of the acidity or alkalinity of urine. The normal pH value is 6.0. The pH color reactions used for comparison usually range from 5 to 9. Five indicates a very acid urine, nine a very alkaline urine. Do not allow a urine specimen to stand at room temperature because bacterial growth will cause an alkaline pH reading.

2. *Protein*. Protein is measured by the dipstick method. A chemical reaction between the reagent on the dipstick and the protein which is present in the urine is interpreted by matching the color reaction to the color code. Values are recorded as negative, 1+, 2+, 3+, etc. Protein is not normally found in urine, and persistent high concentrations of protein indicate proteinuria, which is due to renal disease. To confirm the presence of trace amounts of protein, a backup test using equal parts of sulfosalicylic acid and urine is used. This method will precipitate protein, and the turbidity of the solution is graded as negative, 1+, 2+, 3+, 4+, etc. Occasional positive protein tests may be found with patients taking excessive exercise or having bacterial infections or exposure to cold. The test will not be positive with each successive specimen tested but will be transient.

3. *Glucose*. Glucosuria is the presence of glucose in the urine and may be detected by dipstick methods and/or by Clinitest tablets. The dipstick methods test specifically for glucose, whereas the Clinitest tablets will detect reducing sugars such as lactose, galactose, fructose, or ascorbic acid. Large amounts of ascorbic acid will give a false positive test with the dipstick method. Glucose is not normally present in urine, and its presence is usually investigated by a blood sugar test and possibly by a glucose tolerance test (GTT), a diagnostic blood test for diabetes.

4. *Ketone*. Ketonuria is the presence of ketone bodies in the urine, consisting of acetoacetic acid, beta-hydroxybutyric acid, and acetone. Ketone bodies are formed from the breakdown of fat, and when excessive amounts form, the condition is known as ketosis. Ketone bodies are detected by the reagent dipstick due to a chemical reaction, and the color code is matched. The results are recorded as negative, 1+, 2+, 3+, etc. Ketonuria is associated with uncontrolled diabetes mellitus, starvation, dehydration, exposure to cold, and severe exercise.

5. *Blood*. Blood may be found in the urine as intact RBCs or lysed RBCs which have released their hemoglobin. Hemoglobinuria is the presence of free hemoglobin or its derivatives in the urine and may indicate renal lesions, hemolytic transfusion reaction, extensive burns or injuries, or paroxysmal hemoglobinuria. Hematuria is the presence of intact RBCs. The dipstick will chemically react to hemoglobin, RBCs, and myoglobin (resulting from muscle injury). The color code is matched for reactivity. Any positive test for blood should be correlated to the microscopic examination for RBCs and may be confirmed with occult blood tests such as Occultest, Hematest, guaiac, or benzidine.

6. *Bilirubin.* Bilirubinuria is the presence of bilirubin in the urine and is associated with obstructive jaundice, hepatitis, and cirrhosis. Bilirubin is a normal byproduct of the breakdown of hemoglobin, and is usually processed by the liver into bile which is excreted by the intestines. Normally, bilirubin is not detected in the urine. The dipstick reacts chemically and is matched to the color code. The results are recorded as positive or negative. Positive biliribin tests should be confirmed by Ictotest Reagent Tablets because the sensitivity is greater. Bilirubin is light-sensitive, and the specimen should not be placed in direct light. Precautions should always be taken due to the possibility of hepatitis when a positive bilirubin test is detected.

7. *Urobilinogen.* Urobilinogen is a compound formed by the reduction of bilirubin. Small amounts may normally be present in the urine, but increased amounts are associated with hemolytic anemia, cirrhosis, hepatitis, and hepatic jaundice. The dipstick reacts chemically, and the results are matched to the color code.

MICROSCOPIC EXAMINATION OF URINARY SEDIMENT

The urinary sediment is prepared by centrifuging 15 ml of a well-mixed, fresh, first-voided urine specimen at 2000 rpm for 5 minutes. The sediment is resuspended in 1 ml of urine by pouring off the supernatant. One drop of the sediment suspension is then observed microscopically under the low-power objective with low light to scan for casts. The high-power objective is used to identify white blood cells, red blood cells, casts, crystals, bacteria, or parasites. Normally, the urine will contain a few WBCs, a few epithelial cells, occasional crystals, and rare RBCs. Five to ten high-power fields are observed and the average recorded. The following discussion will be divided into four parts: (1) cells, (2) casts and cylindroids, (3) crystals and amorphous salts, and (4) miscellaneous urine sediment.

Cells

Three cell types are of special importance in the microscopic examination of urinary sediment (Fig. 26-13).

1. *Red blood cells.* RBCs are significant in the urinary sediment except in the case of noncatheterized menstruating females. They appear as refractile, uniform, non-nucleated small cells. A 2 percent acetic acid solution will lyse RBCs and is an excellent differentiation test. Record RBCs as the average number per high-power field after observing five to ten fields.

2. *White blood cells.* Segmented neutrophils will appear round, nucleated, and larger than RBCs. The presence of a few WBCs is normal, but increased numbers indicate urinary infections. WBCs will often appear in large clumps. Record WBCs as the average number per high-power field after observing five to ten fields.

3. *Epithelial cells.* Normally, a few epithelial cells are found in the urine, particularly squamous epithelial cells which are flat, nucleated, and irregular. They arise from the urethra and vagina. Renal epithelial cells are abnormal and appear round with

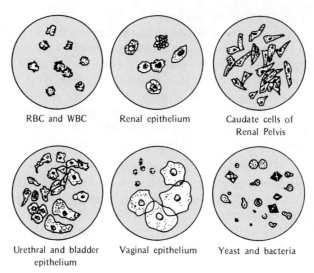

| RBC and WBC | Renal epithelium | Caudate cells of Renal Pelvis |

| Urethral and bladder epithelium | Vaginal epithelium | Yeast and bacteria |

FIGURE 26-13. Cells found in urine. (Courtesy of Ames Company, Inc.)

a large, round nucleus. Other types of epithelial cells will appear larger than WBCs or RBCs. Rarely seen are oval fat bodies which are renal epithelial cells that have undergone fat degeneration and contain refractile fat droplets within the cell. Record the average number of epithelial cells per low-power field after observing five to ten fields.

Casts and Cylindroids

Casts are formed in the renal tubules, usually have two rounded ends, and are composed of mucoprotein (Fig. 26-14). They are highly significant and indicate diseases of the kidney. For proper viewing the microscope should have a very low light, the condenser should be down, and the diaphragm should be closed because casts, particularly hyaline casts, tend to be transparent. The edges of the slide should be observed first and the average number per low-power field reported after five to ten fields have been observed. Cylindroids appear to be similar to casts but have one rounded end and the other end tapering to a long tail.

The following types of casts should be recognized:

Hyaline casts:	Low refractive index, clear cylinders with rounded ends.
Red blood cell casts:	Hyaline casts embedded with RBCs.
White blood cell casts:	Hyaline casts embedded with WBCs.
Epithelial cell casts:	Hyaline casts embedded with epithelial cells.
Granular casts:	Cellular casts that are degenerating. They may appear either in finely granular or coarsely granular forms.
Waxy casts:	The final degenerative state of cellular casts.

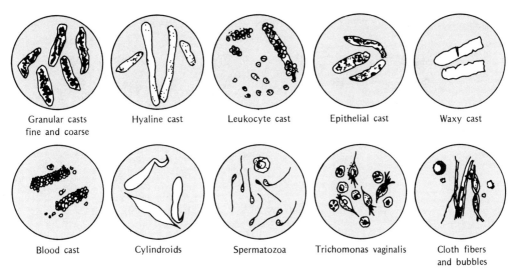

FIGURE 26-14. Casts and artifacts found in urine. (Courtesy of Ames Company, Inc.)

Broad casts: Wider than other casts and may be cellular, granular, or waxy.

Fatty casts: Have lipid or fat droplets and are usually epithelial cell casts.

Crystals and Amorphous Salts

Crystals and amorphous salts are compounds often found during a routine urinalysis and may be classified according to urine pH and the characteristic crystal morphology (Fig. 26-15).

Crystal	pH	Morphology
Calcium oxalate	acid	envelope-shaped crystals; small, colorless
Cystine	acid	hexagonal crystals; colorless and flat
Leucine	acid	yellow, spheroid crystals
Triple phosphate	alkaline	"coffin-lid" shape
Tyrosine	acid	needlelike crystals; usually yellow
Uric acid and urates	acid	vary in shape; usually rosettes, hexagons, or small spheres
Sulfonamides	acid	yellow-brown sheaves

Miscellaneous Urine Sediment Components

Among the components of urine sediment classified as miscellaneous are the following forms:

1. *Bacteria.* Bacteria may appear as cocci (round) or bacilli (rod-shaped). A few

CRYSTALS FOUND IN ACID URINE (X400)

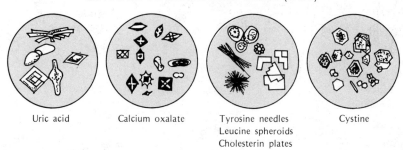

Uric acid   Calcium oxalate   Tyrosine needles   Cystine
                                        Leucine spheroids
                                        Cholesterin plates

CRYSTALS FOUND IN ALKALINE URINE (X400)

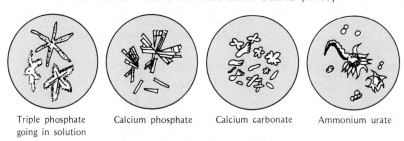

Triple phosphate   Calcium phosphate   Calcium carbonate   Ammonium urate
going in solution

SULFA CRYSTALS

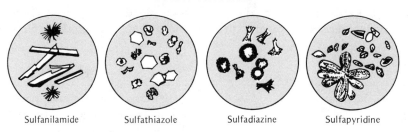

Sulfanilamide   Sulfathiazole   Sulfadiazine   Sulfapyridine

FIGURE 26-15.   Crystals found in urine. (Courtesy of Ames Company, Inc.)

bacteria may represent contaminants, but large numbers indicate a urinary infection.

2. *Yeast.* Yeast cells are refractile, flat, oval bodies which vary in size and have buds. They are often confused with RBCs. Yeast cells are often a vaginal contaminant, but may also be seen in diabetic patients.

3. *Parasites.* Parasites may be identified in the urine but are usually contaminants. The most common parasite seen is *Trichomonas vaginalis*. Trichomonas is a flagellate protozoan and should only be reported when the flagellates are motile. Inactive Trichomonas can easily be confused with leukocytes, and most cases of

Trichomonas vaginalis are accompanied by increased vaginal epithelial cells, leukocytes, and bacteria.

4. *Mucus threads.* Mucus threads may be found in the normal urine, but increased amounts usually indicate urinary tract inflammation.

5. *Spermatozoa.* Spermatozoa may be present in female urine after sexual intercourse and usually are not reported. A few spermatozoa in male urine are normal, but abnormal amounts are significant and should be reported.

6. *Other contaminants.* Talcum powder often resembles calcium oxalate crystals and is often present in pediatric urine specimens.

URINE SPECIMEN COLLECTION

Purpose: To obtain a freshly voided urine specimen for diagnostic laboratory testing.

Equipment: Sterile or nonsterile specimen containers

Procedure	Principle
1. Instruct the patient to collect a urine specimen by voiding into the container provided.	1. Sterile urine specimen containers are preferable to avoid chemical or bacterial contamination. If the patient is to bring in a first-morning specimen, provide the patient with a sterile container to prevent the using of such containers as household bottles.
2. Identify the patient and label the specimen.	2. The specimen should not be labeled on the lid, because during the testing procedure the lids might be mismatched.
3. Have the patient return to the waiting room.	3. Make the patient as comfortable as possible.
4. Record the patient's name on a transfer (KOVA) tube. Agitate the specimen gently and transfer 12 ml of the freshly voided specimen into the KOVA-tube and seal the tube with a KOVA-Kap.	4. Proper identification must be maintained throughout the laboratory testing procedure. Improperly mixed specimens will give invalid results. Sealing the specimen prevents airborne contamination and spillage.
5. Discard the remaining urine.	5. This will prevent spillage.
6. Store the urine specimen at 2° to 8° C for up to 4 hours.	6. It is best to perform laboratory tests on urine specimens within an hour. Refrigeration retards bacterial growth.

The KOVA System

In an effort to control the many variables involved in performing a routine urinalysis, the KOVA-System was developed by ICL Scientific for the standardization of urinalysis (Fig. 26-16). It has been shown that by utilizing the KOVA-System, routine urinalysis can be quite precise and accurate.

A freshly voided specimen is properly agitated, and 12 ml of the urine is poured into a graduated tube and centrifuged at 1500 rpm for 5 minutes. This allows for the formed

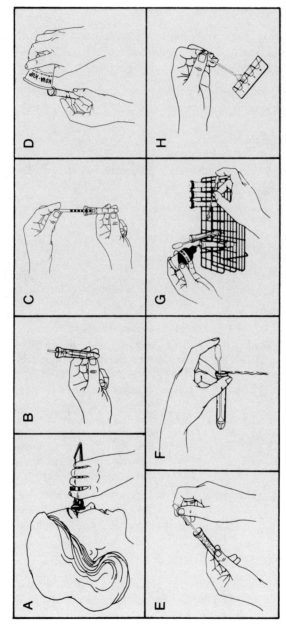

FIGURE 26-16. Procedure for use of the KOVA-System. After the urine specimen is mixed to resuspend sediment, its color and turbidity are recorded. Specific gravity is then measured and recorded by means of a temperature-compensated refractometer (A) or a hydrometer (B). C, Chemical tests are performed using dipsticks and results recorded. D, 12 ml of the specimen are decanted into a graduated KOVA-Tube. This is then centrifuged at 1500 rpm for 5 minutes. After removal from the centrifuge, the KOVA-Petter (E) is placed in the KOVA-Tube, and the supernatant is decanted and discarded (F). G, the KOVA-Petter is withdrawn, and 1 drop of KOVA-Stain is added to the remaining 1 ml of urine and sediment. The KOVA-Petter is reinserted and the specimen is mixed well. H, the KOVA-Petter is squeezed several times to allow the specimen to be drawn in. Then, using the KOVA-Petter, 1 drop of the specimen is transferred to the area adjacent to the appropriate covered chamber on the KOVA-Slide. The specimen should be drawn under the covered examination area by capillary action. The KOVA-Slide is allowed to stand for 1 minute to permit settling. It is then placed on the microscope under the objective. Using the $10 \times$ eyepiece and the $10 \times$ objective, 10 low-power fields are read, followed by 20 high-power fields with the $43 \times$ objective. (Courtesy of ICL Scientific)

elements to fall to the bottom of the KOVA-Tube. The sediment and 1.0 ml of the urine are resuspended using a pipette, or KOVA-Petter. The KOVA-Petter is used to transfer the resuspended urine sediment by capillary action onto a KOVA-Slide for microscopic examination. Each chamber on the slide has a calibrated depth. A microscopic evaluation is performed by observing ten microscopic fields of the urine sediment. The urinary sediment may be stained with KOVA-Stain prior to placement on the KOVA-Slide to enhance cellular elements. The results are recorded on the laboratory slip and on the daily log sheet. A urine control, such as KOVA-Trol, is used to assure that the laboratory test is within limits.

ROUTINE URINALYSIS USING THE KOVA-SYSTEM

Purpose: To examine a urine specimen for macroscopic and microscopic abnormalities.

Equipment: dipsticks (reagent strips)
　　　　　　stopwatch
　　　　　　urine control (KOVA-Trol)
　　　　　　KOVA-Tube
　　　　　　KOVA-Petter
　　　　　　KOVA-Slide
　　　　　　KOVA-Kup
　　　　　　KOVA-Stain
　　　　　　microscope

Procedure	*Principle*
1. Mix the urine specimen.	1. Improperly mixed specimens will cause invalid results.
2. Record the color and appearance.	2. Observe the color and appearance macroscopically.
3. Select a dipstick.	3. Do not touch any reagent area on the dipstick to avoid contamination.
4. Dip the dipstick into the urine, coating all test areas.	4. The contact of the urine with the reagent strips results in chemical reactions which are compared to known color codes on the container.
5. Rest the dipstick on the KOVA-Tube and record results after the proper time lapses.	5. The horizontal position assures that no crossreaction will result between the reagents. A stopwatch is used to monitor the various reading times for the reactions.
6. Interpret the dipstick.	6. The color changes are correlated to the manufacturer's color code index.
7. Record results on the laboratory slip and the daily log sheet.	7. Immediately recording results will prevent errors.
8. Place one drop of urine on the refractometer and record the specific gravity.	8. The refractometer should be wiped clean after use to prevent the urine from drying.

9. Centrifuge the KOVA-Tube.	9. Centrifuge at 1500 rpm for 5 minutes to allow the formed elements to go to the bottom of the tube.
10. Place the KOVA-Petter into the KOVA-Tube and pour off the supernatant.	10. The KOVA-Petter allows for 1 ml of urine to remain in the KOVA-Tube.
11. Add one drop of KOVA-Stain to the KOVA-Tube.	11. The stain is used to enhance the cellular elements.
12. Resuspend the urinary sediment with the KOVA-Petter and place one drop on the KOVA-Slide.	12. The drop of urinary sediment and stain fills the calibrated slide area by capillary action. The specimen must be well mixed.
13. Observe the KOVA-Slide under the low-power objective with subdued lighting and scan the area for casts.	13. Casts, particularly hyaline casts, are difficult to see using a bright light source.
14. Using the high-power objective, identify cellular elements, casts, bacteria, and crystals by observing ten fields and taking the average.	14. The microscopic examination must be correlated to the dipstick results. For example, a large amount of blood should show RBCs in the microscopic examination.
15. Record results on the laboratory slip and and the daily log sheet. Initial the results.	15. Recording the results immediately prevents errors.
16. Discard the urine specimens properly.	16. Specimens may be flushed down the toilet. Special precautions must be taken with any specimens having a high bilirubin because of the possibility of hepatitis.
17. Wash hands.	17. Proper handwashing technique prevents the spread of microorganisms.

Pregnancy Tests

Pregnancy tests are based on the presence of a hormone, human chorionic gonadotropin (HCG), in the serum or urine. Three basic methods are used for pregnancy testing:

1. *Bioassays* using animals such as frogs, rats, rabbits, and mice to demonstrate the presence of HCG were frequently employed prior to 1960.

2. *Immunologic tests* are based on the reaction between HCG found in serum or urine on commercially prepared human chorionic gonadotropin antibody (anti-HCG). These methods are the most commonly used in medical offices.

3. *Radioimmunoassay* (RIA) is a highly sensitive method that can detect minimal amounts of HCG earlier than other methods. Because RIA is a highly sophisticated method and requires expensive laboratory equipment and specialized personnel, it is rarely performed in the medical office. Many reference laboratories use RIA techniques, and medical offices may draw patients' blood samples by venipuncture for transfer to these laboratories. Each reference laboratory will provide special instructions for collection and transportation of laboratory specimens.

IMMUNOLOGIC PREGNANCY TESTS

Many immunologic pregnancy tests are commercially available using either tube test or slide test methods. Slide tests are manufactured by several companies, including Ortho, Hyland, Organon, Roche, and Burroughs Wellcome. These methods employ latex particles as indicators in an indirect or agglutination inhibition test. Anti-HCG, a commercially prepared serum, is incubated with the patient's urine. If HCG is present in the urine, an antibody-antigen immunologic reaction occurs, and the anti-HCG serum will be neutralized. Latex particles which are coated with HCG are then added, and if urinary HCG has neutralized the anti-HCG, no agglutination will occur. Therefore, the test is positive. If neutralization has not occurred, the anti-HCG is free to react with the latex particles, and agglutination takes place. In this case the test is negative.

A second type of slide test is based on the principle of direct agglutination testing and is commercially available from Monchida and Wampole. The latex particles are coated with anti-HCG and are incubated with the patient's urine. If agglutination occurs, the test is positive. If agglutination does not occur, the test is negative. This method is less sensitive than the preceding one.

Tube tests, commercially available from manufacturers such as Wampole, Organon, Ames, Burroughs Wellcome, and Roche, employ hemagglutination-inhibition methods using erythrocytes as indicators. Anti-HCG serum and HCG-coated red blood cells are incubated with patients' urine. If urinary HCG is present, the antiserum will be neutralized and the red blood cells will not agglutinate, but will settle to the bottom of the test tube to form a ring or "doughnut" design. This is reported as a positive test. Patients' urine which does not contain HCG will not neutralize the anti-HCG, and therefore the RBCs will agglutinate and form a mat of cells at the bottom of the tube with no visible ring. This is reported as a negative test. Methods that use red blood cells as indicators are usually more sensitive than those that use latex particles.

Immunologic pregnancy tests are about 95 to 97 percent accurate and can detect low concentrations of HCG early in pregnancy, usually 2 to 3 weeks after the first missed period. The first-morning voided urine specimen should be used for laboratory testing because it is more concentrated. Positive pregnancy tests may result from conditions other than pregnancy, such as malignant tumors of the ovaries or testes, choriocarcinoma, or hydatidiform mole. These conditions usually produce high levels of HCG. Due to the variations in HCG concentrations found in urine specimens, positive and negative controls must be run with each test to ensure accurate readings. Most manufacturers include positive and negative controls with their kits. Sources of error include failure to follow the manufacturer's directions exactly, improper storage of reagents, and interfering substances such as drugs, proteins, and erythrocytes.

BASIC HEMATOLOGY TESTING

Hematology is the study of blood. When properly studied, the various components of blood can reveal specific disease conditions and can serve as indications of the state of body metabolism. Because venipuncture and capillary puncture are simple procedures to perform, blood tests are a frequently ordered diagnostic aid. The medical assistant must have a general knowledge of the blood system and hematology to function successfully within the medical office.

Composition of Blood

Blood is composed of two major parts: cellular elements and plasma (Fig. 26-17).

CELLULAR ELEMENTS

The cellular elements of blood are roughly divided into erythrocytes, leukocytes, and thrombocytes.

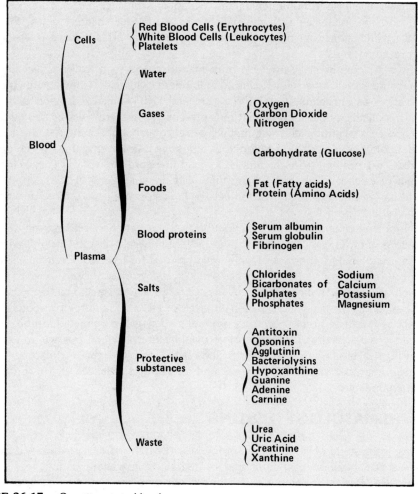

FIGURE 26-17. Constituents in blood.

Erythrocytes, or red blood cells, are cells which contain hemoglobin. The function of hemoglobin is to carry oxygen from the lungs to the tissue cells and transport carbon dioxide and other waste products away from the cells to the lungs. When attached to the hemoglobin molecule, the oxygen is known as oxyhemoglobin and gives arterial blood a bright red color. Once this oxygen is released into the tissues, the blood will travel back to the lungs by way of veins and will have a bluish-black color due to the lower oxygen contents. Many patients become apprehensive when they see the dark bluish-black color of their blood in a test tube. They expect it to have the bright red color of capillary blood which they have seen when their finger has been cut in minor injuries. The medical assistant's job is often to reassure them that the appearance of the blood is normal and, perhaps, to explain briefly the differences in color of arterial and venous blood.

Leukocytes, or white blood cells, function in the role of immunology and defend the body against infection. There are three major types of WBCs which are used for classification when performing a differential count: granulocytes, lymphocytes, and monocytes. A differential count is the percent distribution of the various white blood cells when observing a stained smear of peripheral blood.

1. *Granulocytes* function to phagocytize or engulf bacteria and consist of three types: neutrophils, basophils, and eosinophils.

2. *Lymphocytes* function primarily in antibody production and are formed in lymphoid tissue. They are normally found in higher percentage in children and decrease to about 25 to 35 percent in adults.

3. *Monocytes* function to phagocytize bacteria and are formed mainly in the bone marrow.

Finally, *thrombocytes*, or platelets, are disk-shaped structures that play a major role in blood coagulation.

PLASMA

Plasma is the fluid portion of the blood and functions as a transport medium for the cellular elements. Other metabolic products are transported as well, such as nutrients, waste products, hormones, and antibodies. Plasma is composed of approximately 90 percent water and 10 percent solids.

Hematopoiesis

Hematopoiesis is the production and development of the cellular elements of blood. In performing hematology tests, the medical assistant will examine the formed cellular elements of the blood by studying a stained blood smear of peripheral blood. Although most differential counts will reveal mature cells, occasionally immature cells will be circulated into the peripheral blood due to various disease states. It is necessary for the MA to be able to recognize abnormal or immature cells and to alert the physician. The staining characteristics discussed below are representative of Wright's stain, an eosin and methylene blue stain used for differential counts.

Three major categories of hematopoiesis will be discussed: erythropoiesis, leukopoiesis, and thrombopoiesis (see Fig. 26-18).

Erythropoiesis is the development of erythrocytes. Red blood cells are formed in the bone marrow primarily of the ribs, sternum, and femur. The erythrocyte develops from a rubriblast into a metarubricyte, then into a reticulocyte, and finally into an erythrocyte. The immature cells have a nucleus, and occasionally these nucleated RBCs appear in the peripheral blood. The normal RBC has a life span of 120 days and is a biconcave disk approximately 7 to 8 microns in diameter. When stained, RBCs appear to be pale pink.

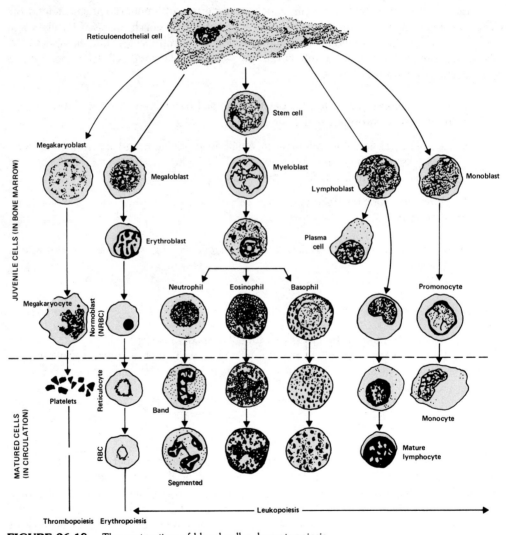

FIGURE 26-18.   The maturation of blood cells—hematopoiesis.

Leukopoiesis is the development of leukocytes. The formation of the different types of leukocytes follows three basic lines of development: granulocytic, lympocytic, and monocytic.

Granulocytic development involves the progression from myeloblast to promyelocyte to myelocyte to metamyelocyte. At this point, the cells can develop into one of the following types of white blood cells:

1. Neutrophils or polymorphonuclear cells (PMNs), which appear when stained to average about 12 microns in diameter, have a pale pink granulated cytoplasm and a darp purple, segmented nucleus usually having three to five lobes connected by strands of chromatin. If the nucleus is undivided, the cell is known as a band or stab and is an immature neutrophil.

2. Eosinophils average about 13 microns in diameter, and, when stained, appear with bright orange granules in the cytoplasm and a purple nucleus, usually with two lobes.

3. Basophils average about 12 microns in diameter, and, when stained, have dark blue-black granules in the cytoplasm with a purple nucleus which is usually indented.

Lymphocytic development involves the progression from lymphoblast to large lymphocyte to small lymphocyte. Lymphocytes will appear in the peripheral blood smear as a dark purple nucleus filling almost the entire cell with a faint blue cytoplasm. They are between 7 and 20 microns in diameter.

Monocytic development involves the progression from a monoblast to a monocyte. Monocytes appear in the peripheral blood smear to be larger than other WBCs, with a gray-blue cytoplasm and a kidney-shaped nucleus. They are between 13 and 25 microns in diameter.

Thrombopoiesis is the development and production of platelets. Platelets involve the progression from megakaryoblast to promegakaryocyte to megakaryocyte to platelet. Platelets or thrombocytes are fragments of the cytoplasm of megakaryocytes. In a thin, peripheral blood smear, platelets appear, when stained, to be pale blue and about 1 to 4 microns in diameter, with approximately 5 to 25 platelets per oil immersion field. The life span of a platelet is approximately 10 days.

Differential Count of White Blood Cells

Four separate steps are involved in performing a complete differential count of white blood cells:

1. Percentage distribution of the different types of WBCs.

2. Estimation of the total leukocyte count.

3. Estimation of platelets.

4. RBC morphology description.

The percentage distribution of the different types of WBCs is calculated by identifying 100 WBCs from a stained smear. They are classified by the staining characteristics discussed earlier. The cells are counted with the aid of a mechanical counter which provides a separate key for each type of white blood cell, and maintains a running total which automatically rings when 100 cells have been recorded. It is often difficult to classify each WBC observed, and if any cell is unidentifiable, the physician should be consulted. WBC abnormal morphology should be noted.

The second part of a differential count is the estimation of the total leukocyte count made from the number of leukocytes seen with the low-power objective. This provides a check on the total WBC count. For example, a patient with a 10,000 count should show approximately twice as many WBC/lpf (WBCs per low power field) as a patient having a 5,000 count.

Thirdly, an estimation of the platelets should be done and reported as increased, decreased, or normal. Five to 25 platelets per oil immersion field is considered a normal range.

The last category is a description of the red cell morphology. RBC morphology is the study of the structure and forms of the individual RBCs observed in the stained smear. Normal RBCs, when stained, are 7 to 8 microns in diameter, round in shape, and have a pink color with a paler central area.

The normal adult range for a differential count is as follows:

Neutrophils	60 to 70%
Eosinophils	1 to 4%
Monocytes	2 to 6%
Basophils	0 to 1%
Lymphocytes	25 to 35%

MAKING A DIFFERENTIAL CELL COUNT

Purpose: To perform a differential count of the percentage distribution of various white blood cells found in the peripheral blood smear.

Equipment: peripheral blood
clean microscope slides
staining rack
Wright's stain
buffer solution
microscope
immersion oil
differential cell counter

Procedure	*Principle*
1. Obtain peripheral blood specimen.	1. Peripheral blood may be obtained from a finger puncture or venous blood. EDTA is the preferred anticoagulant.

2. Label the slide.

2. A numbering system may be used which correlates with the daily log sheet. Positive patient identification must be maintained.

3. Place one drop of blood on the slide about $3/4$ inch from the end of the slide.

3. The drop of blood should be small in order to prepare a thin smear.

4. Place the slide on a flat surface and hold a second slide at a 30- to 45-degree angle against the first slide (see Fig. 26-19A).

4. The second slide spreads the drop of blood and distributes the cells over the slide. An angle greater than 45 degrees results in a thick smear and less than 45 degrees results in a thin smear.

5. The second slide is allowed to touch the drop of blood which will spread along the edge by capillary action (see Fig. 26-19B).

5. This allows an even distribution of the drop of blood.

6. With an even flowing motion spread the drop of blood over the first slide. The blood will be thicker at the beginning and thinner at the end. The work should be done quickly (see Fig. 26-19C).

6. The thin edge is known as the "feathered" edge. This provides an area one cell thick for differential counting. If capillary blood is used, the blood will clot if the process is not done quickly.

7. Allow to air-dry.

7. When cells are allowed to dry quickly, less shrinkage will result.

8. Place the stain on a staining rack and flood the smear with Wright's stain. Allow to stain for 2 to 3 minutes.

8. The Wright's stain is an eosin (acid dye) and methylene blue (basic dye) stain. The timing will vary according to the technique used.

9. Apply the buffer solution to the slide on top of the Wright's stain. A green, metallic sheen should appear. Allow to stain 5 to 7 minutes (see Fig. 26-19D).

9. The timing will vary according to the specific technique.

10. Rinse with distilled water. Wipe the back of the slide with gauze and air-dry in a vertical position (see Fig. 26-19E).

10. Rinsing the slide with distilled water removes the stain and buffer. Wiping the back of the slide prevents the stain from drying on the back, making it difficult to read microscopically.

11. Place one drop of immersion oil in the center of the slide. Place the slide on the microscope stage and focus using the low-power objective. Switch to the oil immersion objective and judge the slide for proper staining. Locate an area appropriate for differential counting, red cell morphology description, and platelet estimation.

11. Using the low-power objective, estimate the total WBC count. Oil immersion increases the resolving power, which is the ability to give a detailed image. An appropriate area for a differential count should be an area where the cells are one layer in thickness near the "feathered" edge. Proper staining characteristics for Wright's stain were given earlier.

12. Perform a differential count using a differential cell counter to classify the WBCs.

12. Count 100 WBCs by systematically scanning the slide. Do not cover the same area. Convert the number of cells in each category to a percentage.

13. Perform a red cell morphology description.

13. The second part of a differential is red cell morphology. Are there abnormal forms, inclusion bodies, or immature red blood cells?

14. Perform a platelet estimation.

14. The third part of a differential is a platelet estimation. Are platelets increased, decreased, or normal? Five to 25 platelets per oil immersion field is a normal range.

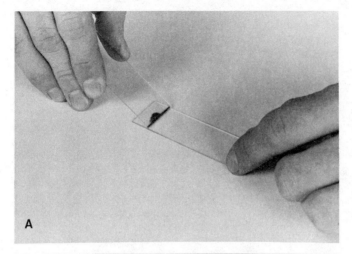

A, Place one drop of blood on the slide about $3/4$ inch from the end of the slide. On a flat surface hold a second slide at a 30- to 45-degree angle against the first slide.

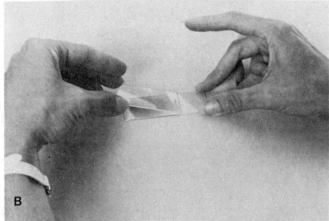

B, Allow the second slide to touch the drop of blood which will spread along the edge by capillary action. With an even, flowing motion spread the blood over the first slide.

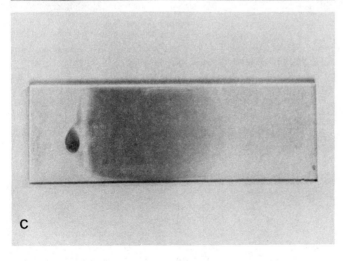

C, The blood will be thicker at the beginning and thinner at the end. The thin portion is known as the "feathered" edge.

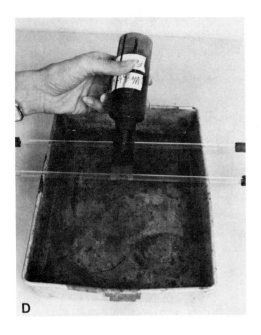

D, Place the slide on a staining rack and flood the smear with Wright's stain. Stain for 2 to 3 minutes. Apply the buffer solution on top of the Wright's stain.

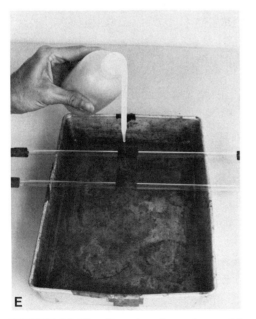

E, Rinse with distilled water. Wipe the back of the slide with gauze and air-dry in a vertical position. Observe under oil immersion and locate areas appropriate for differential counting, red cell morphology, and platelet estimation.

FIGURE 26-19. Procedure for making a differential cell count.

15. Record results on a laboratory request form and the daily log sheet.	15. Records must be properly documented. Always initial the results.
16. Store the slide for reference in a slide box for one week.	16. Maintaining a reference slide box is an excellent way to check laboratory results at a future date.

Terms Used in Abnormal Red Blood Cell Morphology (see Fig. 26-20)

Anisocytosis	Excessive variation in cell size.
Basophilic stippling	Fine blue granules found in RBCs, possibly diagnostic of lead poisoning.
Cabot rings	Loop or figure-eight designs that stain red or blue and are indicative of anemia.
Crenated cells	Cells with a scalloped or notched appearance, due to shrinkage.
Howell-Jolly bodies	Small nuclear fragments in the RBC which stain deep blue.
Hyperchromia	A condition in which cells have increased hemoglobin.
Hypochromia	A condition in which cells have decreased hemoglobin.
Inclusion bodies	Particles such as secretory granules or crystals in the cytoplasm of a cell. Not found in normal RBCs.
Macrocyte	An abnormally large cell (10 to 12 microns in diameter).
Megalocyte	An exceptionally large cell (12 to 25 microns in diameter).
Microcyte	An abnormally small cell (5 microns or less in diameter).
Nucleated RBCs	The number of RBCs containing a nucleus seen in a count of 100 WBCs.
Ovalocytes	Oval-shaped cells, also called elliptocytes.
Poikilocytosis	Abnormal variation in cell shape.
Polychromasia	A condition in which stained cells show bluish shades with tinges of pink.
Reticulocytes	Immature RBCs showing a blue reticulum when stained with methylene blue.
Rouleaux	Rolls of red blood corpuscles having the appearance of stacked coins.
Schistocytes	Fragmented cells, also called helmet cells.
Sickle cells	Crescent-shaped cells occurring in hereditary anemias.

Spherocytes	Small, round, completely hemoglobinated cells.
Target cells	Abnormally thin RBCs with a dark center and a surrounding ring of hemoglobin, occurring in anemia and jaundice.

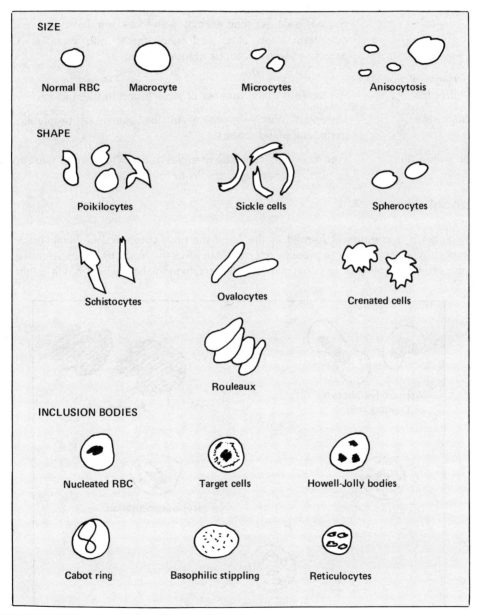

FIGURE 26-20. Abnormal red blood cell morphology.

Terms Used in Abnormal White Blood Cell Morphology (see Fig. 26-21)

Döhle bodies	Cytoplasmic, pale-blue-staining inclusions found in neutrophils, which occur in severe infections and have a nucleus not normally found in the peripheral smear.
Downey cells	Atypical lymphocytes, usually of larger than normal size. The nucleus is denser than normal, with lobes or indentations, and the cytoplasm stains bluer and may appear with vacuoles. Often associated with infectious mononucleosis.
Hypersegmentation of neutrophils	An increase in the number of lobes found in the nucleus.
Smudge cells	Disrupted WBCs appearing in the course of preparation of peripheral blood smears.
Toxic granulation	Fine to coarse dark blue granules in the cytoplasm of neutrophils, occurring in severe infections or inflammations.

Hemoglobin

Hemoglobin is a compound formed in the bone marrow, composed of *heme* (iron and photoporphyrin) and *globin* (a protein). Hemoglobin gives the blood its red appearance and has the ability to combine with oxygen, forming oxyhemoglobin, which has a bright red

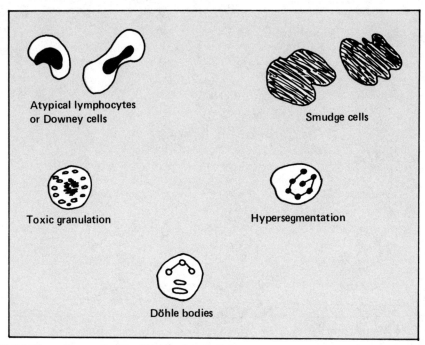

FIGURE 26-21. Abnormal white blood cell morphology.

color. It carries this oxygen to the tissues by way of the arteries. The oxygen is released at the tissue sites, and the reduced hemoglobin, which has a bluish color, is returned to the lungs by the veins.

There are many methods for hemoglobin determination. The cyanmethemoglobin method is a colorimetric procedure. Whole blood reacts with potassium ferricyanide and potassium cyanide (Drabkin's solution) to produce cyanmethemoglobin which has a stable color. The hemoglobin concentration is proportional to the intensity of the color developed. A spectrophotometer at a wavelength of 540 millimicrons is used to measure the absorbance of this color. Standards must be used to set up a standard curve, and quality control must be used for daily calibration.

Other methods using automatic pipettes or the Unopette System supplied by Becton-Dickinson should be employed because cyanmethemoglobin is a poison, and consequently it is dangerous to pipette by mouth. With the Unopette System diluents of cyanmethemoglobin are already aliquoted.

There is a direct relationship between hemoglobin and hematocrit determinations. The hematocrit value should be approximately three times the hemoglobin reading plus or minus two. For example, if the hemoglobin reading were 15 grams, the hematocrit value should be 45 percent, with a range of 43 to 47 percent. The normal range for hemoglobin is 13.3 to 17.7 gm/dl in men, and 11.7 to 15.7 gm/dl in women.

Hematocrit

Hematocrit, or packed cell volume (PCV), is the volume of packed RBCs compared by percentage to the total blood volume. Venous or capillary blood may be used for the micromethod which involves filling capillary hematocrit tubes with the specimen, sealing the tubes, centrifuging for 3 to 5 minutes, and reading the volume of packed RBCs by means of a hematocrit reader. The normal range for hematocrit values is 40 to 54 percent in men, and 37 to 47 percent in women.

THE MICROHEMATOCRIT METHOD

Purpose: To determine the hematocrit—the amount of packed RBCs as a percentage of total blood volume.

Equipment: sterile alcohol swab
sterile gauze pad (2 × 2 inches)
sterile lancet
capillary tube (plain tubes for anticoagulated blood,
heparinized for "finger-stick" blood)
sealing compound

Procedure	Principle
1. Wash hands.	1. Handwashing prevents the spread of micro-organisms
2. Assemble equipment.	2. Equipment readily at hand will facilitate a rapid procedure.

3. Perform a finger puncture. If a venipuncture is utilized, the anticoagulated tube, properly mixed, may be used.

3. Either capillary or venous blood is satisfactory. Plain capillary tubes must be used with anticoagulated specimens. Heparinized capillary tubes must be used with "finger-stick" blood since blood will clot.

4. Fill the capillary tube approximately $3/4$ full by slanting the tube at a 10-degree angle to the finger puncture or the EDTA tube (see Fig. 26-22A).

4. Blood flows into the capillary tube by capillary action.

5. Fill the two capillary tubes.

5. Two specimens processed in duplicate will provide a check for accuracy. Also, if one breaks during centrifugation, it is not necessary to repeat the finger puncture.

6. Seal one end of the tube with Sealease (a commercial sealing compound).

6. Sealing one end prevents the leakage of blood during centrifugation.

7. Place the capillary tube with sealed end facing outward in the microhematocrit centrifuge. Use the other specimen as a balance tube on the opposite side of the centrifuge (see Fig. 26-22B).

7. With the sealed end to the outside, the blood is prevented from spinning out due to the high rate of speed of the centrifuge.

8. Secure the top of the centrifuge. Centrifuge 3 to 5 minutes at 10,000 rpm.

8. The speed of the centrifuge causes the RBCs to become packed on the bottom of the tube. The centrifuge must be calibrated daily with known standards to assure that the speed is not too high and the time not too long for quality results. Many standards are available for manual hematocrit values.

9. The capillary tube is read by means of a hematocrit reader for the percentage of total blood volume (see Fig. 26-22C).

9. The buffy coat is a gray-white interphase area of WBCs found between the RBCs and the plasma. Do not include this area when calculating the hematocrit.

10. Record results on the patient's request and daily log sheet.

10. Maintaining proper records allows for easier correlation of data.

11. Dispose of contaminated materials properly.

11. Proper disposal prevents the spread of microorganisms.

The Hemacytometer

A hemacytometer is a counting chamber utilized in manual microscopic methods for studying the number of cells in a unit volume of specimen per cubic millimeter. The medical office employs the hemacytometer primarily for white cell counts, although it can readily be used for red cell, platelet, sperm, spinal fluid, and eosinophil counts.

The Spencer Bright-Line double-counting chamber with improved Neubauer ruling is the hemacytometer of choice (Fig. 26-23). The glass slide is divided into two separate chambers. Each chamber has a total ruled area measuring 3 mm by 3 mm (9 sq mm). This area is subdivided into nine squares measuring 1 mm by 1 mm. The four corner squares are subdivided into 16 squares measuring 0.25 mm by 0.25 mm. White blood counts are performed using the four corner squares.

The middle square is subdivided into 25 squares measuring 0.2 mm by 0.2 mm.

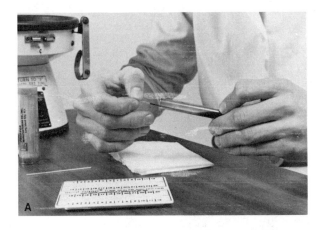

A, Fill the capillary tube approximately $3/4$ full by slanting the tube at a 10-degree angle to the EDTA tube. Seal one end of the tube with Seal-ease.

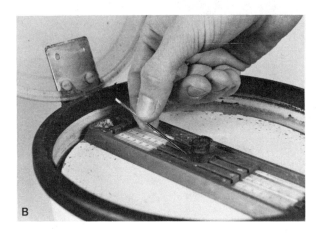

B, Place the filled capillary tube in the microhematocrit centrifuge with the sealed end facing outward. Centrifuge for 3 to 5 minutes at 10,000 rpm.

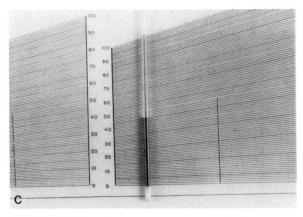

C, The capillary tube is read by means of a hematocrit reader to determine the percentage of packed red blood cells as compared to the percentage of total blood volume. The bottom of the packed RBCs is placed on the 0 mark, and the top of the plasma level is placed at the 100 mark. The junction between the packed RBCs and the plasma is the hematocrit reading.

FIGURE 26-22. The microhematocrit method.

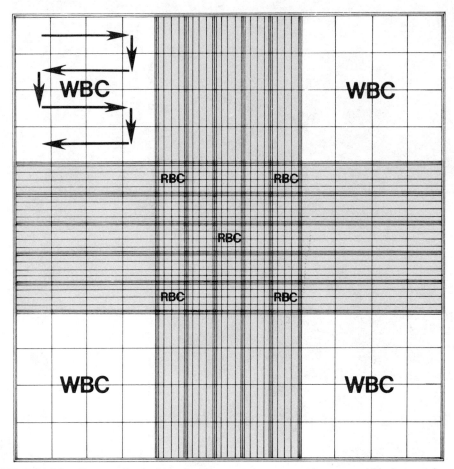

FIGURE 26-23. Spencer Bright-Line double-counting system with improved Neubauer ruling.

These 25 squares are subdivided into 16 squares measuring 0.05 mm by 0.05 mm, which makes a total of 400 tiny squares in the middle counting area. Eighty of the tiny squares, or the four corner squares and the central square, are used for red cell counting.

White cells are counted as shown by the arrows in the upper left corner of Figure 26-23. The movement of the microscopic field during the actual counting is from left to right, down to the next row, then right to left, and down again, until all cells in the counting area are included.

Figure 26-24 is an enlargement of the central red blood cell counting area. This area measures 0.04 sq mm, and is one of the five areas used for red cell counts. To prevent individual cells from being counted twice, cells on the upper and left borders of the counting area are included. but those on the lower and right borders are not. This method is used for all particles being counted by means of a manual counting chamber method.

Cells will appear as small, round dots which are best seen with a low light. The refraction of light will enable the viewer to distinguish between a cell and debris such as dust or

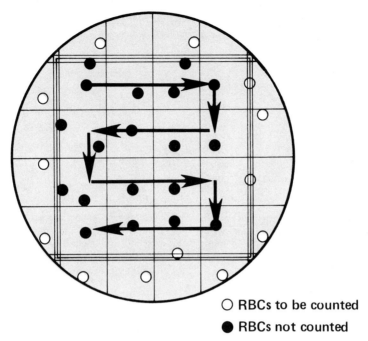

○ RBCs to be counted

● RBCs not counted

FIGURE 26-24. An enlargement of the central red blood cell counting area showing the movement of the microscopic field during the actual counting.

stain sediment. There should be an even distribution of cells in the various counting areas. A difference of no more than 10 cells should be observed between areas. Poor cell distribution may be due to one or more of the following:

1. A dirty cover slip or hemacytometer.

2. Overfilling the counting chamber.

3. Underfilling the counting chamber.

4. Drying of the solution caused by taking too long to count the cells.

5. Bumping or tilting the hemacytometer while focusing with the microscope.

MAKING A MANUAL WHITE BLOOD CELL COUNT

Purpose: To determine the number of WBCs in thousands per cubic millimeter for diagnostic testing.

Equipment: anticoagulant blood specimen (preferably EDTA)
WBC pipettes (2)
hemacytometer

aspirating tube
standard cover glass
WBC diluting fluid
microscope
WBC counter
mechanical shaker

Procedure	*Principle*
1. Assemble equipment.	1. Equipment close at hand allows for the procedure to be performed quickly.
2. Using the aspirating tube attached to a WBC pipette, draw the blood specimen to the 0.5 ml mark. Press the tongue on the opening of the mouthpiece once the 0.5 ml mark is reached. Remove the WBC from the specimen.	2. The aspirating tube provides protection from contamination. Once the 0.5 ml mark is reached, the suction pressure maintained by the tongue will prevent the specimen from dropping below the dilution mark.
3. Remove excess blood with a clean gauze.	3. Do not touch the tip of the blood specimen.
4. Using slow, even mouth suction, draw up the diluting fluid. Tap the bulb of the pipette to keep the white bead below the diluent. Rotate the pipette slowly. Once the diluent has reached 11.0 ml mark, again hold the suction by pressing the tongue on the opening of the mouthpiece.	4. The slow, even motion prevents air bubbles. Rotation of the pipette allows proper mixing of the specimen and diluent. Capillary blood will clot if the dilution procedure is not done quickly.
5. Hold the pipette at a 45° angle, remove aspirating tubing, and immediately place one finger over the top end of the pipette.	5. This will prevent the solution from flowing out.
6. Place on the mechanical shaker for 3 to 5 minutes.	6. Vigorous shaking allows for a properly mixed specimen.
7. Run a second WBC pipette following steps 2 through 6, and place on the shaker.	7. Two separate dilutions offer less chance of dilution errors and will increase accuracy.
8. Place the cover glass on the hemacytometer.	8. The cover glass and the hemacytometer must be clean and dust-free.
9. Remove the pipette from the shaker. Hold the pipette vertically over a piece of gauze, and with finger control at the top of the pipette, allow 3 drops to fall.	9. This allows for the diluting fluid which was in the stem to be removed and the cell suspension in the bulb to move to the tip of the pipette.
10. Plate the hemacytometer using a different dilution pipette for each side. Using finger control, touch the tip of the pipette to the hemacytometer and allow the solution to flow under the cover glass. The ruled area should be covered by capillary action without overfilling.	10. An even flow of the cell suspension allows for even cell distribution. With two dilutions from the same specimen, errors on plating technique are easily recognized. Overfilling shows a pooling of the solution outside the ruled area. Underfilling will show air bubbles. The hemacytometer and cover glass must be wiped, cleaned, and the plating repeated. Inaccurate results will occur with poor plating technique.

11. Cover the hemacytometer with an inverted Petri dish lined with moist filter paper for 2 to 3 minutes.

11. This allows the cells to settle out without drying. Drying will cause the solution to shrink in the ruled area, which will give inaccurate results.

12. Place the hemacytometer on the microscope stage. Use low power and focus on the ruled area. Observe for even cell distribution and count the WBCs, which will appear as round, refractile bodies.

12. Uneven distribution reveals poor plating technique. The diluent contains gentian violet which will lightly stain the WBCs. The diluent also hemolyzes the RBCs so that only WBCs remain.

13. Locate the upper right-hand square. Count the cells in 16 small squares contained in the four large outside squares. Do not count cells on the right and lower borders.

13. Counting cells on the upper and left but *not* on the right and lower borders prevents double counting of a single cell.

14. Count the opposite side of the hemacytometer.

14. Each side should be checked with the other within 20 percent:

> Side 1: 50 cells
> Side 2: 40 cells
> Average: 45 cells

New dilutions should be performed if error is greater than 20 percent. Errors in dilution, plating, and counting are minimized and accuracy increased.

15. Calculate the number of WBCs per cubic millimeter. Multiply the number of cells counted by 50.

15. WBCs/cu mm = count × 10 (depth factor) × $\frac{1}{4}$ (area factor) × 20 (dilution factor) = count × 50. The calculation is based on the depth of the cover glass and hemacytometer, the ruled area actually counted, and the dilution factor used.

16. Record results on the patient's lab request and daily worksheet. Initial the results.

16. Proper records must be maintained.

17. Clean all equipment. Wash pipettes with a suction pump, prime the washer with a detergent, rinse thoroughly with water, and run acetone through the pipettes followed by air suction. Clorox may be used to remove blood stains inside the pipette. Clean the hemacytometer with water or mild soap and a soft, lintless cloth; avoid scratching.

17. Clean equipment is necessary for good pipetting and plating techniques.

Comparisons Between WBC and RBC Manual Cell Counts

The method and principles of red blood cell counts are similar to the procedure described for manual white blood cell counts. The following differences do occur:

	RBC Count	WBC Count
Pipette used	RBC (red bead)	WBC (white bead)
Dilution range	1:100 to 1:1000	1:10 to 1:100
Outstanding marks	0.5, 1.0, 101.0	0.5, 1.0, 11.0

Diluent	Hayem's solution (mercury chloride and sodium sulfate)	2% acetic acid
Blood is drawn to "x" mark	0.5 ml	0.5 ml
Diluent is drawn to "x" mark	101 ml	11 ml
Dilution	1 to 200	1 to 20
Ruled area counted	5 RBC areas	4 WBC areas
Microscope power used	High power	Low power
Calculations	RBC/cu mm = count × 10 (depth factor) × 5 (area factor) × 200 (dilution factor). RBC/cu mm = count × 10,000.	WBC/cu mm = count × 10 (depth factor) × $\frac{1}{4}$ (area factor) × 20 (dilution factor). WBC/cu mm = count × 50.
Normal range	Men: 4.5-6.0 million/cu mm	
	Women: 4.3-5.5 million/ cu mm	5,000 to 10,000/cu mm

Common Sources of Error in Manual Pipetting Techniques

1. Dirty pipettes, cover glass, or hemacytometer.

2. Blood clots during dilution.

3. Air bubbles.

4. Poor plating technique.

5. Blood not drawn exactly to the dilution mark.

6. Overfilling or underfilling the counting chamber.

7. Poor cell distribution.

8. Poor mixing of specimen or of specimen and diluent.

9. Wiping off blood from the tip of the pipette.

10. Not discarding 3 drops prior to plating.

The Unopette System

The Unopette System, developed by the Becton-Dickinson Company, is a disposable pipetting system used for micro-blood specimens in hematology and chemistry. The system consists of a pipette, a pipette shield, and a reservoir with a diaphragm inside the neck (Fig. 26-25).

The reservoir contains various diluents, depending upon the test being done. This system readily adapts itself to manual counting of white cells, red cells, platelets, reticulocytes, and eosinophils, as well as to hemoglobin determinations and dilutions for automated cell counters. The advantages of this system over conventional methods of manual counting should be stressed, including greater accuracy and speed, and standardized expiration

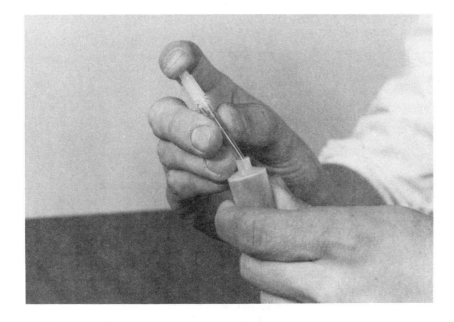

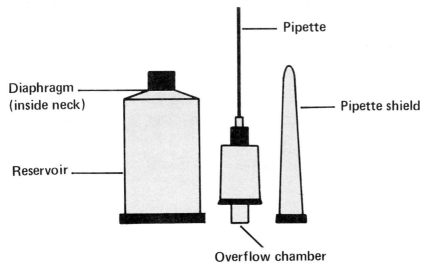

FIGURE 26-25. The Unopette System, consisting of a reservoir containing a diluent; a pipette used to deliver the specimen into the reservoir; and a pipette shield used to puncture the plastic seal of the reservoir and as a cap for the pipette to prevent evaporation.

dating. Since the system is disposable, less time is consumed in equipment cleanup and there is no need for mouth pipetting, which is a health hazard. Because the Unopette System has different dilution values and different areas to be counted with the hemacytometer, instruction packets must be followed closely.

USE OF THE UNOPETTE DISPOSABLE DILUTING PIPETTE

Purpose: To perform a dilution using the Unopette System

Equipment: Unopette System
　　　　　　 cover glass
　　　　　　 hemacytometer
　　　　　　 capillary blood or anticoagulated specimen

Procedure	*Principle*
1. Puncture the diaphragm with the pipette shield.	1. This opens the diluent.
2. Remove the pipette shield. Hold the pipette horizontally and touch it to the blood sample. Wipe off excess.	2. The capillary fills by capillary action. Do not wipe the opening of the capillary or the specimen will be removed, giving inaccurate results.
3. Squeeze the side of the reservoir.	3. This forces air out and will create pressure to draw the specimen into the diluent.
4. Repeat squeezing of the reservoir 2 to 3 times.	4. This will rinse the capillary pipette.
5. Place a finger over the pipette opening and mix.	5. Mixing the diluent and specimen allows for proper dilution and cell distribution.
6. Remove the pipette from the reservoir and invert the pipette, securing it into the reservoir and forming a dropper system.	6. The dropper allows for transfer of the specimen to the counting chamber.
7. Discard 3 to 4 drops. Then plate the hemacytometer by gently squeezing the reservoir. Continue with cell count.	7. This prevents any diluent which remained in the pipette to be plated. Avoid overfilling and underfilling the chamber.
8. Place the pipette shield over the pipette.	8. The shield prevents evaporation and allows storage if indicated by the instructions.
9. Discard the Unopette System properly.	9. Proper disposal prevents the spread of microorganisms.

Complete Blood Count

A complete blood count (CBC) includes seven parameters:

1. White blood cells;
2. Red blood cells;
3. Hemoglobin;
4. Hematocrit;
5. Mean corpuscular volume;
6. Mean corpuscular hemoglobin;
7. Mean corpuscular hemoglobin concentration.

A differential count with RBC morphology and platelet estimation is usually included as well. The first four parameters have been discussed in detail; the last three are mathematical calculations derived from the RBC count and from hemoglobin and hematocrit. They are generally known as red cell indices or constants.

Mean corpuscular volume (MCV) is the average volume of individual RBCs.

$$MCV = \frac{Hct \times 10}{RBC \text{ count in millions/cu mm}}$$

The normal range for MCV is 80 to 94 cubic microns per cell.

Mean corpuscular hemoglobin (MCH) is the hemoglobin content of the average RBC.

$$MCH = \frac{Hgb \times 10}{RBC \text{ count in millions/cu mm}}$$

The normal range for MCH is 27 to 34 picograms (micromicrograms) per cell.

Mean corpuscular hemoglobin concentration (MCHC) is the average hemoglobin concentration per 100 ml of packed RBC expressed as a percentage.

$$MCHC = \frac{Hgb \times 100}{Hct}$$

The normal range for MCHC is 31 to 36 percent.

Many medical offices do not report MCV, MCH, and MCHC values. The RBC indices are used primarily to differentiate the types of anemia and represent an average value that must be correlated to the blood smear interpretation. The medical assistant will find these mathematical calculations to be very useful in studying red blood cell morphology. A low MCH, for example, would alert the MA to look for the presence of hypochromic RBCs.

Automation in Hematology

The medical assistant should be familiar with the basic types of automation in hematology. Some physicians may provide a WBC and RBC counter to decrease the time involved in processing individual tests if a large volume of tests are handled in the office. The MA should be prepared to undertake special training in the operation and maintenance of sophisticated laboratory instruments.

There are basically two types of cell counting systems:

1. The *optical system* counts particles appearing as light on a dark-field illumination which is converted to an electrical impulse by a photomultiplier.

2. The *electrical system* counts particles that are suspended in an electrolyte solution by measuring the resistance of the particles. For example, RBCs and WBCs are poor conductors of electricity and when they pass through an opening that measures voltage there will be a drop represented by each cell. The most commonly used type of electrical system is the Coulter Counter. It provides the seven

parameters entailed in a complete blood count. The WBC, RBC, and MCV counts are performed electrically and the Hgb is done colorimetrically. MCH and MCHC are derived from the other readings.

The medical assistant should be familiar with a Coulter Model S processing card since most reference laboratories will report patient results using this type of format (Fig. 26-26).

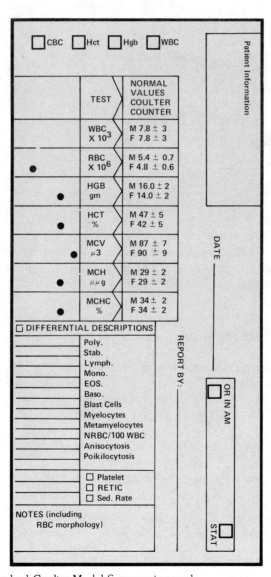

FIGURE 26-26.   Standard Coulter Model S processing card.

APPLICATION EXERCISES

Problem-Solving Activities

1. The patient refuses to have a venipuncture, stating that she fears needles. What is your response?

2. A venipuncture procedure results in the tube filling slowly and only partially. The needle remains in the arm. What is your response?

3. When performing a hemoglobin analysis, you notice that the normal hemoglobin control is not within acceptable limits. What is your response?

4. While performing a venipuncture, you notice that the patient is becoming pale and is perspiring profusely. What is your response?

5. During the patient's visit, you have obtained a urine specimen and completed the testing. Before leaving, the patient asks for the results. What is your response?

6. Upon entering the examining room, the patient is instructed to obtain a midstream "clean-catch" urine sample. She insists that she cannot urinate at the moment and offers you a urine specimen that she had collected at home prior to coming to the office. What is your response?

Practice Activities Related to Laboratory Procedures

Choose partners and upon receiving directions from the instructor, perform the following procedures on one another with proper supervision.

1. Venipuncture

2. Capillary finger puncture

3. Throat culture

4. Gram-staining

5. Routine urinalysis

6. Red blood cell count

7. White blood cell count

8. Hematocrit determination

9. Hemoglobin determination

10. White blood cell differential count

Discuss the results, your feelings, and the problems associated with the procedures.

Practice Activities Related to the Use of the Microscope

1. Demonstrate a microscopic urinalysis count.

2. Demonstrate a manual red blood cell count.

3. Demonstrate a manual white blood cell count.

4. Demonstrate a WBC differential count with RBC morphology, platelet estimation, and estimation of total leukocyte count.

Describe the results and discuss problems encountered with the instructor.

COMPLETING THE LEARNING LOOP

Patients are often confused and unsettled by the vast array of laboratory tests that may be required of them at various times in the course of treatment. In addition to performing basic laboratory procedures accurately and safely, the medical assistant must understand and be able to communicate to patients the purpose and importance of the tests being ordered. Laboratory testing is clearly an immensely valuable facet of the overall diagnostic examination.

The next chapter explores another increasingly important aspect of diagnostic testing—electrocardiography.

BIBLIOGRAPHY

Bailey, R. W., and Scott, E. G.: *Diagnostic Microbiology.* C. V. Mosby, St. Louis, 1970.

Bonewit, K.: *Clinical Procedures for Medical Assistants.* W. B. Saunders, Philadelphia, 1979.

Brown, I. H.: *Lectures for Medical Technologists.* Charles C Thomas, Springfield, Ill., 1964.

Buchanan, R. E., and Gibbons, N. E. (eds.): *Bergey's Manual of Determinative Bacteriology,* ed. 8. Williams & Wilkins, Baltimore, 1974.

Davidsohn, I., and Henry, J. (eds.): *Todd-Sandford Clinical Diagnosis by Laboratory Methods.* W. B. Saunders, Philadelphia, 1969.

Diggs, L. W., Strum, D., and Bell, A.: *Morphology of Human Blood Cells.* Abbott Laboratories, Chicago, 1970.

Helman, E., et al.: *Medical Technology: Board Examination Review,* Vol. 1. Berkeley Scientific Publications, Berkeley, Cal., 1975.

Kark, R., et al.: *A Primer of Urinalysis.* Harper & Row, New York, 1963.

Mukherjee, K. L.: *Review of Clinical Laboratory Methods.* C. V. Mosby, St. Louis, 1979.

Seiverd, C. E.: *Hematology for Medical Technologists,* ed. 4. Lea & Febiger, Philadelphia, 1977.

Settlemire, C., and Hughes, N.: *Microbiology for Health Students.* Reston Publishing, Reston, Va., 1978.

Strand, H.: *An Illustrated Guide to Medical Terminology.* Williams & Wilkins, Baltimore, 1968.

Wallach, J.: *Interpretation of Diagnostic Tests.* Little, Brown, Boston, 1974.

Widmann, F. K.: *Clinical Interpretation of Laboratory Tests,* ed. 8. F. A. Davis, Philadelphia, 1979.

27

ELECTRO-
CARDIOGRAPHY

SPECIFIC OBJECTIVES

Upon completion of this unit you will be able to:

1. Define the terminology applied to electrocardiography.

2. Describe the heart muscle function related to the electrocardiographic procedure.

3. Identify the components of the electrocardiographic cycle.

4. Prepare the patient for the procedure.

5. List and describe the function of the electrocardiograph and its components.

6. Identify the twelve leads and their placement.

7. Operate the electrocardiograph properly and obtain an accurate recording.

8. Identify and correct artifacts.

9. List and describe the marking and mounting procedures.

10. Apply problem-solving techniques to certain types of problems associated with the electrocardiographic procedure.

INTRODUCTION

Since medical assistants are responsible for performing diagnostic tests in the medical office, they will be called upon, in many practices, to record an electrocardiogram (abbreviated EKG or, more often today, ECG). For many physicians a general or comprehensive physical examination includes an ECG evaluation to acquire a normal baseline for future reference and to detect the presence of abnormalities. The medical assistant must acquire the knowledge and skills essential to obtain an accurate ECG reading.

    The information presented in this chapter will enable the MA to perform the electrocardiographic procedure. However, only practice and experience will assure that the task can be performed with confidence and expertise.

APPLIED TERMINOLOGY

Before continuing with an explanation and description of the ECG procedure, it is necessary to introduce the vocabulary associated with electrocardiography. The terms listed below will enhance the medical assistant's understanding of the electrocardiographic procedure.

Alternating current (AC):	A flow of electricity which reverses its electrical direction (as opposed to DC, or battery power).
Arrhythmia:	A cardiac rhythm disturbance.
Artifact:	Electrical activity which interferes with the normal appearance of the ECG cycle recorded on the graph paper.
Baseline:	A flattened horizontal line separating the various waves of the ECG cycle.
Cardiac cycle:	One complete heart beat, combining the contraction and relaxation phases.
ECG cycle:	The cardiac cycle as represented on the graph paper.
Electrocardiogram:	Electrical activity of the heart at a given time, recorded graphically.
Electrocardiograph:	The apparatus which functions to record the electrical activity of the heart.
Electrodes:	Objects, usually metallic, which conduct electricity and are attached to the limbs and chest wall to receive and transmit the electrical impulses of the heart for recording.
Interval:	Another term for wavelength.
P wave:	The electrical impulse emanating from the atria of the heart.

Precordial ECG waves:	Impulses received from electrodes placed on the chest wall.
QRS complex:	Waves of electrical impulse emanating from the ventricle.
Segment:	The area between two waves on an electrocardiogram.
T wave:	The relaxation phase of the ventricles.

ASPECTS OF ELECTROCARDIOGRAPHY

The Medical Assistant's Role

The electrocardiogram is a graphic display of the electrical activity of the heart that is measured and compared with known normal values. A physician is trained to interpret the ECG and to determine the presence, type, location, and severity of the abnormalities. The progress of the patient can then be monitored at certain intervals by repeated ECGs.

As with any other diagnostic tool, the ECG tracing is useful only if the medical assistant presents to the physician a recording that accurately depicts the cardiac activity. To do this, MAs must have an understanding of the normal cardiac function and its relationship to the graphic printout of the ECG. Those who assist must know how to properly set up the machine and prepare the patient to obtain the best possible graphic representation of the patient's cardiac activity. They must be able to recognize and correct any electrical interference and determine whether it originates from the patient, from the machine, or from other electrical devices in the room.

Heart Muscle Function

A brief review of heart muscle function is presented for the purpose of visualization and application. The student is encouraged to refer to Chapter 19 for a more detailed study of the anatomy and physiology of the heart.

The cardiac function relative to the ECG tracing is as follows. The sinoatrial (SA) node located in the right atrium (RA) receives an electrical stimulation that passes throughout both atria, causing them to contract and "squeeze" the blood into the ventricles below. On the ECG this is represented by the P wave. The ventricles then contract to eject blood into the pulmonary and systemic circulation represented by the QRS complex on the ECG tracing. The T wave represents a period of relaxation of the heart muscle before the next cycle. Each QRST is considered one cardiac cycle (Fig. 27-1).

ECG Components

RECORDING PAPER

To understand the significance of the cardiac cycle as represented on the ECG paper, the student must learn the characteristics of the paper and the rate of movement of the paper through the machine. Figure 27-2 is an example of the standard ECG paper.

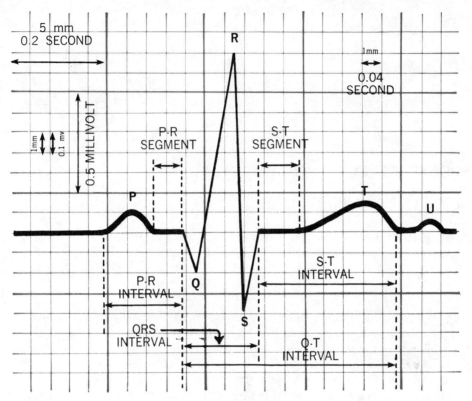

FIGURE 27-1. The QRST complex of an electrocardiogram. (Reproduced from *Taber's Cyclopedic Medical Dictionary*, ed. 14. F. A. Davis, Philadelphia, 1981.)

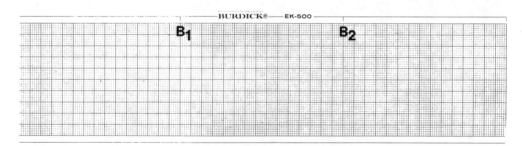

FIGURE 27-2. A sample of electrocardiograph paper.

If one looks carefully at the paper as it moves through the machine, one will discover that the rate of movement is 2.5 cm (25 mm) per second. Each lighter line is 1 mm, and each darker line is 5 mm. The 1 mm squares each represent 0.04 second in time, and each dark square represents 0.20 second. Three-second intervals are represented from B_1 to B_2 in Figure 27-2.

CONTROL PANEL

The position of control dials varies from one model to another, but all machines have the following features (see Fig. 27-3):

1. A *power/run switch*, which turns the machine on or off and sets the paper in motion.

2. A *speed selector*, which runs the paper at 25 or 50 mm per second. The speed selector is generally set at 25 mm/sec for adults. The 50 mm/sec position is used for infants and small children or adults with tachycardia.

3. An *intensity or heat control*, which adjusts for a heavier or lighter stylus.

4. A *position control*, which adjusts stylus position up or down.

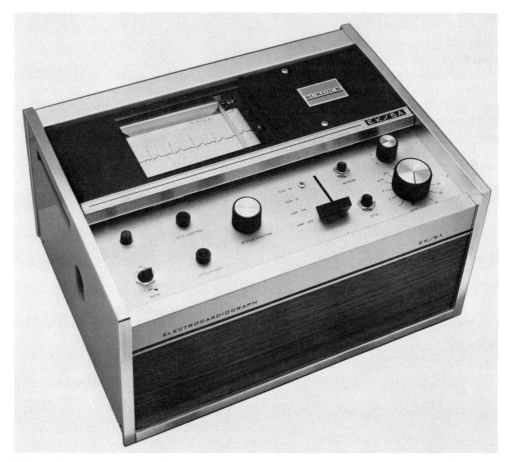

FIGURE 27-3. A medical office electrocardiograph, showing a typical control panel. (Courtesy of the Burdick Corporation)

5. A *sensitivity control,* which adjusts the height of the tracing ($1/2$ = 5 mv; 1 = 10 mv, or 2 = 20 mv). This dial is normally set on 1. If the height of the tracing is so high that the upward and downward deflections do not fit on the paper, the sensitivity control is set on $1/2$. On the other hand, if the complexes are so short that they are barely discernible, the control is set on 2. If it is necessary to adjust to $1/2$ or 2, the selection number should be clearly marked on the tracing to inform the physician of the change, and the standardization button should be depressed at the beginning of the change.

6. A *standardization impulse control,* which should be used at the beginning of each tracing to ensure an accurate, reliable recording. Pressing the standardization button causes 1 millivolt of electricity to enter the machine, which should result in an upward deflection of 10 mm to be recorded on the ECG paper.

7. A *lead marker* (the newer machines may not have this control because it is built into the lead selector and marks automatically).

8. A *lead selector dial* marked STD, I, II, III, ARV, AVL, AVF, V, and CF.

LEADS

The standard electrocardiograph has 12 leads which enable the physician to examine the electrical activity of the heart from three dimensions. This electrical activity is picked up by the electrodes, transmitted through the machine, amplified, and then recorded on the paper.

Five electrodes are used:

RA = right arm

LA = left arm

RL = right leg (also the ground)

LL = left leg

V = chest

These electrodes are connected to the patient with stretchable rubber straps.

Before the electrodes are attached to the patient, an electrolyte-saturated pad must be applied to the electrode to assure conduction of the impulses from the skin to the machine.

The different electrode sites and their associated voltages are defined as follows:

Lead I—right arm to left arm

Lead II—right arm to left leg

Lead III—left leg to left arm

Lead AVR—left arm and left leg to right arm

Lead AVL—left leg and right arm to left arm

Lead AVF—left arm and right arm to left leg

Leads V_1 through V_6 (precordial leads)—left arm and left leg and right arm to one of six electrode sites

The chest electrode placements are as follows (see Fig. 27-4):

V_1—fourth intercostal space at the right sternal border

V_2—fourth intercostal space at the left sternal border

V_3—midway between V_2 and V_4

V_4—fifth intercostal space, midclavicular line

V_5—same level as V_4 at the anterior axillary line

V_6—same level as V_4 and V_5 at the midaxillary line

Leads I, II, and III are called bipolar leads because each lead utilizes two limbs for recording the electrical force of the heart. These leads may also be referred to as standard leads.

Augmented leads are unipolar, recording midpoint positions between the limbs. These include leads AVR, AVL, and AVF. The chest leads V_1, V_2, V_3, V_4, V_5, and V_6 are also unipolar, recording electrical activity of the heart in six areas of the chest wall and an area within the heart itself.

Each lead represents information related to the electrical activity of a specific anatomic

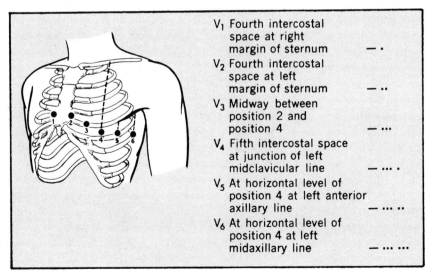

V_1 Fourth intercostal space at right margin of sternum — ·

V_2 Fourth intercostal space at left margin of sternum — ··

V_3 Midway between position 2 and position 4 — ···

V_4 Fifth intercostal space at junction of left midclavicular line — ···· ·

V_5 At horizontal level of position 4 at left anterior axillary line — ··· ··

V_6 At horizontal level of position 4 at left midaxillary line — ··· ···

FIGURE 27-4. Recommended positions for ECG chest leads. (Courtesy of the Burdick Corporation)

area of the heart muscle. The physician interprets the data obtained from each lead separately as well as collectively to determine the condition of the heart.

Patient Preparation

The patient will be lying in the supine position. If the patient has never had an ECG and is apprehensive, explain the procedure and gain the patient's confidence. Make sure that the patient knows that this is a painless procedure. Be certain that the table is large enough, and provide the patient with a pillow under the head and knees. The more comfortable the patient is made, the less likelihood there will be of muscle tremor artifacts.

The room temperature should be comfortable for the patient's state of undress. Arm electrodes are applied to the upper one-third of the arms and to the inner calf of the legs.

The tension of electrodes should be equal and snug but should not restrict circulation. Instruct the patient not to move or talk during the recording. Unplug the electrically operated table or bed and any other unnecessary equipment in the room.

If the patient has oily skin or is very hairy, wipe the area of electrode placement with alcohol before attaching the electrode.

Plug the ECG machine into a properly grounded outlet, but do not pass the cord under the patient's bed or table. Lead wires should follow the patient's body contours and not be allowed to dangle.

Having followed the foregoing instructions, the medical assistant can proceed with the recording of the ECG. If artifacts occur, a check should be made for loose wires, soiled electrodes, improper placement, and improper grounding.

Artifacts

Artifacts are any structures that have unnatural configurations and that interfere with the normal-appearing cardiac cycles. The medical assistant must be able to identify and correct artifact representations as these artifacts, caused by additional electrical activity, will interfere with obtaining a normal representation of the ECG cycles (Fig. 27-5). The most common artifacts are caused by muscle movement, wandering baseline, and alternating current interference.

Muscle tremors, which are characterized by a fuzzy, irregular baseline of the tracing, can often result from both involuntary and voluntary muscular movements. Reassurance is necessary to resolve the patient's probable anxiety and thus help to eliminate the cause of the artifacts. A patient may move voluntarily to adjust position and needs to be reminded of the importance of remaining motionless to assure an accurate tracing. In addition, some patients may be afflicted with a nervous system disorder. In these situations the tracing will need to be interrupted and then reinitiated to accommodate the patient and obtain an accurate tracing.

Wandering baseline artifacts are mechanical in nature. The application and condition of the electrodes are usually faulty. Electrolyte solution that has not been evenly applied may also cause interference. Likewise body creams or other cosmetics and materials already present on the skin may cause disruptive electrical conduction.

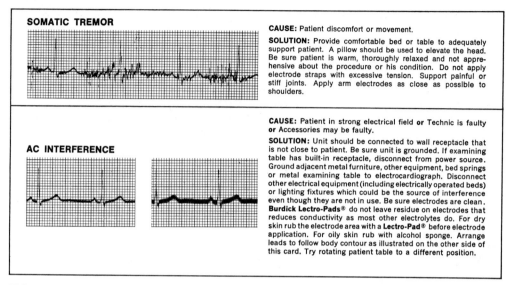

FIGURE 27-5. Common artifacts and their solution. (Courtesy of the Burdick Corporation)

Alternating current artifacts are usually caused by power demand overloads. Other electrical equipment may be competing for the voltage resource. Improper grounding or dangling lead wires could cause electrical interference.

When artifacts cannot be corrected by the medical assistant, they must be reported to the physician as the ECG recording cannot otherwise be continued. The physician can be oriented to the problem if a sample of the artifact is obtained and the lead identified.

A source of interference can be located, in most cases, by (1) running the recording of leads I, II, and III, and (2) examining the recording to determine which two leads have the most interference.

Greatest interference observed	Direction of interference source
Leads I and II	Patient's right arm
Leads I and III	Patient's left arm
Leads II and III	Patient's left leg

ECG Procedure

The stepwise procedure for obtaining an electrocardiogram is outlined below. Careful adherence to the steps and an understanding of the rationale for the techniques will ensure accurate performance of the procedure.

OBTAINING AN ELECTROCARDIOGRAM

Procedure	*Principle*
1. Plug the ECG into a properly grounded outlet.	1. This avoids AC interference which could alter an accurate tracing.
2. Turn the machine on to allow the stylus to warm up.	2. The graph paper is usually coated with a waxy substance. The stylus must be warmed to melt the wax so that the markings can be recorded.
3. Affix electrodes to the patient using electropads next to the patient's skin under the electrode. First place the RA lead on the electropad (or electrolyte gel, if used) on the fleshy part of the right arm. Then connect the LA lead to the left arm and the appropriate leads to the right and left legs on the fleshy portion of the limbs, not over bone. When electrolyte gel or paste is used, a small amount is placed on the limb and the electrode placed over the area and rubbed slightly to distribute the gel on the electrode.	3. Electropads assure conduction of the impulses from the skin to machine.
4. Connect the lead wires to the electrodes and plug them into the machine. Be certain that the RA is connected to the right arm and the LA to the left, etc. (see Fig. 27-6).	4. Accuracy of placement is essential to proper recording.
5. Ground the machine and unplug all unnecessary electrical appliances.	5. This eliminates AC interference which could alter an accurate tracing.
6. Offer reassurance and help the patient to be comfortable. Avoid movement or talking.	6. This eliminates muscle tremor artifacts.
7. Position the lead selector on "Standardize" (STD). Turn recorder selector to "On."	7. This provides a standard for comparison for the height of the tracings.
8. Turn machine selector to "Run."	8. This initiates the recording.
9. Depress the STD and note if the mark as 10 mm high. If it is not, adjust the machine to obtain this height.	9. This is necessary to obtain an accurate recording.
10. Center the stylus, then run leads I, II, III, AVR, AVL, and AVF, allowing 5- to 10-inch strips for each lead. If any bizarre complexes appear that are not caused by interference, make sure to run a long enough strip to record. The height of the standardization measurement must be 10 mm, or two large squares from baseline, to assure acurate recording.	10. These tracings are necessary for a detailed view of the heart. A long strip sample can have tremendous diagnostic potential.
11. Correct any artifacts.	11. This assures an accurate tracing.
12. If the machine does not automatically mark each lead, the following code may be used to mark it:	12. The code identifies different leads for the purposes of accurate mounting and proper diagnosis.

Lead	Code
I	.
II	. .
III	. . .
AVR	.____
AVL	. .____
AVF	. . .____
V_1	____.
V_2	____. .
V_3	____. . .
V_4	____. . . .
V_5	____. . . . .
V_6	____. . . . . .

13. Record the chest leads. Remember that the chest electrode must be moved to six different positions as noted earlier. Turn the machine off between changes of electrode placement.

13. This prevents the stylus from thrashing when the chest leads are moved.

14. Turn off the machine and remove the rhythm strip.

14. This completes the procedure.

15. Remove the electrodes and cleanse the skin with a clean, moistened cloth to remove the electrolyte solution. Repeat the cleansing procedure on the electrode plates.

15. Cleansing is necessary to remove the residue of the electrolyte solution.

16. Write the patient's name, age, sex, height and weight, the date, and list the patient's medications on the recording.

16. This information identifies the tracing and avoids error.

17. Mount the graph, being sure to include any bizarre complexes.

17. All representative segments are monitored to ensure that the proper diagnosis can be established.

18. Assist the patient to a sitting position to await further instruction.

18. The graph may be read by the physician in the office, or sent to another facility for evaluation. The patient should be informed where the results will be made available.

Marking and Mounting Procedures

Mounting procedures depend on the physician's preference and the method and materials being used. There are numerous options. A marking code which identifies the lead for mounting is established by the manufacturer of the ECG machine and materials or by the physician. The code should be catalogued in the procedure manual for reference. In addition, ECG machines are currently available which automatically mark the leads. The incidence of error and demand on the medical assistant's time are thus reduced.

Mounting forms can be purchased or specially designed by the office staff. Two general rules govern mounting procedures:

1. Identify each lead properly and clearly.

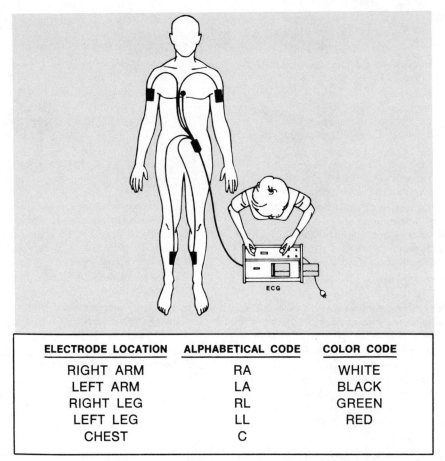

ELECTRODE LOCATION	ALPHABETICAL CODE	COLOR CODE
RIGHT ARM	RA	WHITE
LEFT ARM	LA	BLACK
RIGHT LEG	RL	GREEN
LEFT LEG	LL	RED
CHEST	C	

FIGURE 27-6. Application of electrodes and connection to the electrocardiographic unit. Apply clean electrodes. If paste or gel is used as an electrolyte, electrodes should be washed after each use and scoured frequently. Refer to the chart for the alphabetic or color code of the leads and connect the leads to the proper electrodes. The lead wires should then be arranged to follow the body contour as shown. Note that the power cord points away from the patient. (Courtesy of the Burdick Corporation)

2. Record on the tracing the patient's name, address, age, sex, height and weight, the date, the physician's name, the drugs currently being taken by the patient, and any other information required by the physician.

SUMMARY

The electrocardiogram is a valuable diagnostic tool, and one which is absolutely indispensable to the diagnosis and treatment of heart disease. The ECG procedure requires precise skill and knowledge. The medical assistant who is competent in this procedure will be an immeasurable asset to medical office practice.

APPLICATION EXERCISES

Practice Activities

1. The instructor will demonstrate the ECG procedure and will assign students to participate in the roles of patient and medical assistant. The student in the role of MA will first perform the procedure and then the students will reverse roles.

2. Run a strip for a normal cycle. The student in the patient's role should then talk, breathe deeply, or move to produce an artifact. Continue the tracing. Mark artifacts and identify leads.

Role-Playing Exercises

1. The patient expresses fear of the procedure. What is the assistant's response?

2. The patient is moving about during the procedure. What is the assistant's response?

3. Following the procedure, the patient inquires if the ECG is normal. What is the assistant's response?

4. Before the procedure, the patient asks what the ECG will show. What is the assistant's response?

5. You, as medical assistant, have stopped the machine to correct an artifact. When you restart the machine, you notice that the patient appears apprehensive. You conclude that you must have looked perplexed while correcting the artifact. How should the medical assistant react and respond to the patient?

Problem-Solving Exercises

1. Mrs. Jones has a coughing episode during the procedure.

2. An artifact appears. The patient has been motionless and quiet.

3. The patient is obese. You are not certain that you have correctly placed the leads.

4. The patient's relative wants to remain in the room with the patient during the procedure.

5. The stylus is not marking the cardiac cycle.

COMPLETING THE LEARNING LOOP

It is unlikely that you will ever have your own ECG recorded unless such an experience is offered as a laboratory activity during your training. Thus, if you want to learn about the practical aspects of electrocardiography, you will have to find an older relative who has undergone this kind of testing. If you do find such a person, be sure to ask him about his feelings during the procedure. Most patients experience a good deal of apprehensiveness. This is particularly true of the first such test. Part of the role of the medical assistant is to help the patient deal with these concerns.

BIBLIOGRAPHY

Blowers, M., and Smith, R.: *How to Read an ECG.* Medical Economics, Oradell, N.J., 1977.
Burch, G. E., and Winsor, T.: *Primer of Electrocardiography.* Lea & Febiger, Philadelphia, 1972.
Conover, M. B.: *Understanding Electrocardiography,* ed. 3. C. V. Mosby, St. Louis, 1980.
Goldberger, A. L., and Goldberger, E.: *Clinical Electrocardiography: A Simplified Approach.* C. V. Mosby, St. Louis, 1977.
Hohn, A. R.: *Basic Pediatric Electrocardiography.* Williams & Wilkins, Baltimore, 1974.
Hurst, J. W., and Myerburg, R. J.: *Introduction to Electrocardiography.* McGraw-Hill, New York, 1973.
Laiken, N., et al.: *Electrocardiograms: A Self-Instructional Approach.* Appleton-Century-Crofts, New York, 1978.
Lyon, L. J.: *Basic Electrocardiography Handbook.* Van Nostrand Reinhold, New York, 1977.
Marriott, H. J.: *Practical Electrocardiography.* Williams & Wilkins, Baltimore, 1977.
Reading EKGs Correctly. Intermed Communications, Horsham, Pa., 1975.

CHAPTER 28

RADIOGRAPHY

SPECIFIC OBJECTIVES

Upon completion of this chapter you will be able to:

1. List terms used to describe aspects of radiography.
2. Describe the medical assistant's role related to x-ray procedures.
3. List and explain the components of patient preparation.
4. List the positions used in x-ray procedures.
5. Describe the functions of the x-ray machine, and list and identify the parts.
6. List precautions related to x-ray procedures.
7. Describe x-ray film processing techniques.
8. Apply patient teaching techniques to radiographic procedures.

INTRODUCTION

The medical assistant may be responsible for operating x-ray equipment in the medical office. Although most physicians refer radiographic testing to a hospital or medical center facility, there are physicians who perform basic x-ray procedures in the office. These procedures are usually performed in conjunction with the physical examination. A chest x-ray, for example, may be a routine component of the comprehensive physical examination. In the practice of medical and surgical specialists, the x-ray procedure may be an essential component of almost every examination performed in the office. Therefore, it is necessary for the MA to be able to perform the basic x-ray procedures under the physician's supervision and to understand the basic principles involved.

APPLIED TERMINOLOGY

Certain terms require clarification before continuing with a discussion of radiographic procedure.

Cassette: The container in which x-ray film is placed during a radiographic examination.

Contrast medium: A radioactive substance usually consisting of chemical compounds which can be ingested or injected (as in barium enema and barium swallow), and which is used in radiography to make a particular body structure visible. The substance employed can be air or in tablet, powder, liquid, or gaseous form.

Detail: The clarity and sharpness of an x-ray image.

Fluoroscopy: The use of contrast media with a specialized detection technique for the purpose of viewing internal organs and structures of the body directly. Motion within the body can be observed by being transmitted on a screen coated with fluorescent chemicals.

Oscilloscope: An instrument for visualizing forms associated with body movement, such as heart beat, by means of electrical variations viewed on a fluorescent screen.

Radiography: The use of high-energy radiation to visualize internal body organs and structures. X-rays are passed through the body onto a specially sensitized film which permanently records the image. Fluoroscopy, tomography, and xeroradiography are types of radiographic testing.

Radiolucent: Referring to a structure which is transparent with x-rays.

Radiopaque: Referring to a structure which does not permit the passage of x-rays and therefore is nontransparent.

Radiologist: A physician specialized in the diagnosis and treatment of disease using various forms of radiant energy.

Roentgenologist:	A medical specialist qualified in the use of roentgen rays (x-rays) for diagnosis and treatment.
Tomography:	A type of radiography used to obtain focus on a specific place of the body. The x-ray tube and the photographic plate (parts of the x-ray machine) are rotated on an axis and the selected place remains in focus during the movement. More precise recordings are obtained using tomography when a computer rather than film is used to record the images attained when x-rays pass through the body. Computerized axial tomography scans (CAT scans) were first used in connection with diagnostic studies of the brain. Other applications are now being explored. Highly skilled medical specialists are required for the operation of the CAT scan.
Xeroradiography:	Using a special technique, an electrostatic image of the soft tissue can be projected through the use of x-rays. Mammography is an example of xeroradiography.
X-ray:	Invisible, high-energy electromagnetic waves which have the ability to penetrate solid materials such as body structures.

THE ROLE OF THE MEDICAL ASSISTANT

In certain situations, the medical assistant is likely to be called upon to perform the basic x-ray procedure. More often, however, the MA will not be responsible for performing the procedure, but will prepare and instruct the patient, schedule x-rays, and receive results. In order to carry out these tasks effectively, the medical assistant should acquire a practical understanding of x-ray technology.

PATIENT PREPARATION

The considerations involved in patient teaching apply to radiologic testing. To prepare the patient for the procedure, information must be transmitted from the MA to the patient. An assessment of the patient's ability and willingness to comprehend, his awareness of body functions, and his familiarity with medical procedures is necessary to determine the content of the explanation.

Certain general rules can be applied in briefing patients for diagnostic procedures.

1. Avoid the use of complex medical terms when possible. Use proper terminology but explain it as fully as needed.

2. Encourage the patient and the family to ask questions.

3. Explain the procedure briefly. Emphasize *what* is to be done as well as *how* and *when*. Note certain sensations that the patient may experience in testing.

4. Reinforce the physician's explanation of the rationale for the testing.

5. Give specific instructions both verbally and in writing. *Example:* "Do not eat or drink anything except water for 12 hours. The test is scheduled for 8:00 a.m. in the Radiology Department on the second floor of the hospital."

6. Inform the patient as to when and how he will receive the results.

7. Provide an opportunity for discussion of the patient's fears regarding the procedure.

8. Record the patient's test and the date of exposure to x-ray, and assure the patient that the amount of radiation delivered in his personal history is being monitored.

POSITIONING

The patient's position is determined by the type of x-ray examination required and the specific body part to be visualized. Jewelry and other objects such as hairpins should be removed since the image will be altered by their presence.

The following terms are x-ray positioning references:

1. *Anteroposterior (AP) view:* The anterior aspect of the body faces the x-ray tube, and the posterior aspect faces the film. Any body part can be x-rayed with an AP view. The patient may be placed in a sitting or supine position.

2. *Posteroanterior (PA) view:* The reverse of the AP view.

3. *Lateral view:* The body part is placed on its side to receive the passage of x-rays from one side to the opposite side.

4. *Right lateral (RL) view:* The right side of the body is placed toward the film.

5. *Left lateral (LL) view:* The left side of the body is placed toward the film.

6. *Oblique view:* The body is placed on an angle.

7. *Supine position:* The patient lies on his back.

8. *Prone position:* The patient lies on his abdomen, face down, with his head turned to one side.

The following terms refer to x-ray beam positions:

1. *Axillary:* The beam is directed toward the underarm.

2. *Craniocaudal:* The beam is directed downward from head to toe.

3. *Mediolateral:* The beam is directed from the middle to the side of the part being x-rayed. (The term *supine mediolateral* is used when the patient is in a supine position.)

THE X-RAY MACHINE

The x-ray machine is composed of three parts: (1) the table, (2) the x-ray tube, and (3) the control panel. In the medical office, the x-ray machine may be designed exclusively for chest x-rays. Equipment is now available which is fully automatic. The equipment pictured in Figure 28-1 may be used for various types of x-rays and is representative of a standard machine.

The table is movable and may be placed in various positions and angles, depending on the type of procedure to be performed. The x-ray tube is situated above the table and produces and transmits the x-radiation. The control panel contains knobs for operating the machine. It is positioned behind a specially constructed, lead-lined wall to avoid x-ray contact with the machine operator.

If table-type x-ray equipment is utilized in the office, an x-ray technician will almost always be employed to operate the machine and be responsible for patient management in these procedures.

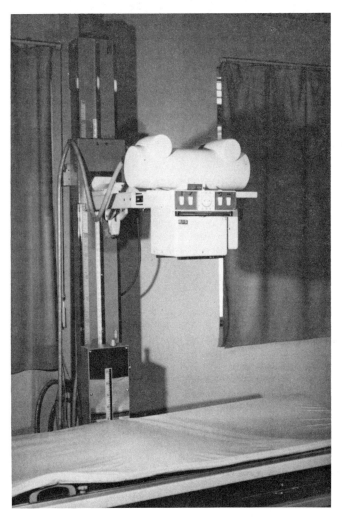

FIGURE 28-1   A standard medical office x-ray machine.

After the patient is properly positioned, the radiographic film is placed underneath the body structure to be x-rayed. The film is supplied in various types of packaging. One type of packaging has each sheet of film inserted between layers of black paper and wrapped together in lightproof paper with a foil backing. The wrapped film sheets are then placed in a box and sealed. The film must be opened in the darkroom to protect it from exposure to light. The film is then placed in a film holder which is lightproof for protection during the actual exposure. When fine details of the image are desired, x-ray film is placed in a cassette with intensifying screens to shorten and intensify the exposure which would be required with the use of x-ray film alone. In this case, the cassette is used in place of the holder. It is an aluminum case with a metal frame which holds two intensifying screens.

Intensifying screens are composed of smooth cardboard or plastic sheeting with special chemical coatings and are fluorescent and highly sensitive to light. There are three common types of screens: (1) "fast" screens which produce high intensification, (2) "average" screens which produce a balance between speed of exposure and definition of the image, and (3) "slow" screens for image sharpness.

Before the film is placed in the machine it must be marked using a method preferred by the physician. The marking identifies the patient's name or code number.

After placing the film in its correct position and maintaining correct patient position, the timing device on the control panel is set to produce an x-ray with a desired exposure time. The x-ray is then taken and the film developed.

X-RAY OPERATING PROCEDURE

The steps outlined in the practical procedure given below can be followed as a guide in operating x-ray equipment. It should be remembered, however, that the physician or x-ray technician will nearly always operate the machine.

MAKING AN X-RAY PHOTOGRAPH

Purpose: To obtain an x-ray image of a body structure or organ.

Procedure	*Principle*
1. Turn on the switch to warm up the machine.	1. Warmup is required for many machines to ensure proper and maximum functioning.
2. In the darkroom, unwrap the film and place in holder (cassette).	2. Avoid exposure to light which would destroy the film's capacity to produce an image.
3. Identify the patient and explain the procedure	3. Identification avoids error and explanation reduces anxiety
4. Position the patient and place the film accordingly.	4. Position depends on what is to be x-rayed. Proper positioning is essential to obtain the desired image.
5. Center the x-ray tube and instruct the patient to remain motionless. Put the guard shield in place.	5. The x-ray tube must be centered to produce the proper image. Moving will blur the film and a second x-ray will be necessary. The guard shield is a lead shield to protect the patient from receiving radiation.

6. Set the timer. The machine is operated according to the manufacturer's or physician's instructions. Observe the patient through the windows of the lead-lined wall.

6. The control panel is positioned behind the lead-lined wall to protect the operator from contact with x-rays.

7. Remove the exposed film and take to the darkroom to unload and develop. Help the patient to a comfortable position and escort him to the waiting room.

7. The film must be handled in the darkroom to avoid exposure to light.

8. If the film has not been previously marked prior to placement, label it immediately.

8. Labeled film can be used in court as a legal document.

9. Process the film. Place the processed film on the viewbox for the physician's interpretation.

9. Using the method preferred, the film is processed to obtain the image. Placing the view on the viewbox is time-saving for the physician.

10. After the film has been interpreted, place the film in a properly labeled envelope and file according to the office policy.

10. Labeling the envelope identifies the film which is filed for future reference. The x-ray is the physician's permanent property.

PRECAUTIONS

Excessive exposure to radiation can cause tissue damage: temporary symptomatic syndromes or even permanent damage to genital and reproductive capacity can result. Certain precautions must be followed to safeguard both the patient and the operator from ill effects.

1. A lead apron is worn by an individual who is positioning or remaining with the patient during the x-ray procedure. While the patient receives a small amount of radiation each time he is x-rayed, the operator or assistant is exposed to daily radiation and would accumulate excessive amounts in a short period of time if unprotected. Lead is used because it absorbs the radiation.

2. Patients should be protected with a lead shield during x-ray of nearby structures.

3. Film badges which detect and record the amount of radiation received must be worn by the operator of the machine and assistants participating in the procedure. (Doses of radiation are measured in *rads*, *rems*, or *roentgens*.)

4. The room in which x-rays are being taken must be specially designed and checked for proper safety measures.

5. The equipment must be kept in good working order and checked routinely by a radiation physicist who is able to detect any radiation leakage in the machinery which would be dangerous both to the patient and the operator.

6. The operator should have routine periodic blood counts performed to detect the presence of blood dyscrasia that may result from excess radiation exposure.

7. The patient should be placed in the appropriate position as determined by the type of x-ray ordered. Retakes expose the patient to unnecessary amounts of radiation.

8. Patients should always be questioned regarding:

   a. The possibility of pregnancy, if applicable.

b. The number and type of x-rays received in the past and the possibility of exposure to radiation in the home, school, or work environment.

c. Adherence to pretest instructions given by the physician or assistant, such as abstaining from food.

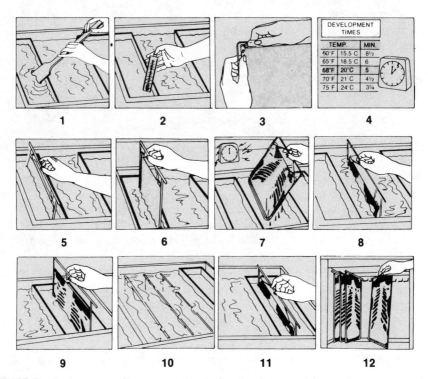

FIGURE 28-2 Steps in x-ray film processing. 1. Stir developer and fixer solutions to equalize their temperature. (Use a separate paddle for each to avoid possible contamination.) 2. Check the temperature of the solutions with an accurate thermometer. Adjust to 68°F (20°C) if possible. 3. Attach the film carefully to a hanger of the proper size. (Attach at lower corners first.) Avoid finger marks, scratches, or bending. 4. Set the timer for the desired period of development, based on the temperature of the developer. Consult the chart on the back of the timer for the correct temperature and time. 5. Immerse the film completely, smoothly, and without pause to avoid streaking, then start the timer. 6. Raise and lower the hanger several times to bathe the film surfaces thoroughly, repeating this once each minute. 7. When the alarm rings, lift out the hanger quickly, then drain the film for a moment into the space between the tanks. 8. Place the film in an acid rinse bath or under running water. Agitate the hanger vigorously, and rinse for 30 seconds. If a water rinse is used, lift the film and drain well. If an acid bath is used, plunge the film immediately into the fixer. 9. Immerse the film and agitate the hanger vigorously. Most films are fixed at 60° to 75°F (15.5° to 24°C) for 5 to 10 minutes in Kodak X-ray Fixer, or for 2 to 4 minutes in Kodak Rapid Fixer. 10. Place the film in a tank of running water with ample space between hangers. Length of time will vary according to the type of film used. 11. If facilities permit, use a final rinse of Kodak Photo-Flo solution to speed drying time and prevent water marks. Immerse the film for about 30 seconds and drain for several seconds. 12. Place the film in a dryer, or on a rack in a current of air. Keep films well separated. When dry, remove films from their hangers and trim the corners to remove clip marks. Insert each film in an identifying envelope. (Drawings courtesy of the Radiography Market Division, Eastman Kodak Company)

X-RAY FILM DEVELOPMENT

Film development occurs in the darkroom. The darkroom permits no natural light. The only artificial light acceptable is a specially designed darkroom light which utilizes a low-wattage bulb. The steps involved in x-ray film processing are pictured and described in Figure 28-2. Either the manual method described or an automatic processor is used. The film solution used in the manual method must be carefully handled and properly maintained. Proper preparation, use, processing, and storage of the film are essential to obtaining high-quality and permanently fixed radiographs.

SPECIFIC RADIOGRAPHIC EXAMINATIONS

The medical assistant will not perform radiographic studies and is not likely to assist with specific radiographic examinations as these are conducted in medical centers by radiologists and specially trained radiologic technicians. However, the MA may be responsible for patient instruction and preparation. The studies listed in Table 28-1 are defined and the patient preparation in which the MA may participate is described. Patient preparation details may be somewhat modified depending on the facility and its administration. As noted in Chapter 19 and 20, all studies ordered by the physician should be contained in the procedures manual with specific instructions included to assist the MA in patient preparation. Brochures or cards should be available and may be designed and written by the MA to give to patients who must undergo x-ray procedures. These materials describe the test, explain why it is required (indications), give instructions for preparation for which the patient is responsible, tell when the results can be expected and how they will be delivered, and attempt to allay general fears related to the radiographic examination.

TABLE 28-1. Common Radiographic Studies

Radiographic Study	Description and Purpose	Patient Preparation
Abdomen study	A flat plate (survey film) is made of the abdomen to detect organ placement and visualization. The test requires approximately 15 minutes.	None
Angiogram	Contrast medium (iodine component dye) is injected into the vessel to be studied through a catheter to examine the condition of the vessel. Used to detect signs or presence of cardiovascular disease. Test requires several hours to perform.	No food or drink is permitted within 4 to 5 hours of the time the procedure is scheduled.
Angiocardiogram	The procedure description above is applicable with the addition of the catheter passage into the heart itself.	Same as for angiogram.

TABLE 28-1. *Continued*

Radiographic Study	Description and Purpose	Patient Preparation
	(Cerebral angiogram is catheter passage through an artery in the neck and into an area of the brain.)	
Arteriogram	The procedure for an angiogram is applicable here; however, an arteriogram specifically studies the condition of an artery or arterial system.	Same as for angiogram.
Barium enema (BE)	Contrast medium (barium sulfate) is instilled in the colon through the enema for the purpose of visualizing the lower intestinal tract to detect any aberrations in normal outline, such as strictures and tumor. The test is also referred to as a lower GI series. The procedure may last 1 hour.	Milk products are avoided because they produce gaseous reactions and phlegm. The patient is ordered NPO (nothing by mouth) after midnight.
Barium meal	Contrast medium of flavored barium sulfate is administered orally to the patient. The outline of the upper gastrointestinal tract can then be visualized. Although the study usually requires an hour, repeat films may be requested at different intervals to observe emptying time of the stomach. Ulcers, inflammation, strictures, and tumors can be detected in the barium meal procedure. The test may require additional time (longer than 1 hour) if the small intestine is also examined. This test is also referred to as an upper GI series. A barium swallow differs from a barium meal in that in a barium swallow a smaller amount of substance is injested and the esophagus is specifically examined. The test requires approximately 15 minutes.	The patient is instructed to remain NPO after supper or after 10 p.m. (whichever is preferred) on the evening before the test is scheduled. No food, drink, or cigarette smoking is permitted on the day of the test as these would obstruct the view and may cause untoward reactions. Barium swallow requires no special patient preparation.

TABLE 28-1. *Continued*

Radiographic Study	Description and Purpose	Patient Preparation
Bone studies	Survey films are made to detect alignment, fracture, and other abnormalities. Requires 10 to 30 minutes depending on body reaction.	None
Bronchogram	Contrast medium (iodine compound) is instilled with the use of a special instrument through the trachea and into the bronchial tree. The general condition of the lungs can be observed. Useful in detecting cancer, abscess, and other disease processes. Usually requires 1 hour.	None
Chest x-ray	X-ray film of the chest is obtained in which lungs and heart can be visualized. Heart size, general condition of lung tissue, and presence of pneumonia can be determined.	None
Cholecystogram	Contrast medium of iodine compound in the form of tablets or granules is ingested by the patient the evening before the scheduled procedure. The outline of the gallbladder can be observed. The pressure of stones, inflammation, and other disease processes can be detected. The study is also referred to as a gallbladder series and usually requires 1 to 2 hours.	A low-fat, light diet is ordered for supper the evening before examination. Tablets or granules are swallowed after supper. The patient then remains NPO with the exception of water in small amounts up to bedtime.
Hysterosalpingogram	Contrast medium of iodine compound is injected into the fallopian tubes and uterus through the vagina. The patency of the tubes can be determined as well as disease processes in the uterus. The time required for the procedure is usually 1 hour.	None required.
Intravenous tests: Kidney, uterus and bladder series (KUB)	A survey film (flat plate) is made if the abdomen is used to study the presence of signs of disease in these organs.	None required.

TABLE 28-1. *Continued*

Radiographic Study	Description and Purpose	Patient Preparation
	Tumors and gas pockets can be detected. When done without the addition of other studies, the procedure requires less than 15 minutes to perform.	
Intravenous Cholangiogram	Contrast medium of iodine compound (dye) is injected intravenously, and the pathway of the dye excretion is followed. The bile ducts can then be observed for signs of disease processes such as stone formation and masses. Usually requires 3 to 4 hours as the films are taken at specified intervals to accommodate excretion patterns	The patient is instructed to remain NPO after midnight the evening before the test until the time scheduled for the procedure.
Intravenous pyelogram (IVP)	Contrast medium of iodine compound (dye) is injected intravenously to observe the pathway of the dye as it is excreted. The outline of the ureter and the urinary bladder is also achieved. Films are taken at intervals requiring approximately 2 hours for completion.	An oral laxative is self-administered by the patient the evening before the test to clear the colon of fecal matter which could obstruct and distort the view desired. A light diet is usually prescribed for supper (low films) the night before. The patient remains NPO after midnight until the scheduled test time, or NPO for 8 hours prior to testing.
Lymphangiogram	Contrast medium of iodine compound (dye) is injected into a lymphatic vessel to determine the general condition of the vessel and to detect obstruction and stricture. The test usually requires 6 hours as the pathways of the lymphatic system are visualized.	None required.
Mammogram	Survey films (flat plates) are made of the breast, with the beam directed at three angles: (1) sitting craniocaudal, (2) sitting axillary, and (3) recumbent mediolateral. Three separate films are required.	None required.

TABLE 28-1. *Continued*

Radiographic Study	Description and Purpose	Patient Preparation
	The breast is examined for presence of masses or lesions. The films are important in the detection of breast cancer. May require up to 1 hour for completion.	
Myelogram	Contrast medium of iodine compound (dye) is injected into the subarachnoid space of the spinal column with the use of a special lumbar puncture needle and syringe. Requires approximately 1 hour.	None required.
Perinasal sinus studies	A flat plate is made of the sinus cavities to detect inflammation or obstruction. Requires approximately 30 minutes.	None
Pneumoarthrogram	Contrast medium of air or other gas is injected into the articular capsule of a joint. The procedure usually requires 1 to 2 hours. The condition of the joint can be determined.	None required.
Pneumoencephalogram	Contrast medium of air or other gas is injected into the ventricle and subarachnoid spaces of the brain, using the lumbar puncture method. Spinal fluid is first withdrawn. The procedure may require 4 hours for completion. Injection of the dye into the subarachnoid spaces for x-ray filming of the brain and spinal cord is termed a pneumoencephalomyelogram.	The patient remains NPO after midnight until the scheduled test time. Headaches are a common side effect.
Scans (nuclear) Skull series	Radioactive substances are injected or instilled (oral or IV) for diagnostic purposes in various parts of the body. A radiosensitive instrument (scanner) outlines the area to be studied and records information by moving across the area. (If a camera is used, it may remain stationary.) In the bone scan, marrow function is studied and anemias	Some scans require special preparation, others do not. Hospitalization may be required.

TABLE 28-1. *Continued*

Radiographic Study	Description and Purpose	Patient Preparation
	can be detected. The progress of metastatic brain tumors can be monitored. Blood flow and cardiac function can be determined. The thyroid scan can detect hyperthyroidism and the presence of nodules. The kidney scan can detect the presence of disease and tumors. Scans usually require 1 hour for completion.	
Stereoscopy	This study is commonly used for skull examination, but may be used elsewhere in the body as well. It is actually a three-dimensional view of the body part observed by using two films taken at different angles and viewed simultaneously through a special device. Used frequently to obtain data on abnormal masses. Time required depends on the part being examined and the objective to be accomplished.	None
Thermography	Heat-sensing techniques in which skin areas appear darker or lighter, depending upon temperature. Lesions or tumors can be detected because temperature elevation of these parts (lightly colored) is represented. Thermography has been most widely used in the detection of breast cancer. The test usually is completed within 1 to 4 hours.	None
Tomography	This method is employed for depth photography of body tissue. By means of a special device, body tissue in front of and behind the part or plane to be examined is blurred so that the structures being studied remain in sharp focus. Cancer detection when	None

TABLE 28-1. *Continued*

Radiographic Study	Description and Purpose	Patient Preparation
	suspected is aided by the use of this procedure. Usually requires 1 hour to complete.	
Tomography Computerized axial (CAT scan)	Computerized axial tomography, or CAT scan, is fast replacing other procedures used to detect the presence of disease in the body, particularly cancerous diseases, and requires specialized machinery and technicians. Varying depths of tissue planes are obtained, which provide the physician with invaluable information regarding the size, shape, and density of tumors. The procedure requires a matter of seconds for completion.	None
Ultrasound	High-frequency sounds (inaudible) bounce off the structure being examined and are recorded, giving valuable information as to tissue density. When an oscilloscope is used to record ultrasonic echoes, the procedure is termed an echogram.	None
Ultrasound Pelvic		Laxative is administered orally just before the examination. The patient drinks 4 to 5 glasses of water 45 minutes prior to the scheduled time. Instruct the patient not to void—the urinary bladder must be full to deflect sound waves.
Ultrasound Abdominal		Oral laxative required for 2 days prior to the test, then no solid food after midnight, or 8 hours before examination.
Ultrasound Renal		Fluid intake of 16 ounces, 1 hour before examination. No voiding.
Ultrasound Thyroid		None required.

TABLE 28-1. *Continued*

Radiographic Study	Description and Purpose	Patient Preparation
Ultrasound Obstetrical		Full urinary bladder is essential. No voiding within 1 hour of examination; 32 to 48 ounces (4 to 6 glasses) of fluid should be ingested 45 minutes prior to examination.

SUMMARY

The medical assistant must have a basic understanding of x-ray technology to be able to give a proper explanation to the patient and to provide assistance to the physician.

Radiography is an important diagnostic tool. Precise techniques must be employed in all aspects of the x-ray procedure. MAs should remain under the physician's supervision in order to safeguard themselves and the patient from the avoidable ill effects working with x-radiation.

APPLICATION EXERCISES

Role-Playing Activities

The instructor will assign the roles of medical assistant and patient.

1. Mrs. Jones experiences fear concerning the x-ray procedure for which she is scheduled. Although she understands the procedure, she is reluctant because of the radiation exposure.

2. Mr. Roberts has never had an x-ray and is confused about the procedure. He is scheduled for a chest x-ray.

3. As medical assistant, you are taking a routine chest x-ray in the office. The patient coughs during the procedure. When you inform him you must repeat the x-ray, he becomes annoyed.

4. Albert is 5 years old and has a possible fracture. He has never had an x-ray. When the physician explains to his mother that an x-ray is necessary, Albert begins to cry. As MA, you are assigned the procedure.

Research and Discussion Activities

1. Mrs. Crawl is scheduled for an upper GI series (barium swallow). Design a teaching plan. What specific information would you include? What considerations? What questions?

2. Mr. Kavat is scheduled for a lower GI series (barium enema). Design a teaching plan. What specific information would you include? What considerations? What questions?

3. Mrs. Annsil is scheduled for a chest x-ray in the office. Design a teaching plan. What specific information would you include? What considerations? What questions?

4. Mr. Anders is scheduled for cholecystography. Design a teaching plan. What specific information would you include? What considerations? What questions?

5. Mrs. Coffey is scheduled for an intravenous pyelogram (IVP). Design a teaching plan. What specific information would you include? What considerations? What questions?

Planning Exercise

Design a general outline for x-ray procedures. You do not have to list the specific tests, but rather identify major content headings.

COMPLETING THE LEARNING LOOP

As a student of the health sciences, you are in a good position to continue to learn about the many aspects of radiographic technology. Like other areas of medicine, the field of radiology is a dynamic one. New advances are constantly being made and new applications discovered. Radiologic testing consequently requires the services of highly trained and specialized professionals. The medical assistant should keep informed of new and changing procedures and should adopt an attitude of respect for and cooperation with these important members of the health care team.

BIBLIOGRAPHY

Baron, J. P.: *A Study Guide for Radiologic Technologists.* Charles C Thomas, Springfield, Ill., 1978.
Cullinan, J. E.: *Illustrated Guide to X-Ray Technique.* J. B. Lippincott, Philadelphia, 1972.
Eastman, J. R.: *Radiographic Fundamentals and Technique Guide.* C. V. Mosby, St. Louis, 1979.
French, R. M.: *Guide to Diagnostic Procedures.* McGraw-Hill, New York, 1975.
Greenfield, G. B., and Cooper, S. J.: *A Manual of Radiographic Positioning.* J. B. Lippincott, Philadelphia, 1973.
Jacobi, C. A., and Paris, D. Q.: *Textbook of Radiologic Technology,* ed. 6. C. V. Mosby, St. Louis, 1977.
Squire, L. F.: *Fundamentals of Radiology.* Harvard University Press, Cambridge, Mass., 1976.
Watson, J. C.: *Patient Care and Special Procedures in Radiologic Technology.* C. V. Mosby, St. Louis, 1974.

THE MEDICAL ASSISTANT AS AN EMERGING MEMBER OF THE HEALTH TEAM

As you have absorbed the material in this text, a fuller awareness of your role as a significant member of the health team should also have emerged. You should now be able to imagine yourself situated in a medical office and performing specific tasks. Although the diversified nature of your role may still seem somewhat overwhelming, the areas of your responsibility can now be understood as interconnected, compatible, and collectively aimed at the objective of providing the highest quality health care to the medical office patient.

The challenge of assuming the professional stature of a medical assistant will require an openness to changing skill demands; the pursuit of continuing education; an involvement in national, state, and local professional associations; the maintenance of certification; and an ongoing personal development.

As you begin to envision yourself as a medical assistant, it is useful to focus upon the fact that medical assisting is a new and dynamic career. Many physicians and other allied health care professionals do not have a clear understanding of what the MA is all about, in terms of skills, training, and expertise. It will largely be up to each of you to educate these individuals, not through lectures or discussions, but through your own daily performance in the role of medical assistant.

Your success as a member of the health care team will be linked to the attitudes which you carry to work with you. MAs who are empathetic, understanding, and inquisitive, and who make a genuine effort to understand the roles of their colleagues in the medical office, will be a positive addition to the office team. MAs who act prudently to facilitate the needs of the physician will soon earn a valued place in the office. MAs who ease the difficulties of patients by listening and counseling effectively will advance the major goals of the medical team.

This book is designed to provide a general introduction; it is clearly not the ultimate resource for all of the functional areas of medical assisting. Thus the completion of this text should be visualized as the beginning, not the end, of your education. You should use the chapter discussions as a guide, while moving toward more complex and technical resource materials relative to both the administrative and clinical aspects of medical assisting.

The career-minded MA should also join and remain an active member of the American Association of Medical Assistants, as well as attending local chapter meetings on a regular basis and reading the professional journals.

The future of medical assisting belongs to those who will assertively act as builders and caretakers of the profession.

APPENDIX

CONTENTS

GUIDE TO ESTIMATED TIMES FOR COMMON MEDICAL OFFICE PROCEDURES

The times given below are approximate and may be adjusted to accommodate physician preference and patient needs.

Procedure	Time in Minutes
Allergy testing	30
Cast change	30
Complete physical examination (CPX)	30-60
with electrocardiogram (ECG)	+15
Dressing change (with drain)	15
Hypertension followup	10-15
Minor surgery	30-60
Office visits*	
brief	5-10
intermediate (for acute illness)	15-20
extended	30+
Patient teaching session/conference	30-60
Pelvis and pap test (P&P)	15-30
Prenatal checkup	15-30
Replacement suturing	30
Suture removal	10-20

*The intermediate visit is the most common. These breakdowns reflect standard manual record-keeping categorizations.

PUNCTUATION PATTERNS IN MEDICAL CORRESPONDENCE

Both open and mixed punctuation patterns are acceptable in office correspondence, provided that consistency of pattern is maintained throughout. Open punctuation is preferred for letters typed in block form.

	Open	*Mixed*	*Difference*
Dateline:	January 28, 1982	January 28, 1982	No difference. The comma is retained in both styles between day and year.
Inside Address:	Mr. John Wilkes 2970 East Lake Road Fairview, Pennsylvania	Mr. John Wilkes 2970 East Lake Road Fairview, Pennsylvania	No difference. No punctuation is used at the ends of lines in either style.
Salutation:	Dear Mr. Wilkes	Dear Mr. Wilkes:	No punctuation is used after the salutation in the open style; a colon or comma is used in the mixed style.
Complimentary Close:	Sincerely	Sincerely,	No punctuation is used in the open form; a comma is always used in the mixed form.
Signature Block Line:	Joseph Caruso	Joseph Caruso	No difference.

MEDICAL WRITING ABBREVIATION GUIDE

The following examples may be of help to the medical assistant in writing original letters or proofreading the physician's correspondence and manuscripts.

Correct Form	Incorrect Form	Rule
Figure 11 illustrates . . .	Fig. 11 illustrates . . .	Avoid beginning a sentence with an abbreviation.
The lesion (Fig. 11) was superficial.	The lesion (Figure 11) was superficial.	Words placed in parentheses may be abbreviated.
Fever, headache, and related signs were present.	Fever, headache, etc. were present.	Avoid use of "etc." in sentences and lists.
Smith and coworkers found that . . .	Smith et al. found that . . .	Avoid use of "et al." to indicate a group of persons except in listing references.
The test took 35 minutes.	The test took 35 min.	Spell out units of time unless they appear in parentheses or in tables.
Nearly 90 percent of the patients experienced relief.	Nearly 90% of the patients experienced relief.	Spell out "percent" unless it appears in parentheses or in tables.
General Medical Supply	Gen. Med. Supply	Avoid abbreviating company names unless the abbreviation *is* the official company name, such as: CIBA; 3M Company; TRW, IBM.
Article IV, Section II	Art. IV, Sec. II	Laws and bylaws are written in full when referred to for the first time. Subsequently they may be abbreviated.
prn; GI; IV	p.r.n.; G.I.; I.V.	Current practice favors omission of periods in medical abbreviations.
Escherichia coli	E. coli	Names for microorganisms may be abbreviated only after a first reference in full.
Professor; General; Senator; Reverend	Prof.; Gen.; Sen.; Rev.	With the exception of Ms., Mrs., Mr., and Dr., full titles are used for business letter salutations. Titles may be abbreviated in envelope blocks and inside addresses.
JAMA; N. Engl. J. Med. (in references)	Journal of the American Medical Association; New England Journal of Medicine	Names of journals are abbreviated in reference lists, but are written in full when they appear in sentences. (Reference example: Nelson, M.A.: Intra-arterial blood pressure. N. Engl. J. Med. 303:35-56, 1982.)

PROOFREADER'S MARKS

New paragraph.

No paragraph.

Insert word, letter or punctiation written in the margin.

Insert material omitted (place caret where insertion is to be made).

Delete matter crossed out.

Insert space.

Close up or delete space.

Delete letter and close up.

Close up, leaving some space.

Put in middle of page or line.

Turn letter or illustration.

Move to left.

Move to right.

Move down.

Move up.

Indent one em.

Align.

Straighten lateral margin.

Transpose or words letters.

Transpose space.

Adjust uneven spacing.

Spread words apart.

Run over to next line.

Run back to preceding line.

Have material continuous.

Period.

Comma.

Apostrophe.

Colon.

Semicolon.

Quotation marks.

Hyphen (-).

En dash (–)

Em dash (—)

Two em dash (——)

Equals sign (=).

Parentheses.

Brackets.

Question to author: OK?

Let it stand.

Set in LOWER case.

Set in capital letters.

Set in small capitals.

Set in roman type.

Set in italic type.

Set in bold face.

Wrong font (wrong size or face).

Use superior figure.

Use inferior figure.

SYMBOLS USED IN MEDICAL WRITING

♏	Minim.	μm	Micrometer.
℈	Scruple.	μ	Micron (common term for micrometer).
℥	Dram.	$\mu\mu$	Micromicron.
f℥	Fluid dram.	+	Plus; excess; acid reaction; positive.
℥	Ounce.	−	Minus; deficiency; alkaline reaction; negative.
f℥	Fluid ounce.		
O	Pint.	±	Plus or minus; either positive or negative; indefinite.
℔	Pound.		
℞	Recipe; take.	#	Number; following a number; pounds.
M	Misce; mix.	÷	Divided by.
a͞a, āa	Of each.	×	Multiplied by; magnification.
A, Å	Angstrom unit.	=	Equals.
C′	Complement.	≅	Approximately equals.
c, c̄	[L. *cum*.]. With.	>	Greater than; from which is derived.
E_0	Electroaffinity.	<	Less than; derived from.
F_1	First filial generation.	≮	Not less than.
F_2	Second filial generation.	≯	Not greater than.
$m\mu$	Millimicron, micromillimeter.	≦	Equal to or less than.
μg	Microgram.	≧	Equal to or greater than.
mEq	Milliequivalent.	≠	Not equal to.
mg	Milligram.	√	Root; square root; radical.
mg. %	Milligrams percent; milligrams per 100 ml.	$\sqrt[2]{}$	Square root.
		$\sqrt[3]{}$	Cube root.
Qo_2	Oxygen consumption.	∞	Infinity.
m-	Meta-.	:	Ratio; "is to."
o-	Ortho-.	::	Equality between ratios; "as."
p-	Para-.	∴	Therefore.
Po_2	Partial pressure of oxygen.	°	Degree.
Pco_2	Partial pressure of carbon dioxide.	%	Percent.
s͞s, ss	[L. *semis*]. One-half.	π	3.1416—ratio of circumference of a circle to its diameter.
	Foot; minute; primary accent; univalent.	□, ♂	Male.
		○, ♀	Female.
	Inch; second; secondary accent; bivalent.	⇌	Denotes a reversible reaction.

PRINCIPAL MEDICAL ABBREVIATIONS

Abbreviation	Latin (unless indicated)	English Definition
ad	ad	to; up to
ad lib.	ad libitum	as desired
AQ	aqueous	water
AV		atrioventricular
av.	(French)	avoirdupois
		average
B.P.		British Pharmacopeia
BUN		blood urea nitrogen
C.		Celsius
		centigrade
		Calorie (kilocalorie)
C.	congius	gallon
ca.	circa	about
CBC		complete blood count
cc.	(French)	cubic centimeter
CDC		Center for Disease Control
cg.	(French)	centigram
cm.	(French)	centimeter
comp.	compositus	compound
CNS		central nervous system
cong.	congius	gallon
contra	contra	against
CSF		cerebrospinal fluid
CV		cardiovascular
d	dexter	right
	dies	day (24 hours)
/d		per day
D&C		dilatation and curretage
def.	defaecatio	defecation
DPT		diphtheria-pertussis-tetanus
dr.	drachma	dram
ECG		electrocardiogram
ECT		electroconvulsive therapy
EEG		electroencephalogram
elix.	(Arabic)	elixir
EMG		electromyogram
emp.	emplastrum	a plaster
ENT		ear, nose, and throat
ESR		erythrocyte sedimentation rate
et	et	and
F.	(proper name)	Fahrenheit
f		female
FDA		Food and Drug Administration
FEV		forced expiratory volume
Fld.	fluidus	fluid
fl. dr.	fluidrachma	fluid dram
fl. oz.	fluidus uncia	fluid ounce
FSH		follicle-stimulating hormone
GI		gastrointestinal
Gm.; gm.	gramme (French)	gram
gr.	granum	grain
Gtt., gtt.	guttae	drops
h	hora	hour
hgb		hemoglobin
hypo	(Greek)	hypodermically
I.M.		intramuscular
inf.	infusum	infusion
inhal.		inhalation
inj.		injection
instill		instillation
I.Q.		intelligence quotient

Abbreviation	Latin (unless indicated)	English Definition
IU		international unit
I.V.		intravenously
kg.	(French)	kilogram
l	litre (French)	liter
lab		laboratory
lb.	libra	pound
LD$_{50}$		lethal dose, median
liq.	liquor	liquid; fluid
m.	(French)	meter
	minimum	minim
		male
MED		minimum effective dose
mEq.		milliequivalent
mg.		milligram
ml.		milliliter
mM		millimole
mm.	(French)	millimeter
mol. wt.		molecular weight
μEq		microequivalent
μg		microgram
no.	numero	number
NPN		nonprotein nitrogen
O.	octarius	pint
OC		oral contraceptive
O.D.	oculus dexter	right eye
O.L.	oculus laevus	left eye
O.S.	oculus sinister	left eye
os.	os; ora	mouth
oz.	uncia	ounce
paren.		parenterally
PBI		protein-bound iodine
per	per	through or by
pH		hydrogen in concentration
ppm		parts per million
pt	pinte (French)	pint
qt.	quartina	quart
rad		radiation absorbed dose
s̄	sine	without
S.	signa	mark
s	sans	without
s.c.	sub cutis	subcutaneously
s.cut.		subcutaneously
SGOT		serum glutamic oxalacetic transaminase
SGPT		serum glutamic pyruvic transaminase
sp. gr.	gravitus	specific gravity
spt.	spiritus	spirit
stat.	statim	immediately
syr.	syrupus	syrup
top.		topically
tr., tinct.	tinctura	tincture
UHF		ultrahigh frequency
ung.	unguentum	ointment
UV		ultraviolet
vin	vinum	wine
vol. %		volume per cent
WBC		white blood count
Wt.	wiht (Old English)	weight
w/v.		weight by volume
×		multiplied by

OTHER MEDICAL ABBREVIATIONS

Abbreviation	Latin Phrase	English Definition
abs. feb.	absente febre	without fever
a.c.	ante cibum	before eating
ad effect.	ad effectum	until effectual
adhib.	adhibendus	to be administered
ad part. dolent.	ad partes dolentes	to the painful parts
adst. feb.	adstante febre	when fever is present
ad us.	ad usum	according to custom
ad us. ext.	ad usum externum	for external use
ag. feb.	aggrediente febre	when the fever increases
alt. dieb.	alternis diebus	every other day
alt. hor.	alternis horis	every other hour
alt. noc.	alternis nocte	every other night
aq.	aqua	water
bal.	balneum	bath
bal. sin.	balneum sinapis	mustard bath
bis in 7d.	bis in septem diebus	twice a week
BP		blood pressure
c̄	cum	with
cat.	cataplasma	a poultice
cito disp.	cito dispensetur	let it be dispensed quickly
c.m.	cras mane	tomorrow morning
c.m.s.	cras mane sumendus	to be taken tomorrow morning
c.n.	cras nocte	tomorrow night
cont. rem.	continuetur remedia	let the medicines be continued
c.v.	cras vespere	tomorrow night
cyath.	cyathus	glassful
cyath. vinos.	cyathus vinosus	wineglassful
d	da	give
d	dies	day
/d		daily
decub.	decubitus	lying down
donec alv. sol. ft.	donec alvus soluta fuerit	until bowels are open
dur. dolor.	durante dolore	while pain lasts
en., enem.		enema
exhib.	exhibeatur	let it be given
h.n.	hoc nocte	tonight
hor. som, h.s.	hora somni	at bedtime
in d.	in dies	daily
mod. praesc.	modo praescripto	as prescribed
mor. dict.	more dicto	in the manner directed
mor. sol.	more solito	in the usual manner
n.b.	nota bene	note well
noct.	nocte	night
noxt.	noxte	night
p.a.a.	parti affectae applicetur	let it be applied to the affected region
post. cib. or p. c.	post cibum	after meals
p.r.	per rectum	through the rectum
p.r.n.	pro re nata	as needed
p.v.	per vaginam	through the vagina
Q.h.	quaque hora	every hour
Q. 2h.		every two hours
Q. 3h.		every three hours
q.i.d.	quater in die	four times a day
q.l.	quantum libet	as much as is wanted
q.p.	quantum placeat	at will
q.s.	quantum sufficiat	a sufficient quantity, as much as may be needed
quotid.	quotidie	daily
s.a. or sec. a.	secundum artem	by skill
semih.	semihora	half an hour
s.o.s.	si opus sit	if necessary
st.	stet, stetem	let it (them) stand

Abbreviation	Latin Phrase	English Definition
sum.	sumat, sumendum	let him take, to be taken
s.v.	spiritus vini	alcoholic spirit
s.v.v.	spiritus vini vitis	brandy
T.		temperature
tere	tere	rub
tere bene	tere bene	rub well
t.i.d.	ter in die	three times daily
t.i.n.	ter in nocte	three times a night
ur		urine

Reproduced from *Taber's Cyclopedic Medical Dictionary*, ed. 14. F.A. Davis, Philadelphia, 1981.

COMMON MEDICAL PREFIXES AND SUFFIXES

a-, an. Negative.
a-, ab-, abs-. Away from.
ad-, -ad. Toward.
-aemia. Blood.
aer-. Air.
-aesthesia. Sensation.
-algesia, algia. Suffering; pain.
algi-. Pain.
all-. Other.
amb-. Both; on both sides.
amph-. Around; on both sides.
ana-, an-. Up.
angio-. Relating to blood or lymph vessels.
ante-. Before.
anti-. Against.
apo-. From; opposed.
-ase. Enzyme.
aut-, auto-. Self.
bi, bis-. Twice; double.
brachy-. Short.
brady-. Slow.
cac-, caco-. Bad; evil.
cat, cata, cath-. Down.
-cele. A tumor; a cyst; a hernia.
cent-. Hundred.
cephal-. Relating to a head.
chrom-, chromo-. Color.
-cide. Causing death.
circum-. Around.
co, com, con-. Together.
contra-. Against.
cyst-, -cyst. Bag; bladder.
-cyte. A cell.
dacry-. Tears.
dactyl-. Fingers.
de-. From; not.
deca-. Ten.
deci-. Tenth.
demi-. Half.
dent-. Relating to the teeth.
derma-. The skin.
di-. Double; apart from.
dia-. Through; between; asunder.
dipla, diplo-. Double.
dis-. Negative; double; apart; absence of.
-dynia. Pain.
dys-. Difficult; bad.
ec, ecto-. Out; on the outside.
-ectomy. A cutting out.
ef, es, ex, exo-. Out.
-emesis. Vomiting.
-emia. Blood.
en-. In, into.
endo-. Within.
entero-. Relating to the intestine.
ento-. Within.
epi-. Upon.
-esthesia. Sensation.
eu-. Well.
ex-, exo-. Out.

extra-. On the outside; beyond.
fore-. Before; in front of.
-form. Form.
-fuge. To drive away.
galact, galacto-. Milk.
gaster, gastro-. The stomach; the belly.
-gene, -genesis, -genetic, -genic. Production; origin; formation.
glosso-. Relating to the tongue.
-gog, gogue. To make flow.
-gram. A tracing; a mark.
-graphy. A writing; a record.
hem, hemato-. Relating to the blood.
hemi-. Half.
hepa-, hepar-, hepato-. Liver.
hetero-. Other; indicating dissimilarity.
holo-. All.
homo, homeo-. Same; similar.
hydra, hydro-. Relating to water.
hyp, hyph, hypo-. Under.
hyper-. Over; above; beyond.
hypo-. Under.
-iasis. Condition; pathological state.
idio-. Peculiar to the individual or organ.
ileo-. Relating to the ileum.
in-. In; into; not.
infra-. Beneath.
inter-. Between.
intra, intro-. Within.
-ism. Condition; theory.
iso-. Equal.
-itis. Inflammation.
-ize. To treat by special method.
juxta-. Near.
karyo-. Nucleus; nut.
kata-, kath-. Down.
kera-. Horn; indicates hardness.
kinesi-. Movement.
-kinesis. Motion.
lact-. Milk.
laparo-. The loin; relating to the loin or abdomen.
laryng, laryngo-. The larynx.
latero-. Side.
lepto-. Small; soft.
leuko-. White.
-lite, -lith. A stone; a calculus.
lith-. A stone.
-logia, -logy. Science of; study of.
-lysis. Setting free; disintegration.
macro-. Large; long; big.
mal-. Bad; poor; evil.
med-, medi-. Middle.
mega, megal-. Large; great.
-megalia, megaly. Large; great; extreme.
melan-, melano-. Black.
mes-, meso-. Middle.
meta-. Beyond; over; between; change, or transposition.
-meter. Measure.

metra, metro-. The uterus.
micro-. Small.
mio-. Less; smaller.
mono-. Single.
multi-. Many.
my, myo-. Muscle.
myel, myelo-. .Marrow.
myxa, myxo-. Mucus.
neo-. New.
nephr, nephra, nephro-. Kidney.
neu, neuro-. Nerve.
niter, nitro-. Nitrogen.
non-, not-. No.
nucleo-. Nucleus.
ob-. Against.
oculo-. The eye.
-ode, oil. Form; shape; resemblance.
odont-. A tooth.
-oid. Form; shape; resemblance.
oligo-. Few.
-oma. A tumor.
omo-. Shoulder.
o-. An egg; ovum.
oophoron-. Ovary.
opisth-. Backward.
orchid-. Testicle.
ortho-. Straight; normal.
os-. A mouth; a bone.
-osis. Condition; disease; intensive.
oste, osteo-. A bone.
-ostomosis, ostomy. To furnish with a mouth
   or an outlet.
-otomy. Cutting.
oxy-. Sharp; acid.
pachy-. Thick.
pan-. All; entire.
para-. Alongside of.
path-, -path, -pathy. Disease; suffering.
-penia. Lack.
per-. Excessive; through.
peri-. Around.
-phobia. Fear.
-phylaxis. Protection.
-plasm. To mold.
-plastic. Molded; indicates restoration of lost or
   badly formed features.

-plegia. A stroke.
plur-. More.
pneu-. Relating to the air or lungs.
poly-. Much; many.
post-. After.
pre-. Before.
pro-. Before; in behalf of.
proto-. First.
pseud-, pseudo-. False.
psych-. The soul; the mind.
py-, pyo-. Pus.
re-. Back; again.
retro-. Backward.
-rhage, -rhagia. Hemorrhage; flow.
-rhaphy. A suturing or stitching.
-rhea. To flow; indicates discharge.
sacchar-. Sugar.
sacro-. Sacrum.
salping, salpingo-. A tube; relating to a fallopian tube.
sarco-. Flesh.
sclero-. Hard; relating to the sclera.
-sclerosis. Dryness; hardness.
-scopy. To see.
semi-. Half.
-stomosis, -stomy. To furnish with a mouth or
   outlet.
sub-. Under.
super, supra-. Above.
syn-. With; together.
tele-. Distant; far.
tetra-. Four.
thio-. Sulfur.
thyro-. Thyroid gland.
-tomy. Cutting.
trans-. Across.
tri-. Three.
-trophic. Relating to nourishment.
tropho-. Relating to nutrition.
uni-. One.
-uria. Relating to the urine.
urino, uro-. Relating to the urine or urinary
   organs.
vaso-. A vessel.
venter, ventro-. The abdomen.
xanth-. Yellow.

GLOSSARY OF LATIN MEDICAL WORDS

abacus, -ī. *m.* Shelf.
abdōminālis, -e. Abdominal.
abdūcēns, -ntis. Leading or drawing from (the median line); applied also to 6th pair of cranial nerves.
aberrāns, -ntis. Wandering.
abstractum, -ī. *n.* Abstract.
accessōrius, -a, -um. Accessory.
accidō, -ere, -cidī. Occur; happen.
ācer, ācris, ācre. Sharp; severe.
acervulus, -ī. *m.* (Lit., little heap), acervulus.
acētābulum, -ī. *n.* (Lit., vinegar cup), the bony cuplike cavity of the hip joint; acetabulum.
acētās, -ātis. *m.* Acetate.
acētum, -ī. *n.* Vinegar.
acidum, -ī. *n.* Acid.
acinus, -ī. *m.* A terminal compartment or secreting portion of a gland; acinus.
acusticus, -a, -um. Auditory.
acūtus, -a, -um. Acute.
adeps, adipis. *m.* and *f.* Fat; lard.
adjūtor, -ōris. *m.* Helper; assistant.
adjuvō, -āre, -jūvī, -jūtus. Aid; assist.
adsum, -esse, -fuī. Be present.
aeger, -gra, -grum. Sick.
aegrōtus, -a, -um. Sick.
āēr, āëris. *m.* Air.
aeternus, -a, -um. Eternal.
aether, -is. *m.* Ether.
āla, -ae. *f.* Wing.
ālāris, -e. Winglike; alar.
albicāns, -ntis. Whitening; white.
albūgineus, -a, -um. White.
albulus, -a, -um. Whitish.
albus, -a, -um. White.
alcoholicus, -a, -um. Alcoholic.
aliquandō. Sometimes.
alius, -a, -ud. Other.
aloina, -ae. *f.* Aloin.
alter, -tera, -terum. Other.
altus, -a, -um. High.
alūmen, -inis. *n.* Alum.
alvus, -ī. *f.* Belly, or its contents.
amārus, -a, -um. Bitter.
amīcus, -ī. *m.* Friend.
āmissiō, -ōnis. *f.* Loss.
āmissus, -ūs. *m.* Loss.
ammōnium, -ī. *n.* Ammonium.
amygdala, -ae. *f.* Almond.
anaestheticus, -a, -um. Producing insensibility; anesthetic.
anastomoticus, -a, -um. Anastomosing.
ānellus, -ī. *m.* Ring.
angulus, -ī. *m.* Angle.
anima, -ae. *f.* Breath; life.
anīsum, -ī. *n.* Anise.
ānnulāris, -e. Ringlike; annular.
ānnulus, -ī. *m.* Ring.
anterius, -a, -um. Anterior.
antīcus, -a, -um. Foremost.
antidōtum, -ī. *n.* Antidote.
antimōniālis, -e. Of antimony; antimonial.
antimōnium, -ī. *n.* Antimony.

antipyreticus, -a, -um. Reducing the temperature; antipyretic.
antisepticus, -a, -um. Destroying germ life; antiseptic.
antitrāgus, -ī. *m.* A conical eminence opposite the tragus, q.v.; antitragus.
antīquus, -a, -um. Ancient.
aperiēns, -ntis. Laying open; laxative; aperient.
appellō, -āre, -āvī, -ātus. Call.
aptē. Aptly.
apud. Near.
aqua, -ae. *f.* Water.
aqueductus, -ūs. *m.* A canal; aqueduct.
aquōsus, -a, -um. Watery.
arbor, -oris. *f.* Tree.
arceō, -ēre, -uī, -tus. Ward off.
arcuātus, -a, -um. Curved like a bow.
arcus, -ūs. *m.* A bow; arch.
āreola, -ae. *f.* Small area, especially around the nipple.
argentum, -ī. *n.* Silver.
arōmaticus, -a, -um. Aromatic.
arsenicum, -ī. *n.* Arsenic.
arsenis, -itis. *m.* Arsenite.
artēria, -ae. *f.* Artery.
articutāris, -e. Articular.
articulō, -āre, -āvī, -ātus. Articulate.
artus, -ūs. *m.* Joint.
ascendēns, -ntis. Ascending.
asepticus, -a, -um. Free from putrefactive matter; aseptic.
asper, -a, -um. Rough.
astrictus, -a, -um. Bound up.
astūtus, -a, -um. Shrewd; artful.
atropīna, -ae. *f.* Active principle of belladonna; atropine.
attollēns, -ntis. Raising up; elevating.
attrāhēns, -ntis. Drawing to or towards.
audītōrius, -a, -um. Auditory.
aurantium, -ī. *n.* Orange.
auricula, -ae. *f.* Auricle.
auris, -is. *f.* Ear.
axis, -is. *m.* (Lit., that about which a body turns), 2nd cervical vertebra; axis.
balneum, -ī. *n.* Bath.
basīlāris, -e. Basilar.
basis, -is. *f.* Base.
bene. Well.
benignus, -a, -um. Mild; benign; not malignant.
berberis, -idis. *f.* Barberry.
bibō, -ere, bibī. Drink.
bicarbonās, -ātis. *m.* Bicarbonate.
biceps, -cipitis. Two-headed.
bifidus, -a, -um. Cleft.
biliaris, -e. Pert. to or conveying bile; bilary.
bīnī, -ae, -a. Two each.
bismuthum, -ī. *n.* Bismuth.
bitartrās, -ātis. *m.* Bitartrate.
bonus, -a, -um. Good.
borās, -ātis. *m.* Borate.
brachiālis, -e. Of the arm; brachial.
brāchium, -ī. *n.* Arm.

brevis, -e. Short.
brōmidum, -ī. *n.* Bromide.
būbula, -ae. *f.* Beef.
būccinātor, -ōris. *m.* The trumpeter muscle; buccinator.
bulbus, -ī. *m.* Bulb.
caecus, -a, -um. Blind.
calamus, -ī. *m.* Reed.
calcaneum, -ī. *n.* The heelbone (os calcis).
calcium, -ī. *n.* Calcium.
calidus, -a, -um. Hot.
callōsus, -a, -um. Hard, tough.
calor, -ōris. *m.* Heat.
calumba, -ae. *f.* Calumba.
calvārium, -ī. *n.* The skullcap.
calx, -cis. *f.* Lime.
calyx, -icis. *f.* Cup; calyx.
camphora, -ae. *f.* Camphor.
camphorātus, -a, -um. Camphorated.
canāliculus, -ī. *m.* Small duct or canal.
canālis, -is. *m.* Canal.
canīnus, -a, -um. Of a dog, canine.
canis, -is. *m.* and *f.* Dog.
cānitiēs, -ēī. *f.* A gray color, hoariness.
cannabis, -is. *f.* Hemp.
cantharis, -idis. *f.* Spanish fly.
canthus, -ī. *m.* The corner or angle of the eye.
capiō, -ere, cēpī, captus. Take.
capitulum, -ī. *n.* A knob or protuberance of bone received into a concavity of another bone.
capsicum, -ī. *n.* Cayenne pepper; capsicum.
capsula, -ae. *f.* A small box; capsule.
carbō, -ōnis. *m.* Carbon; coal; charcoal.
carbolicus, -a, -um. Carbolic.
carbonās, -ātis. *m.* Carbonate.
cardamōmum, -ī. *n.* Cardamom.
careō, -ēre, -uī, -itus. Need; want.
carneus, -a, -um. Fleshy.
carpus, -ī. *m.* Wrist.
cartilāginōsus, -a, -um. Cartilaginous.
cartilāgo, -inis. *f.* Cartilage.
caruncula, -ae. *f.* A little piece of flesh; caruncle.
cataplasma, -atis. *n.* Poultice; cataplasm.
catharticus, -a, -um. Cathartic.
cauda, -ae. *f.* Tail.
caudātus, -a, -um. Having a tail; caudate.
causa, -ae. *f.* Cause.
causō, -āre, -āvī, -ātus. Cause.
cavernōsus, -a, -um. Hollow; cavernous.
cavitās, -ātis. *f.* Cavity.
cavus, -a, -um. Hollow.
celeriter. Quickly.
centrālis, -e. Central.
centrum, -ī. *n.* Center.
cephalalgia, -ae. *f.* Headache.
cērātum, -ī. *n.* Waxed dressing; cerate.
cerātus, -a, -um. Waxed.
cerevisa, -ae. *f.* Beer.
certus, -a, -um. Sure; certain.
cēterus, -a, -um. Other.
charta, -ae. *f.* Medicated paper.
chartula, -ae. *f.* Small paper (powder).
chirāta, -ae. *f.* Chirata.
chīrurgia, -ae. *f.* Surgery.
chīrurgus, -ī. *m.* Surgeon.
chlōral. *n.* Chloral.

chlōrās, -ātis. *m.* Chlorate.
chlōridum, -ī. *n.* Chloride.
chlōrōformum, -ī. *n.* Chloroform.
choledochus, -ī. *m.* Holding or receiving bile.
chorda, -ae. *f.* Cord.
chronicus, -a, -um. Chronic.
chylum, -ī. *n.* Chyle.
cibus, -ī. *m.* Food.
cicātrōsus, -a, -um. Full of scars, scarred.
ciliāris, -e. Ciliary.
cinchōna, -ae. *f.* Cinchona.
cinchonīna, -ae. *f.* Cinchonine.
cinereus, -a, -um. Ash-colored.
cinnamōmum, -ī. *n.* Cinnamon.
circulāris, -e. Circular.
circulatiō, -ōnis. *f.* Circulation.
circulus, -ī. *m.* Circle.
circum. Around.
circumdō, -dare, -dedī, -datus. Surround.
citō. Promptly; quickly.
citrās, -ātis. *m.* Citrate.
clārus, -a, -um. Clear, distinguished.
claudus, -a, -um. Lame.
clāvus, -ī. *m.* A corn, usually on the toes.
cludō, -ere, -sī, -sus. Shut; close.
cochlea, -ae. *f.* (Lit., snail shell), spiral cavity of the internal ear; cochlea.
cochleāre, -is. *n.* Spoon.
codeina, -ae. *f.* An alkaloid of opium; codeine.
coeliacus, -a, -um. Relating to the stomach; celiac.
colicus, -a, -um. Of or pert. to the colon.
collateriālis, -e. Collateral.
collum, -ī. *n.* Neck.
colocynthis, -idis. *f.* Colocynth.
color, -ōris. *m.* Color.
cōlum, -ī. *n.* Large intestine; colon.
columna, -ae. *f.* Column.
comes, -itis. *m.* Companion.
commissūra, -as. *f.* A joining; commissure.
communicāns, -ntis. Communicating.
commūnis, -e. Common.
compōnō, -ere, -posuī, -positus. Compound.
conarium, -ī. *n.* A synonym for the pineal gland; conarium.
concha, -ae. *f.* (Lit., a shell), hollow part of the external ear; concha.
confectiō, -ōnis. *f.* Confection.
conium, -ī. *n.* Poison, hemlock; conium.
conīveō, -āre, -nīvī. Blink; half close.
conjectūra, -ae. *f.* Guess.
contineō, -ēre, -tinuī, -tentus. Contain.
contrāhō, -ere, -xī, -ctus. Draw together; contract.
contusiō, -ōnis. *f.* Bruise.
cōnus, -ūs. *m.* Cone.
convalescō, -ere, -valuī. Regain health.
cor, cordis. *n.* Heart.
cornicula, -ae. *f.* Little horn.
cornu, -ūs. *n.* Horn; horn-shaped process.
corōna, -ae. *f.* Crown.
coronārius, -a, -um. Encircling like a crown; coronary.
corpus, -oris. *n.* Body.
corrōsīvus, -a, -um. Corrosive.
corrugātor, -ōris. *m.* A muscle which wrinkles; corrugator.

cortex, icis. *m.* and *f.* Bark; rind; external layer; cortex.
costa, -ae. *f.* Rib.
craniālis, -e. Cranial.
crās. Tomorrow.
crassus, -a, -um. Gross; large.
creasōtum, -ī. *n.* Creasote.
crēber, -bra, -brum. Frequent.
crēdō, -ere, -credidī, -creditus. Trust; believe.
crēta, -ae. *f.* Chalk.
cribriformis, -e. Sievelike; cribriform.
cribrōsus, -a, -um. Having holes like a sieve.
crista, -ae. *f.* Crest; comb of a cock (gallus).
crūrālis, -e. Of the leg; crural.
crūreus, -a, -um. Of the leg.
crūs, crūris. *n.* The leg.
crusta, -ae. *f.* Crust.
cubēba, -ae. *f.* Cubeb.
cubitum, -ī. *n.* Elbow.
cuboideus, -a, -um. Cubelike; cuboid.
cum. With.
cuneiformis, -e. Wedge-shaped; cuneiform.
cūra, -ae. *f.* Care.
cūrō, -āre, -āvī, -ātus. Treat; cure.
cutis, -is. *f.* Skin.
decem. Ten.
deciduus, -a, -um. That which falls off.
decoctum, -ī. *n.* Decoction.
deferēns, -ntis. Bearing away.
defessus, -a, -um. Tired; wearied.
deformāns, -ntis. Deforming.
deformitās, -ātis. *f.* Deformity.
demonstrō, -āre, -āvī, -ātus. Show; prove.
dēns, dentis. *m.* Tooth.
dentātus, -a, -um. Toothed; dentate.
depressor, -ōris. *m.* That which depresses; depressor.
descendēns, -ntis. Descending.
dexter, -tra, -trum. Right.
diabeticus, -a, -um. Diabetic; one having diabetes.
diabolus, -ī. *m.* Devil.
dīcō, -ere, -dixī, dictus. Say.
diēs, -ēī. *m.* Day.
difficilis, -e. Difficult.
digitus, -ī. *m.* Finger.
digitus pedis. A toe.
dilātor, -ōris. *m.* That which dilates; dilator.
dilūtus, -a, -um. Dilute.
dimidius, -a, -um. Half.
discipulus, -ī. *m.* A learner; pupil; student.
diū. For a long time.
diureticus, -a, -um. Diuretic.
dividō, -ere, -vīsī, -vīsus. Divide.
dō, dare, dedī, datus. Give.
doctus, -a, -um. Learned.
dolor, -ōris. *m.* Pain.
dolōrōsus, -a, -um. Painful.
domicilium, -ī. *n.* Abode.
dorsālis, -e. Of the back; dorsal.
dorsum, -ī. *n.* Back.
dosis, -is. *f.* Dose.
drachma, -ae. *f.* Dram.
dustus, -ūs. *m.* Duct.
dulcis, -e. Sweet.
duo, duae, du. Two.
dūrus, -a, -um. Hard.

dyspepticus, -a, -um. Dyspeptic; a dyspeptic.
edō, -ere, -ēdi, -ēsus. Eat.
efferēns, -ntis. Bearing out or away; efferent.
effervescēns, -ntis. Boiling up.
elegāns, -ntis. Elegant.
ēluviēs, -ēī. *f.* Discharge.
emeticus, -a, -um. Causing vomiting; emetic.
ēminentia, -ae. *f.* Eminence.
emō, -ere, -ēmī, emptus. Buy.
empiricus, -ī. *n.* Quack; empiric.
emplastrum, -ī. *n.* Plaster.
ensiformis, -e. Sword-shaped; ensiform.
eō, īre, īvī, itus. Go.
epilepsia, -ae. *f.* Epilepsy.
epiploicus, -a, -um. Relating to the epiploön (omentum).
equīnus, -a, -um. Of a horse; equine.
ergota, -ae. *f.* Ergot.
errō, -āre, -āvī, -ātus. Wander; err.
ērudītus, -a, -um. Learned; educated; erudite.
et. And.
et-et. Both-and.
ethmoidālis, -e. Ethmoid.
etiam. Even.
euonymus, -ī. *m.* Wahoo; Euonymus.
eupatōrium, -ī. *n.* Boneset; eupatorium.
excessus, -ūs. *m.* Departure.
excīdō, -ere, -īdī, -īsus. Cut out; excise.
excitō, -āre, -āvī, -ātus. Excite.
expectatiō, -ōnis. *f.* Expectation.
experimentum, -ī. *n.* Experiment.
expressiō, -ōnis. *f.* Expression.
exsiccātus, -a, -um. Dried out.
exsudō, -āre, -āvī, -ātus. Sweat out; exude.
externus, -a, -um. External.
extractum, -ī. *n.* Extract.
faciēs, -ēī. *f.* Face; countenance.
faciō, -ere, fēcī, factus. Make.
falx, -cis. *f.* Sickle (a sickle-shaped process).
familia, -ae (or **as**). *f.* Family.
fasciculus, -ī. *m.* A small bundle of fibers.
febrifuga, -ae. *f.* Agent that reduces fever; febrifuge.
febris, -is. *f.* Fever.
fēmina, -ae. *f.* Woman.
femorālis, -e. Of the thigh; femoral.
fenestra, -ae. *f.* Window; an opening in the wall of the tympanum.
ferē. Almost.
ferrum, -ī. *n.* Iron.
fibrilla, -ae. *f.* Filament; fibril.
fibrōsus, -a, -um. Fibrous.
fides, -eī. *f.* Faith; trustworthiness.
fīdus, -a, -um. Faithful; trustworthy.
filia, -ae. *f.* Daughter.
filius, -ī. *m.* Son.
filix, -icis. *f.* Fern.
fimbria, -ae. *f.* fringe.
fimbriātus, -a, -um. Fringed; fimbriated.
finiō, -īre, -īvī, -ītus. End; finish.
fiō, fierī, factus. Be made.
fissūra, -ae. *f.* Cleft; fissure.
flavus, -a, -um. Yellow.
flexilis, -e. Flexible.
flōs, flōris. *m.* Flower.
fluidus, -a, -um. Fluid.
flūmen, inis. *n.* River.

fluō, -ere, fluxī, fluxus. Flow.
fluor, -ōris. *m.* Flux; flow.
foetidus, -a, -um. Offensive, fetid.
folium, -ī. *n.* Leaf.
folliculus, -ī. *m.* A small secretory sac; follicle.
fons, -ntis, *m.* Fountain; spring.
formō, -āre, -āvī, -ātus. Form.
fornicātus, -a, -um. Arched.
fornix, -icis. *m.* Arch; vault; fornix.
fortis, -e. Strong; brave.
fossa, -ae. *f.* Ditch; depression; fossa.
fovea, -ae. *f.* Small pit; depression.
fractus, -a, -um. Broken.
fragilitās, -ātis. *f.* Brittleness.
frēnum, -ī. *n.* A bridle; a membranous fold; frenum.
frigidus, -a, -um. Cold.
fructus, -ūs. *m.* Fruit.
frumentum, -ī. *n.* Corn; grain.
frustum, -ī. *n.* Piece; bit.
functiō, -ōnis. *f.* Execution; normal action; function.
fuscus, -a, -um. Brown.
fūsiformis, -e. Spindle-shaped; fusiform.
gallus, -ī. *m.* Cock.
ganglioniformis, -e. Ganglionlike.
gelsemium, -ī. *n.* Gelsemium; yellow jasmine (root).
gemellus, -a, -um. Paired; twin.
gena, -ae. *f.* The cheek.
geniōhyoglossus, -ī. *m.* Muscle attached to chin, hyoid bone and tongue.
gentiāna, -ae. *f.* Gentian.
genu, -ūs. *n.* Knee.
genus, generis, *n.* Kind.
germinātīvus, -a, -um. Germinative; germinal.
glabrus, -a, -um. Smooth.
glaciēs, -ēī. *f.* Ice.
globus, -ī. *m.* Globe.
glomerulus, -ī. *m.* Small ball or tuft of vessels; glomerule.
glūteus, -a, -um. Of the buttock; gluteal.
glycerīnum, -ī. *n.* Glycerin.
glycerītum, -ī. *m.* Glycerite.
glycyrrhiza, -ae. *f.* Licorice.
gracilis, -e. Slender; graceful.
granulōsus, -a, -um. Granular.
granum, -ī. *n.* Grain.
gratus, -a, -um. Agreeable; pleasing.
gubernāculum, -ī. *n.* (Lit., a helm), applied to fetal cord directing descent of testes; gubernaculum.
gummi. Gum.
gustō, -āre, -āvī, -ātus. Taste.
gutta, -ae. *f.* Drop.
gyrus, -ī. *m.* Circle; ring; convolution (of the brain).
habeō, -ēre, -uī, -itus. Have.
habitō, -āre, -āvī, -ātus. Inhabit.
hallex, -icis, or **hallux, -ucis.** *f.* The great toe.
harmonia, -ae. *f.* Harmony, "suture of harmony."
helix, -icis. *f.* Outer ring of the external ear; helix.
hemisphericus, -a, -um. Hemispherical.
hēpar, hepatis. *n.* Liver.
herba, -ae. *f.* Herb.

herī. Yesterday.
hiātus, -ūs. *m.* Opening; aperture.
hīc, haec, hoc. This.
hilāris, -e. Cheerful.
hīlus, -ī. *m.* Small fissure or depression.
hippocampus, -ī. *m.* (Lit., sea horse), applied to two convolutions of brain (major and minor); hippocampus.
homo, -inis. *m.* Man.
horribilis, -e. Horrible.
hūmānus, -a, -um. Human.
hūmor, -ōris. *m.* Fluid; humor.
hydrargyrum, -ī. *n.* Mercury.
hydrastis, -is. *f.* Golden seal (root); hydrastis.
hyoideus, -a, -um. Hyoid.
Hyoscyamus, -ī. *m.* Henbane; Hyoscyamus.
īdem, eadem, idem. Same.
ignārus, -a, -um. Ignorant.
iliacus, -a, -um. Of or pert. to the flanks or ilium; iliac.
ille, illa, illud. He; she; it.
immōbilis, -e. Immovable.
immōbilitas, -ātis. *f.* Immobility.
impar, -is. Without a mate or fellow.
impediō, -īre, -īvī, -ītus. Hinder; check; prevent.
imperītus, -a, -um. Unskilled.
impūrus, -a, -um. Impure.
īmus, -a, -um. Lowest.
incisūra, -ae. *f.* Groove or notch.
Indicus, -a, -um. Indian.
infans, -ntis. *m.* and *f.* Infant.
inflammatiō, -ōnis. *f.* Inflammation.
infraspinātus, -a, -um. Beneath the spine (of the scapula); infraspinate.
infūsum, -ī. *m.* Infusion.
ingressus, -ūs. *m.* Entrance.
innominātus, -a, -um. Unnamed; innominate.
intermittō, -ere, -mīsī, -missus. Intermit.
internōdium, -ī. *n.* Space between two joints; internode.
internus, -a, -um. Inner.
interpositus, -a, -um. Placed between.
intertragicus, -a, -um. Between the tragus, q.v., and antitragus.
intestīnum, -ī. *n.* Intestine.
intumescentia, -ae. *f.* An enlargement; intumescence.
inveniō, -īre, -vēnī, -ventus. Find; discover.
inversiō, -ōnis. *f.* Inversion.
iodidum, -ī. *n.* Iodide.
ipecacuanha, -ae. *f.* Ipecac.
ipse, ipsa, ipsum. Himself; herself; itself.
iris, iridis. *f.* Iris.
is, ea, id. He; she; it.
iter, itineris. *n.* Way; passageway.
jecur, jecinoris. *n.* Liver.
jūcundē. Happily; pleasantly.
jūglans, juglandis. *f.* Walnut.
jugulāris, -e. Jugular.
jūniperus, -ī. *f.* Juniper tree.
juvenis. *m.* and *f., adj.,* and *subst.* Young; a youth.
labium, -ī. *n.* Lip.
lacer, -a, -um. Lacerated; mutilated.
lacrima, -ae. *f.* Tear.
lacrimālis, -e. Pert. to tears; lacrimal.

lactās, -ātis. *m.* A salt of lactic acid; lactate.
lactiferus, -a, -um. Milk-bearing; lactiferous.
lacus, -ūs. *m.* Lake; basin; reservoir.
lamella, -ae. *f.* Layer.
lamina, -ae. *f.* Thin plate; layer.
lāna, -ae. *f.* Wool.
lassus, -a, -um. Weary.
laterālis, -e. Lateral.
lātus, -a, -um. Broad.
laudō, -āre, -āvī, -ātus. Praise.
lavandula, -ae. *f.* Lavender.
lavō, -āre, -āvī, -ātus or lavi, lautus. Wash.
laxātor, -ōris. *m.* A muscle that loosens; relaxer.
legō, -ere, -lēgī, lectus. Bring together; collect.
leniō, -īre, -īvī, -ītus. Calm; soothe; assuage.
lenticulāris, -e. Lentil-shaped (double-convex); lenticular.
lentus, -a, -um. Sticky.
letifer, -a, -um. Deadly.
levis, -e. Light.
lienālis, -e. Of the spleen.
ligamentōsus, -a, -um. Ligamentous.
ligamentum, -ī. *n.* Ligament.
lignum, -ī. *n.* Wood.
limbus, -ī. *n.* Border; band; fringe.
līmitāns, -ntis. Limiting.
limon, -ōnis. *f.* Lemon.
linea, -ae. *f.* Line.
lingua, -ae. *f.* Tongue.
linguālis, -e. Of the tongue; lingual.
linimentum, -ī. *n.* Liniment.
linum, -ī. *n.* Flax.
liquidus, -a, -um. Liquid.
lobulus, -ī. *m.* Lobule.
lobus, -ī. *m.* Lobe.
longitudinālis, -e. Longitudinal.
longus, -a, -um. Long.
lotiō, -ōnis. *f.* Wash; lotion.
lucidus, -a, -um. Clear; transparent.
lumbālis, -e. Of the loins; lumbar.
lumbus, -ī. *m.* Loin.
lūnula, -ae. *f.* Small crescent; lunula.
lupulīna, -ae. *f.* Yellow powder from the scales of the hop; lupulin.
luteus, -a, -um. Yellow.
luxatiō, -ōnis. *f.* Dislocation.
lympha, -ae. *f.* Chyle; lymph.
mācerō, -āre, -āvī ātus. Soak; macerate.
magister, -trī. *m.* Teacher; master.
magnus, -a, -um. Large; great.
māla, -ae. *f.* The cheekbone.
malignus, -a, -um. Malignant.
malus, -a, -um. Bad.
mandibulum, -ī. *n.* A jaw.
māne. *n.* Morning.
manūbrium, -ī. *n.* (Lit., a handle, hilt), upper part of sternum; manubrium.
manus, -ūs. *f.* Hand.
massa, -ae. *f.* Mass.
masticō, -āre, -āvī, -ātus. Chew.
mastoideus, -a, -um. Nipplelike: mastoid.
mater, -tris. *f.* Mother.
māteria, -ae. *f.* Materials.
māternus, -a, -um. Maternal.
matrix, -īcis. *f.* Source; origin.
maxilla, -ae. *f.* Jawbone; jaw.
meātus, -ūs. *m.* Opening; passage.

mediānus, -a, -um. Middle; median.
medicāmen, -inis. *n.* Drug.
medicāmentārius, -a, -um. Medicated.
medicāmentum, -ī. *n.* Drug.
medicātus, -a, -um. Medicated.
medicīna, -ae. *f.* Medicine.
medicus, -ī. *m.* Physician; doctor.
medius, -a, -um. Middle.
membrāna, -ae. *f.* Membrane.
membrum, -ī. *n.* Member.
memoria, -ae. *f.* Memory.
mentha, -ae. *f.* Mint.
mentum, -ī. *n.* Chin.
mesentericus, -a, -um. Of the mesentery; mesenteric.
metus, -ūs. *m.* Fear.
mīles, -itis. *m.* Soldier.
minerālis, -e. Mineral.
misceō, -ēre, miscuī, mixtus. Mix.
miser, -a, -um. Poor; wretched.
mistūra, -ae. *f.* Mixture.
mītis, -e. Mild.
mitto, -ere, mīsī, missus. Send.
mobilis, -e. Movable.
mobilitās, -ātis. *f.* Mobility.
modiolus, -ī. *m.* (Lit., a small measure), hollow cone in the cochlea of the ear, modiolus.
molāris, -e (mola, mill). The grinder teeth; molar.
molliō, -īre, -īvī, -ītus. Soften; mitigate.
mollis, -e. Soft.
mollitīes, -ēī. *f.* Softness.
mons, -ntis. *m.* Mountain.
montānus, -a, -um. Of a mountain; mountain.
monticulus, -ī. *m.* Small eminence.
morbus, -ī *m.* Disease.
mordeō, -ēre, momordī, morsus. Bite.
moritūrus, -a, -um. About to die.
morphīna, -ae. *f.* Morphine.
morrhua, -ae. *f.* A genus of fishes, including the cod; cod.
mors, mortis. *f.* Death.
morsus, -ūs. *m.* Bite.
mortarium, -ī. *n.* Mortar.
mōtor, -ōris. *m.* That which moves; mover.
moveō, -ēre, mōvī, mōtus. Move.
mox. Presently; soon; directly.
mucilāgō, -inis. *f.* Mucilage.
mucōsus, -a, -um. Mucous.
mulceō, -ere, mulsi, mulsus. Soothe; allay.
multifidus, -a, -um. Many-clefted.
multus, -a, -um. Much; many.
muriāticus, -a, -um. Muriatic.
musculus, -ī. *m.* Muscle.
mūtātiō, -ōnis. *f.* Change.
myristica, -ae. *f.* Nutmeg.
myrtiformis, -e. Shaped like the myrtle leaf or berry; myrtiform.
nāris, -is. *f.* Nostril.
nāsus, -ī. *m.* Nose.
natō, -āre, -āvī, -ātus. Swim; float.
natūra, -ae. *f.* Nature.
nauta, -ae. *m.* Sailor.
naviculāris, -e. Boat-shaped; navicular.
neglectus, -a, -um. Neglected.
nemō, -inis. *m.* and *f.* No one.
nervus, -ī. *m.* Nerve.

nescio, -īre, -īvi, -ītus. Not know; be ignorant of.

neurilemma, -atis. *n.* Nerve sheath.

nictitāns, -ntis. Winking.

nil. Nothing.

nimium. Too often.

nisi. Unless.

nitrās, -ātis. *m.* Nitrate.

nitricus, -a, -um. Nitric.

nitrōsus, -a, -um. Nitrous.

nōmen, -inis. *m.* Name.

nōminō, -āre, -āvī, -ātus. Name.

nōn. Not.

nondum. Not yet.

nōnus, -a, -um. Ninth.

nosco, -ere, nōvī, nōtus. Learn; know.

novem. Nine.

novus, -a, -um. New.

nox, noctis. *f.* Night.

nucha, -ae. *f.* Nape of neck.

nullus, -a, -um. No; none.

numerus, -ī. *m.* Number.

nunc. Now.

oblīquus, -a, -um. Oblique.

oblongātus, -a, -um. Oblong.

octō. Eight.

oculus, -ī. *m.* Eye.

officīna, -ae. *f.* Office.

officinālis, -e. Officinal.

oleorēsīna, -ae. *f.* Oleoresin.

oleum, -ī. *n.* Oil.

olfactōrius, -a, -um. Olfactory.

omentum, -ī. *n.* Epiploon; omentum.

omnis, -e. Every; all.

operculum, -ī. *n.* (Lit., a cover or lid), applied to a group of convolutions in the cerebrum, between the two divisions of the fissure of Sylvius.

ophthalmicus, -a, -um. Of the eye; ophthalmic.

oppōnēns, -ntis. Opposing.

opticus, -a, -um. Optic.

opus, operis. *n.* Work.

orbita, -ae. *f.* The cavity which lodges the eye; orbit.

ordō, -inis. *m.* Row.

orificium, -ī. *n.* Opening.

orior, -īrī, ortus. Arise.

ōs, ōris. *n.* Mouth.

os, ossis. *n.* Bone.

ossiculum, -ī. *n.* Small bone.

ostium, -ī. *n.* An opening.

ovālis, -e. Egg-shaped; oval.

oxalās, -ātis. *m.* A salt of oxalic acid, oxalate.

oxidum, -ī. *n.* Oxide.

palātum, -ī. *n.* Palate.

palpēbra, -ae. *f.* Eyelid.

pālus, -ūdis. *f.* Marsh; swamp.

pancreāticus, -a, -um. Pancreatic.

papillāris, -e. Resembling or covered with papillae; papillary.

pār, paris. *n.* A pair.

parasiticus, -a, -um. Parasitic.

paries, -iētis. *m.* Wall.

parō, -āre, -āvī, -ātus. Prepare.

pars, partis. *f.* Part.

partus, -ūs. *m.* Parturition; childbirth.

parvus, -a, -um. Small.

pater, -tris. *m.* Father.

patheticus, -a, -um. That which moves the passions; a name given to the 4th pair of nerves.

patria, -as. *f.* Fatherland; country.

paucus, -a, -um. Few.

pectinātus, -a, -um. Resembling the teeth of a comb; pectinate.

pectineus, -a, -um. Comblike.

pectiniformis, -e. Comblike.

pectus, pectoris. *n.* Breast; bosom.

pellūcidus, -a, -um. Transparent.

pensō, -āre, -āvī, -ātus. Weigh.

pepsīnum, -ī. *n.* Pepsin.

percolō, -āre, -āvī, -ātus. Filter; strain.

perforō, -āre, -āvī, -ātus. Bore through; perforate.

periculōsus, -a, -um. Dangerous.

perītus, -a, -um. Skilled.

peronēus, -a, -um. Relating to the fibula; peroneal.

persōna, -ae. *f.* Person.

perspiratōrius, -a, -um. Relating to perspiration; perspiratory.

pēs, pedis. *m.* Foot.

petō, -ere, -īvī, -ītus. Seek.

petrolātum, -ī. *n.* Petrolatum; vaseline.

petrōsus, -a, -um. Rocklike; petrous.

pharmacopoeia, -a. *f.* Pharmacopoeia.

phiala, -ae. *f.* Vial.

philosophis, -ī. *m.* Philosopher.

phosphās, -ātis. *m.* A salt of phosphoric acid; phosphate.

phrenicus, -a, -um. Of the diaphragm; phrenic.

physostigma, -atis. *n.* Calabar bean; physostigma.

piger, -gra, -grum. Lazy.

pigmentum, -ī. *n.* Pigment.

pilula, -ae. *f.* Pill.

pilus, -ī. *m.* Hair.

pineālis, -e. Resembling a pine cone; pineal.

pinna, -ae. *f.* (Lit., feather), pavillion of the ear; pinna.

piper, piperis. *n.* Pepper.

piperītus, -a, -um. Pepper, peppery.

pistillum, -ī. *n.* Pestle.

pituitārius, -a, -um. (pituita, phlegm or mucus), pituitary (applied to a reddish-gray body occupying the sella turcica of the sphenoid bone from a former erroneous belief that it discharged mucus into the nostrils).

pius, -a, -um. Tender.

pix, picis. *f.* Pitch.

plantāris, -e. Relating to the sole of the foot; plantar.

plānus, -a, -um. Flat; level; smooth.

plexus, -a, -um. Network; plexus.

plica, -ae. *f.* Fold.

plumbum, -ī. *n.* Lead.

poculum -ī. *n.* Cup.

pollex, -icis. *f.* The thumb.

pomum, -ī. *n.* Apple.

pons, pontis. *m.* Bridge.

poples, poplitis. *m.* Ham of the knee; popliteal space.

poplitēus, -a, -um. Relating to the ham; popliteal.

populus, -ī. *m.* People.
portō, -āre, -āvī, -ātus. Carry.
portiō, -ōnis. *f.* Portion.
porus, -ī. *m.* Channel; canal.
post. Behind; after.
posteā. Afterward.
posticus, -a, -um. Hindmost.
potēns, -ntis. Powerful.
potiō, -ōnis. A drink; draught.
potō, -āre, -āvī, -ātus. Drink.
potus, -ūs. *m.* Drink.
praeparō, -āre, -āvī, -ātus. Prepare.
praeparatiō, -ōnis. *f.* Preparation.
praeputium, -ī. *n.* Foreskin; prepuce.
praescrībō, -ere, -scripsī, -scriptus. Prescribe.
praescriptum, -ī. *n.* Prescription.
praesēns, -ntis. Present.
praestāns, -ntis. Excellent.
pressiō, -ōnis. *f.* Pressure.
primus, -a, -um. First.
princeps, -ipis. The first; chief; principal.
privō, -āre, -āvī, -ātus. Deprive.
prō. For; in behalf of.
processus, -ūs. *m.* A prominence; process.
profundus, -a, -um. Deep.
pronātor, -ōris. *m.* A muscle which turns the palm of the hand downward; pronator.
properō, -āre, -āvī, -ātus. Hasten.
proprius, -a, -um. One's own; special; proper.
prudēns, -ntis. Prudent.
pterygium, -ī. *n.* An eye disease; pterygium.
publicus, -a, -um. Public.
puella, -ae. *f.* Girl.
pugnō, -āre, -āvī, -ātus. Fight.
pulcher, -chra, -chrum. Beautiful.
pulmo, -ōnis. *m.* Lung.
pulmonālis, -e. Of the lungs; pulmonary.
pulverō, -āre, -āvī, -ātus. Powder; pulverize.
pulvis, pulveris. *m.* Powder.
punctum, -ī. *n.* Point.
puniō, -īre, -īvī, -ītus. Punish.
pūpilla, -ae. *f.* Pupil (of eye).
pupillāris, -e. Pupillary; applied to a delicate membrane which covers the pupil of the eye in the fetus.
purgātīvus, -a, -um. Purgative.
purificātus, -a, -um. Purified.
pūrus, -a, -um. Pure.
pyramidālis, -e. Pyramidal.
pyramis, -idis. *f.* Pyramid.
pyriformis, -e. Pear-shaped; pyriform.
quadrātus, -a, -um. Four-sided; square.
quadriceps, -cipitis. Four-headed.
quadrigeminus, -a, -um. Fourfold; four.
quaestiō, -ōnis. *f.* Question.
quam. Than.
quartus, -a, -um. Fourth.
quatuor. Four.
quatuordecim. Fourteen.
que. And.
quinīna, -ae. *f.* Quinine.
quis, quae, quid. Who; which; what.
quondam. Formerly.
quoque. Also.
quot. How many.
radiālis, -e. Of the radius; radial.
radiātus, -a, -um. Radiated.

rādix, -īcis. *f.* Root.
ramus, -ī. *m.* Branch.
rārō. Rarely.
rārus, -a, -um. Rare.
recens. Recently.
recipiō, -ere, -cēpī, -ceptus. Take.
recreō, -āre, -āvī, -ātus. Refresh.
rectus, -a, -um. Straight.
reductio, -ōnis. *f.* A bringing back.
reflexus, -a, -um. Turned back; reflected.
relevō, -āre, -āvī, -ātus. Relieve.
remedium, -ī. *n.* Remedy.
remittō, -ēre, -mīsī, -missus. Send back; remit.
removeō, -ēre, -mōvī, -mōtus. Remove.
rēn, rēnis. *m.* (usually pl.), kidney.
rēnalis, -e. Of the kidney; renal.
reperiō, -īre, -perī, -pertus. Find.
reprimō, -ēre, -pressī, -pressus. Check; repress.
requiesco, -ēre, -ēvī, -ētus. Rest.
rēs, reī. *f.* Thing.
rēsīna, -ae. *f.* Resin.
rēspīrātiō, -ōnis. *f.* Respiration.
rēte, -is. *n.* Net.
reticulāris, -e. Like a net; reticular.
retrāhēns, -ntis. Drawing back; retracting.
rheumatismus, -ī. *m.* Rheumatism.
ricinus, -ī. *m.* (Lit., a tick, which the seeds resemble), the castor oil plant (Ricinus communis).
rima, -ae. *f.* Slit; cleft.
rogō, -āre, -āvī, -ātus. Ask.
rosa, -ae. *f.* Rose.
rostrum, -ī. *n.* Beak.
rotundus, -a, -um. Round.
ruber, -bra, -brum. Red.
rubor, -ōris. *m.* Redness.
rūga, -ae. *f.* A wrinkle; fold.
rumex, -icis. *m.* and *f.* Sorrel.
sabulum, -ī. *n.* Sand.
saccharātus, -a, -um. Saccharated.
saccharum, -ī. *n.* Sugar.
sacciformis, -e. Saclike.
saccus, -ī. *m.* A sack or bag.
saepe. Often.
sal, -is. *m.* and *f.* Salt.
salicīnum, -ī. *n.* Salicin.
salicylās, -ātis. *m.* Salicylate.
salix, -īcis. *f.* Willow.
sānābilis, -e. Curable.
sanguis, -guinis. *m.* Blood.
sānitās, -ātis. *f.* Healing.
sānō, -āre, -āvī, -ātus. Heal; cure.
sapientia, -ae. *f.* Wisdom.
sapō, -ōnis. *m.* Soap.
sartōrius, -ī. *m.* The tailor's muscle; sartorius.
scāla, -ae. *f.* Ladder.
scalēnus, -a, -um. Of unequal sides.
scaphoideus, -a, -um. Boat-shaped; scaphoid.
schola, -ae. *f.* (Lit., leisure given to learning), school.
scientia, -ae. *f.* Knowledge; science.
scilla, -ae. *f.* Squill.
sciō, -īre, -īvī, -ītus. Know.
scrībō, -ēre, scripsī, scrīptus. Write.
scriptōrius, -a, -um. Of a writer; writer's.
secundus, -a, -um. Second.

sed. But.
sēdes, -is. *f.* Seat.
segmentum, -ī. *n.* Segment.
sella, -ae. *f.* Saddle.
sēmicirculāris, -e. Semicircular.
sēmiellipticus, -a, -um. Semielliptical.
sēmilunāris, -e. Semilunar.
sēmimembranōsus, -a, -um. Semimembranous.
seminālis, -e. Seminal.
sēmis, sēmissis. *m.* Half.
sēmitendinōsus, -a, -um. Semitendinous.
senectus, -tūtis. *f.* Old age.
senex, senis. *m.* Old man.
senilitās, -ātis. The feebleness of old age; senility.
sentiō, -īre, -sī, -sus. Feel.
septem. Seven.
sequestrum, -ī. *n.* A portion of dead bone; sequestrum.
sermō, -ōnis. *m.* Conversation.
serrātus, -a, -um. Notched like a saw; serrated.
servus, -ī. *m.* Servant; assistant.
sesamoideus, -a, -um. Like a sesame seed; sesamoid (bone developed in a tendon).
seu. Whether.
signō, -āre, -āvī, -ātus. Write; direct.
similō, -āre, -āvī, -ātus. Simulate.
simplex, -icis. Simple.
sināpis, -is. *f.* Mustard.
sitis, -is. *f.* Thirst.
solitārius, -a, -um. Solitary.
somnificus, -a, -um. Sleep-producing.
somnus, -ī. *m.* Sleep.
sopor, -ōris. *m.* Deep sleep.
spectrum, -ī. *n.* Image.
spēs, speī. *f.* Hope.
sphenoideus, -a, -um. Wedge-shaped; sphenoid.
spīna, -ae. *f.* (A thorn), a process on the surface of a bone; the backbone.
spinālis, -e. Spinal.
spinōsus, -a, -um. Spiny.
spirālis, -e. Spiral.
spiritus, -ūs. *m.* Spirit.
splēnius, -a, -um. Resembling the spleen; applied to a muscle of the back and neck.
spongiōsus, -a, -um. Spongy.
squamōsus, -a, -um. Scaly; squamous.
stapēdius, -ī. *m.* A muscle acting upon the stapes; stapedius.
stertor, -ōris. *m.* Snoring.
stomachālis, -e. Stomachic.
stomachus, -ī. *m.* Stomach.
stramōnium, -ī. *n.* Jamestown weed; stramonium.
stria, -ae. *f.* Stripe; stria.
striātus, -a, -um. Striped; striated.
struō, -ēre, -xī, -ctus. Arrange.
strychnīna, -ae. *f.* Strychnine.
subacetās, -ātis. *m.* Subacetate.
subanconeus, -a, -um. Under the elbow.
subitō. Suddenly.
subitus, -a, -um. Sudden.
sublīmis, -e. Deep.
submuriās, -ātis. *m.* Submuriate.
subnitras, -ātis. *m.* Subnitrate.
subscapulāris, -e. Under the scapula; subscapular.

substantia, -ae. *f.* Substance.
subsultus, -ūs. *m.* A jumping; a twitching.
succus, -ī. *m.* Juice.
sudor, -ōris. *m.* Sweat.
sulcus, -ī. *m.* Furrow.
sulphās, -ātis. *m.* Sulfate.
sulphonal. Sulfonal.
sulphuricus, -a, -um. Sulfuric.
sum, esse, fui. Be.
sūmō, -ēre, -psi, -ptus. Take.
supercilium, -ī. *n.* Eyebrow.
superficialis, -e. Superficial.
superficiēs, -ēī. *f.* Surface.
suppositōrium, -ī. *n.* Suppository.
supraspinātus, -a, -um. Above the spine (of scapula); supraspinate.
suspensōrium, -ī. *n.* That which suspends.
suspensōrius, -a, -um. Suspensory.
sustentaculum, -ī. *n.* A prop; support.
sutūra, -ae. *f.* Seam; suture.
sympatheticus, -a, -um. Sympathetic.
symptōma, -atis. *n.* Symptom.
synoviālis, -e. Synovial.
tabacum, -ī. *n.* Tobacco.
taenia, -ae. *f.* A band.
taenia semicirculāris, a layer in the cerebrum; also a genus of intestinal worms, the tapeworm.
talus, -ī. *m.* The heel.
tam. So.
tapētum, -ī. *n.* (**tapēte,** carpet, tapestry), a lining membrane; also, the radiating fibers of the corpus callōsum.
taraxacum, -ī. *n.* Dandelion root; taraxacum.
tarsus, -ī. *m.* Ankle.
tartaricus, -a, -um. Tartaric.
tartrās, -ātis. *m.* Tartrate.
tetōrium, -ī. *n.* A covering.
tectōrius, -a, -um. Protecting; covering.
tegō, -ēre, -xī, -ctum. Cover; protect.
temporālis, -e. Temporal.
tempus, -oris. *n.* Time.
tenax, -ācis. Holding fast; tenacious.
tendineus, -a, -um. Tendinous.
tendō, -ēre, tetendī, tentus. Stretch; reach.
tendō, -dinis. *m.* Tendon.
teneō, -ēre, -uī, -tus. Keep; hold.
tener, -a, -um. Delicate; tender.
tensor, -ōris. *m.* Stretcher; tensor.
tentō, -āre, -āvī, -ātus. Test, try.
tentōrium, -ī. *n.* A tent; covering.
tenuis, -e. Thin; small.
tepidus, -a, -um. Lukewarm.
terebinthina, -ae. *f.* Turpentine.
teres, -etir. Rounded; smooth.
tergum, -ī. *n.* Back.
terminus, -ī. *m.* End.
tertius, -a, -um. Third.
theobrōma, -ātis. *n.* Cacao (food of the gods).
thoracicus, -a, -um. Thoracic.
thyroideus, -a, -um. Having the shape of an oblong shield; thyroid.
tiglium, -ī. *n.* The specific name of the croton oil plant.
tinctūra, -ae. *f.* Tincture.
tonicus, -a, -um. Tonic.
tonsilla, -ae. *f.* Tonsil.

torcular, -āris. *n.* A wine press.
trachealis, -e. Tracheal.
tractō, -āre, -āvī, -ātus. Handle.
tragus, -ī. *m.* Small nipple in front of external auditory meatus, so called because sometimes covered with hair; tragus.
transversālis, -e. Transverse.
transversus, -a, -um. Transverse.
trapezoideus, -a, -um. Like a trapezium; trapezoid.
trauma, -atis. *n.* Injury; wound.
trēs, tria. Three.
triangulāris, -e. Triangular.
triceps, -ipitis. Three-headed.
trigeminus, -a, -um. Three-fold.
trigīnta. Thirty.
trigōnum, -ī. *n.* Triangle.
triquetrus, -a, -um. Three-cornered; triangular.
trochiscus, -ī. *m.* Troche.
tuba, -ae. *f.* (Trumpet), tube.
tuber, -eris. *n.* Swelling, protuberance.
tuberculum, -ī. *n.* A protuberance; tubercle.
tubulus, -ī. *m.* Small tube.
tubus, -ī. *m.* Tube.
tunica, -ae. *f.* Coat; covering.
tussiō, -īre, -īvī, -ītus. Cough.
tūtāmen, -minis. *n.* Means of defense; a protection.
tūtō. Safely.
tympanicus, -a, -um. Of the tympanum; tympanic.
ubi. Where.
ulna, -ae. *f.* Larger bone of forearm; ulna.
ulnāris, -e. Of the ulna; ulnar.
uncia, -ae. *f.* Ounce.
unciformis, -e. Hooked.
uncinātus, -a, -um. Hooked; uncinate.
unguentum, -ī. *n.* Ointment.
unguis, -is. *m.* Nail.
ūnus, -a, -um. One.
urbānus, -a, -um. Of the city; urbane.
urīna, -ae. *f.* Urine.
uriniferus, -a, -um. Urine-bearing; uriniferous.
usque. Continuously; constantly.
uterīnus, -a, -um. Of the uterus; uterine.
ūtilis, -e. Useful.
uvula, -ae. *f.* A small appendix or tubercle; uvula.
uxor, -ōris. *f.* Wife.
vaginālis, -e. Sheathlike; vaginal.
valeriānās, -ātis. *m.* Valerianate.
valetūdō, -inis. *f.* Health.
validus, -a, -um. Strong; sturdy; healthy.
valvula, -ae. *f.* Valve.
vās, vāsis. *n.* Vessel.

vasculōsus, -a, -um. Vascular.
vasculum, -ī. *n.* Small vessel.
vastus, -a, -um. Extensive; large.
vegetābilis, -e. Vegetable.
vehiculum, -ī. *n.* Vehicle.
vel. Either.
vēlum, -ī. *n.* Veil.
vēna, -ae. *f.* Vein.
vendō, -ēre, vendidī. Sell.
veneficus, -ī. *m.* Poisoner.
venēnum, -ī. *n.* Poison.
venōsus, -a, -um. Venous.
venter, -tris. *m.* Belly.
ventriculus, -ī. *m.* Ventricle.
vērātrum, -ī. *n.* Hellebore; veratrum.
vermiformis, -e. Wormlike.
veru, -ūs. *n.* A spit (for roasting upon); used only in **verumontanum,** a longitudinal ridge in the floor of the male urethra.
verus, -a, -um. True.
vesica, -ae. *f.* Urinary bladder.
vesicatōrium, -ī. *n.* Blister.
vesicula, -ae. *f.* Vesicle.
vesiculāris, -e. Full of vesicles or cells; vesicular.
vestibulāris, -e. Relating to the vestibule of the ear; vestibular.
vetus, veteris. Old.
vigilō, -āre, -āvī, -ātus. Watch.
vīgintī. Twenty.
villus, -ī. *m.* Tuft of hair; villus.
vinculum, -ī. *n.* Link; chain.
vinum, -ī. *n.* Wine.
vir, virī. *m.* Man.
viridis, -e. Green.
vīs, vīs, pl. vīres, -ium. *f.* Force; power.
viscus, -eris. *n.* Any internal organ of the body.
visiō, -ōnis. *f.* Vision.
vīsus, -ūs. *m.* Vision.
vīta, -ae. *f.* Life.
vitellus, -ī. *m.* Yolk.
vitreus, -a, -um. Resembling glass; vitreous.
vocālis, -e. Vocal.
vocō, -āre, -āvī, -ātus. Call.
vola, -ae. *f.* Palm of the hand (sole of the foot).
vorticōsus, -a, -um. Resembling an eddy or whirlpool.
vulnerō, -āre, -āvī, -ātus. Wound.
vulnus, vulneris. *n.* A wound.
vultus, -ūs. *m.* Countenance.
zincum, -ī. *n.* Zinc.
zingiber, -eris. *n.* Ginger.
zōna, -ae. *f.* Zone; belt.
zōnula, -ae. *f.* Little zone, or belt; zonule.

GREEK AND LATIN
SINGULARS AND PLURALS

Singular	Plural	Singular	Plural
addendum	addenda	focus	foci
aden	adena	fornix	fornices
adenoma	adenomata	fossa	fossae
ala	alae	glans	glandes
albacans	albacantes	gonad	gonades
amygdala	amygdalae	gonococcus	gonococci
antenna	antennae	gyrus	gyri
antiad	antiades	ilium	ilia
antrum	antra	keratosis	keratoses
apertura	aperturae	labium	labia
apex	apices	lamina	laminae
aponeurosis	aponeuroses	loculus	loculi
appendix	appendices	locus	loci
aqua	aquae	medium	media
arcus	arcus	mucosa	mucosae
ascaris	ascarides	naevus	naevi
ascus	asci	nodus	nodi
atrium	atria	nox	noxa
axis	axes	os	ora
bacillus	bacilli	ovum	ova
bacterium	bacteria	papilla	papillae
bronchus	bronchi	pathema	pathemata
bulla	bullae	pes	pedes
bursa	bursae	petechia	petechiae
cactus	cacti	pilula	pilulae
cadaver	cadavera	polypus	polypi
calcaneum	calcanea	ramus	rami
calculus	calculi	septum	septa
calix	calices	sequestrum	sequestra
cantharis	cantharides	serosa	serosae
canthus	canthi	spasmus	spasmi
cornu	cornua	spectrum	spectra
corpus	corpora	speculum	specula
crisis	crises	sperma	spermata
cuniculus	cuniculi	stoma	stomata
dens	dentes	sudamen	sudamina
diagnosis	diagnoses	sulcus	sulci
diaphoreticus	diaphoretici	tarsus	tarsi
diastema	diastemata	tela	telae
digitus	digiti	tinctura	tincturae
dorsum	dorsi	toxicosis	toxicoses
echolatus	echolati	typha	typhae
enema	enemata	ulcus	ulcera
ensis	enses	varix	varices
epididymis	epididymides	vas	vasa
esthesis	estheses	vesicula	vesiculae
fibroma	fibromata	vis	vires
filix	filices	viscus	viscera
filum	fila	vomica	vomicae
flagellum	flagella	zygoma	zygomata

LATIN AND ROMAN NUMERALS

1	unus	1st	primus
2	duo	2nd	secundus
3	tres	3rd	tertius
4	quattuor	4th	quartus
5	quinque	5th	quintus
6	sex	6th	sextus
7	septem	7th	septimus
8	octō	8th	octāvus
9	novem	9th	nōnus
10	decem	10th	decimus
11	ūndecim	11th	ūndecimus
12	duodecim	12th	duodecimus
13	tredecim	13th	tertius decimus
14	quattuordecim	14th	quartus decimus
15	quīndecim	15th	quīntus decimus
16	sēdecim	16th	septus decimus
17	septendecim	17th	septimus decimus
18	duodēvīgintī	18th	duodēvīcēsimus
19	ūndēvīgintī	19th	ūndēvīcēsimus
20	vīgintī	20th	vīcēsimus
21	vīgintī ūnus, *or* ūnus et vīgintī	21st	vīcēsimus primus, *or* prīmus et vīcēsimus
22	vīgintī duo, *or* duo et vīgintī	22nd	vīcēsimus secundus, *or* duo et vīcēsimus
28	duodētrīgintā	28th	duodētrīcēsimus
29	ūndētrīgintā	29th	ūndētrīcēsimus
30	trīgintā	30th	trīcēsimus
40	quadrāgintā	40th	quadrāgēsimus
50	quīnquāgintā	50th	quīnquāgēsimus
60	sexāgintā	60th	sexāgēsimus
70	septuāgintā	70th	septuāgēsimus
80	octōgintā	80th	octōgēsimus
90	nōnāgintā	90th	nōnāgēsimus
100	centum	100th	centēsimus
101	centum ūnus, *or* centum et ūnus	101st	centēsimus prīmus, centēsimus et prīmus
102	centum duo, *or* centum et duo	102nd	centēsimus secundus, centēsimus et secundus
200	ducentī	200th	ducentēsimus
300	trecentī	300th	trecentēsimus
400	quadringentī	400th	quadringentēsimus
500	quīngentī	500th	quīngentēsimus
600	sēscentī, *or* sexcenti	600th	sēscentēsimus
700	septingentī	700th	septingentēsimus
800	octingentī	800th	octingentēsimus
900	nōngentī	900th	nōngentēsimus
1,000	mīlle	1,000th	mīllēsimus
2,000	duo mīllia	2,000th	bis mīllēsimus
10,000	decem mīllia	10,000th	decies mīllēsimus
100,000	centum mīllia	100,000th	centiēs mīllēsimus

A line placed over a letter increases its value one thousand times.

1	I	6	VI	11	XI	40	XL	90	XC
2	II	7	VII	12	XII	50	L	100	C
3	III	8	VIII	15	XV	60	LX	500	D
4	IV	9	IX	20	XX	70	LXX	1000	M
5	V	10	X	30	XXX	80	LXXX	2000	MM

5000	$\bar{\text{V}}$
10,000	$\bar{\text{X}}$
100,000	$\bar{\text{C}}$
1,000,000	$\bar{\text{M}}$

INSURANCE VOCABULARY

Assignment of insurance benefits. Authorization granted to the insurance company by an insured individual to pay policy benefits to another individual.

Attending physician. The physician ultimately in charge or the overseer of the patient's care.

Authorization to release information. Signed permission given by the patient, authorizing the physician to release privileged information.

Benefits. Services provided under the insurance agreement.

Carrier. The agent designated by the policy-holder to process claims. The carrier can be a commercial company or, in the case of Medicare, a federal agency.

Certification of eligibility. Written verification of the policy-holder's entitlement to benefits.

Claimant. The individual making a formal request to receive payment or benefits as mandated by the insurance policy.

Claim form. A written statement listing services rendered, usually signed by both the physician and the patient. Payment is made on the basis of the information provided on the form.

Claim payments. Payments made by the insurance company, under terms of the agreement, to the insured (the patient) as reimbursement or to the physician for services rendered.

Co-insurance. Payment for services shared by the insurance company and the insured.

Coverage. Benefits forthcoming to the insured, stated in the insurance plan.

Effective date. The date on which coverage can be granted and the contractual agreement is binding.

Eligibility rules. Specific criteria, stated in the insurance plan, indicating when benefits may be granted, to whom, and for how long.

Eligible members. Those individuals in a family or group plan who qualify, by reason of their relationship, for benefits stated in the plan.

Exclusions (Exceptions). Occasions specified by the policy for which there is no coverage.

Expiration date. The date on which coverage can no longer be granted; termination of the contract.

Explanation of benefits. The statement that accompanies benefit payment, describing in detail how the amount of payment was calculated.

Extended care. Health care provided by a facility other than a hospital that specializes in long-term care.

Fee (or Benefit) schedules. The policy statement listing specified amounts to be paid for specified services.

Group plan. An insurance policy providing coverage to a number of individuals who share premium costs. Companies may share premium costs as well.

Income limit. 1. The maximum income an individual can earn and still be eligible for insurance benefits. 2. The maximum amount of income protection to which the insurance company will agree in the contract.

Indemnity allowance (or schedule). The fee amount to be paid by the insurance plan. Coverage differences which are less than the physician's fee are the patient's responsibility.

Individual insurance plan. An insurance policy purchased by an individual who accepts full responsibility for premium payment.

Inpatient. The hospital patient receiving room and board.

Insuring clauses. Statements in the policy that specify the terms and conditions of coverage and benefits.

Manual of procedures. The insurance company's instructions for interpreting its plans and processing the related forms.

Maximum benefit. The dollar amount of benefits that the insurance company will pay for processed claims in any one year.

Outpatient. A patient receiving hospital treatment without room and board.

Participating physician. A physician member of a group or organization providing health care, such as Blue Shield.

Pre-existing condition. An abnormal physical or mental condition existing prior to the date on which the policy becomes effective.

Primary physician. The physician who first cares for the patient.

Physician's profile. The physician's statement of the patient's general health status following a comprehensive physical examination.

Referring physician. The physician who recommends another physician to the patient. The term may also be used when speaking of the physician who authorized the patient's hospital admission.

Release of information. A form signed by the patient, granting permission to the physician to release medical information to the insurance company.

Retroactive. Made effective to an earlier date.

Rider. An amendment to an original policy statement which increases, decreases, or excludes certain aspects of coverage.

Schedule of allowances. A list of specified amounts to be paid by the insurance company for medical services.

Subscriber. The insured representing the family unit in the insurance agreement.

Termination date. The date on which insurance protection and coverage cease.

Time limit. The time in which a claim must be filed in order to receive benefits.

Usual and customary. Normal or average charges or fees for services rendered.

MEDICAL LAW VOCABULARY

Assault. An expressed threat to do bodily harm.

Battery. Body contact that is unauthorized.

Board of Medical Examiners. The licensure board of the American Medical Association which is responsible for suspending or revoking a physician's license to practice medicine.

Breach. A violation of law, promise, or duty.

"Captain of the Ship" doctrine. The legal doctrine which holds that a physician is in complete charge of those individuals present and those providing assistance during and until the conclusion of an operative procedure.

Committee. A term used to refer to the guardian of a mentally incompetent individual.

Consent. The agreement, authorization, or permission which allows the physician to act upon the patient's body.

Consent implied in action. Permission given nonverbally but evidenced in the patient's activity, such as the patient's keeping an appointment for x-ray testing.

Consent implied in emergency. Permission given nonverbally but evidenced in the urgency of the patient's condition when the patient cannot clearly respond. Consent is implied for life-saving measures. It is deemed reasonable that an individual would give permission for any procedure required to save his life.

Consent implied in law. Consent implied in emergency and consent of parent or guardian are also termed consent implied in law as legal statutes govern their use.

Consent of parent or guardian. Written permission given by the parent or guardian to the physician so that he may act upon the body of the parent's or guardian's charge.

Criminal offense. An act for which there is no legal support, such as the practice of medicine by an unlicensed person.

Damages. The approximated money equivalent for a detriment or damage sustained by the plaintiff.

Defamation. Written or oral statements or representations that attack the character of an individual, resulting in an unfavorable impression or unjust actions.

Defendant. The individual being prosecuted or being sued.

Direct liability. The term used to describe a suit which charges the physician with willful or negligent acts performed during the rendering of his services.

Discreet disclosure. The principle which allows the physician to elect not to disclose all information relating to the patient's condition as long as no form of consent is elicited.

Dying declaration. Statements made by an individual approaching death, which are witnessed and can be used legally in a court action.

Emancipated minor. A person who is not of legal age but is married and therefore has legal rights and responsibilities.

Endorsement. The term used to describe the acceptance by some states of the National Board of Medical Examiners certification in lieu of a state licensure examination for the practice of medicine.

ENT specialist. A physician who is Board-certified to practice medicine relating to diseases of the ear, nose and throat.

Excess damages. The term used to refer to the circumstances in which an individual is responsible for the payment of damages which exceed the amount covered by the insurance policy.

Express consent. Written permission, authorization, or agreement given by a relative of the deceased for the performance of an autopsy on the deceased.

Expert witness. A professional (physician) who testifies against another professional (physician) in the legal determination of negligence or malpractice.

Fee-splitting. An arrangement in which a physician-specialist charges the patient a fee and then returns a portion of the fee to the referring physician. This act may result in the suspension or revocation of the physician's license to practice medicine.

Fraud. Deceit or misrepresentation used for the purpose of obtaining unfair advantage.

"Good Samaritan" statute. The statute which protects the physician from legal action for the treatment of an accident victim requiring emergency care.

Implied (or Oral) contract. The contractual agreement which pertains to the physician-patient relationship and usually begins when the patient first visits the medical office and the physician lays his hand upon the patient for the purpose of examination.

Informed consent. Agreement, authorization, or permission which, to be legally valid, necessitates the physician's sharing information in the following five areas before a procedure can be performed:
1. The nature of the illness and why it necessitates treatment.
2. The nature of the proposed treatment, the details of the procedure and who will perform the procedure.
3. The risks or consequences and their probability of occurrence.
4. Alternative treatment methods and the reasons for their appropriateness or inappropriateness related to this illness.
5. Reasonable expectations for recovery and chances for failure.

Insanity. A legal term used to describe an individual who is mentally incompetent and therefore not legally responsible for his actions. An individual must be declared insane by a court of law.

Law of contracts. The legal framework for unwritten agreements between two parties, as between physician and patient. To be binding, such agreements must satisfy four requisites:
1. Manifestation and assent must be shown. The individual must request the services of the physician, and the physician must accept the responsibility to render care.
2. The legal subject matter of the agreement must bear upon the relationship between physician and patient.
3. The patient and physician must be of legal age and sound mental capacity.
4. Consideration must exist. This term refers to the assumption that the patient will pay for the services rendered.

Liable. Legally responsible for one's actions.

Liability suit. A legal action taken when one individual (the plaintiff) seeks damages from another (the defendant). A breach of the defendant's legal obligation is presumed by the plaintiff.

Licensed physician. A physician who has passed a state licensure examination and has been determined to be competent to practice medicine.

Majority. The age at which one's full civil rights are granted.

Malfeasance claim. A malpractice claim charging that the physician wrongfully treated the patient, thus committing a wrongful act. An example would be the surgical removal of a healthy organ.

Malpractice. Dereliction of professional skill through carelessness, ignorance, or intent, which results in undesirable consequences of the treatment rendered. Malpractice claims fall into one of three categories: malfeasance, misfeasance, and nonfeasance.

Medical practice acts. Legal statutes which govern the practice of medicine.

Minority. The age at which one's full civil rights cannot be granted and during which the parent or guardian is granted the right of jurisdiction.

Misfeasance claim. A malpractice claim involving the wrongful manner of an act, as when a physician is alleged to have performed a procedure incorrectly, although the procedure itself was rightful.

Moral turpitude. Acts or actions of an immoral or shameful nature.

Nonfeasance claim. A malpractice claim charging the physician with failure to act in accordance with duty or necessity.

Plaintiff. The individual seeking legal resolution (damages) and initiating legal action (suit).

Professional fee. Payment due from the patient for professional services. Medical fees are determined with the aid of geographic averages and the fee schedule recommendations of the AMA.

Professional liability insurance. Insurance available to health professionals which can be obtained for protection from monetary loss when legal action is taken against them.

Proximate cause. In order for negligence to be proved and liability charged, the injury to the patient could not have occurred without the physician's action, thus establishing the proximate, or direct, cause.

Reciprocity. The granting of licensure without medical examination in one state to a physician who has successfully passed the medical board examination in another state in which the requirements meet or surpass those in the state granting reciprocity.

Registration fee. The fee that is paid periodically to the Board of Medical Examiners to maintain the licensure to practice.

Re-registration. Periodic payment of the registration fee.

Res ipsa loquitur. (Latin "The thing speaks for itself.") A doctrine applied to malpractice cases to assist in the determination of negligence. There are several requirements for the application of res ipsa loquitur:

1. The consequences of treatment must be out of the ordinary; that is, not within the normal range of expectations. It must be proved that "the thing speaks for itself" and occurred solely as a result of the physician's negligence.
2. The physician must be directly or vicariously liable for the action.
3. The patient must be free of making any contribution to the consequences through his own actions.

Respondeat superior. (Latin "Let the one higher up answer for it.") Respondeat superior places responsibility on the physician for the liability of others in his employ. The physician is ultimately responsible for the wrongful acts of others, be they physicians who are junior partners, office staff members, or those assisting him in surgery.

Standards of care. This term refers to the qualifications of the physician who serves as expert witness. The expert witness must occupy a position in which the same quality of care (techniques and procedures) is expected as that maintained by the defendant.

Statute. A legal doctrine set forth by a legislative body for the purpose of governing specific acts.

Statute of fraud. The doctrine bearing upon the failure of the patient or his agent to pay the physician's fee when agreement had been assumed.

Statute of limitations. A statute restricting the time period in which a claim may be prosecuted. For instance, in some states, legal action cannot be initiated for treatment received when three years have lapsed from the time of treatment.

Suit. The act of seeking legal resolution in the form of damages in a court of law.

Tort. Any wrongful act (not involving breach of contract) for which civil or legal action can be initiated.

Vicarious liability. The physician's responsibility for the wrongful acts committed by others in his employ or under his supervision.

MEDICAL ETHICS VOCABULARY

Abortion (criminal). The termination of pregnancy for reasons other than medical and lawful.

Amniocentesis. Withdrawal of a sample of amniotic fluid from the uterine cavity by means of a needle inserted into the abdomen.

Artificial insemination. The introduction of seminal fluid from a donor into the female reproductive organs.

Atopogenics. The term assigned to highly controversial studies in biological engineering for such purposes as the development of "genetically superior" offspring.

Cloning. The term used to refer to experiments in biological engineering concerned with genetic duplication of individual organisms through asexual reproduction, as by cellular stimulation.

Code of medical ethics. Guidelines for the moral conduct of physicians.

Confidentiality. The term referring to the responsibility of all health professionals to safeguard the privacy of patient records, files, and discussions.

Eugenics. The applied science of genetics which deals with efforts to improve the hereditary qualities of a species.

Euthanasia. The "merciful killing" of another human being, usually deemed to be terminally ill, and often at his own request.

Genotype. The aggregate of genes that constitutes the individual's biological heredity.

Hippocratic Oath. The oath concerning ethical professional behavior taken by physicians and attributed to the Greek physician, Hippocrates (460?–377? B.C.).

Medical ethics. The application of a moral code of behavior to medical practice.

Morality. The evaluation of human conduct in terms of the inherent rightness and wrongness of human actions.

Phenotype. The appearance, structure, and functional state which the body has at a given moment in time. (Phenotype is dependent on genotype.)

Psychoanalysis. The technique, originated by Sigmund Freud, that explores and interprets past experiences to enable the patient to make personality adjustments. A specially trained psychoanalyst leads the patient through the course of treatment.

Psychosurgery. Surgical intervention for the purposes of altering behavior.

Psychotherapy. Therapeutic intervention, such as group and individual counseling, for the purpose of altering behavior.

Spontaneous abortion. The natural termination of a pregnancy; another term for miscarriage.

Sterilization. Any procedure by which an individual is made incapable of reproduction, such as by castration, vasectomy, or salpingectomy (surgical removal of the uterine tube).

Therapeutic abortion. The termination of a pregnancy for specific medical reasons.

Tubal ligation. The surgical tying or binding of the fallopian tubes as a contraceptive measure.

Vasectomy. The surgical removal of the ductus deferens (the excretory duct of the testis), or a portion of it, sometimes performed as a contraceptive measure.

INDEX

An *A* indicates placement in the Appendix.
A *t* indicates a table.